Health Promotion in Health Care – Vital Theories and Research

Gørill Haugan • Monica Eriksson
Editors

Health Promotion in Health Care – Vital Theories and Research

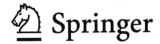

Springer

Editors
Gørill Haugan
Department of Public Health
and Nursing
NTNU Norwegian University
of Science and Technology
Trondheim
Norway

Monica Eriksson
Department of Health Sciences
University West
Trollhättan
Sweden

Faculty of Nursing and Health Science
Nord University
Levanger
Norway

This book is an open access publication.
ISBN 978-3-030-64012-5   ISBN 978-3-030-63135-2   (eBook)
https://doi.org/10.1007/978-3-030-63135-2

This Springer imprint is published by the registered company Springer Nature Switzerland AG
The registered company address is: Gewerbestrasse 11, 6330 Cham, Switzerland

Introduction to This Book

High Ages: A Success That Signifies Health Challenges

As we all are aware of, there is a demographic shift toward an older population worldwide. The segment of people aged 80 years and more is growing rapidly and those aged 100+ are growing fastest [1]. This is a sign that we have succeeded in some ways. This shift started in high-income countries. However, for the first time in history, people can expect to live until their 60s and beyond globally [2]. During the period from 2015 and 2050, the proportion of those 60 years and more will nearly double from 12 to 22%; by 2050 individuals aged 60 years and older is expected to total two billion, up from 900 million in 2015 [2]. Currently, low- and middle-income countries are experiencing the greatest demographic change; hence, all countries are now facing major challenges to ensure that their health and social systems are ready to make the most of this demographic shift [2, 3]. Age is an aim in life and not a disease. Still, with high ages, several diseases appear; now our task is to ensure that the extra years are worth living. Hence, with a steadily growing older population, the world faces a growing need of health care. In the years to come, health promotive initiatives enhancing well-being and coping in the population will become ever more important. Accordingly, this book provides novel knowledge in the field of health promotion in the health care services from various parts of the world; Africa, America, Asia, Australia, and Europe are represented.

Today, the medical perspective and treatment approaches are highly developed giving emphasis to save lives from severe illnesses and injuries. This is good. However, a great number of patients, both in hospitals and in the municipality health care, suffer from a lack of holistic oriented health care and support. Their illness is treated, but they feel scared, helpless, and lonely, experiencing meaninglessness and low quality of life. Several patients with chronic or long-term conditions (heart and lung diseases, cancer, rheumatologic diseases, dementia, diabetes, long-term intensive care patients, palliative patients, mental disorders, etc.) fight and must cope with a heavy symptom burden and life challenges on their own at home. These people are asking for social support, empowerment, patient education (salus education), guidance, hope, meaning, dignity, and coping strategies in order to manage their life situation. Human beings are whole persons consisting of different dimensions; individuals comprise of a wholeness of body-mind-spirit which cannot be separated in a body, a mind, and a spirit; these three parts are totally integrated performing in close interaction. Thus, a holistic physical-psychological-social-spiritual model of health care is required to provide high-quality and effective health care. Health promotion and the salutogenic perspective on health are holistic. In the years to come, health promotive initiatives will become ever more important. Accordingly, learning how to reorient the health care sector in a health promotion direction is highly needed.

Health promoting approaches are resource-oriented focusing on the origin of health along with people's abilities and capacities for well-functioning and well-being. The health promotion field is based in the salutogenic health theory representing an area of knowledge and learning, a way of relating to others, and a way of working in a health promoting manner. In the salutogenic perspective, health is a movement on a continuum between ease and disease. In this approach, no one is categorized as healthy or diseased; we are all somewhere between the imaginary poles of total wellness and total illness. Every person, even if severely diseased, has health, and health promotion is about strengthening the health. Either by changing the ways we work or by changing the environment or educate the person in question how he or she can work to strengthen his/her health. The salutogenic approach seems useful for reorienting the health care systems around the globe. Therefore, this book entailing three parts comprehends the salutogenic health theory as a model of health and a life orientation, representing a vital theoretical basis for the health promotion field, along with the salutogenic theoretical framework.

Health Promotion in the Health Care Services (Part I)

First, in Part I, we provide the historical and theoretical basis for health promotion in the health care (Chap. 1), followed by a presentation of the salutogenic health theory and its potential in reorienting the health care services in a health promotion direction (Chap. 2) as well as ethical perspectives on health promotion (Chap. 3). Hence, Part I elaborates on the need for reorienting the health services in a health promotion direction. Both hospitals and the municipality health care services should be based on the health promotion perspective and an integrated understanding of pathogenesis-salutogenesis. This goes for acute as well as chronic illness and conditions. The arguments include efficiency, effectiveness of the health care services, along with beneficial outcomes for the patients, their families and the societies. Health care is expensive and challenging; all the efforts put into it should pay off as much as possible. A health care which along with the medical treatment and care, also aims at supporting/promoting patients' health by means of identifying and supporting their health resources, will result in better patient outcomes; shorter stays in hospitals, less re-hospitalization, better coping at home, more well-being indicating increased public health and smaller health care budgets. Hence, re-orienting the health services to provide health promoting health care, will not merely remove a disease, but provide more health, well-being, and coping. A more abundant outcome!

Moreover, health services are first and foremost about health. Thus, this overarching aim—and not only diseases—should be leading principles and visible in the organizational structures, leadership and management philosophy, the working culture, and in the health care of individuals and the families. The health care sector should be led toward the aim of treating illness accompanied by actively promotion of people's health. Moreover, the health care services should not only be responsible for the development of health-promoting working environments but be in the forefront of such developments in the societies. Hospitals, nursing homes, homecare, etc. should represent health-promoting work places, facilitating well-being and peoples' experiences of their work situation as comprehensible, manageable, and meaningful. Still, all countries have much left on their "to-do-list" toward such a reorientation of the health services. Hence, knowledge about development and the implementation of health promotion strategies in the health care is highly welcome and much needed in the years to come.

Vital Salutogenic Resources for the Health Services (Part II)

The second part of this book gives the reader an updated overview on significant salutogenic concepts representing resources for health promotion and well-being. The selected salutogenic concepts are relevant for the health services, globally. *Sense of coherence* (Chap. 4) kicks off Part II, representing a corner stone in the salutogenic health concept. A growing body of evidence has shown that sense of coherence—that is, an individual's perception of one's life situation as comprehensible, manageable, and meaningful—is strongly related to health, wellbeing and coping in all segments of the human population; young as well as old people, healthy, as well as individuals having diseases. Thus, this book suggests that the dimensions of comprehensibility, manageability, and meaningfulness should be generally addressed in the health services. If people are going to be *flourishing* individuals (Chap. 5), meaning that they lead flourishing lives going well, coping well, and thriving well, sense of coherence is a vital basis. The salutogenic concept of flourishing represents a living goal and an understanding that people, despite physical or mental illnesses, can lead happy and well-functioning lives. Such ideas provide us *hope* (Chap. 6)—which also represents a salutogenic concept and resource for health, well-being, and coping. Hope entails positive energy, vitality, and power to strive for whatever one wants in life and is therefore a significant sign of health.

Human beings are not only a physical body and a mind, but physical-emotional-social-spiritual/existential entities, or an integrated wholeness of body-mind-soul. Thus, human beings need to experience *dignity* (Chap. 7); suffering results from not attending to an individual's dignity. Thus, dignity is a vital aspect of patients' health and should therefore be addressed in health care. If dignity is overseen, most often the individual loses her sense of *meaning-in-life* (Chap. 8). Without dignity and meaningfulness, life does not seem worth living, and the *inner strength* and *willpower* to fight for health, recovery, etc. will be drained and deprived (Chaps. 8 and 18). The salutogenic concept of *self-transcendence* (Chap. 9) represents a vital resource for well-being and coping, specifically among vulnerable populations such as the seriously ill, palliative patients, mentally ill, nursing home residents, and terminal patients. However, self-transcendence is also seen to be fundamental to healthy people's well-being and coping such as nursing students and home-dwelling older people. Thus, the dimensions of inter-personal and intra-personal self-transcendence along with the sense of coherence dimensions might be useful as a map to assess which health promoting resources are present in an individual's life. The core of self-transcendence is connectedness, outwardly, inwardly, upwardly, and backwardly (one's past). *Connectedness* is also a salutogenic resource, facilitating health, well-being, as well as meaningfulness, hope, and joy-of-life, and is a vital aspect of the nurse–patient relationship and the interaction between these two.

While assessing the patient's situation, both bodily, emotionally, socially, functionally, and spiritually/existentially, the *nurse–patient interaction* (Chap. 10) is a necessary tool. However, the nurse–patient interaction is not only a tool for valid and reliable assessment, but a salutogenic resource for well-being and health by itself. By means of attentional and influencing competences, health care personnel can positively impact on long-term nursing home patients' anxiety and depression, as well as joy-of-life, hope, meaning-in-life, self-transcendence, and *social support* (Chap. 11). Indeed, social support is seen to be related with loneliness and mortality among older people in nursing homes, representing a vital salutogenic resource. Social support (Chap. 11), *efficacy* (Chap. 12), and *empowerment* (Chap. 13) are all interrelated salutogenic resources embedded in the nurse–patient interaction.

Health Promotion in Different Contexts (Part III)

Based on the health promotion perspective and these vital salutogenic resources, Part III in this book presents different health promotion approaches to several patient groups. Part III sets out with focusing on families having a newborn baby (Chap. 14), which represents an important and existential experience in parents' lives having huge impact on the family health and the baby's health. A healthy population starts with a healthy and well-functioning family raising healthy children. An individual's health is highly dependent on childhood conditions, both physically and mentally. In all countries, the aim is to facilitate a flourishing population (Chap. 15), despite chronic illnesses (Chap. 16), cancer (Chap. 17), long-term intensive care treatment (Chap. 18), and heart failure (Chap. 19).

The segment of older people is increasing, resulting in many people 80 years an older being treated for various diseases in hospitals. Being 80+ and treated in a hospital setting represents a specific vulnerable state (Chap. 20). While treating older people medically in hospitals, their specific vulnerability must be considered in every aspect; if overseen, the health services will fail and create more illness and suffering than they relieve or solve, which of course is a great pity!

In an international perspective, part three focuses on palliative care in an African context of Uganda (Chap. 21) as well as on age care in a middle-income context of Turkey (Chap. 22). Health promotion as a central idea in palliative care as well as elderly care should be further developed along with efficient symptom management and pain relief. In Turkey, the care of old people is mainly handled by the families. As the Turkish society develops toward a modern organization of both genders partaking in the work life, health promoting strategies caring for the elders, as well as the female caretakers will be important. In Singapore, researchers have operationalized the salutogenic health theory into diverse health promotion programs; the SHAPE study (Chap. 23) and the intergenerational e-health literacy program (Chap. 24) interestingly demonstrate ideas about how to promote people's health as part of the municipality public health services. Finally, the number of individuals having dementia is heavily increasing worldwide, representing a huge challenge in all countries. Hence, health promotion initiatives are strongly needed in the care for people having dementia (Chap. 25) as well as their families.

The last chapter (Chap. 26) sums it all up, pointing forwards to the future challenges. With the aim of reorienting the health services in a health promoting direction, still much work remains worldwide. This book intends to serve these coming reorienting processes. This edited scientific anthology represents a vital contribution to university educations in the health sciences. Currently, a collection in between two binders of the central salutogenic theoretical framework and empirical research on health promoting assets in the health system is missing. This edited scientific anthology meets the need for a substantial overview of vital salutogenic theories/concepts in health care, along with knowledge on health promotion research related to different patient populations.

This book represents a vital contribution to university education globally; the target group is bachelor students in nursing as well as other health professions (occupational therapists, physiotherapists, radiotherapists, social care workers, etc.) and master students in nursing and health sciences. This book also provides an overview for PhD students, clinicians, and researchers in the field of health science and health promotion. The fact that all authors are in the forefront and widely published in their specific field, work as professors (educators and researchers) in health/social care, representing different parts of the world (Africa, America, Australia, Asia, Europe), and different countries (Australia, Belgium, China, Norway, Uganda, USA, Singapore, Sweden, Turkey) gives this book a broad audience and thus a broad influence.

We as the editors of this scientific anthology providing ideas and perspectives on how to reorient the health care system, wish and hope for this book to be extensively used. Therefore, we afford this anthology as an open access easily reached for everyone.

We are grateful and want to thank all the contributors for their interesting and important manuscripts included here. Also, we are thankful to the NTNU Publiseringsfondet, and NTNU Deparment of Public Health Nursing for supporting the open access of this book.

Trondheim, Norway   Gørill Haugan
Levanger, Norway
Trollhättan, Sweden   Monica Eriksson

References

1. HOD. St.meld. nr. 25: Mestring, muligheter og mening. Framtidas omsorgsutfordringer. Omsorgsplan 2015. In: HOD, [Ministry of Health and Care Services] editor. Oslo: www.odin.dep.no; 2005–2006.
2. WHO. World Report on Ageing and health. World Health Organization; 2018. https://www.who.int/news-room/fact-sheets/detail/ageing-and-health [updated 5 Feb 2018].
3. Kinsella K, He W. An Aging World: 2008. Washington, DC: U.S. Department of Health and Human Services National Institutes of Health National Institute on Aging. U.S. Department of Commerce Economics and Statistics; 2009. Contract No.: Report No.: P95/09-1.

Contents

About the Editors

Gørill Haugan graduated as a registered nurse (RN) in 1984 and holds a PhD in health science. Haugan has worked as an academician since 1989 and thus educated a great number of nursing and health care students at all levels. Currently, she works as a professor in health and nursing science at NTNU Department of Public Health and Nursing, Faculty of Medicine and Health in Norway, and professor II at Nord University, Faculty of Nursing and Health science. Professor Haugan is supervising bachelor theses in nursing care, along with PhD and master's projects focusing on different aspects of nursing and global health, collecting data in Norway as well as in Nepal and Uganda. Furthermore, she is supervising assistant professors in achieving competence as associate professor at NTNU and Nord University. Haugan is widely published internationally, with more than 140 scientific publications in the field of health promotion among different populations such as older people, long-term intensive care patients, adolescents and postnatal women, as well as nursing students and health care workers. She is the main editor of three different scientific anthologies (including this one) focusing on health promotion in health care. In particular, she has investigated the influence of nurse–patient interaction, self-transcendence, hope, meaning-in-life, sense of coherence, joy-of-life and spirituality on individual's well-being and quality of life, as well as developed and validated several measurement models central to nursing and health care. Haugan leads several research projects in various fields including various populations and evaluates research proposals for funding in Norway. She collaborates with researchers at different universities in Norway, Belgium, the Netherlands, Poland, Turkey, Sweden, Finland, Singapore, Uganda, Nepal, Malta, and the USA.

Monica Eriksson is associate professor in social policy (health promotion) at Åbo Akademi University Vasa, Finland. Current position as Senior Professor in public health and health promotion in the Department of Health Sciences, University West, Trollhättan, Sweden. Former Head of the Center on Salutogenesis, University West. Member of the Global Working Group on Salutogenesis 2007–2018. Defended a doctoral thesis in 2007, a systematic research synthesis, based on more than 450 scientific papers on studies using Antonovsky's sense of coherence scale, titled "Unravelling the Mystery of Salutogenesis" (Eriksson 2007). Now continuing the analysis and following salutogenic research up to date. Main research focuses on salutogenesis in public health and health promotion research and practice where peoples' abilities and resources are essential for health and well-being. The most recent research is on salutogenic factors for sustainable working life for nurses. Previously worked as a hospital-based social worker, operative director of an umbrella organization for people with disabilities, later as the Nordic investigator of mobility of people with disabilities. "My clinical experience and practice has convinced me the resource perspective of public health and health promotion is the way forward for both research and effective interventions."

Part I

Introduction to Health Promotion

An Introduction to the Health Promotion Perspective in the Health Care Services

1

Gørill Haugan and Monica Eriksson

Abstract

Currently, the world faces a shift to an older population. For the first time in the history, now most people can expect to live into their 60s and beyond. Within this trend of people living longer, many grow very old; 80, 90 and 100 years. Today, 125 million people are 80 years or older; the proportion of ≥80 years increases the most. Age is not an illness, still most chronically ill are older people. Consequently, all countries in the world face major challenges to ensure that their health and social systems are ready to make the most of this demographic shift. Globally, finding new and effective ways to improve people's health is crucial. Thus, in the years to come, health promotive initiatives will become ever more important. Accordingly, learning how to reorient the health care sector in a health promotion direction is highly needed. The salutogenic approach seems useful for such a reorientation.

Salutogenesis is a resource-oriented theoretical approach which focuses on the origin of health along with people's abilities and capacities for well-functioning and well-being. Salutogenesis is an area of knowledge and learning, a way of relating to others, and a way of working in a health-promoting manner. From the salutogenic point of view, health is a movement on a continuum between ease and dis-ease. In this approach, no one is categorized as healthy or diseased; we are all somewhere between the imaginary poles of total wellness and total illness.

This chapter, as well as this book, comprehend the salutogenic health theory as a model of health and a life orientation, representing a vital theoretical basis for the health promotion field. Accordingly, this chapter presents some important points in the development of the health promotion field, followed by the core principles and strategies of health promotion and the promising potential of the salutogenic health theory.

G. Haugan (✉)
Department of Public Health and Nursing, NTNU Norwegian University of Science and Technology, Trondheim, Norway

Faculty of Nursing and Health Science, Nord University, Levanger, Norway
e-mail: gorill.haugan@ntnu.no,
gorill.haugan@nord.no

M. Eriksson
Department of Health Sciences, University West, Trollhattan, Sweden
e-mail: monica.eriksson@hv.se

Keywords

Health promotion · Salutogenesis · Demographic trends · Non-communicable diseases · Reorienting the health services

© The Author(s) 2021
G. Haugan, M. Eriksson (eds.), *Health Promotion in Health Care – Vital Theories and Research*,
https://doi.org/10.1007/978-3-030-63135-2_1

1.1 Introduction

1.1.1 Demographic Trends

Currently, the world faces a shift to an older population; 125 million people are now aged 80 years or older [1]. While this shift started in high-income countries (e.g. in Japan 30% of the population are already over 60 years old), it is now low- and middle-income countries that are experiencing the greatest change. Today, for the first time in the history, most people can expect to live into their 60s and beyond [2]. Between 2015 and 2050, the proportion of the world's population over 60 years will nearly double from 12% to 22%; by 2050, the world's population aged 60 years and older is expected to total two billion, up from 900 million in 2015 [1, 2]. All countries in the world face major challenges to ensure that their health and social systems are ready to make the most of this demographic shift [1]. Within this trend of people living longer, many grow very old; 80, 90 and 100 years. Today, 125 million people are 80 years or older; the proportion of ≥80 years increases the most.

Thus, it is important to ensure that the extra years of life are worth living, despite chronic illnesses and loss of functionality. This is of great importance not only to the individual elderly, but also to the families, the local community and the municipality. However, there is little evidence showing that older adults today have better health than their parents had in their older years. Age is no disease; however, most chronically ill people today are older people. Increased age is followed by an increased incidence of functional and chronic comorbidities and diverse disabilities [3], which for many leads to the need for medical treatment and different levels of nursing care. Accordingly, the WHO's Action Plan on Aging and Health [4] highlights a global need of systems for providing long-term care to meet the needs of older people globally.

All countries face major challenges to ensure that their health and social systems are ready to make the most of these demographic shifts [2]. For instance, in the North Africa and the Middle East, due to very rapid demographic ageing, the estimated number of people with dementia is expected to grow exponentially, two million people in 2015 rising to four million in 2030 and ten million in 2050 [2], an increase of 329% from 2015 through to 2050, the second fastest in the world. Currently, North Africa and the Middle East are estimated to have the highest age-standardized prevalence globally [5].

The increasing burden due to cancer and other non-communicable diseases poses a threat to human development, which has resulted in global political commitments reflected in the Sustainable Development Goals as well as the World Health Organization (WHO) Global Action Plan on Non-Communicable Diseases. Between 2006 and 2016, the average annual age-standardized incidence rates for all cancers combined increased in 130 of 195 countries or territories, and the average annual age-standardized death rates decreased within that timeframe in 143 of 195 countries or territories [6]. Thus far, few countries have been able to overcome this challenge. Nevertheless, in the US cancer incidence (for all cancer sites combined) rates have decreased among men and were stable among women. Overall, there continue to be significant declines in cancer death rates among both men and women. With early detection and treatment people survive cancer and are living with several side effects [7].

Heart failure (HF) is a global pandemic affecting about 38 million people and is a growing health problem worldwide [8–10]. Even though the incidence of HF is stable, the prevalence is going to rise because of the ageing population and improvements in treatment [11, 12]. The HF condition is common in both developing and developed countries; the switch towards a Western lifestyle in developing countries may be contributing to a real HF pandemic. Consequently, HF health expenditures are considerable and will increase dramatically with an ageing population. HF is one of the most common causes of hospitalization and readmission [13–16]. The prevalence, incidence, mortality and morbidity rates reported show geographic variations, depending on the different aetiologies and clinical characteristics observed among patients with HF. The risk factors for HF are multifactorial and complex, and there is no known prevention other than treatment of the risk factors, such as hypertension, diabetes and obesity; whereas prevention and early treatment strategies (i.e. early revascularization) appear to be effective in reducing the risk and severity of acute myocardial infarction [17].

Moreover, today depression is the most common psychological disorder, affecting about 121 million people in all ages worldwide. WHO states that depression is the leading cause of disability as measured by Years Lived with Disability (YLDs) and the fourth leading contributor to the global burden of disease. By the year 2020, depression is projected to reach the second place in the ranking of Disability Adjusted Life Years (DALY) calculated for all ages.

This demographic development will have consequences both economically, socially, culturally and politically [18]. The health care systems around the globe will face great challenges in the years to come. Health promotive initiatives will become ever more important; not only for people with physical and mental disabilities and older persons living at home or in care facilities, but also among the healthy population in supporting them to stay healthy. Facing these demographic trends, finding new and effective ways to improve people's health globally is imperative. Health promotion should be a vital part of the health care systems.

1.1.2 The Background of Health Promotion

WHO has for a long time promoted a common approach to health policy by developing a series of targets for improved health status, i.e. *the Health for All Strategy—Targets for Health for All* [19]. Several health conferences have been arranged by WHO. Two of the most significant conferences were arranged in Alma Ata in 1978, resulting in the Alma-Ata Declaration, which emerged as a milestone of the twentieth century in the field of public health [20]. The second was arranged in Ottawa, Canada, where 200 del-

egates from 38 nations came together and made a commitment to health promotion; based on the Alma-Ata Declaration, the Ottawa Charter for health promotion was born [21]. This charter defined health promotion as '*the process of enabling people to increase control over, and to improve, their health. To reach a state of complete physical mental and social wellbeing, an individual or group must be able to identify and to realize aspirations, to satisfy needs, and to change or cope with the environment*' [22]. The Ottawa Charter became a core policy document and a cornerstone in establishing the health promotion field [23].

The Lancet—University of Oslo (UiO) Commission of Global Governance for Health stated that '*health is a precondition, outcome, and indicator of a sustainable society, and should be adopted as a universal value and shared social goal and political objective for all*' [24]. According to Samdal and Wold [23], health promotion is a modern ideology and strategy to improve public health. It represents a reorientation of public health from addressing individual risk factors of health or risk behaviours toward targeting determinants of health and empowering individuals and communities to participate in improving the health of their communities [25, 26].

'*Health promotion is positive and dynamic. It opens up the field of health to become an inclusive social, rather than an exclusive professional activity. It represents a broadening of perspectives in relation to health education and to prevention as a whole*' ([27], p. 3). In these words, the former Chair of the Editorial Board of Health Promotion International introduced this new scientific journal in 1986. She was one of the key persons strongly and deeply involved in the discussions of the content of health promotion and how health promotion differs from public health and disease prevention. Some of the key notions of these discussions were summarized in a document by the WHO European Office [28]; Scriven and Orme described this publication as the emergence of health promotion as a major movement [21].

1.1.3 The Core Principles and Strategies of Health Promotion

Health is seen as a resource of everyday life, not the objective of living. Health is a positive concept emphasizing social and personal resources, as well as physical capacities. The prerequisites for health as the fundamental conditions and resources are peace, shelter, education, food, income, a stable ecosystem, sustainable resources, social justice and equity [22]. Three basic principles for health promotion work from the Ottawa Charter: *advocate, enable and mediate.*

- *Advocate:* Political, economic, social, cultural, environmental, behavioural and biological factors can all favour health or be harmful to it. Health promotion action aims at making these conditions favourable through advocacy for health [22].
- *Enable:* Health promotion focuses on achieving equity in health. Health promotion action aims at reducing differences in current health status and ensuring equal opportunities and resources to enable all people to achieve their fullest health potential. This includes a secure foundation in a supportive environment, access to information, life skills and opportunities for making healthy choices. People cannot achieve their fullest health potential unless they are able to take control of those things which determine their health [22].
- *Mediate:* The prerequisites and prospects for health cannot be ensured by the health sector alone. Professional and social groups and health personnel have a major responsibility to mediate between differing interests in society for the pursuit of health [22].

The Ottawa Charter clearly stated that a major aim of health promotion is to achieve equity in health by enabling all people to achieve their fullest health potential. To achieve this goal, five core strategies for health promotion action were identified:

1. Build a healthy public policy.
2. Create supportive environments.
3. Strengthen community action.
4. Develop personal skills.
5. Reorient health services.

These principles have stood the test of time, and the first four actions are developing well. However, the principle of 'reorienting health services' has until recently been given less attention. Available evidence guiding the health care services into a more health-promoting direction is still scarce. What does it mean to reorient health services? According to the Ottawa Charter [22], it means that the responsibility for health promotion in health services is shared among individuals, community groups, health professionals, health service institutions and governments. They must work together toward a health care system which contributes to the pursuit of health. Health services need to embrace an expanded mandate which is sensitive to and respects cultural needs. This mandate should support the needs of individuals and communities for a healthier life and open channels between the health sector and broader social, political, economic and physical environmental components. Reorienting health services also requires stronger attention to health research as well as changes in professional education and training. This must lead to a change of attitude and organization of health services, which refocuses on the total needs of the individual as a whole person.

In the special supplement of Health Promotion International entitled 'The Ottawa Charter for Health Promotion 25 years on', a panel of diverse commentators reviewed progress and opportunities. Authors agreed that there had been slow progress in making health promotion a core business for health services, and there was a need to reframe, reposition and renew efforts. One proposal was to focus on reorienting the system itself—not just the delivery of services—by health promotion leaders engaging more actively in system development [29]. In an Editorial in *Health Promotion International*, John Catford claimed that it is time to reorient health services

[30]. He expressed that at the time of Ottawa in 1986 the conferees agreed that '*The role of the health sector must move increasingly in a health promotion direction, beyond its responsibility for providing clinical and curative services*' ([30], p. 1). What has happened after Ottawa? Twenty-three years later '*there still seems to be an urgency towards the empowerment of patients to truly take control over a hospital environment that too often seems counter to their health*' ([31], p. 106). This echoed earlier comments that '*across the world there appears to have been stubborn resistance to systematic change in health care services, and only limited examples of effective and sustainable health services reorientation*' [32]. Thompson, Watson and Tilford come to the same conclusion after summarizing the efforts done 30 years after the Ottawa ([33], p. 73): '*Although its principles have been widely applauded, opportunities to transfer these principles into the radical changes and practical solutions needed globally to improve health have been missed. Nevertheless, it is argued that the Ottawa Charter retains its relevance to the present day and that all policy makers and professionals working to promote positive health should revisit and take heed of its principles*'.

The WHO Regional Office for Europe has further developed basic guiding principles for health promotion work ([34], pp. 4–5) which should be characterized by the following principles:

- Empowering (enabling individuals and communities to assume more power over the personal, socioeconomic, and environmental factors that affect their health).
- Participatory (involving all concerned at all stages of the process).
- Holistic (fostering physical, mental, social and spiritual health).
- Equitable (guiding by a concern for equity and social justice).
- Sustainable (bringing about changes that individuals and communities can maintain once initial funding has ended).
- Multistrategy (using a variety of approaches and methods).

An editorial entitled 'Turn, turn, turn: time to reorient health services' in the *Health Promotion International* journal ([30], p. 3) emphasized a changed way of working from 'downstream' acute repair—to 'upstream' health improvement and from patient compliance—to consumer control and centredness. This way of working can be visualized by using 'health in the river of life' as a metaphor for health promotion [35].

The river as a metaphor of health development (Fig. 1.1) has often been used. According to Antonovsky, it is not enough to promote health by avoiding stress or by building bridges keeping people from falling into the river. Instead, people have to learn to swim [36]. Lindström and Eriksson (2010) presented Salutogenesis in the context of health promotion research, using a new analogue of a river, 'Health in the River of Life'. The river of life is a simple way to demonstrate the characteristics of medicine (care and treatment) and public health (prevention and promotion) shifting the perspective and the focus from medicine to public health and health promotion toward population health.

The aim of this anthology is to describe and clarify health promotion in the context of health care settings. By doing so, we argue that the most appropriate theoretical foundation for health promotion in health care is the salutogenic theory of health by Antonovsky [36–38]. An integration of salutogenesis in health care could be a way to reorient health services in line with the Ottawa Charter for health promotion [22].

1.1.4 The Salutogenic Theory as the Foundation of Health Promotion

In many countries, health promotion has been primarily a field of practice and less a field of research [23]. The Ottawa conference in 1986 established the health promotion field, while the Jakarta conference in 1997 started a discussion of theory-driven approaches and evidence in this field. Throughout the two decades following the Ottawa conference, the health promotion

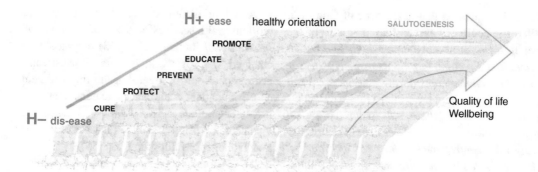

© Begt Lindstrom, Monica Erikson, Peter Wikström

Fig. 1.1 Health in the River of Life. (Published with permission from Folkhälsan Research Center, Helsinki, Lindström & Eriksson ([35], p. 17))

field has developed from a practice and policy field to also include a stronger theory and research field. There is currently a strong drive toward research-based practice in this field building on numerous evaluations of practices and programmes that have been developed and implemented in the course of these years ([23], p. 7). Samdal and Wold ([23], p. 9) provided an overview of theories relevant to health promotion; at the individual level, numerous concepts and theories in behavioural sciences contribute to the identification of conditions and processes that enable people to develop the personal skills necessary to make healthy choices. Vital psychological phenomena found to influence healthy choices are beliefs, knowledge, self-efficacy, skills, roles, attitudes and values. Important psychosocial concepts include social support, social cohesion, interpersonal stress, significant others and social norms. Social influence processes on health are explained by social psychological theories, such as social learning theory (social cognitive theory), the theory of planned behaviour, the self-determination theory, the social reproduction perspective and various socialization theories (e.g. ecological systems theory). In her lecture, 'The history and the future: towards a new public health' at the conference Next Health in Trondheim, Kickbusch [39] described how people involved in the Ottawa conference were influenced by

various theories, both health theories (Antonovsky, Illich, Lalonde) and sociological theories (Giddens, Mead, Foucault). However, the theoretical base for health promotion came in the cloud of more practical health work.

Just before the Ottawa conference in 1986, a special meeting was held in Copenhagen hosted by the WHO Regional Office for Europe. Aaron Antonovsky was invited and participated in the meeting and discussions. Nonetheless, the salutogenic theory did not appear in the formulations of the Ottawa Charter. Tamsma and Costongs ([40], p. 45) from the EuroHealthNet partnership stated that even if much evidence has been generated about the value of health promotion to health systems efficiency, outcomes and sustainability, yet the health (care) sector itself has been unable to adopt a systematic health promotion perspective and integrate it into broader systems and governance. The wide gap between the worlds of promoting health and curing disease remains. The reorientation of health sectors is where least progress from the Ottawa Charter principles can be noted. To conclude, there is still much work to do to implement health promotion into the health care sector in general, and the salutogenic theory and perspective in particular. Therefore, this book provides knowledge on health promotion and the potential role of salutogenesis in order to reorient the health care sector in a health promotion direction.

1.1.4.1 The Ontology of Salutogenesis

Ontology is the study of reality [41]. What do we know about the ontological background of salutogenesis? In his second book, *Unraveling the Mystery of Health* [36], Antonovsky described how he perceived the world. Two important things stand: (1) he saw man in interaction with his environment and (2) chaos and change as normal states of life. The former calls for system theory thinking where the focus is on the individual in a context [42, 43]. By the latter, Antonovsky perceived daily life as constantly changing; a heterostatic as opposed to a homeostatic state. For the individual, the challenge is to manage the chaos and find strategies and resources available for coping with the changes in everyday life. As a medical sociologist, he distinctly expressed systems theory thinking, this was a natural way for Antonovsky to perceive the world: seeing humans as part of and in interaction with the environment and context.

1.1.4.2 The Epistemology of Salutogenesis

Epistemology is the study of knowledge [44]. Going back to Antonovsky's writings [36, 37], little insight into his thoughts about knowledge generating and learning is provided. As far as we know, he did not manifest an epistemological basis for salutogenesis, neither describing his view of how knowledge in general arises nor how learning can be meaningful in the salutogenic framework. It appears that he was preoccupied with examining and describing how a strong SOC may have an impact on perceived health. A search in different databases provides little response [43]. Epistemologically, salutogenesis can be conceived as a constant learning process as shown in Fig. 1.2.

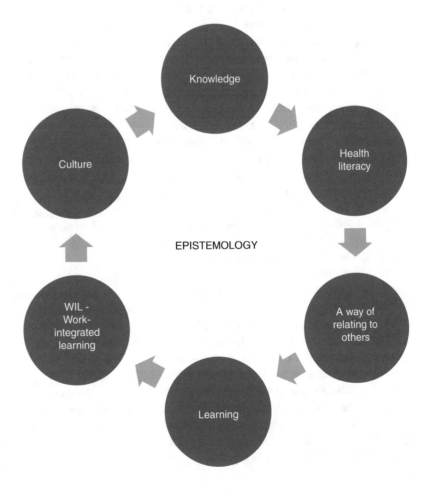

Fig. 1.2 Salutogenesis from an epistemological perspective. (With permission from: Eriksson M. The Sense of Coherence in the Salutogenic Model of Health. In: Mittelmark MB, Sagy S, Eriksson M, Bauer G, Pelikan J, Lindström B, et al., editors. The Handbook of Salutogenesis. New York: Springer; 2017. p. 91–6)

Figure 1.2 portrays that knowledge supports the movement toward the ease pole of the ease/dis-ease continuum (Fig. 1.3), while knowledge increases health literacy, which facilitates development in the ways one relates to one's world. The process of relating to others produces learning, and the knowledge gained from practice expands one's area of knowledge. In the course of daily life, this integrated learning process is continuous. The concept of work-integrated learning (WIL) is a new concept describing distinctive aspects of pedagogics and learning processes in health care settings [45]. The core of the salutogenic theory is to maintain and even develop health; this happens here and now in the context and culture where people live. To relate to health promotion and the Ottawa Charter for health promotion [22], culture becomes a resource in everyday life.

1.1.4.3 Health as a Process in an Ease/ Dis-Ease Continuum

According to Antonovsky, health is the movement on a continuum between (H+, Fig. 1.3) ease and dis-ease (H-, Fig. 1.3) [46]. He referred to the ability to comprehend the whole situation and the capacity to use the resources available as the *sense of coherence (SOC)*. This capacity was a combination of peoples' ability to assess and understand the situation they were in, to find a meaning to move in a health-promoting direction, also having the capacity to do so—that is, comprehensibility, meaningfulness and the manageability, to use Antonovsky's own terms [43, 47]. In such an approach, no one is categorized as healthy or diseased. Since we are all somewhere between the imaginary poles of total wellness and total illness, the whole population becomes the focus of concern. Even the fully robust, energetic, symptom-free, richly functioning individual has the mark of mortality: he or she wears glasses, has moments of depression, comes down with flu and may also have yet non-detectable malignant cells. Even the terminal patient's brain and emotions may be fully functional. The great majority of us are somewhere between the two poles. The idea of movement along an ease/disease continuum is illustrated in Fig. 1.3.

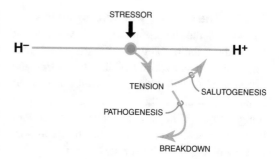

Fig. 1.3 The ease/dis-ease continuum [36, 37]. (Published with permission from Folkhälsan Research Center, Helsinki, Bengt Lindström, Monica Eriksson, Peter Wikström [35])

Antonovsky assumed that we constantly are exposed to changes and events that may be considered as stressors. This may involve major life events such as when someone in the family falls ill, changes in the family (e.g. a divorce) or changes in the workplace (organizational changes or unemployment). Theories on stress and coping are mainly focused on the concept of control. However, the concept of control is not central in the salutogenic theory. According to Antonovsky, who can control life? To use Antonovsky's own words, the salutogenic view of stress and coping includes the following:

> … *life is inherently full of stressors, with life-situation stressor complexes by far deserving most of our attention if we wish to understand either health or disease. Focusing on health, I expressly rejected the implicit assumption that stressors are inherently pathogenic. Their health consequences can only be understood if we understand the coping process* ([48], p. 48)

1.1.4.4 The Key Concepts of the Salutogenic Theory

Three key concepts form the salutogenic theory: (1) sense of coherence and (2) generalized and (3) specific resistance resources (described more in detail in Part I, Chap. 2 and Part II, Chap. 4).

Sense of coherence (SOC): Based on the interviews with Israeli women about health and how they were able to adapt to life events they went through, an important factor emerged: the sense of coherence. It reflects a person's view of life and capacity to respond to stressful situations. The original definition by Antonovsky [36] is as follows:

> SOC is a global orientation that expresses the extent to which one has a pervasive, enduring though dynamic feeling of confidence that (1) the stimuli from one's internal and external environments in the course of living are structured, predictable, and explicable; (2) the resources are available to one to meet the demands posed by these stimuli; and (3) these demands are challenges, worthy of investment and engagement. (p. 19)

Behind a global orientation, SOC is a way of viewing life as structured, manageable, and meaningful. At least three dimensions form the SOC: comprehensibility, manageability and meaningfulness. It is a personal way of thinking, being and acting, with an inner trust, which leads people to identify, benefit, use, and re-use the resources at their disposal [49].

Generalized and Specific Resistance Resources (GRR and SRR): Along with the SOC, the other key concepts in the salutogenic theory are the resistance resources [36, 37], including generalized resources (potentially available for engagement in a wide range of circumstances) and specific resources (particular resources relevant to particular circumstances). The resistance resources are of a different nature: among others genetic and constitutional, psychosocial, cultural and spiritual, material and a preventive health orientation [47]. Resistance resources exist at the individual, the group (family), the subculture and the whole society levels ([37], p. 103) and represent the prerequisites for developing a strong SOC.

1.1.5 Salutogenesis Is More Than the Measurement of the SOC

Salutogenesis is an area of knowledge and learning, a way of relating to others and a way of working in a health-promoting manner [43]. First and foremost, salutogenesis is a resource-oriented approach focusing on health and on people's abilities and capacities. Currently, there is extensive research that focuses on the resources of individuals, groups, and communities; this includes much more than the measurement of the SOC. Today, we talk about salutogenesis as a model of health and a life orientation (the SOC) [50], as well as the salutogenic conceptual framework. Salutogenesis now represents an umbrella concept with many different theories and concepts with salutogenic elements and dimensions [35]. Several of these concepts are highlighted in this anthology in Chaps. 4–18 and shown in bold fonts in Fig. 1.4.

Certain trends in the salutogenic research can be identified. These are (1) the translation and validation of the original SOC questionnaires (29 and 13 items), to other languages than English, (2) the use of the SOC questionnaires in different areas of research, (3) the term theory is more frequently used instead of idea of health and health model. What is a theory? The development of a theory begins with an idea, continues via various models, development of questionnaires, testing in empirical practice, systematically synthesize research, new instruments and insights. When all these steps take place in a systematic order, a theory arises. Such a development can be seen according to the salutogenic theory. Further, (4) development of programmes and interventions aiming at strengthening the SOC among patients and professionals and (5) the use of the SOC questionnaire for the evaluation of the effectiveness of interventions. The SOC questionnaire has been used in different areas compared to when the research began. Examples of new areas are oral health, health behaviour and work–life research. Currently, a tendency to move from only measuring SOC to applying salutogenic principles into practice when programmes and interventions are planned in various settings can be seen; such promising approaches among different populations in the health care are presented in Part III of this book; examples are the SHAPE intervention among older community-dwelling people (Chap. 23), the inter-generational platform intervention study in Singapore (Chap. 24), nurse–patient interaction as a health promotion approach in nursing homes (Chap. 10) and the

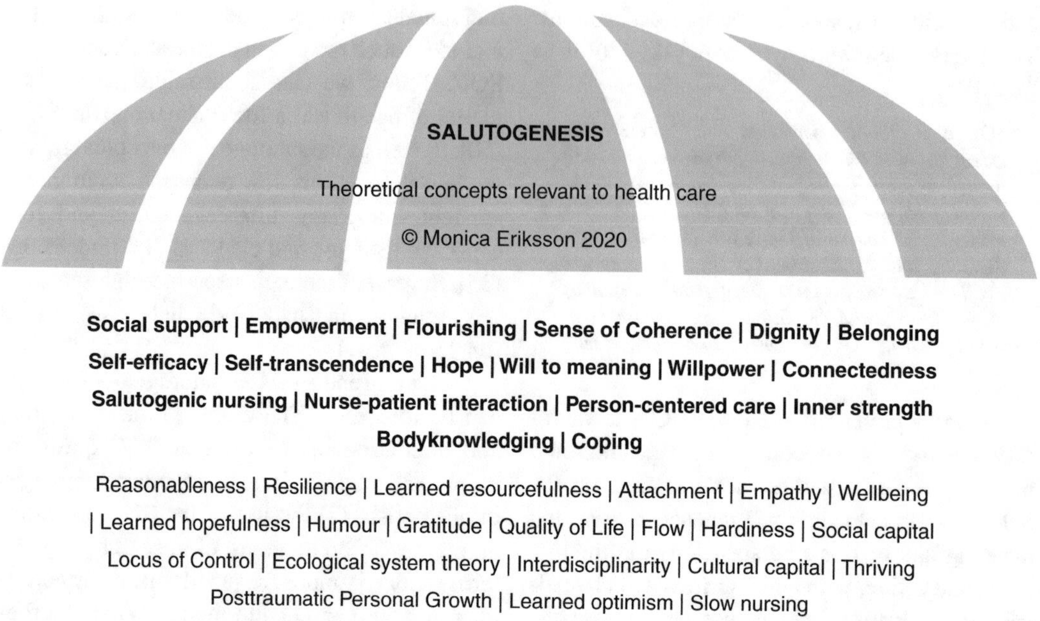

SALUTOGENESIS

Theoretical concepts relevant to health care

© Monica Eriksson 2020

**Social support | Empowerment | Flourishing | Sense of Coherence | Dignity | Belonging
Self-efficacy | Self-transcendence | Hope | Will to meaning | Willpower | Connectedness
Salutogenic nursing | Nurse-patient interaction | Person-centered care | Inner strength
Bodyknowledging | Coping**

Reasonableness | Resilience | Learned resourcefulness | Attachment | Empathy | Wellbeing
| Learned hopefulness | Humour | Gratitude | Quality of Life | Flow | Hardiness | Social capital
Locus of Control | Ecological system theory | Interdisciplinarity | Cultural capital | Thriving
Posttraumatic Personal Growth | Learned optimism | Slow nursing

Fig. 1.4 Salutogenesis. Theoretical concepts relevant to health care

bodyknowledging among chronical ill (Chap. 16). This implies that along the original SOC questionnaires, a range of different questionnaires have been developed and validated for use in the field of health promotion research. This is promising. As presented earlier in this chapter, due to the demographic development worldwide, the health care systems in all countries will face great challenges in the years to come. Facing the demographic trends, finding new and effective ways to improve people's health globally is imperative. Hence, health promotive initiatives will become ever more important worldwide.

References

1. Kinsella K, He W. An Aging World: 2008. Washington, DC: U.S. Department of Health and Human Services National Institutes of Health National Institute on Aging, U.S. Department of Commerce Economics and Statistics; 2009. Contract No.: Report No.: P95/09–1.
2. WHO. World report on ageing and health. Geneva: WHO; 2018. https://www.who.int/news-room/fact-sheets/detail/ageing-and-health. Accessed 5 Feb 2018.
3. WHO. Global status report on non-communicable diseases. 2010. http://www.who.int/chp/ncd_global_status_report/en/index.html. Accessed 23 Aug 2012.
4. WHO. Global strategy and action plan on ageing and health. IGO LCB-N-S, editor. Geneva: World Health Organization; 2017.
5. Prince M, Wimo A, Guerchet M, Ali G-C, Wu Y-T, Prina M. World Alzheimer Report 2015: The Global Impact of Dementia. An analysis of prevalence, incidence, cost and trends. London: Alzheimer's Disease International; 2015.
6. Global Burden of Disease Cancer Collaboration, Fitzmaurice C, Akinyemiju TF, et al. Global, regional, and national cancer incidence, mortality, years of life lost, years lived with disability, and disability-adjusted life-years for 29 Cancer Groups, 1990 to 2016: a systematic analysis for the Global Burden of Disease Study. JAMA Oncol. 2018;4(11):1553–68.
7. Cronin KA, Lake AJ, Scott S, Sherman RL, Noone AM, Howlader N, et al. Annual report to the nation on the status of Cancer, part I: National Cancer Statistics. Cancer. 2018;124(13):2785–800.
8. Ponikowski P, Anker S, AlHabib K, Cowie M, Force T, Hu S, et al. Heart failure: preventing disease and death worldwide. ESC Heart Fail. 2014;1(1):4–25.
9. Heidenreich P, Trogdon J, Khavjou O, Butler J, Dracup K, Ezekowitz M, et al. Forecasting the future of cardiovascular disease in the United States: a policy statement from the American Heart Association. Circulation. 2011;123(8):933–44.
10. Reyes E, Ha J, Firdaus I, Ghazi A, Phrommintikul A, Sim D, et al. Heart failure across Asia: same health-

care burden but differences in organization of care. Int J Cardiol. 2016;2016(223):163–7.

11. Rajadurai J, Tse H, Wang C, Yang N, Zhou J, Sim D. Understanding the epidemiology of heart failure to improve management practices: an Asia-Pacific perspective. J Card Fail. 2017;23(4):327–39.

12. Richards A, Lam C, Wong R, Ping C. Heart failure: a problem of our age. Ann Acad Med Singapore. 2011;40(9):392–3.

13. Bundkirchen A, Schwinger R. Epidemiology and economic burden of chronic heart failure. Eur Heart J Suppl. 2004;6:D57–60.

14. Kannel W. Incidence and epidemiology of heart failure. Heart Fail Rev. 2000;5(2):173–7.

15. Ng T, Niti M. Trends and ethnic differences in hospital admissions and mortality for congestive heart failure in the elderly in Singapore, 1991 to 1998. Heart. 2003;89(8):865–70.

16. Santhanakrishnan R, Ng T, Cameron V, Gamble G, Ling L, Sim D, et al. The Singapore heart failure outcomes and phenotypes (SHOP) study and prospective evaluation of outcome in patients with heart failure with preserved left ventricular ejection fraction (PEOPLE) study: rationale and design. J Card Fail. 2013;19(3):156–62.

17. Savarese G, Lund LH. Global public health burden of heart failure. Card Fail Rev. 2017;3(1):7–11.

18. United Nations. World Population Ageing: 1950–2050. New York: United Nations, Department of Economic and Social Affairs; 2002. www.un.org/esa/population/publications/worldageing19502050.

19. WHO. Targets for health for all 2000. Copenhagen: WHO Regional Office for Europe; 1986b.

20. WHO. Primary health care: report of the international conference on primary health care Alma-Ata, USSR. Geneva: WHO; 1978.

21. Scriven A, Orme J, editors. Health promotion—professional perspectives. New York: Palgrave/The Open University; 2001.

22. WHO. The Ottawa charter for health promotion: an international conference on health promotion. The Move towards a New Public Health. Copenhagen: WHO; 1986c.

23. Samdal O, Wold B. Introduction to health promotion. In: Wold B, Samdal O, editors. An ecological perspective on health promotion systems, settings and social processes. Sharjah: Bentham Science; 2012. p. 3–10.

24. The Lancet–University of Oslo Commission on Global Governance for Health. The political origins of health inequity: prospects for change. Lancet. 2014;383:630–67.

25. Kickbusch I. The contribution of the World Health Organization to a new public health and health promotion. Am J Public Health. 2003;93(3):383–8.

26. Mittelmark MB, Kickbush I, Rootman I, Scriver A, Tones K. Health promotion. In: Heggenhougen K, Quah S, editors. International encyclopedia of public health. San Diego, SD: Academic Press; 2008. p. 225–39.

27. Kickbusch I. Introduction to the journal. Health Promot Int. 1986;1(1):3–4.

28. WHO. Health promotion. A discussion document on the concept and principles. Copenhagen: WHO Regional Office for Europe; 1986a.

29. Ziglio E, Simpson S, Tsouros A. Health promotion and health systems: some unfinished business. Health Promot Int. 2011;26:ii216.

30. Catford J. Turn, turn, turn: time to reorient health services. Health Promot Int. 2014;29(1):1–4.

31. De Leeuw E. Have the health services reoriented at all? Health Promot Int. 2009;24(2):105–7.

32. Wise M, Nutbeam D. Enabling health systems transformation: what progress has been made in re-orienting health services? Promot Educ. 2007;2:23–7.

33. Thompson S, Watson M, Tilford S. The Ottawa charter 30 years on: still an important standard for health promotion. Int J Health Promot Educ. 2018;56(2):73–84.

34. Rootman I, Goodstadt M, Hyndman B, McQueen D, Potvin L, Springett J, et al., editors. Evaluation in health promotion principles and perspectives. Copenhagen: World Health Organization; 2001.

35. Lindström B, Eriksson M. The Hitchhiker's guide to Salutogenesis. Salutogenic pathways to health promotion. Folkhälsan Research Center: Helsinki; 2010.

36. Antonovsky A. Unraveling the mystery of health. How people manage stress and stay well. San Fransisco: Jossey-Bass; 1987.

37. Antonovsky A. Health, stress, and coping: new perspectives on mental health and physical wellbeing. San Francisco, CA: Jossey-Bass; 1979.

38. Mittelmark MB, Sagy S, Eriksson M, Bauer GF, Pelikan JM, Lindström B, et al., editors. The handbook of Salutogenesis. New York: Springer; 2017.

39. Kickbusch I. The history and the future: towards a new public health. Trondheim: Next Health; 2014.

40. Tamsma N, Costongs C. Promoting health and Wellbeing in the context of the United Nations sustainable development agenda, on behalf of the EuroHealthNet partnership, EuroHealthNet, Brussels. Belg Scand J Publ Health. 2018;46:44–8.

41. Heil J. From an ontological point of view. Gloucestershire: Clarendon; 2005.

42. Antonovsky A. The life cycle, mental health and the sense of coherence. Isr J Psychiatry Relat Sci. 1985;22(4):273–80.

43. Eriksson M. The sense of coherence in the Salutogenic model of health. In: Mittelmark MB, Sagy S, Eriksson M, Bauer G, Pelikan J, Lindström B, et al., editors. The handbook of Salutogenesis. New York: Springer; 2017. p. 91–6.

44. Epistemology AR. A contemporary introduction to the theory of knowledge. New York: Routledge; 2011.

45. Pennbrant S, Svensson L. Nursing and learning—healthcare pedagogics and work-integrated learning. Higher Educ Skills Work Based Learn. 2018;8(2):179–94.

46. Antonovsky A. The structure and properties of the sense of coherence scale. Soc Sci Med. 1993;36:969–81.
47. Lindström B, Eriksson M. Salutogenesis. J Epidemiol Community Health. 2005;59(6):440–2.
48. Antonovsky A. Can attitudes contribute to health? Advances. J Mind Body Health. 1992;8(4):33–49.
49. Eriksson M, Lindström B. Antonovsky's sense of coherence scale and the relation with health: a systematic review. J Epidemiol Community Health. 2006;60(5):376–81.
50. Mittelmark MB, Bauer G. The meanings of Salutogenesis. In: Mittelmark MB, Sagy S, Eriksson M, Bauer G, Pelikan J, Lindström B, et al., editors. The handbook of Salutogenesis. New York: Springer; 2017. p. 7–13.

The Overarching Concept of Salutogenesis in the Context of Health Care

2

Geir Arild Espnes, Unni Karin Moksnes, and Gørill Haugan

Abstract

Two concepts that widely impact on our ways to work with health is *health promotion* and *salutogenesis* (For a quick overview of the concept of salutogenesis, read Lindström B. & Eriksson M. (2010). The Hitchhiker's Guide to Salutogenesis. Folkhälsan Research Center). The concept of health promotion was voted for use by the participants of World Health Organization (WHO) general assembly in 1978. And after 8 years, the concept of health promotion was filled with content by the WHO meeting in Ottawa in 1986. Meanwhile, salutogenesis as a concept was constructed of the Israeli scientist Antonovsky during the 1970s. It can be said that both health promotion and salutogenesis grew out of a wanting to understand health development rather than understanding health as a variable tied to the presence or absence of disease developments. This chapter concentrates on discussing the use of the salutogenic framework on the understanding of health care situations.

G. A. Espnes (✉)
Department of Public Health and Nursing, NTNU Norwegian University of Science and Technology, Trondheim, Norway

NTNU-Center for Health Promotion Research, Trondheim, Norway
e-mail: geirae@ntnu.no, geir.arild.espnes@ntnu.no

U. K. Moksnes
Department of Public Health and Nursing, NTNU Norwegian University of Science and Technology, Trondheim, Norway

NTNU-Center for Health Promotion Research, Trondheim, Norway

Faculty of Nursing and Health Science, Nord University, Levanger, Norway
e-mail: unni.moksnes@ntnu.no

G. Haugan
Department of Public Health and Nursing, NTNU Norwegian University of Science and Technology, Trondheim, Norway

Faculty of Nursing and Health Science, Nord University, Levanger, Norway
e-mail: gorill.haugan@ntnu.no, gorill.haugan@nord.no

Keywords

Health · Health promotion · Salutogenesis · Resources · Pathogenesis · Treatment

2.1 Salutogenesis: Turning Health Concerns from Solely be Occupied with What Gives Disease to What Gives Health

Salutogenesis has become a frequently used word or concept in the health domain, and especially within the public health and health promotion

G. Haugan, M. Eriksson (eds.), *Health Promotion in Health Care – Vital Theories and Research*,
https://doi.org/10.1007/978-3-030-63135-2_2

area (see [1]). But where does the word come from? And what does this concept mean? This chapter sets out to reveal the answer to both these questions and also to investigate how the understanding of health can be encompassed in health care and disease treatment.

The WHO Ottawa Charter [2] almost 35 years ago clearly defined that health is "...a resource for everyday life ... A positive concept emphasizing social and personal resources, as well as physical capacities ... To reach a state of complete physical, mental and social well-being." This explanation of what health is gave a whole new understanding of the rationale for what brings health instead of the sole pursuit of the reasons of a disease or how to prevent diseases. These two equally old concepts of health promotion and salutogenesis sometimes are deemed the "starting shot" for the new challenge of enhancing health rather than explaining and preventing disease. A new aera had begun.

Salutogenesis was first used as a concept of health by the Israeli medical sociologist Aron Antonovsky. In the 1960s, Antonovsky studied female survivors from the Second World War's German concentration camps who by then had become grandmothers. What he found was remarkable. A number of the Jewish grandmothers, now living in Israel, had not only survived the concentration camps, but also been able to live a good flourishing life, with good mental and physical health, in spite of the horrors in the camps. Antonovsky stated that even if only a few would have lived through the horrors and still were able to live a flourishing life that would be most remarkable and should be subject to thorough studies in search for the overarching question; what is the origin of good health? One of Antonovsky's deviations from pathogenesis was to reject the dichotomization into categories of diseased or healthy. Antonovsky stated that disease, stressors, and unpredictability are part of life and can never be controlled completely. The interesting question that came to his mind was: how can we survive in spite of all this? The answer to this was understood as the individual's sense of coherence and ability to identify and use generalized and specific resistance resources.

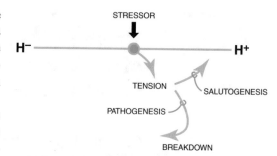

Fig. 2.1 The ease dis-ease continuum. (Published with permission from Folkhälsan Research Center, Helsinki, Lindström & Eriksson [3])

One of the keys to the salutogenic approach was to describe health as a continuum between "total health (H+) and total absence of health" (H−) or the "ease – dis-ease continuum" (see below Fig. 2.1).

At any time, each of us can be placed on this continuum [4]. Stressors can upset our position, and we come under tension. Here are two options: either the pathogenic forces overtake us and we break down or we regain our health through SOC and move toward H+. The important point is to focus on what moves an individual toward the ease pole of the continuum, regardless of where the individual is initially located. By the continuation of his studies, Antonovsky presented a few distinct characteristics of what gave good health to people, as well as developed a new health theory of "salutogenesis." The name of "salutogenesis" was constructed by combining the Latin word Salut (health—or to your health) with the Greek word Genesis (origin). Salutogenesis has become an interesting concept for scientists and practitioners from a wide range of backgrounds who had been in search for an approach to study what brings health. Especially, the movement for health promotion research and work has shown great interest.

For many years, WHO had enquired for a reorientation in health care representing the use of both the resource (salutogenesis) and the treatment paradigms (pathogenesis) as complementary in health care. The health promotion approach had surfaced as an alternative to disease prevention, keeping health as a target rather than avoidance of disease on the WHO 1978 World

Conference in Alma Ata. After 8 years of intensive work to establish an understanding of health promotion and the need for an alternative to disease prevention across the world, the Ottawa Charter on Health Promotion was launched in the WHO World Conference in Ottawa 1986 [2], and the health social anthropologist that had led the work became notoriously famous. Her name is Ilona Kickbusch.

The Ottawa Charter became the answer to the request for a reorientation of the world's health care systems. One can claim that there is quite an unrealized potential in health care to be more protective and promotive of health. However, the Ottawa Charter was in lack of a theoretical model or theoretical approach to back its ideas. Since salutogenesis was developed as a paradigm in opposition to the "pathogenic orientation which suffuses all western medical thinking" ([5], p. 13), it had to be considered a health promotion concept. In his brief 1996 paper in the journal *Health Promotion International*, Antonovsky challenged the health promotion field to adopt salutogenesis as a health promotion theory.

In principle, applying salutogenesis as a health theory in the health promotion field could mean to restrict the leading pathogenic orientation in health care practice (research and policy) and complement or change it by a salutogenic orientation in everyday practice and research. It also became evident that Antonovsky had come up with a theoretical basis for the concept of salutogenesis, and the underlying concept of "Sense of Coherence" which explains what brings good health. The next part of this chapter dives further into the key concepts of Antonovsky's salutogenic health model, namely sense of coherence and resistant resources.

2.2 The Sense of Coherence and Resistant Resources

As stated above, Antonovsky introduced the salutogenic model as a new possible paradigm for health research [5]. In a lecture at Berkley in 1993 [6], he defined the concept of salutogenesis as "the process of movement toward the health end of a health ease/dis-ease continuum" and defined the life orientation concept of sense of coherence (SOC) as follows:

> "… a global orientation that expresses the extent to which one has a pervasive, enduring though dynamic feeling of confidence that one's internal and external environments are predictable and that there is a high probability that things will work out as well as can reasonably be expected." [7]

Accordingly, salutogenesis is understood to describe the process of enabling individuals, groups, organizations, and societies to emphasize on abilities, resources, capacities, competences, strengths, and forces in order to create a strong SOC; that is, to perceive life as comprehensible, manageable, and meaningful which represent three central components in SOC. Recent research shows this model is an effective approach to positive health development in a life course perspective [1]. However, the potential of this model has not been fully explored in health promotion practice and research [1].

The salutogenic model includes three central concepts: generalized resistance resources (GRRs), specific resistant resources (SRR), and the above-mentioned SOC. The GRRs are of both external and internal characters; people have at their disposal resources of both internal and external characters which make it easier for them to manage life [4]. Specific resistance resources, on the other hand, are optimized by societal action in which health promotion has a contributing role, for example, the provision of supportive social and physical environments [1].

The GRRs are of any character ranging from material to virtual and spiritual dimensions of the mind, processes, and psychological mechanisms. The main thing is that people are able to use the GRRs for their own good and for health development. The GRRs, characterized by underload–overload balance and participation in shaping outcomes (empowering processes), provide a person with sets of meaningful and coherent life experiences, which in turn create a strong SOC [1].

While GRRs are the prerequisites for developing a strong SOC, the capability to use GRRs is based on people's SOC, a concept that has been shown to be of key importance in health research, correlating positively with good health outcomes, quality of life, and most psychological measures of well-being [1]. Today, there are hundreds of articles referring to the SOC in individuals and groups, as well as population studies that demonstrate the strength of this concept and phenomenon. Antonovsky stated that people's SOC is mainly developed in childhood and early adulthood. However, new research points to the fact that SOC is a continuous process throughout the entire life [1]. The perception of coherence is based on cognitive, behavioral, and motivational factors which are improved by raising the awareness of the population, empowering the population and engagement in areas which are meaningful to the population.

2.3 Salutogenesis in Health Care Settings

The health care sector is still primarily defined by a pathogenic paradigm, and the health care system is most often anticipated as the system of struggle against pathological developments, or as Antonovsky expressed it "health care or more correctly the disease care system" ([5], p. 12). The health care area has therefore often been seen as challenging for the application and implementation of a salutogenic approach. To understand the challenge completely, one needs to ask what is the essence in the challenge of integrating these newer, more modern, and comprehensive health perspectives into health care?

The health care sector intends to professionally manage illness by trying to prevent or cure diseases, or if this is not possible, at least to offer care for chronic patients and palliative care. However, the contribution of health promotion is still marginal in the health care sector. Reorientation of health services, as demanded by the Ottawa Charter [2], has not yet happened in accordance to the expectations [8, 9]. There is still quite an unrealized potential in health care to be more protective and promotive of positive health. Further, also salutogenesis has quite an unrealized potential for being more evidence

based in reference to preserving and promoting health in different patient groups living with disease and infirmity. In his 1996 publication [5], Antonovsky suggested that the appeal of the full salutogenic model for those engaged in health promotion cannot be on the grounds of powerfully demonstrated efficacy in producing significant health-related change outcomes. It can be understood that to release the unreleased potential of using the salutogenic framework in health care, the only way to test the potential and effectiveness is to start using it in different health care settings. A relevant question today is, therefore, how far has the change toward a more protective and promotive approach in health care come since Antonovsky wrote this statement, and are there any differences between different health care settings?

First things first. Salutogenesis—the newer and more focused concept—has been introduced by Antonovsky into health promotion, which represents an older and broader concept, field, and movement. As pointed to above, Antonovsky [5] underlined that "the basic flaw of the field (of health promotion) is that it has no theory." Thus, he proposed "the salutogenic orientation… as providing a direction and focus to this field." He also stated that "the salutogenic model is useful for all fields of health care. In its very spirit, however, it is particularly appropriate to health promotion." Hence, health promotion in health care definitely has the blessings of Antonovsky. Therefore, we have to clarify how the salutogenic orientation or model and its related construct of SOC can be integrated into health care, directly or via (re-)orienting health promotion in health care indirectly.

2.4 What Can Salutogenesis Mean for Health Care, Across Settings?

In health care settings, the salutogenic paradigm can be used for two purposes: either to guide health promotion interventions in health care practice across settings or to (re)orient health care research as such. For this, the salutogenic paradigm offers specific concepts, assumptions, and instruments. According to Pelikan [10], three quite different conceptual forms can be distinguished: (1) a salutogenic orientation, (2) a salutogenic model, and (3) the construct of the SOC and a methodologically sound way to operationalize it. These three forms first have to be specified in more detail, to be applied later to the whole field of health care and later for specific settings. For that, health care has to be understood as a complex of a strongly interrelated professional practice, with clinical research and supporting policy. Therefore, applying salutogenesis in health care successfully cannot just be done by introducing salutogenesis in health care practice; there is also a need for a change in underlying health care policy.

2.4.1 The Salutogenic Orientation and Health Care

The first and most broad form of salutogenesis, a salutogenic orientation, is described by three assumptions: (a) the human system is subject to unavoidable processes toward an unavoidable final death. Therefore, the necessity of adaptation or coping with accompanying tension that may result in stress is universal and not the exemption. (b) A continuum model, which sees each and all of us somewhere along a health ease/dis-ease continuum. Therefore, a dichotomization into healthy and sick is not very helpful. (c) The concept of salutary factors or health-promoting factors are shown to actively promote health, which represents better health rather than just being low on risk factors (see [5], p. 14). Therefore, both risk and salutary factors have to be attended.

From these three assumptions follow implications for health promotion. A salutogenic orientation as the basis for health promotion directs both research and action efforts: (1) to encompass all persons, wherever they are on the continuum, and (2) to focus on salutary factors, which (3) relate to all aspects of the person instead of focusing on a particular diagnostic category as in curative medicine or (even) in preventive medicine.

Applying these assumptions and implications to health care practice would mean, again according to Pelikan [10], that (1) since a salutogenic orientation encompasses all individuals independently of their position on the ease/dis-ease continuum, health care should not only just care for the health of its patients, but take responsibility for the health of its staff and the health of citizens as well (however, dichotomous classification of individuals into those who have some specific disease or not, is unavoidable for doing curative medicine on patients); (2) in relation to these three groups of patients, health care staff, and citizens, not only their risk factors have to be dealt with or fought by health care, but also possible health-promoting (salutary) factors have to be enhanced in curative, preventive, protective, and promotive practice; (3) a holistic approach, including all sides and aspects; physical, mental, spiritual/existential, and social aspects of a person have to be taken into account in dealing with all people affected by health care.

In principle, to apply these assumptions on health care sounds plausible and rational, but three aspects need to be fulfilled: firstly, to realize a policy change of the mandate of health care is necessary; secondly, to understand that the traditional diagnostic and therapeutic repertoire of health care has to be widened; and thirdly, a radical change of clinical understanding and application is implied. The last of these three might be especially difficult since part of the spectacular medical success rests on focusing on a narrow biomedical model.

2.4.2 The Salutogenic Model

A second way of understanding salutogenesis in relation to health care settings is to understand Antonovsky's specific and rather complex salutogenic model ([7], see Chap. 7)). Within this model, the concept of GRRs is introduced as "a property of a person, a collective or a situation which, as evidence or logic has indicated, facilitated successful coping with the inherent stressors of human existence" ([5], p. 15). This model has not been further explored, even if major psychosocial, genetic, and constitutional GRRs are specified within this model [11]. There is, however, a possibility via scientific scrutinization of a wider view of this complex model encompassing large societies and a possibility to further explore the model as an underlying understanding for policy and society interventions.

In some countries, like Norway, we have through the last years seen a growing number of practical interventions in public health and health care that has been based in the general salutogenic model or other resource-based models [12]. It has also been observed how practical salutogenic work solutions have been used in health care among young in schools [13], for elderly both in nursing homes [14] and as an intervention approach in care situations among elderly outside nursing homes [15]. These new studies make their ways into health planning and health policy, but now also increasingly in care and health care. It might seem like the change in orientation that De Leeuw [8] was asking for slowly is appearing. How central researchers in the area of salutogenesis research sees the future developments is spelled out in two central publications: (1) the Handbook of Salutogenesis from 2016 [16] and (2) in the 2019 article entitled "Future directions for the concept of salutogenesis: a position article" [17].

2.4.3 The Sense of Coherence and Health Care Settings

If one utilizes the salutogenic model in health care (see above), the GRRs specified in detail in the salutogenic health model would have to be more adequately taken into account in health care practice and research, as well as in policy documents describing research activities and practices. The model and its implications make much sense for health care in different settings and afford a more holistic and complex outlook and a widening of diagnostic and therapeutic methods applied.

The third most focused form of salutogenesis, the specific construct of SOC which has been introduced as a central factor in the salutogenic model of health, is defined as:

a generalized orientation toward the world which perceives it, on a continuum, as comprehensible, manageable and meaningful ([5], p. 15).

Antonovsky further stated that

The strength of one's SOC, I proposed, was a significant factor in facilitating the movement toward health. This construct answers what do all these GRRs have in common, why do they seem to work. What united them, it seemed to me, was that they all fostered repeated life experiences which, to put it at its simplest, helped one to see the world as 'making sense', cognitively, instrumentally and emotionally ([5], p. 15).

Here Antonovsky introduced the SOC as a moderator or mediator of other determinants of health rather than a specific determinant of health. "What matters is that one has had the life experiences which lead to a strong SOC; this in turn allows one to "reach out," in any given situation and apply the resources appropriate to that stressor. "The strength of one's SOC is shaped by three kinds of life experiences: consistency, underload-overload balance, and participation in socially valued decision making. The extent of such experiences is molded by one's position in the social structure and by one's culture.. ." ([5], p. 15).

Is there one pivotal argument of how the SOC can be introduced into health care? A thought experiment:

Being ill and becoming a patient in professional health care is often a rather threatening life experience for people and being a health care professional is a rather demanding job. Therefore, using the SOC concept for making the health care context and the culture as far as possible consistent, underload–overload balanced, and participatory for patients, health care staff, and visitors could be an adequate argument and way to make health care systems more salutogenic driven, generally. This is possible, since "social institutions in all but the most chaotic historical situations can be modified to some degree" ([5], p. 15). A different way to think about this, is to work with the possible feasibility, effectiveness, and efficiency in developing salutogenic "standards" [18] and make institutional contexts more salutogenic. Even if Antonovsky assumed that one's SOC cannot be radically transformed, he left it open that the SOC could be shaped and strengthened, so that it in turn can push people towards health [15]. Therefore, in reference of patients' situation, improving SOC by increasing their health literacy among an array of other coping resources could become an explicit goal of chronic disease management.

2.5 Conclusions

The salutogenic perspective has clearly a potential to be applied in the health care across settings in relation to health promoting interventions for the health of patients, staff, and citizens, and in supporting health-promoting structures and cultures of health care institutions for better everyday practice and policy.

As we have pointed to in this chapter, there are some very important implications for utilizing the salutogenic approach and model as a way to work in health care settings. The field or setting will need (1) to encompass all persons, wherever they are on the ease/(dis)ease continuum and (2) to focus on known salutary factors, which (3) relate to all aspects of the person rather than solely focusing on a particular diagnostic medical category or criteria.

There is, of course, as for most other concepts and theories, a clear need for further research, no doubt. Especially research focusing on the salutogenic model and on the specific role of SOC as a predictor, mediator, or moderator is needed. Moreover, research shaped to lead to a better conceptual clarity and application of more complex research designs, especially on the link between SOC and other aspects of health than subjective and mental health, as well as on the impact of health care setting functioning are required.

Take Home Messages
- The WHO Ottawa Charter clearly defines that health is a "…a resource for everyday life… A positive concept emphasizing social and personal resources, as well as physical capacities…."
- The Israeli medical sociologist Aron Antonovsky presented a few distinct characteristics of what gave good health to people, as

well as developed a new health theory termed "salutogenesis." The name of "salutogenesis" was constructed by combining the Latin word Salut (health) with the Greek word Genesis (origin).
- WHO has for many years demanded for a reorientation in health care representing the use of both the resource (salutogenesis) and the treatment (pathogenesis) paradigms as complementary in health care. The Ottawa Charter became the answer to the request for a reorientation of the world's health care systems; there is still quite an unrealized potential in health care to be more protective and promotive of positive health.
- Applying salutogenesis as a health theory in the health promotion field could mean to restrict the leading pathogenic orientation in health care practice (research and policy) and complement or change it by a salutogenic orientation in everyday practice and research.
- Salutogenesis as a concept is understood to describe the process of enabling individuals, groups, organizations, and societies to emphasize abilities, resources, capacities, competences, strengths, and forces to create a sense of coherence; that is, to perceive life as comprehensible, manageable, and meaningful.
- The salutogenic model includes three central concepts: generalized resistance resources (GRRs), specific resistance resources (SRR), and sense of coherence (SOC).
- In health care settings, the salutogenic paradigm can be used for two purposes: either to guide health promotion interventions in health care practice across settings or to (re)orient health care research as such. For this, the salutogenic paradigm offers specific concepts, assumptions, and instruments.

References

1. Mittelmark MB, Sagy S, Eriksson M, Bauer GF, Pelikan JM, Lindström B, et al., editors. The handbook of Salutogenesis. New York: Springer; 2017.
2. WHO. The Ottawa charter for health promotion—World 1986. 1986. http://www.who.int/healthpromotion/conferences/previous/ottawa/en/.

3. Lindström B, Eriksson M. The Hitchhiker's guide to Salutogenesis. Folkhälsan Research Center, Health Promotion Research Programme and the IUHPE Global Working Group on Salutogenesis. ISBN: 978–952-5641-34-9; 2010.

4. Antonovsky A. Unraveling the mystery of health: how people manage stress and stay well. San Francisco: Jossey-Bass; 1987.

5. Antonovsky A. The salutogenic model as a theory to guide health promotion. Health Promot Int. 1996;11(1):11–8.

6. Antonovsky A. The salutogenic approach to aging. Lecture held in Berkeley. January 21, 1993.

7. Antonovsky A. Health, stress, and coping: new perspectives on mental health and physical wellbeing. San Francisco, CA: Jossey-Bass; 1979.

8. De Leeuw E. Have the health services reoriented at all? Health Promot Int. 2009;24(2):105–7.

9. Wise M, Nutbeam D. Enabling health systems transformation: what progress has been made in *reorienting* health services? Promot Educ. 2007;2:23–7.

10. Pelikan JM. The application of Salutogenesis in healthcare settings. In: Mittelmark MB, Sagy S, Eriksson M, Bauer GF, Pelikan JM, Lindström B, et al., editors. The handbook of Salutogenesis. New York: Springer; 2017.

11. Mittelmark M, Bull T. The salutogenic model of health in health promotion research. Glob Health Promot. 2013;20(2):30–8.

12. Lillefjell M, Magnus E, Knudtsen MS, Wist G, Horghagen S, Espnes GA, Maass REK, Anthun S. Governance for public health and health equity: The Trøndelag model for public health work. Scand J Public Health. 2018;46(22):37–47. https://doi.org/10.1177/1403494818765704.

13. Moksnes UK, Espnes GA. Sense of coherence in association with stress experience and health in adolescents. Int J Environ Res Public Health. 2020;17:3003.

14. Rinnan E, Andre B, Drageset J, Garåsen H, Espnes GA, Haugan G. Joy of life in nursing homes: a qualitative study of what constitutes the essence of joy of life in elderly individuals living in Norwegian nursing homes. Scand J Caring Sci. 2018;32(4):1468–76.

15. Seah B, Espnes GA, Ang ENK, Lim JY, Kowitlawakul Y, Wang W. Achieving healthy ageing through the perspective of sense of coherence among senior only households: a qualitative study. Aging Ment Health. 2020:1–10. https://doi.org/10.1080/13607863.2020.1725805.

16. Espnes GA. Salutogenesis: the editors discuss possible futures. In: Mittelmark MB, Sagy S, Eriksson M, Bauer GF, Pelikan JM, Lindström B, et al., editors. The handbook of Salutogenesis. New York: Springer; 2017.

17. Bauer GF, Roy M, Bakibinga P, Contu P, Downe S, Eriksson M, Espnes GA, Jensen BB, Canal DJ, Lingström B, Mana A, Mittelmark MB, Morgan AR, Pelikan JM, Saboga-Nunes L, Sagy S, Shorey S, Vandraager L, Vinje HF. Future directions for the concept of salutogenesis: a position article. Health Promot Int. 2020;35(2):187–95.

18. Dalton C, McCartney K. Salutogenesis: a new paradigm for pervasive computing in healthcare environments? In: Conference: 5th international conference on pervasive computing technologies for healthcare, pervasive health, 2011, Dublin; 2011. https://doi.org/10.4108/icst.pervasivehealth.2011.246064.

The Ethics of Health Promotion: From Public Health to Health Care

3

Berge Solberg

Abstract

Health promotion is often been associated with altering social arrangement in order to improve the health of citizens—the domain of public health. Ethical aspects of health promotion then is generally discussed in terms of a public health ethics. In this chapter, I start out with some classical ethical and political dilemmas of health promotion in public health before I move into the ethics of health promotion in health care. I argue that empowerment, better than any other value, may serve as the ethical foundation for health promotion in health care. I further claim that empowerment may serve as the ethical bridge between health promotion in health care and health promotion in public health.

Keywords

Ethics · Empowerment · Autonomy Paternalism · Nudging · Health · Positive freedom · Salutogenesis · Agency

3.1 Introduction

Even though 'health promotion' probably has been defined again and again in this book, we still need to pay attention to the definition before we start talking about ethics. 'Health promotion is the process of enabling people to increase control over, and to improve, their health. To reach a state of complete physical, mental and social well-being, an individual or group must be able to identify and to realize aspirations, to satisfy needs, and to change or cope with the environment'. These are some of the first sentences in the Ottawa charter for Health Promotion from 1986 [1]. Taken in isolation, they may suggest that health promotion mainly has to do with the well-being of individual persons and patients. If that is the case, an ethics of health promotion seems to be some variants of an ethics of health care.

If we, however, focus on the first sentence of the charter, we can notice that it says that 'this conference was primarily a response to growing expectations for a new *public health movement* around the world'. Health promotion is here associated with public health. In a paper with the telling title *How to Think about Health Promotion Ethics*, Carter et al. define an ethics of health promotion in this way: 'We consider the normative ideal of health promotion to be that aspect of public health practice that is particularly concerned with the equity of social arrangements: it imagines that social arrangements can be altered

B. Solberg (✉)
Department of Public Health and Nursing, The Norwegian University of Science and Technology (NTNU), Trondheim, Norway
e-mail: berge.solberg@ntnu.no

G. Haugan, M. Eriksson (eds.), *Health Promotion in Health Care – Vital Theories and Research*,
https://doi.org/10.1007/978-3-030-63135-2_3

23

to make things better for everyone, whatever their health risks, and seeks to achieve this in collaboration with citizens. This raises two main ethical questions. First: what is a good society? And then: what should health promotion contribute to a good society?' [2]. If they are correct, an ethics of health promotion seems to be some variants of an ethics of public health.

An ethics of health promotion belongs to both spheres. In many ethical discussions, public health has been a natural framework. The ethical questions are clearly recognizable on this arena. But already in the Ottawa charter, there is a call for *reorienting the health services* in the direction of health promotion. In this chapter, we take a roundabout way. We start with some basic concepts of political philosophy that gives us a framework for the discussion. Then we take a look at some of the typical ethical dilemmas of health promotion in public health, before we end up with articulating an ethics of health promotion within health care.

3.2 The Two Concepts of Liberty: Two Concepts of Health?

A deep discussion on the ethical justifiability of health promotion in a society needs to start with some considerations on the relation between the individual and the society. A person's view on the legitimacy and the need for health promotion will very often reflect his political position. Both libertarians and communitarians will be concerned with freedom and choice, but different concepts of freedom will be applied. For libertarians, only freedom from an intrusive and paternalistic state will be genuine freedom. For communitarians, only freedom to realize your potential will amount to genuine freedom. These are the 'two concepts of liberty' that Isaiah Berlin talked about in his famous paper from 1958 [3].

Negative freedom means that you are free, as long as you are left to do whatever you want to do without interference from others (except from harming other people). The more other people, the society and the state interfere with your life, the less freedom you have. Low taxes give you more freedom than high taxes, because the former interferes less with your life than the latter. Individuality and liberty must be protected from the community. Negative freedom is often referred to as 'freedom *from…*'.

Positive freedom means the freedom to pursue and realize your interest and priorities in your life. If I am really interested in an academic career, but cannot afford education, then my freedom is limited, even though the state has not interfered with my wishes. Rather the opposite would be true; the fact that the state has not provided opportunities for free education makes me less free than I could have been. Defenders of positive freedom very often argue that the negative concept of liberty is naive and insufficient [4]. Positive freedom is the rationale for the welfare state and the idea that everybody should have equal opportunity to participate in the different practices of a society. The focus is very often systemic: Individuality and liberty are dependent on a strong community. Positive freedom is often referred to as 'freedom *to…*'.

The positive concept of liberty has substantial resemblance with the concept of health applauded in health promotion. Central in the theory of health promotion is the term *salutogenesis*, coined by Aaron Antonovsky [5], where he saw the origins of health in the factors causing well-being and meaning. While health understood as the absence of disease would amount to a *negative* understanding of health, health understood in the tradition of health promotion is a positive one. Like positive liberty, health is here understood as a concept of realization and capabilities: It means being able to realize a biological potential, realize aspirations, to satisfy needs and to change or cope with the environment—again to quote the Ottawa charter.

In the same way that there exist two fundamentally different concepts of liberty, it seems fair to claim that there exist two fundamentally different concepts of health. Health promotion is based on a positive concept, where health, like freedom, is something that can be realized given the proper context. The positive concept of health, like the positive concept of liberty, stresses the importance of others for the individual's realization of his or her potential. This brings us onto some reflections on the relation between health and responsibility.

3.3   Poor Health and Responsibility

In a libertarian model, the individual should be free to make good or bad health choices. Knowledge, attitudes, will power, character, values, habits and more are factors that affect the decision individuals take. These are factors that we think we should be held responsible for. On that background, we are responsible for the health choices we make. To hold individuals responsible for their actions is of intrinsic value—it is the fundamental prerequisite for treating people as autonomous individuals.

At the same time, we know, as a fact, that the society has a huge impact on the individual's health. Access to clean water, sanitation facilities, safe housing, vaccines and a good health care system are of course basic elements in the public health of a society, but the social elements of health go far beyond this. The way a society is politically 'rigged' determines in a deep sense the health of its inhabitants. Education and income are the most prominent *social determinants of health* [6]. A society with small social inequalities produces healthier individuals than a society with large social inequalities. The more a society manage to distribute education and income in an egalitarian way (where people are treated as equals), the better the health of its citizen will be. In the same way, adverse experiences in a person's biography, like sexual child abuse, seem to be a life-course social determinant of adult health [7]. In this explanation of good and poor health, individual character and will power play a minor role. The social structure as well as the social context of upbringing and socialization plays a major role. Politics plays a major role.

The danger of the libertarian model is that health is 'individualized'. The true social determinants of health are masked by an ideology that says that everything starts and ends with the will of the individual. The danger of the communitar-

ian model is that health is 'socialized'. Individual responsibility disappears, autonomy disappears, and individuals in poor health are 'victimized'— they are regarded as victims of an unfair society.

Luckily, we do not have to choose between the libertarian and the communitarian model. There are insights from both of them in the *salutogenic model of health*. A central concept in the salutogenic model of health is *sense of coherence*. How healthy we feel and how healthy choices we make depend to a certain degree on whether we regard the hardships of our lives as comprehensible, manageable and meaningful [8]. Social context plus individual agency are both inescapable in this model.

3.4   Health Choices: What Interference Is Ethically Justified?

The most typical ethical dilemma in public health ethics is that of state interference in choices concerning the health of people. According to the theory of negative liberty, it is of highest value that the state does not interfere with the freedom of people. People should be left alone.

However, from a positive concept of liberty and health—what Carter et al. denote as a *capability point of view*—interference could be justified. Peoples' most important interest is probably not to be left alone, because '…they have a moral stake in that environment providing them with real opportunities, including the opportunity to be healthy' [2].

Informing people through public health campaigns is one of the most classical ways of trying to help people taking good and healthy choices. There is nothing inherently unethical with information campaigns, if the information given is honest and correct. But one problem with them is that results are moderate, probably because education programmes have often failed to acknowledge the limitations of health education or the complex relationship between health communication and behaviour change, according to Gill and Boylan [9]. In order to make them more effective, there is a temptation to move beyond factual and objective information and use instruments that make a strong appeal to emotions, like for instance the use of fear and disgust in anti-tobacco campaigns. While this may have a bigger effect than information, it also increases the risk of stigmatization. As Lupton claims, there is a substantial risk that such campaigns may '…reinforce negative attitudes towards already disadvantaged and marginalized individuals and social groups' [10].

A less stigmatizing but maybe more coercive way of trying to improve public health is to tax products that contribute to poor health and disease, like tobacco, alcohol, sugar and fat. Such taxation might contribute to more 'real opportunities' for people to choose healthy, in the sense that unhealthy choices will not continue to be a cheap option. The coercive element here is that if you put really high taxes on some products, it will be too expensive for people to buy regularly.

An even more coercive strategy is to ban certain products or ban the use of certain products. Many countries today have a law on smoking, where smoking is banned in public buildings and transportation, restaurants, offices, etc. Systematic reviews suggest a considerable medical benefit from such legislation [11, 12]. There are many practical challenges with taxation of as well as a ban on certain products, such as equal treatment of different products and the risk of increased trade leakage to more liberal jurisdictions nearby. But deeper than that is the challenge that we cannot necessarily ban everything we may find unhealthy from our society. The characteristics of a liberal societies is that we allow people to choose the way they will live their lives, as long as this freedom of choice do not harm others, or significantly reduce others freedom of choice. This freedom of choice is regarded as an intrinsic value and as a common good in liberal democracies. A totalitarian regime could easily ban tobacco, Happy Meal, Toblerone and alcohol. But in liberal democracies, such laws would be considered a violation of some of our dearest values. This creates a tension between values. You have to carefully balance the two.

But how could laws against smoking in public indoor areas be introduced in liberal democracies if it violated fundamental liberal values? The answer is that these laws were introduced in the first place *to safeguard the work environment*. Nobody should be a victim of 'passive smoking'. The justification of these laws was not that health trumped freedom of choice, but rather that the choice of smokers to smoke, threatened the freedom of choice of others (the choice of not smoking/not inhaling nicotine) in these buildings. In that sense, *freedom of choice* was the justification for banning the freedom to smoke indoors. The paradox, however, is that even though these laws were not motivated by health promotion, the consequences have probably been huge in terms of health.

Some scholars do, however, defend coercive strategies in a liberal democracy. Sarah Conley is one of them. People are generally prone to cognitive bias, says Conley. We make bad decisions because we are tempted, we lack will power and we have a bad means-end thinking. That makes it hard for us to reach our ultimate goals. Coercing people to do what is good for them is in this sense is respectful, because people then will reach their ultimate goals [13].

Is Conley's position compatible with a health promotion view? On the one hand, health promotion is based on empowering and enabling people to realize their health potential. Coercion and prohibitions do not seem to have a place here. On the other hand, some types of addiction may be so hard to ignore and overcome that prohibitions ('you are not allowed to smoke here') actually could be the only thing that may help a person resist the craving for a cigarette. From such a perspective, law limiting and prohibiting smoking may help a person to get in control and in charge of his or her health. Although bans and prohibitions seldom would have a place within the paradigm of health promotion, we cannot absolutely rule out that such strategies may play a role in empowering and enabling people to live the lives that they really want to live.

Conley's position, though, is challenging from a liberal perspective. As Jonathan Pugh has argued that it would be very problematic if it becomes impossible for agents to choose some action that poses a risk to their health without them being accused of making a cognitive error in weighing their values [14]. Are all smokers today making a cognitive error when they choose to smoke? Could we ban smoking in general on the assumption that the ultimate goal of all smokers is to quit smoking? Probably the answer is no. People have different values and people weigh their values differently. That means that some smokers have no ultimate goal of quitting smoking. For them, coercive paternalism will become highly illiberal and not enabling them to live more in accordance with ultimate goals and values.

3.5 Promoting Health Without Taking Away Choices

An increasingly popular strategy for promoting healthy choices is 'nudging'. Nudging or 'friendly pushing' is, according to Thaler and Sunstein, about changing the choice *architecture* [15]. No choices will be taken from you, no one will be coerced, nothing will be prohibited, but the choices will look a little bit different than before. When choices are nudged, they have been designed in order to raise the likelihood that you make *the good* choice. In a friendly way, you are pushed in the direction of what is good for you.

A simple example of nudging is to place fruit and vegetables in the middle of where you enter the groceries store. This makes it impossible to get into the store without feeling the call of buying fruits and vegetables. You still have the freedom to choose not to buy these healthy products, but it is more difficult to drop it, compared to a choice architecture where vegetables and fruit are hidden at the very back wall of the store.

Nudging can be scaled up to include more fundamental aspects of health. In cities, we can take some of the driving lanes and transform them to bike-cycle lanes. This will probably create more cyclists and less drivers and contribute to better health, better environment and less traffic. Still, no choices are removed. You can take your car and drive to work if you prefer that. But,

the choice of driving to work is not that attractive anymore while the choice of cycling to work has become much more attractive. You have been nudged towards cycling.

Nudging can be even more scaled up. Urban planning can be done with health promotion as a central perspective. A typical example is so-called age-friendly cities and communities where it is easy to participate when you age, easy to stay connected, stay healthy as well as to receive adequate support. The goal is to 'promote healthy and active ageing and a good quality of life for their older residents' [16]. In such cities, no choice is taken away from you (you can still choose not to participate), but the good choices are much easier and more attractive to make, compared with other cities. When you live in such a city, you will be nudged towards active participating, regularly exercising, healthy food, healthy transportation and healthy work environment—all these will be options that represent more attractive choices than the unhealthy ones.

3.6 Is Nudging Ethical from a Health Promotion View?

Nudging could be an effective mean to improve personal as well as public health. There are, however, two typical objections: First, nudging can be accused for being essentially paternalistic. Second, nudging can be accused for being essentially manipulative. If these accusations are valid, nudging seems to be a bad strategy for health promotion.

Paternalism (from Latin pater = father) means that somebody else (a father figure) knows what is good for you. Medical paternalism is an example of something we today consider as an ethical problem because we think that the patient knows best what is good for him or her. Nudging in health promotion presupposes that somebody knows what is best for you and organizes the possible choices in such a way that you will make the 'right' choice. Clearly there is a paternalist element in this, in the same way that coercive strategies for health promotion are paternalistic. In addition, the paternalism is partly hidden. That makes nudges more problematic than coercive strategies, where the paternalism is open for everybody to see.

At the same time, it is important to note that choice is not abandoned. We are still within the liberal zone. This is why nudging has been labelled 'liberal paternalism'. Whether paternalism in a given situation is acceptable or problematic depends on whether a certain good is commonly shared, or rather a contested good. Good candidates for nudging presuppose high agreement. To nudge people to eat more fruits and vegetables is not very controversial. There is a general agreement in the society that eating more fruits and vegetables is good for us. To nudge people to read more in the Bible is controversial. There is no general agreement in the society that we should read more in the Bible. When nudging is about means and goals that most people can agree upon, paternalism may not be that problematic.

The second objection was that nudging is manipulative. When we buy more vegetables and fruits because these groceries are placed at the entry, most of us are not conscious that the shop has chosen this setup in order to influence our behaviour. As we said, this presupposes a hidden paternalism. But in addition, the rearrangement of the choice architecture plays with our brain. We are to a certain degree manipulated. This is problematic. We do not like to be deceived. We like transparency. And far worse, while buying more vegetable seems to be a rather innocent consequence of manipulation, there are of course regimes that want to use these techniques for bad purposes if they really influence our cognition [17]. Maybe we then need to be careful with introducing nudges if they are inherently manipulative?

There is clearly an element of behaviour manipulation involved in nudging. This is problematic from an ethics of health promotion, since the concept of health within this tradition is so clearly linked to enabling and empower people to improve their health. If we are solely manipulated to make better choices, the agency disappears—we do not seem to be in charge or in control of the choices we make.

There are however ways to defend nudging as an ethical health promoting strategy: First, people can be oriented about the changes of the choice architecture and why it is done. In that way, nudges become transparent. Second, Thaler and Sunstein stress that nudgers—those that are nudged—should be better off, *judged by themselves* [15]. People can also be included in decision processes about which products, actions and lifestyles that is best fitted for nudging. That takes away some of the paternalist critique and let nudges become democratic. Finally, we should remember that manipulation of our brain is something that the consumer industry has been doing through commercials for decades. Using nudging for public health promotion—for the common good—and not for private enrichment, serves a higher goal. With that reminder health-promoting nudges might become legitimate and important.

3.7 Health Promotion in Health Care Vs. Public Health

When we shift the focus from health promotion in public health to health promotion in health care, all the goals we have been talking about are still valid. Enabling people to increase control over, and to improve, their health is of course of utmost importance. Furthermore, to be able to cope well for instance with a chronic disease would be central in health promotion in health care.

Still, there are some differences. The political dimension of public health is not that distinct within health care. What makes a difference within health care would be the doctor–patient relation, the nurse–patient relation as well as the systemic approach to continuous follow-up of patients. It is in the relational aspect of health care, then, that we find the key to the ethical dimension of health promotion in health care.

Some of the same ethical discussions that we find in public health, though, is also found within health care. One of them is the discussion on nudging that recent years also have entered the field of health care. Nudging in a clinical setting would mean that doctors rearrange the 'choice architecture' in such a way that is more likely that the patient will make what the doctor consider as the right choice. In the anthology Nudging Health from 2016, arguments for and against clinical nudging are discussed thoroughly. Clinical nudging was also the subject for a special issue in the *American Journal of Bioethics* in 2013. Here Shlomo Cohen suggested that nudging in health care offers 'an important new paradigm' and has the potential to 'overcome the classical dilemma between paternalistic beneficence and respect for autonomy' [18].

I will not dive deep into this special discussion. But since I expressed a positive attitude to nudging as a tool for health promotion in public health, I should say something about my view on nudging in a clinical context. Nudging in a clinical setting, is in my view, far more ethical problematic than nudging in a public health setting. This is due to the manipulative and deceptive element of nudging. In the former discussion, I agreed that there is such a manipulative element. But I also gave reason for how this manipulative element can be reduced as well as legitimated. In a clinical setting, I agree with the criticism raised by Søren Holm that 'deceptive nudging in a personal relationship may undermine trust much more quickly than deceptive nudging from institutions that by definition are known to act strategically to pursue societal goals' [19]. What we are really interested in the clinical setting cannot be reduced to health, but rather the process of creating health, what Lindström and Eriksson have called healthy learning [20].

The risk of undermining trust by nudging 'the right choice' is one important criticism of clinical nudging. But almost equally important is the question whether we can talk of 'the right choice' in health care. Seen from a health promotion view, this is far more complicated. This takes us to some of the fundamental value discussions in health care today.

3.8 The Shortcomings of an Ethics of Autonomy in Health Care

For many decades, there has been focus on one prominent value in medical ethics and health care ethics in the western world—patient auton-

omy. Already in the 1980s, a leading text book in medical ethics wrote that although '…*the physician's primary obligation is to act for the patient's medical benefit (..) autonomy rights have become so influential that it is today difficult to find clear affirmations of traditional models*' [21]. The focus on patient autonomy came as a reaction to medical paternalism and the attitude that the doctor always knows best for you. People and patients must be allowed to decide for themselves.

Why autonomy should be considered such an important value in health care is not obvious. Medical knowledge is an expert field where doctors and nurses usually know a lot more than their patients. Patients obviously need healing and caring, but not that obviously choices. While choices are of utmost importance in many fields of society, choices are any way only offered within a limited range in health care—your medical doctor always decide what treatments to choose between. Some critics have claimed that the presence of a choice does not in itself ensure empowerment of patients and that the whole focus on patient autonomy is delusional and 'does not reflect what is really at stake in health care settings' [22].

It is here that health promotion in health care enters the value field. Health promotion is not concerned with choices per se, but with health. However, with the underlying definition of health as salutogenesis, health promotion offers a comprehensive value system where also patient autonomy can find its proper place. Below we will explain how.

3.9 Empowerment as the Basis for Health Promotion in Health Care

Sense of coherence, meaning, is, as we noted earlier, a vital aspect of health promotion. As Eriksson and Lindström have pinpointed, sense of coherence is '…an important disposition for people's development and maintenance of their health' [23]. For a patient to be able to benefit from a treatment, he must be able to see for instance how a certain lifestyle change or a follow-up make sense and can fit into her life. He must of course be informed about every aspect of the treatment, but equally important he must feel he is able to cope with the task, manage the disease and comprehend all aspects of the situation. To promote health in health care means enable patients to be in charge or in control of their patient role. Patients must be educated, but they must also be ascribed trust, optimism, hope and responsibility. Nurses and doctors must be interested in the patient's biography and social context, in order to contribute to the coping, the control and the sense of coherence. That entails an empathic and holistic approach to patients.

There is a single word for all of this, a word that is far more important in health care than autonomy. That word is empowerment. Health promotion in health care is genuinely about empowerment. From a focus on empowerment, many other values can easily be derived, values like holism, empathy, autonomy and user involvement. An ethics of health promotion in health care is genuinely an ethics of empowerment. What difference does it make if we shift the main ethical focus to empowerment instead of autonomy in health care?

Empowering patients and persons means to enable people to participate or perform in a certain practice or role. A patient can formally be declared autonomous, and she might also be offered choices, but if she is not able to transform the choices and the information into her own life project, then the term autonomy does not seem to do the job. Neither from the point of view of health personnel, does this term do the job: Nurses and doctors can be taught that their ethical duty is to respect patient autonomy, but what does that mean? Does it mean that nurses should encourage patients to have independent 'opinions' on the treatment offered? If so, why would that be an ethical ideal?

Empowerment, on the other hand, is a value that can do the job. Empowerment addresses the importance of *agency*—the importance of being a person or patient that as far as possible leads his life from the inside, copes with the hardships of his life and integrates medical events into a meaningful biographical story. Unlike autonomy,

empowerment directly instructs nurses and doctors on what their ethical obligation towards patients are. In the words of Koelen and Lindström, the role of the professional '...is to support and provide options that enable people to make sound choices, to point to the key determinants of health, to make people aware of them and enable people to use them. In this enabling process it is important to help people to see a correspondence between their efforts and the outcomes thereof. It includes guiding clients through change processes in a successful way, that positively influences feelings of control' [24]. Doctors and nurses should do whatever they can to enable the patient to become this *agent* that can cope, master and feel coherence. And why should they do it? Because this is what health is about.

The fundamental ethical idea of salutogenesis could basically be formulated as a variant of the old slogan saying that it is not what happens to you, but how you react to it matters. A patient may have a severe disease, but his health could still be considered good if he considers his life meaningful, he is capable of coping with the disease, and he has some feeling of well-being. Promoting health in this sense should be the ultimate ethical goal of health care, because this goal would be valid independent of whether we talk about curative treatment, chronic diseases, palliation or end-of-life care. Exactly *how* health can be promoted through patient empowerment is not the topic of this chapter of the book. We have confined ourselves to a mild warning against *nudging* in health care in contrast to public health.

Having reached the conclusion that empowerment represents the ethical ideal for health promotion in health care, we can now look back on our discussions on public health ethics. Are there anything that suggest that empowerment is less relevant as an ethical ideal for health promotion outside health care? In my view, the answer is no. Even though some would suggest that the ultimate goal of a society would be to reduce the burden of disease, this would not be the most satisfying answer. Also, in public health, the ultimate goal should be to create a society where citizens can flourish, cope, realize their potential and aspirations, feel coherence and have a high degree of well-being. This is what health is about. And this is what health promotion should care about—either in health care or in public health.

3.10 Conclusion

Ethical issues in health promotion has often been discussed with regard to public health issues. In the same way as two fundamentally different concept of liberty defines the political debates in our societies, in the same way two corresponding concepts of health define the public health debates. Health promotion is premised on a positive concept of health, where the society and the community play a major part for individuals to realize their potential for living and leading a healthy life. Nudging is an ethically contested but also interesting tool for how to promote health in our society, but probably less valid within health care. An ethical reading of health promotion in health care tells us that one of the most fundamental values we should adhere to is empowerment. Empowerment guides health personnel in a very direct way towards their ethical mission. This concept should replace the focus on patient autonomy as the core value of western health care.

Take Home Messages
- There is an important ethical difference between a positive and a negative concept of health.
- Interfering in people's life in order to enable them to make better health choices judged by themselves is ethically justified.
- Nudging is a very interesting tool for health promotion in public health, but should be used with caution within health care, due to the deceptive aspect that may undermine trust in care relations.
- Empowering patient within health care or empowering citizens within public health, to better be able to cope, control, find meaning and reach well-being, seems to be the most superior ethical call and vision for health promotion.

- The prominent position of patient autonomy within health care should be replaced by the principle of empowerment—it better directs health personnel to their ethical task, and it better suits the ethical needs of patients.

References

1. The Ottawa charter for Health Promotion. First International Conference on Health Promotion, Ottawa, 21 November 1986 [Internet]. https://www.who.int/healthpromotion/conferences/previous/ottawa/en/index1.html. Accessed 1 May 2020.
2. Carter SM, Cribb A, Allegrante JP. How to think about health promotion ethics. Public Health Rev. 2012;34(1):1.
3. Berlin I. Two concepts of liberty. In: Four essays on liberty. London: Oxford University Press; 1969. p. 118–72.
4. Taylor C. What's wrong with negative liberty. In: Philosophy and the human sciences—philosophical papers, vol. 2. Cambridge: Cambridge University Press; 1985. p. 211–29.
5. Antonovsky A. Health, stress and coping. San Francisco: Jossey-Bass; 1979.
6. Marmot M. Social determinants of health inequalities. Lancet. 2005;365(9464):1099–104.
7. Greenfield EA. Child abuse as a life-course social determinant of adult health. Maturitas. 2010;66(1):51–5.
8. Eriksson M. The sense of coherence in the Salutogenic model of health. In: Mittelmark MB, Sagy S, Eriksson M, et al., editors. The handbook of Salutogenesis. Cham: Springer; 2017.
9. Gill TP, Boylan S. Public health messages: why are they ineffective and what can be done? Curr Obes Rep. 2012;1:50–8.
10. Lupton D. The pedagogy of disgust: the ethical, moral and political implications of using disgust in public health campaigns. Crit Public Health. 2015;25(1):4–14.
11. Jones MR, Barnoya J, Stranges S, Losonczy L, Navas-Acien A. Cardiovascular events following smoke-free legislations: an updated systematic review and meta-analysis. Curr Environ Health Rep. 2014;1:239–49.
12. Faber T, Kumar A, Mackenbach J, Millett C, Basu S, Been J. Effect of tobacco control policies on perinatal and child health: a systematic review and meta-analysis. Lancet Public Health. 2017;2(9):e420–37.
13. Conley S. Coercive paternalism in health care: against freedom of choice. Publ Health Ethics. 2013;6(3):241–5.
14. Pugh J. Coercive paternalism and back-door perfectionism. J Med Ethics. 2014;40(5):350.

15. Tahler R, Nudge SC. Improving decisions about health, wealth and happiness. New Haven: Yale University Press; 2008.

16. WHO Global Network for Age-friendly Cities and Communities [Internet]. https://www.who.int/ageing/projects/age_friendly_cities_network/en/. Accessed 1 May 2020.

17. Wilkinson TM. Nudging and manipulation. Polit Stud. 2013;61:341–55.

18. Cohen S. Nudging and informed consent. Am J Bioeth. 2013;13(6):3–11.

19. Holm S. Context matters—why nudging in the clinical context is still different. Am J Bioeth. 2019;19(5):60–1.

20. Lindström B, Eriksson M. From health education to healthy learning: implementing salutogen-esis in educational science. Scand J Public Health. 2011;39(Suppl 6):85–92.

21. Beauchamp TL, Childress JF. Principles of bioethics, vol. 272. New York: Oxford University Press; 1989.

22. Agledahl KM, Førde R, Wifstad Å. Choice is not the issue. The misrepresentation of healthcare in bioethical discourse. J Med Ethics. 2011;37:212–5.

23. Eriksson M, Lindström B. Antonovsky's sense of coherence scale and the relation with health: a systematic review. J Epidemiol Community Health. 2006;60:376–81.

24. Koelen MA, Lindström B. Making healthy choices easy choices: the role of empowerment. Eur J Clin Nutr. 2005;59(Suppl 1):S10–6.

Part II

Central Health Promotion Concepts and Research

Sense of Coherence

4

Unni Karin Moksnes

Abstract

This chapter introduces the concept of sense of coherence which is a core concept in the salutogenic model defined by Aron Antonovsky. The salutogenic model posits that sense of coherence is a global orientation, where life is understood as more or less comprehensible, meaningful, and manageable. A strong sense of coherence helps the individual to mobilize resources to cope with stressors and manage tension successfully with the help of identification and use of generalized and specific resistance resources. Through this mechanism, the sense of coherence helps determine one's movement on the health ease/dis-ease continuum. Antonovsky developed an instrument named Orientation to Life Questionnaire to measure the sense of coherence which exists in two original versions: a 29-item and a 13-item version. This chapter presents the measurement of the sense of coherence and the validity and reliability of the 13-item scale. It gives a brief overview of empirical research of the role of sense of coherence in association with mental health and quality of life and also on sense of coherence in different patient groups including nursing home residents, patients with coronary heart disease, diabetes, cancer, and mental health problems. It also briefly discusses the implications of using salutogenesis in health care services and the importance of implementing this perspective in meeting with different patient groups. The salutogenic approach may promote a healthy orientation toward helping the patient to cope with everyday stressors and integrate the effort regarding how to help the patient manage to live with disease and illness and promote quality of life.

Keywords

SOC · Resistance resources · Salutogenesis
Health promotion · Nursing

U. K. Moksnes (✉)
Department of Public Health and Nursing,
NTNU Norwegian University of Science
and Technology, Trondheim, Norway

NTNU-Center for Health Promotion Research,
Trondheim, Norway

Faculty of Nursing and Health Science,
Nord University, Levanger, Norway
e-mail: unni.moksnes@ntnu.no

4.1 Introduction

Aron Antonovsky introduced the key concept of sense of coherence as part of the salutogenic model in the book *Health, Stress and Coping* in 1979. Salutogenesis focuses on what are the sources for people's resources and capacity to create health as distinct from, and yet a complementary perspective to pathogenesis, focusing on risk for disease, which traditionally had been the leading focus in research [1, 2]. One of Antonovsky's deviations from pathogenesis was to reject the dichotomization into categories of sick or well and instead understand health as an ease/dis-ease continuum; a horizontal line between total absence of health (H−) and total health (H+) [3] (Fig. 4.1). We are all more or less ill or well at any given point in time and consequently positioned on different places on this health continuum during the life course. The important point is to focus on what moves an individual toward the ease-pole of the continuum, regardless of where he/she was initially located with a focus on what promotes health, well-being, and quality of life. The interesting question stated by Antonovsky was therefore what explains movement toward the health end of the ease/dis-ease-continuum? His answer to this salutogenic question was formulated in terms of sense of coherence (SOC) and generalized resistance resources (GRR) and specific resistance resources (SRR) [4, 5]. The salutogenic theory posits that life experiences shape the SOC. This capacity is a prerequisite for peoples' ability to move in the positive direction on the health continuum and is a combination of peoples' ability to assess and understand the situation they are in, to find a meaning to move in a health-promoting direction, and also having the capacity to do so [4, 5].

When Antonovsky introduced salutogenesis, it was originally aimed to be a stress theory. Antonovsky saw stress as a natural and inevitable part of life, assuming that life was challenging and health being continuously threatened by ubiquitous stressors [1, 2, 6]. Stressors place a load on us, which causes tension. However, tension and strain are considered as potentially health promoting, rather than as inevitably health damaging, depending on the individual ability to identify and use GRRs to cope adequately with stressors. Antonovsky was interested in the explanation for why some people, regardless of major stressful situations, manage to stay healthy, and live good lives, while others

do not [7]. This may involve major life events such as experience of acute and serious illness, changes in the family, or changes in the workplace. The frequency, intensity, and duration of the stressor(s) are all factors that affect the individual's ability to cope adequately. Three potential reactions and outcomes of stress are (1) being neutral against the stressors, (2) being able to manage stress for the movement toward the health end, and (3) being unable to manage stress which leads to a breakdown expressed in terms of diseases and death [2] (see Fig. 4.1). Under the influence of stressors, the individual experiences tension and is constantly challenged to adapt to the stressor and to identify and use personal and environmental GRRs to cope adequately with the stressor(s). The individual's ability to identify and use GRRs affects the individual's ability to cope adequately with the stressor, which further affects health, that is, where the individual is positioned on the ease/dis-ease continuum [4, 5].

Antonovsky referred to the ability to comprehend the whole situation, and the capacity to identify and use the resources available, as the SOC [1, 3]. As a medical sociologist, Antonovsky saw the individual in continuous interaction with the context and daily life as something in constant change. For the individual, the challenge is to manage the stimuli and find strategies and resources available for coping with the changes in everyday life and manage complexity. Complexity may lead to conflicts but also offers opportunities for different and flexible choices, possibilities for adapting to change. It becomes

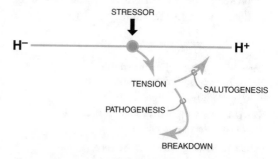

Fig. 4.1 The ease/dis-ease continuum. (Published with permission from Folkhälsan Research Center, Helsinki, Lindström & Eriksson [3])

vital how the individual can manage this chaos. SOC is the term Antonovsky introduced as an opportunity to manage and adapt to life's chaos. The primary focus is on the dynamic interaction between health promoting factors and stressors in human life and how people can move to the healthier end of the ease/dis-ease continuum. SOC is proposed to be a significant variable in affecting this movement [2, 5].

4.2   The Concept of Sense of Coherence

The concept sense of coherence (SOC) is defined as *"a global orientation that expresses the extent to which one has a pervasive, enduring though dynamic feeling of confidence that 1) the stimuli deriving from one's internal and external environments in the course of living are structured, predictable, and explicable, 2) the resources are available to one to meet the demands posed by these stimuli; and 3) these demands are challenges, worthy of investment and engagement"* ([2], p. 19). These three components, termed *comprehensibility, manageability,* and *meaningfulness* are thought to be highly interrelated but separable, forming the SOC (Fig. 4.2). *Comprehensibility* is the cognitive component and refers to the degree to which the individual sense that information that concerns themselves, the social environment, and the context is not only understandable but also ordered, structured, and consistent. However, perceiving events as comprehensible does not mean that they are completely predictable or without difficulty; the point is that stimuli experienced are explicable and

logic. *Manageability* is the "instrumental" component and refers to the extent to which individuals perceive that available resources are at their disposal and sufficient to adequately cope with the demands. *Meaningfulness* is the motivational component and refers to the extent to which individuals feel that certain areas of life are worthy of time, effort, personal involvement, and commitment [2, 3, 6]. All the three dimensions interact with each other. According to Antonovsky, the most important component is meaningfulness, which he thought was the driving force in life. When the individual perceives at least some of life's problems and demands as worthy of commitment and engagement, that also gives a greater sense of the two components of comprehensibility and manageability as well. However, this statement has been discussed. In a study of myocardial infarction patients, this hypothesis was rejected, showing that the dimension of comprehensibility was more important than meaningfulness for changes in SOC [8].

The three components in the SOC concept are strongly connected and reflect an individual resource and life orientation that enables the individual to reflect on its external and internal resources in order to cope with stressors and the ability to resolve tension in a health-promoting way [6]. Further, the life orientation of SOC is a way of thinking, being, and acting as a human being, which gives direction in life. The SOC concept also reflects a person's view of life and capacity to respond to stressful situations, which leads people to identify and mobilize the GRR at disposal [1, 2, 6]. Antonovsky saw the individual in interaction with the context. However, Antonovsky stressed that the salutogenic theory

Fig. 4.2 Dimensionality of the construct of sense of coherence

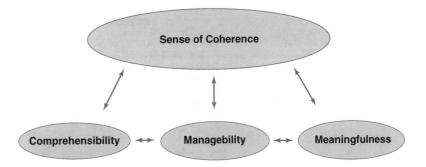

and its key concept, SOC, also can be applied at a collective level, and not only with a focus on the individual level [6].

4.3 Generalized Resistance Resources (GRRs)

Along with the concept of SOC, a key concept in the salutogenic theory/model is the role of generalized and specific resistance resources [1, 2], which are seen as important prerequisites for the development of SOC. Antonovsky promoted that generalized resistance resources (GRR) and specific resistance resources (SRR) are not exchangeable concepts. Others seem to agree that the distinction is not particularly important [9]. As though most focus has been given to the role of GRR in the literature, that will also be the focus in this chapter.

Overall, the term generalized resistance resources (GRR) was established by Antonovsky [1, 2] and constitutes the assets and characteristics of a person, a group, or a community that facilitate the individual's abilities to cope effectively with stressors and that contribute to the development of the individual's level of SOC [2]. Consequently, higher levels of GRRs are associated with stronger SOC. Resources fall into three basic (but interrelated) domains: those that enhance comprehensibility, those that enhance manageability, and those that enhance meaning-fulness. Because the person and the environment will always interact, it is not possible to identify all possible GRRs. Therefore, Antonovsky formulated the following definition that provides a criterion to identify GRRs: *"every characterization of a person, group or environment that promotes effective management of tension"* ([1], p. 99). Resistance resources may exist at the individual, the group, in the subculture, and at the whole society levels ([1], p. 103). Antonovsky's [1, 2] illustration of GRR is given in Fig. 4.3, and such resources may include the following factors: (1) physical and genetic (strong physic, strong immune system, genetic strength); (2) material resources (e.g., money, accommodation, food); (3) cognitive and emotional (knowledge, intelligence, adaptive strategies for coping, emotional intelligence); (4) ego identity (positive perception of self); (5) valuative and attitudinal (coping strategies characterized by rationality, flexibility foresight); (6) interpersonal-relational (attachment, social support from friends and family); (7) macro sociocultural aspects (culture, shared values in society).

The initial GRR resources [1] may be perceived as manifested within the life experiences. Four types of life experiences are assumed to contribute to the SOC developmental process during the course of growing up: *consistency, load balance, participation in shaping outcomes,* and *emotional closeness* [10]. Experiences of *consistency* in an individual's life provide the

Fig. 4.3 Illustration of generalized resistance resources (Source: Antonovsky, 1979 [1], p. 103)

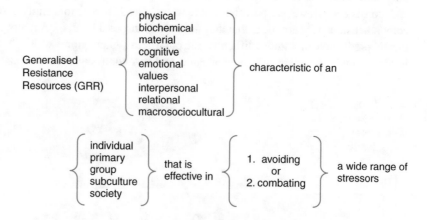

and thus preventing tension from being transformed into stress

basis for the comprehensibility component of the SOC [4, 10, 11]. Consistency refers to the extent to which messages were clear and that there were order and structure from experienced stimuli rather than chaos. The second life experience, *load balance*, refers to the extent to which one experienced overload or underload in the balance between the demands experienced and one's resources to cope. Load balance is important for the manageability component of SOC. The third life experience including participation in *shaping outcomes* refers to the extent to which the individual perceives autonomy, has impact in deciding her/his fate, and is not under pressure of others. Participation in shaping outcomes provides the basis for the meaningfulness component. The fourth life experience, *emotional closeness*, refers to the extent to which one feel consistent emotional bonds and a sense of belonging in social groups of which one was a member [10, 11]. A person with a strong SOC is able to mobilize GRRs to promote effective coping. This resolves tension in a health-promoting manner and leads toward the salutary health end of the health ease/dis-ease continuum [6]. SOC and different GRRs work together in a mutual interplay. The more GRRs people are conscious of, able to mobilize and make use of, the stronger SOC. A stronger SOC will in turn help people mobilize more of their resources, leading to better health and well-being.

Antonovsky divided resistance resources into GRR, which are resources that have wide-ranging utility to facilitate effective salutary tension management, while SRRs have situation-specific utility in particular situations of tension [1]. As described by Mittelmark et al. [9], the relationship between GRR and SRR is that via the SOC, the GRRs enable one to recognize, pick up, and use SRR in ways that keep tension from turning into debilitating stress. For example, Sullivan [12] makes a differentiation, stating that nursing is a GRR, while the nurse providing help with a particular problem is an SRR. Hence, supportive environments may include both GRR and SRR, but they have distinctions in reference to specificity. When being confronted with a special stressor, a strong SOC enhances one's ability to recognize and activate the most appropriate SRR from those that may be available. A study investigating the role of different SRRs and GRRs in informal caregivers originating from themselves and their care recipients as dyads showed the necessity of living in a well-functioning relationship which enabled dyads to solve challenges through cooperation and use of SRRs/GRRs (e.g., mutual understanding of the situation, good communicative skills, and enjoying togetherness) [13]. These resistance resources were important to be able to resolve the challenges they encountered, that is, through cooperation and use of their specific dyadic tension management. The study suggests that good past and present relationships wherein the dyad can use SRRs/GRRs might facilitate the dyad's adaptation to the caregiving situation [13].

4.4 Assessment of Sense of Coherence

Antonovsky developed the Orientation to Life Questionnaire (OLQ) to operationalize SOC. The questionnaire exists in two forms: a long version consisting of 29 items and a short 13-item version [2]. The OLQ has been translated in several languages and seems to be a cross-culturally valid, reliable, and feasible instrument, especially in adult samples [3, 7].

According to Antonovsky [2, 7], the OLQ comprises one general factor of SOC with three correlated components of comprehensibility (five items), manageability (four items), and meaningfulness (four items). However, previous validation studies have shown that the factor structure of the scale is complex and seems to measure a multidimensional rather than a one-dimensional construct [3, 7]. Following from that, Antonovsky maintained that on theoretical grounds, one should avoid lifting out individual dimensions in order to examine them separately. Studies investigating the factor structure of the 13-item OLQ based on exploratory and confirmatory approaches in adult and older populations have shown support for a three-factor structure [14–17], a second-order three-factor structure [14,

18–20], and a one-factor structure [21]. Accordingly, the construct validity of the OLQ-13 does not seem to be clear in reference to that different factor structures are evident in different populations. It may also be a question whether the items included in the instrument adequately represent the construct of SOC and that there may be variations in how the items are understood across different cultures and age groups. Validations of the factor structure in adolescent populations are less investigated, but previous studies have found support for a one-factor structure in a sample of Swedish adolescents [22] and three-factor structure in Norwegian adolescents [23]. While many translations of the OLQ and the research that has used it have given confidence that the SOC construct is measurable, the substance of the SOC construct needs to be further explored. This may include using the salutogenic model and qualitative methods investigating the core of the SOC components of comprehensibility, manageability, and meaningfulness [3].

4.5   Sense of Coherence in Association with Health and Quality of Life

A strong SOC is associated with good health, especially mental health and quality of life in different groups and populations [24–27]. Further, a strong SOC is associated with positive perceived health [24, 28] and is found to be inversely and strongly related to psychological problems like symptoms of anxiety and depression [24]. SOC is positively related to other health resources, such as optimism, hardiness, resilience, and coping. Individuals with a strong SOC also show more positive health behavior, with less use of alcohol, being a non-smoker, better oral health care [29–31] and more healthy food choice [32]. The SOC construct has been questioned regarding the weak relationship with physical health contrary to mental health [3, 33, 34]. The weak correlation to physical health may not be surprising since SOC mainly focuses on the mental, social, and spiritual ability to manage life [35]. The SOC construct has also been criticized for being too close

to the construct of mental health, suggesting they overlap [35]. The lack of evidence of the stability of SOC over time has also been criticized. Antonovsky [2] claimed that SOC like personality traits develops during childhood and early adulthood and becomes stabilized in the period of early adulthood. The SOC seems to be relatively stable over time, at least for people with an initial strong SOC [27, 36]. However, the SOC seems to be stronger with age and continues to develop over the whole life span [3, 27].

4.6   Sense of Coherence and Health in Different Patient Groups

4.6.1   Nursing Home Residents

Long term care facilities, including nursing homes, provide most institutional care for older people in many western countries. Moving to a nursing home results from numerous losses, illnesses, disabilities, loss of functions and social relations, and approaching mortality; all of which increase an individual's vulnerability and distress. In particular, loneliness and depression are identified as risks to the emotional and social well-being of older people [37, 38]. Thus, an important core function of health care professionals is to support everyday living, health, well-being, and quality of life [39]. Studies that have investigated the role of SOC in nursing home residents have found support for that SOC is an important component of functioning in old age. SOC has been shown to be associated to better health-related quality of life among nursing home residents [40, 41]. Stronger SOC also relates to lower emotional and social loneliness among nursing home residents [37, 42]. The challenge for health professionals is to help residents to reduce mental health problems and emotional and social loneliness and to strengthen their SOC. Promoting respectful and present nurse–patient interaction, acknowledging the individual as a person, might be a crucial resource in relation to nursing home patients' health and well-being.

4.6.2 Coronary Heart Disease (CHD)

Studies on SOC in coronary heart disease (CHD) patients is important in reference to their ability to cope with their life situation. A study of Bergman et al. [43] showed that the level of SOC seems to be relatively stable among patients who had suffered from myocardial infarction; although there were significant individual variations over the years. A longitudinal study of Silarova et al. [44] have shown that SOC is a predictor of mental and physical health-related quality of life of patients with CHD at 12- to 28-month follow-up and in female myocardial infarction survivors [45]. Stronger SOC has been shown to be associated with better health behavior related to physical activity [8, 46] and quality of life in patients after myocardial infarction [8, 47]. A study of Bergman et al. [43] which investigated the components of SOC in myocardial patients showed that comprehensibility was the most important component of SOC changes for 2 years after a myocardial infarction. Coping has been emphasized as an important factor in explaining differences between patients' perceptions of their life situations when affected by a life-threatening disease. Although SOC does not refer to a specific type of coping strategy, it comprises factors that may be regarded as a basis for successful coping with stressors. Hence, a positive outcome from a stressor is primarily dependent on successful management of the stressor and the presence of strong SOC. Within the dimensions of a strong SOC, critically ill patients may be able to show better ability to cope and to manage their lives after discharge from hospital by supporting their SOC.

4.6.3 Diabetes

The prevalence of diabetes is rapidly increasing; this is the case especially for type 2 diabetes. Given that type 2 diabetes is partly preventable, it is important to identify not only physical and health behavioral risk factors but also psychological risk factors that can promote coping and good health. Previous studies have shown that a strong SOC has been associated with more positive health behavior change [48] related to physical activity and food choices, which are factors relevant in the development of type 2 diabetes. Antonovsky did not use the concept "health behavior" but used a related concept "*a health orientation,*" that served as a GRR. Combined with other GRRs, a healthy orientation serves as a prerequisite for the development of a strong SOC [2]. Study findings have shown that patients with type 2 diabetes report lower SOC than a control group of patients without diabetes, and especially men [49]. The relationship between SOC and the incidence of diabetes was prospectively studied among Finnish male employees (5827 at baseline) [50], showing that a weak SOC was associated with a 46% higher risk of diabetes ($\leq$50 years of entry). This association was significant, independent of age, education, marital status, psychological distress, self-rated health, smoking status, binge drinking, and physical activity. Studies have also shown that patients with type 1 diabetes that report stronger SOC also show better metabolic control than those with weaker SOC, through adherence to self-care behaviors related to food choices and physical activity [51, 52].

4.6.4 Cancer

For most people, receiving a cancer diagnosis often causes severe distress. Therefore, working on supporting the patient's coping resources in order to promote positive psychological adjustment is important. The concept of SOC has been studied in individuals with various forms of cancer and moreover, in survivors of various forms of cancer, SOC is a strong predictor of quality of life [53, 54] and fewer symptoms of anxiety and depression [55]. In breast cancer patients, reports of stronger SOC relate to higher quality of life [53, 54, 56] through better emotional functioning and less fatigue and pain [53]. Further, stronger SOC is associated with less report of stress, distress [57, 58], and more positive coping strategies such as direct action and relaxation [54]. However, cancer patients are reported to score lower on SOC than the general population [56].

4.6.5 Mental Health

According to WHO, depression is one of the leading causes of disease burden in terms of disability. Although some people only suffer a single episode of depression, the high prevalence together with the associated impairment of functioning and socioeconomic consequences underscores the need to understand this illness fully. The experience of having a serious illness such as depression affects the individual's quality of life and requires significant adaptation by the patient and his/her family in order to cope. Research shows the significance of the salutogenic approach in mental health promotion, including various mental health problems [59]. One buffering component may be the individual's perception of SOC. In a 4-year and a 1-year follow-up study of people with major depression, SOC was shown to increase significantly as patients recovered after therapy [60, 61]. SOC is also found to predict life satisfaction in people with chronic mental health problems [62], and stronger SOC is found to be associated with reduced risk of psychiatric disorders during a long time period [63].

4.7 Implications for Practice

The WHO Ottawa Charter for health promotion [64] states that health is created and lived by people within the settings of their everyday life where they learn, work, play, and love. Salutogenesis has been applied to guide health promotion research and practice in various settings, however, mainly in everyday life settings. A central question is therefore what implications salutogenesis and related concepts have for practice in the health care setting?

With advances in medical technology and improvement in the living standard globally, the life expectancy of people is increasing worldwide [65]. Meanwhile, we also see an increasing prevalence of non-communicable diseases and chronic illnesses in the population [66]. With more advanced medical technology and medical treatment, more people survive from serious diseases but that also leads to that more people will have to learn to live with different chronic impairments in their everyday life. A new life situation is demanding and requires adaptation in many life areas for the individual. The preferences, or what is evaluated as valuable in life changes in meeting with illness, therefore, the experience of quality of life is a highly individual matter. At the same time, most people have a unique ability to adapt to and cope with inevitable life situations, and our expectations change according to life's realities. Here, health care personnel have a great responsibility in identifying possibilities for change and help the patient to cope with a new life situation. These aspects also challenge the health care sector's provision of efficient primary health care and long-term care, where more responsibility is given to the health care sector in the community/municipality.

The salutogenic perspective can be used to guide health promotion interventions in health care practice and to (re)orient health care practice [67]. The health care sector is generally a challenging area for applying salutogenesis and to reorient in a health-promoting direction, as the focus is and should be disease treatment. The reorientation of the health care services in a health-promoting direction therefore seems to be the least systematically developed, implemented, and evaluated key action of the five action areas outlined in the Ottawa Charter. The goal of implementing the salutogenic perspective is therefore that salutogenesis can be a complementary perspective to the pathogenic perspective where these perspectives interact in the planning and implementation of actions. In meeting with all patient groups, and especially with patients living with chronic diseases, health professionals need to focus on the patient's salutary resources as well as focusing on how to diminish and reducing risk factors. Further, it is important that the individual is seen in holistic terms, interacting with his/her daily life context. One of the central aspects implies promoting a more active patient role, where the health care professionals empower the patient to activate the use of knowledge and clarification of resources and needs in the planning of health care needed. An important role of health professionals is to identify the patient's experiences and prerequisites and help the patient to identify and activate resistance resources, in order to promote coping with everyday life challenges. This challenges the health care personnel's ability to work holistically with the patient's resources and needs and to see the patient as an equal partner in the planning of health care. This approach is important in order to integrate the resources and efforts needed regarding how to help the patient mange lives' challenges and promote quality of life.

In reference to intervention work, using salutogenesis as a basis for providing health-promoting interventions is found to be effective, e.g., toward strengthening SOC in patients living with long-term illness [68–70]. For instance, in patients with severe mental disorders, a combination of perspectives in order to provide holistic nursing is found to be important; this includes applying salutogenic knowledge about living a good and meaningful life in addition to knowledge anchored in the biomedically dominated understanding of mental illness [70]. Consequently, mental health care services should offer education programs with a complementary perspective on mental health, denoted "salus education" [70]. This implies a shift in practice to identify and build upon each individual's assets, strengths, and competence and support the person in managing his or her condition in order to gain a meaningful, constructive sense of being a part of a community [70]. The focus is not only how to combat and survive disease, but to help and "educate" people to "swim in the river of life."

4.8 Conclusion

This chapter has given an introduction to salutogenesis and the concept of sense of coherence (SOC) and generalized and specific resistance resources (GRR/SRR). It has also presented empirical research on assessment of SOC with use of the Orientation to Life Questionnaire developed by Antonovsky. The chapter has presented empirical research on the central role of SOC as a personal coping resource and life orientation in relation to health and quality of life in different populations and patient groups. Today, we can talk about salutogenesis more as a salutogenic umbrella and assets apprach with many different concepts with salutogenic elements and dimensions besides SOC [35]. The application of salutogenesis as a perspective guiding work in the health care settings seems to be vital and important as a complementary approach to the biomedical paradigm, since it is about implementing salutogenesis into a territory which is still predominantly dominated by the biomedical paradigm. Salutogenic thinking also seems to have good potential to be applied in health promoting interventions, and in supporting health promoting work in health care institutions for better everyday practice and quality of life for patiens [67].

Take Home Messages

- Sense of coherence is an important concept within salutogenesis and is considered as a personal coping resources and life orientation, where life is understood as more or less comprehensible, meaningful, and manageable.
- A strong sense of coherence helps the individual to mobilize resources to cope with life stressors and manage tension successfully with help of identification and use of generalized and specific resistance resources.
- Antonovsky developed the 29-item and a shorter 13-item version of the Orientation to Life Questionnaire (OLQ) to measure the sense of coherence.
- The OLQ scale has been translated in several languages and seems to be a cross-culturally valid and reliable instrument. Criticism of the SOC concept covers the multidimensionality of the concept. The substance of the SOC construct needs to be further explored.
- In health care, salutogenesis can be used to guide health promotion interventions in health care practice and/or to (re)orient health care services into a more health-promoting direction.

References

1. Antonovsky A. Health, stress and coping. San Fransisco: Jossey-Bass; 1979.
2. Antonovsky A. Unraveling the mystery of health. How people manage stress and stay well. San Francisco: Jossey-Bass; 1987.
3. Eriksson M, Mittelmark MB. The sense of coherence and its measurement. In: Mittelmark M, et al., editors. The handbook of Salutogenesis. Cham: Springer; 2017.
4. Bauer GF, Roy M, Bakibinga P, Contu P, Downe S, Eriksson M, et al. Future directions for the concept of salutogenesis. Health Promot Int. 2020;35(2):187–95.
5. Mittelmark MB, Bauer GF. The meanings of Salutogenesis. In: Mittelmark M, et al., editors. The handbook of Salutogenesis. Cham: Springer; 2017.
6. Eriksson M. The sense of coherence in the Salutogenic model of health. In: Mittelmark M, et al., editors. The handbook of Salutogenesis. Cham: Springer; 2017.
7. Eriksson M, Lindström B. Validity of Antonovsky's sense of coherence scale—a systematic review. J Epidemiol Community Health. 2005;59(11):460–6.
8. Bergman E, Malm D, Karlsson JE, Berterö C. Longitudinal study of patients after myocardial infarction: sense of coherence, quality of life, and symptoms. Heart Lung. 2009;38(2):129–40.
9. Mittelmark MB, Bull T, Daniel M, Urke H. Specific resistance resources in the salutogenic model of health. In: Mittelmark M, et al., editors. The handbook of Salutogenesis. Cham: Springer; 2017.
10. Sagy S, Antonovsky H. The development of the sense of coherence: a retrospective study of early life experiences in the family. Int J Aging Hum Dev. 2000;51(2):155–66.
11. Idan O, Eriksson M, Al-Yagon M. The Salutogenic model: the role of generalized resistance resources. In: Mittelmark M, et al., editors. The handbook of Salutogenesis. Cham: Springer; 2017.
12. Sullivan GC. Evaluating Antonovsky's Salutogenic model for its adaptability to nursing. J Adv Nurs. 1989;14(4):336–42.
13. Wennerberg MM, Lundgren SM, Eriksson M, Danielson E. Me and you in caregivinghood—dyadic resistance resources and deficits out of the informal caregiver's perspective. Aging Ment Health. 2019;23(8):1041–8.
14. Ding Y, Bao L, Xu H, Hallberg IR. Psychometric properties of the Chinese version of sense of coherence scale in women with cervical cancer. Psychooncology. 2012;21(11):1205–14.
15. Drageset J, Haugan G. Psychometric properties of the orientation to life questionnaire in nursing home residents. Scand J Caring Sci. 2016;30(3):623–30.
16. Gana K, Garnier S. Latent structure of the sense of coherence scale in a French sample. Personal Individ Differ. 2001;31(7):1079–90.
17. Lajunen T. Cross-cultural evaluation of Antonovsky's orientation to life questionnaire: comparison between Australian, Finnish, and Turkish young adults. Psychol Rep. 2019;122(2):731–47.
18. Feldt T, Lintula H, Suominen S, Koskenuvo M. Structural validity and temporal stability of the 13-item sense of coherence scale: prospective evidence from the population-based HeSSup study. Qual Life Res. 2007;16(3):483–93.
19. Naaldenberg J. Tobi H. van den esker F. Vaandrager L. psychometric properties of the OLQ-13 scale to measure sense of coherence in a community-dwelling older population. Health Qual Life Outcomes. 2011;23(9):37.
20. Richardson CG, Ratner PA, Zumbo BD. A test of the age-based measurement invariance and temporal stability of Antonovsky's sense of coherence scale. Educ Psychol Meas. 2007;67(4):679–96.
21. Hittner JB. Factorial invariance of the 13-item sense of coherence scale across gender. J Health Psychol. 2007;12(2):273–80.
22. Hagquist C, Andrich D. Is the sense of coherence-instrument applicable on adolescents? A latent trait analysis using Rasch-modelling. Personal Individ Differ. 2004;36(4):955–68.
23. Moksnes UK, Haugan G. Validation of the orientation to life questionnaire in Norwegian adolescents. Construct validity across samples. Soc Ind Res. 2014;119(2):1105–20.
24. Eriksson M, Lindström B. Antonovsky's sense of coherence scale and the relation with health: a systematic review. J Epidemiol Community Health. 2006 May;60(5):376–81.
25. von Humboldt S, Leal I, Pimenta F. Sense of coherence, sociodemographic, lifestyle, and health-related factors in older adults' subjective well-being. Int J Gerontol. 2015;9(1):15–9.
26. Länsimies H, Pietilä AM, Hietasola-Husu S, Kangasniemi M. A systematic review of adolescents' sense of coherence and health. Scand J Caring Sci. 2017 Dec;31(4):651–61.
27. Nilsson KW, Leppert J, Simonsson B, Starrin B. Sense of coherence and psychological well-being: improvement with age. J Epidemiol Community Health. 2010 Apr;64(4):347–52.
28. Honkinen PL, Suominen SB, Välimaa RS, Helenius HY, Rautava PT. Factors associated with perceived health among 12-year-old school children. Relevance of physical exercise and sense of coherence. Scand J Public Health. 2005;33(1):35–41.
29. Elyasi M, Abreu LG, Badri P, Saltaji H, Flores-Mir C, Amin M. Impact of sense of coherence on oral health behaviors: a systematic review. PLoS One. 2015;10(8):e0133918.
30. Garcia-Moya I, Jimenez-Iglesias A, Moreno C. Sense of coherence and substance use in Spanish adolescents. Does the effect of SOC depend on patterns of substance use in their peer group? Adicciones. 2013;25(2):109–17.
31. Mattila ML, Rautava P, Honkinen PL, Ojanlatva A, Jaakkola S, Aromaa M, Suominen S, Helenius H,

Sillanpää M. Sense of coherence and health behaviour in adolescence. Acta Paediatr. 2011;100(12):1590–5.

32. Lindmark U, Stegmayr B, Nilsson B, Lindahl B, Johansson I. Food selection associated with sense of coherence in adults. Nutr J. 2005;28(4):9.

33. Flensborg-Madsen T, Ventegodt S, Merrick J. Sense of coherence and physical health. A review of previous findings. ScientificWorldJournal. 2005;25(5):665–73.

34. Endler PC, Haug TM, Spranger H. Sense of coherence and physical health. A "Copenhagen interpretation" of Antonovsky's SOC concept. ScientificWorldJournal. 2008;20(8):451–3.

35. Lindström B, Eriksson M. The Hitchhiker's guide to Salutogenesis: salutogenic pathways to health promotion (research report no. 2). Helsinki: Helsinki Folkhälsan Research Center, Health Promotion Research IUHPE Global Group on Salutogenesis; 2010.

36. Hakanen JJ, Feldt T, Leskinen E. Change and stability of sense of coherence in adulthood: longitudinal evidence from the healthy child study. J Res Pers. 2006;41(3):602–17.

37. Drageset J, Espehaug B, Kirkevold M. The impact of depression and sense of coherence on emotional and social loneliness among nursing home residents without cognitive impairment—a questionnaire survey. J Clin Nurs. 2012;21(7-8):965–74.

38. Drageset J, Eide GE, Ranhoff AH. Depression is associated with poor functioning in activities of daily living among nursing home residents without cognitive impairment. J Clin Nurs. 2011;20(21-22):3111–8.

39. Haugan G, Moksnes UK, Espnes GA. Nurse-patient interaction: a resource for hope in cognitively intact nursing home patients. J Holist Nurs. 2013;31(3):152–63.

40. Drageset J, Nygaard HA, Eide GE, Bondevik M, Nortvedt MW, Natvig GK. Sense of coherence as a resource in relation to health-related quality of life among mentally intact nursing home residents—a questionnaire study. Health Qual Life Outcomes. 2008;21(6):85.

41. Drageset J, Eide GE, Nygaard HA, Bondevik M, Nortvedt MW, Natvig GK. The impact of social support and sense of coherence on health-related quality of life among nursing home residents—a questionnaire survey in Bergen, Norway. Int J Nurs Stud. 2009;46(1):65–75.

42. Lundman B, Aléx L, Jonsén E, Norberg A, Nygren B, Santamäki Fischer R, Strandberg G. Inner strength—a theoretical analysis of salutogenic concepts. Int J Nurs Stud. 2010;47(2):251–60.

43. Bergman E, Malm D, Ljungquist B, Berterö C, Karlsson JE. Meaningfulness is not the most important component for changes in sense of coherence. Eur J Cardiovasc Nurs. 2012;11(3):331–8.

44. Silarova B, Nagyova I, Rosenberger J, Studencan M, Ondusova D, Reijneveld SA, van Dijk JP. Sense of coherence as an independent predictor of health-related quality of life among coronary heart disease patients. Qual Life Res. 2012;21(10):1863–71.

45. Norekvål TM, Fridlund B, Moons P, Nordrehaug JE, Saevareid HI, Wentzel-Larsen T, Hanestad BR. Sense of coherence—a determinant of quality of life over time in older female acute myocardial infarction survivors. J Clin Nurs. 2010;19(5–6):820–31.

46. Myers V, Drory Y, Gerber Y. Sense of coherence predicts post-myocardial infarction trajectory of leisure time physical activity: a prospective cohort study. BMC Public Health. 2011;19(11):708.

47. Ekman I, Fagerberg B, Lundman B. Health-related quality of life and sense of coherence among elderly patients with severe chronic heart failure in comparison with healthy controls. Heart Lung. 2002;31(2):94–101.

48. Nilsen V, Bakke PS, Rohde G, Gallefoss F. Is sense of coherence a predictor of lifestyle changes in subjects at risk for type 2 diabetes? Public Health. 2015;129(2):155–61.

49. Merakou K, Koutsouri A, Antoniadou E, Barbouni A, Bertsias A, Karageorgos G, Lionis C. Sense of coherence in people with and without type 2 diabetes mellitus: an observational study from Greece. Ment Health Fam Med. 2013;10(1):3–13.

50. Kouvonen AM, Väänänen A, Woods SA, Heponiemi T, Koskinen A, Toppinen-Tanner S. Sense of coherence and diabetes: a prospective occupational cohort study. BMC Public Health. 2008;6(8):46.

51. Ahola AJ, Saraheimo M, Forsblom C, Hietala K, Groop PH. The cross-sectional associations between sense of coherence and diabetic microvascular complications, glycaemic control, and patients' conceptions of type 1 diabetes. Health Qual Life Outcomes. 2010;29(8):142.

52. Ahola AJ, Mikkilä V, Saraheimo M, Wadén J, Mäkimattila S, Forsblom C, Freese R, Groop PH. Sense of coherence, food selection and leisure time physical activity in type 1 diabetes. Scand J Public Health. 2012;40(7):621–8.

53. Gerasimcik-Pulko V, Pileckaite-Markoviene M, Bulotiene G, Ostapenko V. Relationship between sense of coherence and quality of life in early stage breast cancer patients. Acta Med Litu. 2009;16(3–4):139–44.

54. Sarenmalm E, Browall M, Persson LO, Fall-Dickson J, Gaston-Johansson F. Relationship of sense of coherence to stressful events, coping strategies, health status, and quality of life in women with breast cancer. Psychooncology. 2013;22(1):20–7.

55. Gustavsson-Lilius M, Julkunen J, Keskivaara P, Lipsanen J, Hietanen P. Predictors of distress in cancer patients and their partners: the role of optimism in the sense of coherence construct. Psychol Health. 2012;27(2):178–95.

56. Bruscia K, Shultis C, Dennery K, Dileo C. The sense of coherence in hospitalized cardiac and cancer patients. J Holist Nurs. 2008;26(4):286–94.

57. Gustavsson-Lilius M, Julkunen J, Keskivaara P, Hietanen P. Sense of coherence and distress in cancer patients and their partners. Psychooncology. 2007;16(12):1100–10.

58. Winger JG, Adams RN, Mosher CE. Relations of meaning in life and sense of coherence to distress in cancer patients: a meta-analysis. Psychooncology. 2016;25(1):2–10.

59. Langeland E, Vinje HF. The significance of Salutogenesis and well-being in mental health promotion: from theory to practice. In: Keyes C, editor. Mental well-being. Dordrecht: Springer; 2013.

60. Skärsäter I, Langius A, Agren H, Häggström L, Dencker K. Sense of coherence and social support in relation to recovery in first-episode patients with major depression: a one-year prospective study. Int J Ment Health Nurs. 2005;14(4):258–64.

61. Skärsäter I, Rayens MK, Peden A, Hall L, Zhang M, Agren H, Prochazka H. Sense of coherence and recovery from major depression: a 4-year follow-up. Arch Psychiatr Nurs. 2009;23(2):119–27.

62. Langeland E, Wahl AK, Kristoffersen K, Hanestad BR. Promoting coping: salutogenesis among people with mental health problems. Issues Ment Health Nurs. 2007;28(3):275–95.

63. Kouvonen AM, Väänänen A, Vahtera J, Heponiemi T, Koskinen A, Cox SJ, Kivimäki M. Sense of coherence and psychiatric morbidity: a 19-year register-based prospective study. J Epidemiol Community Health. 2010;64(3):255–61.

64. WHO. The Ottawa Charter for health promotion. Geneva: WHO; 1986. https://www.who.int/healthpromotion/conferences/previous/ottawa/en/.

65. WHO. Ageing and health 2018. Geneva: WHO; 2018. https://www.who.int/news-room/fact-sheets/detail/ageing-and-health.

66. WHO. Noncommunicable diseases country profiles 2018. Geneva: World Health Organization; 2018. https://www.who.int/nmh/publications/ncd-profiles-2018/en/

67. Pelikan JM. The application of Salutogenesis in healthcare settings. In: Mittelmark M, et al., editors. The handbook of Salutogenesis. Cham: Springer; 2017.

68. Heggdal K, Lovaas BJ. Health promotion in specialist and community care: how a broadly applicable health promotion intervention influences patient's sense of coherence. Scand J Caring Sci. 2018;32(2):690–7.

69. Johansson BA, Pettersson K, Tydesten K, Lindgren A, Andersson C. Implementing a salutogenic treatment model in a clinical setting of emergency child and adolescent psychiatry in Sweden. J Child Adolesc Psychiatr Nurs. 2018;31(2–3):79–86.

70. Mjøsund NH, Eriksson M, Espnes GA, Vinje HF. Reorienting Norwegian mental healthcare services: listen to patients' learning appetite. Health Promot Int. 2019;34(3):541–51.

A Salutogenic Mental Health Model: Flourishing as a Metaphor for Good Mental Health

5

Nina Helen Mjøsund

Abstract

This chapter focuses on a salutogenic understanding of mental health based on the work of Corey Keyes. He is dedicated to research and analysis of mental health as subjective well-being, where mental health is seen from an insider perspective. *Flourishing* is the pinnacle of good mental health, according to Keyes. He describes how mental health is constituted by an affective state and psychological and social functioning, and how we can measure mental health by the *Mental Health Continuum—Short Form* (MHC-SF) questionnaire. Further, I elaborate on Keyes' *two continua model of mental health and mental illness*, a highly useful model in the health care context, showing that the absence of mental illness does not translate into the presence of mental health. You can also read about how lived experiences of former patients support Keyes dual model of mental health and mental illness. This model makes it clear that people can perceive they have good mental health even with mental illness, as well as people with perceived poor or low mental health can be without any mental disorder.

The cumulative evidence for seeing mental disorder and mental health function along two different continua, central mental health concepts, and research significant for health promotion are elaborated in this chapter.

Keywords

Mental health · Mental health promotion · Flourishing · Mental health continuum short form · MHC-SF · Two continua model Salutogenesis · Complete mental health Positive mental health · Well-being

5.1 Introduction

This chapter is about mental health. Mental health is explained from a salutogenic perspective. This is an asset- and resource-oriented approach, which is explained with Corey Keyes' theoretical model of mental health [1–3], where mental health is understood as the presence of feelings and functioning, and not the absent of illness. The *two continua model of mental health* [3, 4] contributes to an understanding of mental health relevant in health care services by incorporating knowledge about diseases (pathogenesis) and complements this with the knowledge about health and well-being (salutogenesis).

N. H. Mjøsund (✉)
Division of Mental Health and Addiction, Department of Mental Health Research and Development, Vestre Viken Hospital Trust, Drammen, Norway
e-mail: nina.helen.mjosund@vestreviken.no

G. Haugan, M. Eriksson (eds.), *Health Promotion in Health Care – Vital Theories and Research*,
https://doi.org/10.1007/978-3-030-63135-2_5

Years ago, WHO [5] introduced a definition of health praised as well as criticized from many perspectives. However, it can be seen as a definition including situations a person is eager to achieve and situations a person is eager to avoid. "Health is a state of complete physical, mental and social well-being and not merely the absence of disease and infirmity" ([5], p. 1). Health has different meanings to different people. Green and Tones [6] say it so strikingly:

> ...health is one of those abstract words, like love and beauty, that mean different things to different people. However, we can confidently say that health is, and has always been, a significant value in people's lives ([6], p. 8).

To focus on mental health by separating it from health in its totality might be artificial due to the risk of losing the sight of health's complexity and composition. Mjøsund et al. [7] argue that perceived mental health, and physical, emotional, social, and spiritual aspects of health reciprocally influence each other. It seems that the phenomenon of mental health is especially fragile from being separated from the totality of health. However, a conscious theoretical attention to one of the aspects of health while remembering its connectedness to the other aspects might facilitate a deeper understanding and more targeted clinical intervention to promote it.

In a society with a dominant awareness on illness and disease prevention, people need useful knowledge to care for and promote their mental health, as well as physical, spiritual, and social health. Academics and scholars need theories and models to study mental health, and health professionals and health promoters need an extensive knowledge base to perform evidence-based interventions for quality enhancement in clinical practices. Scientists claim to adapt a pragmatic approach accepting various conceptualizations of health because it remains unlikely that we arrive at consensus on a health definition for health promotion research [8].

Findings from lived experiences of inpatient care in the project *Positive Mental Health—From What to How* [9] shed light on some elements of the mental health and Keyes' dual model of mental health [2]. In this qualitative research project, the meanings of mental health and mental health promotion were explored from the perspective of persons with former and recent patient experiences [7].

5.2   Mental Health

Nearly two decades ago, Corey Keyes, PhD in sociology [1], suggested to operationalize mental health as a syndrome of symptoms of positive feelings and positive functioning in life. Mental health is about an individual's subjective well-being; the individuals' perceptions and evaluations of their own lives in terms of their affective state, and their psychological and social functioning [1]. Inspired by salutogenesis, mental health is viewed as the presence of positive states of human capacities and functioning in cognition, affect, and behavior [3].

Hence, the more dominant view of mental health as the absence of psychopathology was questioned by Keyes [3]. While still holding this view, Keyes needed to employ the *DSM-3* [10] approach as a theoretical guide for the conceptualization and the determination of the mental health categories and the diagnosis of mental health [1]. These terms, more often used in diagnosing mental disorders, rather than health, were used with a conscious aim [1, 4, 11]. Keyes chooses to utilize *DSM-3*, its established reputation and familiarity, as a tool aiming to place the domain of mental health on equal footing with mental illness [1]. The measurement of mental health was done in the same way as psychiatrist measures common mental disorders, as for example a major depressive episode [12]. The concepts (syndromes, symptoms, and diagnosis) are familiar for nurses and for multidisciplinary professionals in health care services, as well as for patients and their relatives, which is a pedagogic beneficial when health promotion models and theories are used to guide interventions in clinical practice.

Mjøsund [9] contributes to the knowledge base of health promotion by investigating experiences of mental health among persons with mental disorders. This study explored how mental health was perceived by former patients [7], and the experiences of mental health promotion efforts in an inpatient setting [13]. The methodology Interpretative Phenomenological Analysis [14] was applied on 12 in-depth interviews. Apart from the participants, an advisory team of five research advisors either with a diagnosis or related to a family member with severe mental illness was involved at all stages of the research process as part of the extensive service user involvement applied in the project [15, 16].

5.2.1   Mental Health as a Syndrome of Symptoms

Keyes [1] operationalizes mental health as a syndrome of symptoms, based on an evaluation or declaration that individuals make about their lives. The syndrome of symptoms of positive feelings and positive functioning in life included psychological, social, and emotional well-being [1], make up the family tree of mental health, which is portrayed in Fig. 5.1.

How you are feeling about life includes (1) emotional well-being—and how you are functioning is about, (2) psychological well-being, and (3) social well-being. The division of subjective well-being consists in this way of two compatible traditions: the Hedonic tradition, focusing on the individual's feelings toward life, and the Eudaimonic tradition that equates mental health with how human potential, when cultivated, results in functioning well in life [3, 17]. Emotional well-being consists of perceptions of happiness, interest in life, and satisfaction with life [18]. Where happiness is about spontaneous reflection on pleasant and unpleasant affects in one's immediate experience, the life satisfaction represents a more long-term assessments of one's life [2]. The Hedonic approach equals emotional well-being as it frames happiness as positive emotions and represent the opinion that a good life is about feeling good or experiencing more moments of good feelings [12]. In contrast to the emotional well-being, psychological well-being is about the individual's self-report about the quality with which they are functioning [2]. Psychological and social well-being are rooted in

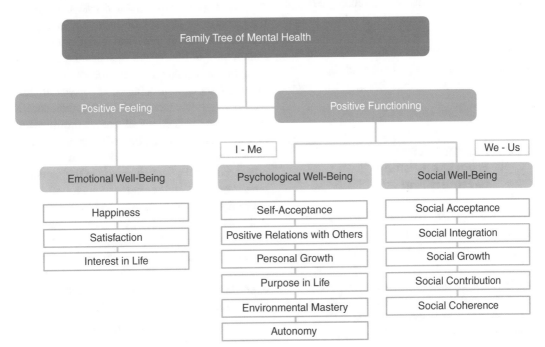

Fig. 5.1   The family tree of mental health. (Reproduced with permission from a lecture given by C. Keyes in Drammen, Norway, 13th of December 2010)

the Eudaimonic tradition which claims that happiness is about striving toward excellence and positive functioning, both individually and as a member of the society [2]. Eudaimonia frames happiness as a way of doing things in the world and represents the opinion that a good life is about how well individuals cultivate their abilities to function well or to do good in the world [12]. Psychological well-being is conceptualized as a private phenomenon that is focused on the challenges encountered by the individual; it is about how well an individual functions in life [12]. Social well-being represents a more public experience related to the individual social tasks in their social structures and communities [2]. Social well-being is about how well an individual is functioning as a citizen and a member of a community [12]. An important distinction between psychological and social well-being is that the former represents how people view themselves functioning as "I" and "Me," while the latter represents how people view themselves functioning as "We" and "Us" [17].

The level of mental health is indicated when a set of symptoms of emotional well-being combined with symptoms of psychological and social well-being at a specific level are present for a specified duration [1, 2]. This constellation of symptoms coincides with the individual's internal and subjective judgment of their affective state and their psychological and social functioning.

5.2.2 Mental Health: From Languishing to Flourishing

Mental health can be conceptualized along a continuum and subdivided into three conditions or levels: languishing, moderate, and flourishing mental health [1]. To be flourishing is to be filled with positive emotions and to be functioning well psychologically and socially. Flourishing has emerged to be a term describing the optimal state of mental health [19]. Languishing is to be mentally unhealthy, which is experienced as being stuck, stagnant, or that life lacks interest and

engagement [2]. Further, languishing can be described as emptiness and lack of progress, the feeling of a quiet despair that parallels accounts of life as hollow, empty, a shell, or a void. Individuals diagnosed as neither flourishing nor languishing are considered to have moderate mental health [1]. To be diagnosed as having flourishing, moderate or languishing mental health, three dimensions or symptoms of emotional well-being, six of psychological well-being, and five dimensions of social well-being are assessed [18]. A state of mental health is indicated when a set of symptoms at a specific level are present or absent for a specified duration, and they coincide with distinctive cognitive and social functioning [1].

5.2.3 Measuring Mental Health: The Mental Health Continuum Short Form

The self-administered questionnaire Mental Health Continuum—Short Form (MHC-SF) was developed to assess mental health based on individuals' responses to structured scales measuring the presence or absence of positive effects (happiness, interest in life, and satisfaction), and functioning in life, which includes the measurement of the two dimensions: psychological well-being and social well-being [1, 18]. Psychological well-being is characterized by the presence of intrapersonal reflections of one's adjustment to and outlook on life and consists of six dimensions: self-acceptance, positive relations with others, personal growth, purpose in life, environmental mastery, and autonomy. Social well-being epitomizes the more public and social criteria and consists of social coherence, social actualization, social integration, social acceptance, and social contribution [17]. Individuals who are flourishing or languishing must exhibit, respectively, high or low levels on at least seven or more of the dimensions [1]. Keyes [18] explains:

To be diagnosed with flourishing mental health, individuals must experience 'every day' or 'almost every day' at least one of the three signs of hedonic wellbeing and at least six of the eleven signs of positive functioning during the past month. Individuals who exhibit low levels (i.e., 'never' or 'once or twice' during the past month) on at least one measure of hedonic wellbeing and low levels on at least six measures of positive functioning are diagnosed with languishing mental health. Individuals who are neither flourishing nor languishing are diagnosed with moderate mental health ([18], p. 1).

The MHC-SF is constructed to be interpreted by both a continuous scoring, sum 0–70, and a categorical diagnosis of flourishing, moderate mental health or languishing. The questionnaire has been translated to many languages and applied in different cultures across many continents, such as Europe [20], Africa [17], Australia [21], South-America [22], North-America [23, 24], and Asia [25, 26]. Recently, the structure and application were evaluated for cross-cultural studies, involving 38 nations [27]. The MHC-SF shows good internal reliability, consistency, and convergent and discriminant validity in respondents between the age of 18 and 87 years [20] and across the lifespan [28]. The MHC-SF is claimed to be valid and reliable for monitoring well-being in student groups [29], as well as in both clinical (affective disorders) and nonclinical groups [30]. Moreover, the MHC-SF has also been used as the outcome in intervention studies [31, 32].

5.2.4 Flourishing: The Pinnacle of Good Mental Health

The term flourishing gives associations to something we want to achieve, a state where we are thriving, growing, and unfolding, and I have vitality, energy, and strength. The concept of flourishing has mostly been used in the field of positive psychology and sociology. Although the concept is considered to be relevant in nursing practice and research, it is still virtually absent in the nursing literature [19]. According to Keyes, flourishing is the pinnacle of good mental health; he chose to use the term flourishing to be clear that he was talking about mental health and not merely the absence of mental illness [12]. An evolutionary concept analysis of flourishing claimed that flourishing is still an immature concept, however with a growing evidence of flourishing as a district concept [19]. This concept analysis was based on four common conceptual frameworks of flourishing. The framework with most information available and most cited was presented by Keyes [1]. Additionally, the frameworks of Diener and Diener et al. [33, 34], Huppert and So [35], and Seligman [36] were included in this concept analysis [19]. The authors request further multidisciplinary research to establish standard operational and conceptual definitions and to develop effective interventions [19].

5.2.5 Perceived Mental Health: A Dynamic Movement on a Continuum

Former inpatients described mental health as an ever-present aspect of life; moreover, mental health was perceived as a dynamic phenomenon, a constantly ongoing movement, or process like walking up or down a staircase [7]. The movement was affected by experiences in the emotional, physical, social, and spiritual domains of life and accompanied by a sense of energy. Figure 5.2 shows that mental health is expressed both verbally and by body language, and in everyday life, mental health was experienced as a sense of energy and as increased or decreased well-being [7].

It is interesting that the participants living with the consequences of severe mental disorders were not talking about the absence of illness, pathological conditions, and disorder symptoms when they described their perception of mental health and mental health promotion [7]. The salutogenic understanding of Keyes [3] claiming that mental health is the presence of feelings and functioning, a state of human capacities, was supported by how the participants perceived mental health.

The understanding of mental health as a process and movement, like walking up or down a spiral staircase—equivalent to a continuum—is previously confirmed by a study of young people [37]. Talking about the experience of being in different positions on the mental health staircase,

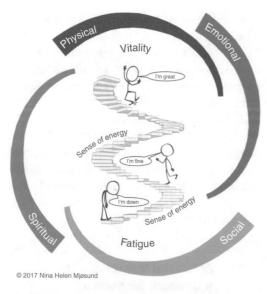

© 2017 Nina Helen Mjøsund

Fig. 5.2 Perceived mental health. (Reproduced with permission from Mjøsund NH. Positive mental health—from what to how. A study in the specialized mental health care service. Trondheim: Norwegian University of Science and Technology, Faculty of Medicine and Health Sciences, Department of Public Health and Nursing; 2017)

the exploration of the participants' accounts and their descriptions clearly indicated a vertical movement in accordance with Keyes' [1] continuum of mental health. The perception of the phenomenon of mental health as an ever present aspect of life, a part of being human [7], is of significance. Mental health was perceived as a quality of daily life, not characterized by quantitative entities such as numbers, but rather as good or bad, up or down, poor or strong. Mental health being experienced as constantly present in life and a part of being could be a contradiction to the early work of Keyes, when he described flourishing as the presence of mental health and languishing as absence of mental health [1]. More recently, [3, 12, 38] languishing is denoted as the absence of positive mental health or "the lowest level of mental health" [39]. Based on the participants' way of speaking about the position "low in the staircase" [7], and Keyes' description of high, moderate, and low mental health, Fig. 5.3 visualizes the levels of mental health.

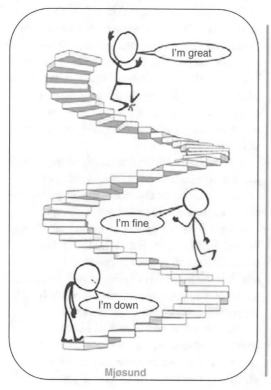

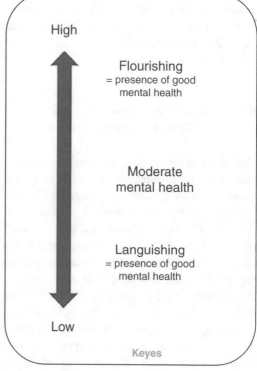

© Nina Helen Mjøsund 2021

Fig. 5.3 Mental health as moving up and down a staircase—equivalent to Keyes' continuum of mental health

Mjøsund et al. [7] claim that a sense of energy was a salient marker of perceived mental health. The sense of energy influenced experiences of mental health in the emotional, physical, spiritual, and relational domains of life. The feeling of energy was proportional with the position on the staircase; while low or down on the staircase, the sense of energy was described as "like starting a shaky engine with a flat battery." The participants described how this lack of mental and physical energy was associated with difficulties initiating and completing any activities [7]. This is in line with Keyes' [1] descriptions of flourishing including the presence of enthusiasm, aliveness, vitality, and an interest in life, associated with a sense of energy. Lack of energy and motivation as a result of mental disorders has been identified by patients as a barrier to integrating healthy lifestyles [40]. An assessment of the sense of energy, in collaboration with the patient, might form the basis for interventions aiming to "push or pull" into an activity or advising rest. Both the interventions have been described by Lerdal [41]. The sense of energy should be investigated more in depth and its relationship with mental health and mental disorders needs further research in order to inform the health promotion knowledge base.

The use of lay language in order to break down barriers between stakeholders in health promotion and health care is encouraged [42]. Having dialogs about taking a step or moving in the staircase of mental health is one way of operationalizing mental health into lay language for all people. Visualizing theoretical models might increase the possibility to grasp the content, as well as the usefulness in clinical practice can be promoted. Illustrations might enhance insight and shared understanding that is significant in health promotion initiatives aiming to increase empowerment (Figs. 5.1, 5.2, 5.3 and 5.4).

5.3   The Two Continua Model

The two continua model includes the presence of human capacities and functioning as well as the assessment of disease or infirmity [3, 4]. The contemporary dominant perspective in mental health care is on treating diseases and illness. Therefore, theories, models, and concepts which can help to facilitate mental health promotion are required. The dual continua model includes related but distinct dimensions of both mental health and mental illness [11, 28, 43, 44]. The illustration of the two continua model of health (Fig. 5.4.) reproduced from Keyes [3] visualizes the conceptualized definition of health along the vertical line and the continuum of mental illness along the horizontal line.

This dual model of mental health and mental illness goes well with WHO's [5] definition of health and is particular significant for health professionals in health care settings. The classical myth of Asclepius, the God of Medicine, and his two daughters Hygeia and Panacea gave rise to complementary concepts and approaches to health. The daughters represents two different points of view enlightening the distinction between the definitions of health and illness [6]. The daughter Hygeia represented a salutogenic approach symbolizing the virtue of wise living and well-being. Salutogenesis comes from the Latin word "salus" which means health and is considered as a state of human capacities and functioning. Health is the natural order of things, a positive attribute to which human beings are entitled if they govern their life wisely. Panacea represented the pathogenic approach, which considers health as the absence of disease and illness [3].

With Hygeia and Panacea in mind, it becomes clear that it is possible to have good mental health even with mental illness, and one can have poor or low mental health without mental illness. This concurs with accounts from persons living with mental disorders [7]. In the field of recovery, the influence of positive mental health has been studied in a sample of persons with mood and anxiety disorders [45] and individuals during recovery from drug and alcohol problems [46]. Moreover, the absence of mental illness does not equal the presence of mental health and revealing that the causes of mental health are often distinct from those understood as the causes for mental illness [43], and the conditions that protect against mental disorders do not automatically promote the

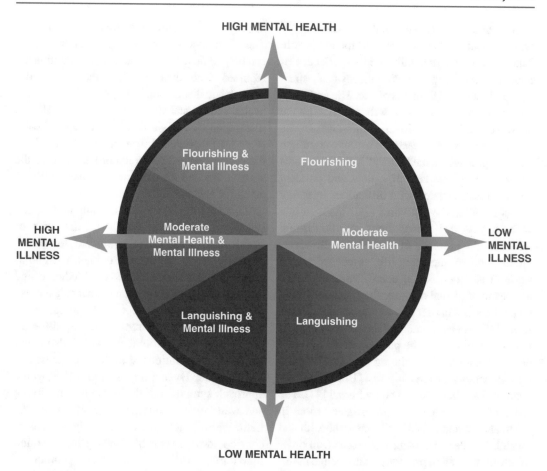

Fig. 5.4 The dual-continua model. (Reproduced with permission from Keyes CLM. Mental Health as a Complete State: How the Salutogenic Perspective Completes the Picture. In: Bauer GF, Hämmig O, editors. Bridging Occupational, Organizational and Public Health: A Transdisciplinary Approach. London: Springer; 2014. p. 179–92)

presence of positive mental health [3]. There seems to be cumulating evidence that mental disorders and mental health function along two different continua that are only moderately interrelated [4, 20, 28].

There is a growing interest for studying the relationship between mental health and mental illness in various environments, including work settings and psychosocial work conditions [47]. MHC-SF has been found to be valid and reliable for monitoring well-being in both clinical (patients with affective disorders) and nonclinical samples [30]. The prevalence of flourishing among individuals with schizophrenia spectrum disorders has been studied in Hong Kong [48].

Psychiatric outpatients with major mental illness have lower rates of well-being compared to controls, although about one-third is seen to be flourishing [49]. Screening of levels of mental health complements mental disorders screening in the prediction of suicidal behavior and impairment of academic performance among college students [50]. High level of mental health seems to protect against the onset of mental disorders (mood, anxiety, and substance abuse disorders) [51] or function as a resilience resource [52]. A study examined the presence and correlates of well-being measured by MHC-SF and psychopathology in a sample of female patients with eating disorders, as well as the level of mental health compared with the general population [53]. Less research has been done in treatment settings and hospitals; however, one study provides evidence for the psychometric properties of the MHC-SF in a primary care youth mental health setting, and they claim that the MHC-SF's three-factor structure is valid for use in mental health care [54].

Health promotion in health care should take a holistic approach, also anchored in the WHO's [5] definition of health, meaning the salutogenic orientation complementing the pathogenic orientation in contemporary health care services. I claim that the two continuum model provides theoretical tools which are useful in the development of health promotion interventions in the health care context; this model is equalizing treatment and care of disorders and the promotion of health. Having the dual continua model in mind, the protection of mental health is not to be confused with protections against mental disorders. I would like to emphasize the differentiation between the protection of mental health (something positive) and the protection against mental illness (something negative). The perception of what is positive or negative depends on the context and culture and might differ from one person to another. However, in this chapter, the terms positive and negative are used simply to illustrate the difference in purpose. In clinical practice of health disciplines such as nursing, it is relevant to have theoretical models to guide in customizing the care to the individual situation of the person. Patients and health care providers may utilize this framework to focus on the mental illness status, as well as the persons' level of mental health [44]. Keyes' conceptual framework maps on to themes emerging from narratives about recovery from mental illness [55] and can be a model to bridge mental illness with positive mental health in processes of recovery [56].

The findings presented by Mjøsund et al. [7] give support to the promotion and protection of mental health as described in the two continua model [2], which brings the continuum of mental illness and the continuum of mental health into the same picture (Fig. 5.4). This corresponds to the experiences presented by the participants and interpretation of their accounts led to an under-

standing of an everyday life where they perceived illness and health as intertwined, but also dissimilar [7]. They have been diagnosed with a mental disorder, *but they are not their diagnosis*, life is also mental health and well-being. The recognition of the duality of mental health and mental illness require major changes for current clinical practice in health care dominated by the pathogenic approach. Health promotion and mental health promotion should have a more dominant position in today's health care systems. Complementing health promotion and the protection of good mental health with treatment and prevention against disorder and illness should be given equal consciousness and resources based on the evidence base. In the words of Keyes, "…*what lowers the bad does not necessarily increase the good*" (Personal communication on 12th of July 2015).

5.4   Flourishing: Significant in Salutogenic Mental Health Promotion

Some perspectives on the opportunities and prospects for a further salutogenic development of mental health promotion in the health care might be relevant. In line with Keyes [3], I claim that research using absence of illness as an outcome as well as mental health promotion interventions with a purpose to restore health understood as absent of illness or to protect against disease are wrongly labeled as salutogenic. Even the father of the term salutogenesis, Aaron Antonovsky [57, 58], might be understood as influenced by this way of thinking in some of his writings. In my view, this is the main difference between Antonovsky's salutogenic model of health and Keyes' dual continua model of mental health. Antonovsky gives a conceptual definition of the health ease/dis-ease continuum as a multifaceted state or condition of the human organism:

> A person's location at a given point in time, on this continuum, can be described by the person's particular profile on four facets: pain (felt by the individual), functional limitations (felt by the individual), prognostic implications (defined by

health authorities) and action implication (seen by such authorities as required) ([58], p. 65).

This definition of health leads us to recognize a person's location on the healthy end of continuum, when these negative facets are missing. Based on this, I claim that Antonovsky did not define health as something present or positive, rather the absence of something negative. This is in line with Antonovsky's own remark:

> The health ease / dis-ease, or breakdown, continuum as presented here essentially seems to formulate the most desirable health category in negative terms; an absence of pain, no functional limitation, and so forth ([58], p. 67).

In a later paper from 1985, however, Antonovsky defined mental health as somewhat more than the absence of something negative:

> Mental health, as I conceive it, refers to the location, at any point in the life cycle, of a person on a *continuum* which ranges from excruciating emotional pain and total psychological malfunctioning at one extreme to a full, vibrant sense of psychological wellbeing at the other ([59], p. 274).

A salutogenic orientation will focus on the achievement of successful coping, which facilitates movement toward that end of the mental health continuum which is a vibrant sense of psychological well-being. Antonovsky proposed relevant issues and questions to be answered by health promoters. Understanding how people move from the use of unconscious psychological defence mechanism toward the use of conscious coping mechanisms is where the emphasis lies, from rigidity in a defensive structure to the capacity for constant and creative inner readjustment and growth, from a waste of emotional energy toward its productive use, from emotional suffering toward joy, from narcissism toward giving of oneself, and from exploitation of others toward reciprocal interaction [59].

However, it is important to underline that the salutogenic orientation is much more than the salutogenic model of health [60]. Eriksson ([60], p. 103) suggests to use the metaphor of an umbrella to underline that salutogenesis is more than Antonovsky's salutogenic model of health. Salutogenesis is an umbrella concept of theories and concepts about assets for health and well-being, including salutogenic elements and dimensions [61]. The editors of *The Handbook of Salutogenesis* discuss possible futures of the salutogenic orientation, and Georg Bauer states:

> If we narrowly follow Antonovsky's conceptualization, salutogenesis is about coping with miserable life situations or about "surviving the toxic river of life" - leaving little space for looking at the bright side of life. Applying salutogenesis to positive health development - or joyful swimming in the river of life - is urgently needed ([60], p. 442).

5.5   Conclusion

In summary, I claim that Keyes' model of mental health is an important contribution to the salutogenic orientation and the knowledge base of health promotion. In this model, mental health is defined by the presence of subjective well-being [1], which is in line with the lived experiences of former patients, who perceived mental health as an ever-present aspect of life [7]. Keyes has also given important contribution to the health promotion field by his two continua model of mental health and mental illness in the same context. Splitting the phenomenon of mental health and the phenomenon of mental illness into two separate, although related, phenomena is a meaningful and useful way of understanding health and illness for patients, relatives, and health care professionals in the context of health care services.

Take Home Messages

- Mental health is an ever-present aspect of life.
- Mental health is about subjective well-being; the individuals' perceptions and evaluations of their own lives in terms of their emotional state and their psychological and social functioning.
- Flourishing, as a term, describes the optimal state of mental health.
- Mental Health Continuum—Short Form (MHC-SF) is a structured scale that can quantify mental health.
- The two continua model of mental health and mental illness includes the presence of human

capacities and functioning as well as the assessment of disease or infirmity.

- Based on the understanding of mental health and mental illness as two continua, it is possible to have good mental health with mental illness and have poor or low mental health without mental illness.
- The absence of mental illness does not equal the presence of mental health, substantiating that the causes of mental health are often distinct processes from those understood as the risks for mental illness and disorder.
- There is cumulating evidence that mental illness and mental health function along two different continua with only moderate correlation.
- The evidence-based salutogenic models of mental health and the two continua model of mental health and mental illness made by Corey Keyes are significant knowledge for health promotion.

Acknowledgments   The author would like to thank Vestre Viken Hospital Trust, Department of Mental Health Research and Development for making it possible to write this chapter. Magnus Lien Mjøsund, thank you for reviewing the language and for assisting in fine-tuning of the figures.

References

1. Keyes CLM. The mental health continuum: from languishing to flourishing in life. J Health Soc Behav. 2002;43(2):207–22.
2. Keyes CLM. Promoting and Protecting positive Mental health: early and often throughout the lifespan. In: Keyes CLM, editor. Mental well-being: international contributions to the study of positive mental health. Dordrecht: Springer; 2013. p. 3–28.
3. Keyes CLM. Mental health as a complete state: how the Salutogenic perspective completes the picture. In: Bauer GF, Hämmig O, editors. Bridging occupational, organizational and public health: a transdisciplinary approach. London: Springer; 2014. p. 179–92.
4. Keyes CLM. Mental illness and/or mental health? Investigating axioms of the complete state model of health. J Consult Clin Psychol. 2005;73(3):539–48. https://doi.org/10.1037/0022-006X.73.3.539.
5. WHO. WHO definition of Health. Preamble to the Constitution of the World Health Organization as adopted by the International Health Conference, New York, 19–22 June, 1946; signed on 22 July 1946 by the representatives of 61 States and entered into force on 7 April 1948. ed: Official Records of the World Health Organization, no. 2, p. 100; 1946.
6. Green J, Tones K. Health promotion: planning and strategies. Los Angeles: Sage; 2010.
7. Mjøsund NH, Eriksson M, Norheim I, Keyes CLM, Espnes GA, Vinje HF. Mental health as perceived by persons with mental disorders—an interpretative phenomenological study. Int J Ment Health Promot. 2015;17(4):215–33. https://doi.org/10.1080/1462373 0.2015.1039329.
8. Mittelmark MB, Bull T. The salutogenic model of health in health promotion research. Glob Health Promot. 2013;20(2):30–8. https://doi.org/10.1177/1757975913486684.
9. Mjøsund NH. Positive mental health—from what to how. A study in the specialized mental healthcare service. Trondheim: Norwegian University of Science and Technology, Faculty of Medicine and Health Sciences, Department of Public Health and Nursing; 2017.
10. American Psychiatric Association. Diagnostic and Statistical Manual of Mental Disorders 3rd ed. Washington, DC: American Psyciatric Assocition. 1987.
11. Keyes CLM. Promoting and protecting mental health as flourishing: a complementary strategy for improving national mental health. Am Psychol. 2007;62(2):95–108. https://doi.org/10.1037/0003-066X.62.2.95.
12. Keyes CLM. Why flourishing? In: Harward DW, editor. Well-being and higher education. A strategy for change and the realization of education's greater purpose. Washington, DC: Bridging Theory to Practice; 2016. p. 8.
13. Mjøsund NH, Eriksson M, Espnes GA, Vinje HF. Reorienting Norwegian mental healthcare services: listen to patients' learning appetite. Health Promot Int. 2018;day012:11. https://doi.org/10.1093/heapro/day012.
14. Smith JA, Flowers P, Larkin M. Interpretative phenomenological analysis: theory, method and research. London: Sage; 2009.
15. Mjøsund NH, Eriksson M, Espnes GA, Haaland-Øverby M, Jensen SL, Norheim I, et al. Service user involvement enhanced the research quality in a study using interpretative phenomenological analysis: the power of multiple perspectives. J Adv Nurs. 2017;73(1):265–78. https://doi.org/10.1111/jan.13093.
16. Mjøsund NH, Eriksson M, Haaland-Øverby M, Jensen SL, Kjus S, Norheim I, et al. Salutogenic service user involvement in nursing research: a case study. J Adv Nurs. 2018;74(9):2145–56. https://doi.org/10.1111/jan.13708.
17. Keyes CLM, Wissing M, Potgieter JP, Temane M, Kruger A, Van Rooy S. Evaluation of the mental health continuum-short form (MHC-SF) in setswana-speaking south Africans. Clin Psychol Psychother. 2008;15(3):181–92. https://doi.org/10.1002/cpp.572.

18. Atlanta: Brief description of the mental health continuum short form (MHC-SF) [database on the Internet]. 2009. https://www.aacu.org/sites/default/files/MHC-SFEnglish.pdf. Accessed 25 Oct 2019.

19. Agenor C, Conner N, Aroian K. Flourishing: an evolutionary concept analysis. Issues Ment Health Nurs. 2017;38(11):915–23. https://doi.org/10.1080/016128 40.2017.1355945.

20. Lamers SM, Westerhof GJ, Bohlmeijer ET, ten Klooster PM, Keyes CLM. Evaluating the psychometric properties of the mental health continuum-short form (MHC-SF). J Clin Psychol. 2011;67(1):99–110. https://doi.org/10.1002/jclp.20741.

21. Hides L, Quinn C, Stoyanov S, Cockshaw W, Mitchell T, Kavanagh DJ. Is the mental wellbeing of young Australians best represented by a single, multidimensional or bifactor model? Psychiatry Res. 2016;241:1–7. https://doi.org/10.1016/j.psychres.2016.04.077.

22. Lupano Perugini ML, de la Iglesia G, Castro Solano A, Keyes CLM. The Mental Health Continuum-short form (MHC-SF) in the Argentinean context: confirmatory factor analysis and measurement invariance. Eur J Psychol. 2017;13(1):93–108. https://doi.org/10.5964/ejop.v13i1.1163.

23. Orpana H, Vachon J, Dykxhoorn J, Jayaraman G. Measuring positive mental health in Canada: construct validation of the Mental Health Continuum-short form. Health Promot Chronic Dis Prev Can. 2017;37(4):123–30. https://doi.org/10.24095/hpcdp.37.4.03.

24. Gallagher MW, Lopez SJ, Preacher KJ. The hierarchical structure of well-being. J Pers. 2009;77(4):1025–50. https://doi.org/10.1111/j.1467-6494.2009.00573.x.

25. Guo C, Tomson G, Guo J, Li X, Keller C, Söderqvist F. Psychometric evaluation of the Mental Health Continuum-short form (MHC-SF) in Chinese adolescents—a methodological study. Health Qual Life Outcomes. 2015;13(1):198. https://doi.org/10.1186/s12955-015-0394-2.

26. Rogoza R, Truong Thi KH, Różycka-Tran J, Piotrowski J, Żemojtel-Piotrowska M. Psychometric properties of the MHC-SF: an integration of the existing measurement approaches. J Clin Psychol. 2018;74(10):1742–58. https://doi.org/10.1002/jclp.22626.

27. Żemojtel-Piotrowska M, Piotrowski JP, Osin EN, Cieciuch J, Adams BG, Ardi R, et al. The mental health continuum-short form: the structure and application for cross-cultural studies—a 38 nation study. J Clin Psychol. 2018;74(6):1034–52. https://doi.org/10.1002/jclp.22570.

28. Westerhof GJ, Keyes CLM. Mental Illness and Mental health: the two continua model across the lifespan. J Adult Dev. 2010;17(2):110–9. https://doi.org/10.1007/s10804-009-9082-y.

29. Johnson BA, Riley JB. Psychosocial impacts on college students providing mental health peer support. J Am Coll Health. 2019:1–5. https://doi.org/10.1080/07448481.2019.1660351.

30. Ferentinos P, Yotsidi V, Porichi E, Douzenis A, Papageorgiou C, Stalikas A. Well-being in patients with affective disorders compared to nonclinical participants: a multi-model evaluation of the Mental Health Continuum-short form. J Clin Psychol. 2019;75(9):1585–612. https://doi.org/10.1002/jclp.22780.

31. Fledderus M, Bohlmeijer ET, Smit F, Westerhof GJ. Mental health promotion as a new goal in public mental health care: a randomized controlled trial of an intervention enhancing psychological flexibility. Am J Public Health. 2010;100(12):2372. https://doi.org/10.2105/AJPH.2010.196196.

32. Santini ZI, Meilstrup C, Hinrichsen C, Nielsen L, Koyanagi A, Krokstad S, et al. Formal volunteer activity and psychological Flourishing in Scandinavia: findings from two cross-sectional rounds of the European social survey. Soc Curr. 2018;6(4):2329496518815868. https://doi.org/10.1177/2329496518815868.

33. Diener E. The science of Well-being: the collected works of Ed Diener. Social indicators research series 37. New York: Springer Science & Business Media; 2009.

34. Diener E, Wirtz D, Tov W, Kim-Prieto C, Choi DW, Oishi S, et al. New Well-being measures: short scales to assess flourishing and positive and negative feelings. Soc Indic Res. 2010;97(2):143–56. https://doi.org/10.1007/s11205-009-9493-y.

35. Huppert FA, So TTC. Flourishing across Europe: application of a new conceptual framework for defining well-being. Soc Indic Res. 2013;110(3):837–61. https://doi.org/10.1007/s11205-011-9966-7.

36. Kobau R, Seligman MEP, Peterson C, Diener E, Zack MM, Chapman D, et al. Mental health promotion in public health: perspectives and strategies from positive psychology. Am J Public Health. 2011;101(8):e1–9. https://doi.org/10.1177/10253823050120020103x.

37. Shucksmith J, Spratt J, Philip K, McNaughton R. A critical review of the literature on children and young people's views of the factors that influence their mental health. Edinburgh: NHS Health Scotland; 2009.

38. Keyes CLM. Mental well-being: international contributions to the study of positive mental health. Dordrecht: Springer; 2013.

39. Iasiello M, van Agteren J, Keyes CLM, Cochrane EM. Positive mental health as a predictor of recovery from mental illness. J Affect Disord. 2019;251:227–30. https://doi.org/10.1016/j.jad.2019.03.065.

40. Verhaeghe N, De Maeseneer J, Maes L, Van Heeringen C, Annemans L. Health promotion in mental health care: perceptions from patients and mental health nurses. J Clin Nurs. 2013;22:1569–78. https://doi.org/10.1111/jocn.12076.

41. Lerdal A. A concept analysis of energy. Its meaning in the lives of three individuals with chronic illness. Scand J Caring Sci. 1998;12(1):3–10.

42. International Health Promotion Hospitals and Health Services. The New Haven recommendations on partnering with patients, families and citizens to enhance performance and quality in health promoting hospitals and health services clinical. Health Promot. 2016;6(1):1–15.

43. Keyes CLM, Dhingra SS, Simoes EJ. Change in level of positive mental health as a predictor of future risk of mental illness. Am J Public Health. 2010;100(12):2366–71. https://doi.org/10.2105/AJPH.2010.192245.

44. Keyes CLM. The next steps in the promotion and protection of positive mental health. Can J Nurs Res. 2010;42(3):17–28.

45. Schotanus-Dijkstra M, Keyes CLM, de Graaf R, ten Have M. Recovery from mood and anxiety disorders: the influence of positive mental health. J Affect Disord. 2019;252:107–13. https://doi.org/10.1016/j.jad.2019.04.051.

46. McGaffin BJ, Deane FP, Kelly PJ, Ciarrochi J. Flourishing, languishing and moderate mental health: prevalence and change in mental health during recovery from drug and alcohol problems. Addict Res Theor. 2015;23(5):351–60. https://doi.org/10.3109/16066359.2015.1019346.

47. Fan JK, Mustard C, Smith PM. Psychosocial work conditions and mental health: examining differences across mental illness and well-being outcomes. Ann Work Expos Health. 2019;63(5):546–59. https://doi.org/10.1093/annweh/wxz028.

48. Chan RCH, Mak WWS, Chio FHN, Tong ACY. Flourishing with psychosis: a prospective examination on the interactions between clinical, functional, and personal recovery processes on well-being among individuals with schizophrenia spectrum disorders. Schizophr Bull. 2018;44:778–86. https://doi.org/10.1093/schbul/sbx120.

49. Stanga V, Turrina C, Valsecchi P, Sacchetti E, Vita A. Well-being in patients with schizophrenia, mood and personality disorders attending psychiatric services in the community. A controlled study. Compr Psychiatry. 2019;91:1–5. https://doi.org/10.1016/j.comppsych.2019.02.001.

50. Keyes CLM, Eisenberg D, Perry GS, Dube SR, Kroenke K, Dhingra SS. The relationship of level of positive mental health with current mental disorders in predicting suicidal behavior and academic impairment in college students. J Am Coll Health. 2012;60(2):126–33. https://doi.org/10.1080/07448481.2011.608393.

51. Schotanus-Dijkstra M, ten Have M, Lamers SMA, de Graaf R, Bohlmeijer ET. The longitudinal relationship between flourishing mental health and incident mood, anxiety and substance use disorders. Eur J Public Health. 2017;27(3):563–8. https://doi.org/10.1093/eurpub/ckw202.

52. Trompetter HR, de Kleine E, Bohlmeijer ET. Why does positive mental health buffer against psychopathology? An exploratory study on self-compassion as a resilience mechanism and adaptive emotion regulation strategy. Cogn Ther Res. 2017;41(3):459–68. https://doi.org/10.1007/s10608-016-9774-0.

53. de Vos JA, Radstaak M, Bohlmeijer ET, Westerhof GJ. Having an eating disorder and still being able to flourish? Examination of pathological symptoms and well-being as two continua of mental health in a clinical sample. Front Psychol. 2018;9:2145. https://doi.org/10.3389/fpsyg.2018.02145.

54. Donnelly A, O'Reilly A, Dolphin L, O'Keeffe L, Moore J. Measuring the performance of the Mental health continuum-short form (MHC-SF) in a primary care youth mental health service. Ir J Psychol Med. 2019;36(3):201–5. https://doi.org/10.1017/ipm.2018.55.

55. Slade M. Mental illness and well-being: the central importance of positive psychology and recovery approaches. BMC Health Serv Res. 2010;10(1):26. https://doi.org/10.1186/1472-6963-10-26.

56. Provencher HL, Keyes CLM. Complete mental health recovery: bridging mental illness with positive mental health. J Public Ment Health. 2011;10(1):57–69. https://doi.org/10.1108/17465721111134556.

57. Antonovsky A. Unraveling the mystery of health: how people manage stress and stay well. San Francisco: Jossey-Bass; 1987.

58. Antonovsky A. Health, stress, and coping. San Francisco: Jossey-Bass; 1979.

59. Antonovsky A. The life cycle, mental health and the sense of coherence. Isr J Psychiatry Relat Sci. 1985;22(4):273–80.

60. Mittelmark MB, Sagy S, Eriksson M, Bauer GF, Pelikan JM, Lindström B, et al. The handbook of Salutogenesis. Cham: Springer International Publishing AG; 2017.

61. Lindström B, Eriksson M. The Hitchhiker's guide to salutogenesis: salutogenic pathways to health promotion. Helsinki: Folkhälsan; 2010.

Hope: A Health Promotion Resource

6

Tone Rustøen

Abstract

Hope is a phenomenon many nurses and patients are concerned about. One of the reasons for this interest may be that many patients today live with chronic illnesses, and hope is something positive and focuses on the future and opportunities. Hope is a way of feeling, thinking, and influencing one's behavior. The way we view our health and health-related challenges are assumed to impact on hope. Hope is forward-looking, realistic, and multi-dimensional. It is a resource for health and health-promoting processes and can be considered a salutogenic resource and construct. This chapter highlights what hope means during illness, what research has so far been concerned with, how hope can be assessed, and how nurses can strengthen hope in patients.

Keywords

Definitions of hope · Hope measurement · Hope interventions

T. Rustøen (✉)
Division of Emergencies and Critical Care, Department of Research and Development, Oslo University Hospital HF, Oslo, Norway

Faculty of Medicine, Institute of Health and Society, University of Oslo, Oslo, Norway
e-mail: tone.rustoen@medisin.uio.no

6.1 The Significance of Hope for Patients with Long-Lasting Illnesses

Patients with a variety of illnesses describe the importance of hope when being ill or feeling threatened in essential areas of life. A Swedish nurse, Eva Benzein, interviewed people with cancer who received palliative home care about hope [1]. Participants in this study described hope of being cured even though they knew they were seriously ill, hope of living as normally as possible, the importance of the presence of affirmative relationships (family and friends, health professionals or of a more spiritual nature), and a reconciliation with life and death. Everyone expressed that their lives changed dramatically when they learned that no curative treatment was possible. They expressed that they wanted to find a meaning in their situation and expressed that if hope disappears you have nothing. Even if this study is some years old, Benzein's study is central in this research field presenting palliative patient's experiences of hope clearly and interestingly.

Worldwide, the number of intensive care unit admissions and survivors after treatment in intensive care is increasing [2, 3] due to an aging population and advances in critical care medicine. Several patients admitted to an intensive care unit have a chronic condition. When being critically ill the future can be uncertain both related to survival, recovery, and daily functioning. A former intensive care patient shared her experiences as critically ill, describing hope to be essential for her recovery [4]. Possibly, an ICU patient's goal is to maintain one's hope during serious illness and recovery. Little research is done on hope in ICU patients.

Hope is an effective coping strategy for patients in demanding life situations [5]; it provides adaptive power for getting through difficult situations and achieving meaning and desired goals [1, 6]. It is described to generate energy, often described as "will," with a motivational quality [5]. It can be a resource that provides strength to master a disorder. It has also been shown that hope is central to one's quality of life [7]. Erich Fromm argues that hope is absolutely essential to life [8].

Hope is also described to act as a psychosocial resource to deal with chronic illness experiences in a meta-analyses about hope in those above 60 years with chronic illnesses [9]. In this meta-analyses the participants explained that a sense of self, feelings of control, relationships with others, and quality of life were associated with hope. Accordingly, hope is part of the generalized resistance resources, important for health promotion and for salutogenic nursing.

6.2   Theoretical Perspectives of Hope

First, this chapter shows some central and frequently used definitions of hope, followed by a description of spheres and dimensions of hope. All these three descriptions of hope contribute to a deeper understanding of the essence of hope as a salutogenic construct and perceived experience.

6.2.1   Definitions of Hope

Hope is a complex phenomenon that is studied in several disciplines. It is also defined as a basic confidence in and feeling that there is a way out of one's difficulties [10]. Joyce Travelbee defined hope as a mental state characterized by the desire

to reach a goal, combined with some degree of expectation that this goal is achievable [11]. Hope is also defined as a positive motivational state based on setting goals and thinking about ways to reach them [12, 13]. The hope literature emphasizes both the emotional and the cognitive aspects.

Dufault and Martocchio [14] published a definition of hope 30 years ago, and this definition is still often referred to. They defined hope as "a multidimensional dynamic life force characterized by a confident yet uncertain expectation of achieving a future good which, to the hoping person, is realistically possible and personally significant" (p. 380). This definition emphasizes that hope represents a dynamic life force. There are strengths in hope, understood as forces to move forward even if you face resistance. Dufault and Martocchio also show the versatility of hope and that hope should be both realistic and important. That hope should be realistic is also emphasized by Travelbee [11]. Fromm [8] wrote that "hope is neither passive waiting nor is it unrealistic forcing of circumstances that cannot occur" (p. 22). He also stated that there is "no sense in hoping for that which already exists or for that which cannot be" (p. 22). Many definitions of hope as the one given by Dufault and Martocchio [14] have in common that hope is considered to be forward-looking, realistic, and multidimensional.

Farran and colleagues [15] have conducted a literature review of studies about hope. Based on this review, hope is defined as follows:

Hope constitutes an essential experience of the human condition. It functions as a way of feeling, a way of thinking, a way of behaving, a way of relating to oneself and one's world. Hope has the ability to be fluid in expectations, and in the event that the desired object or outcome does not occur, hope can still be present. (p. 6)

Through the definitions and descriptions of the content of hope, it emerges that hope is a way of feeling and thinking which influences one's behavior. Within the hope literature, there is a debate about whether hope is a more or less stable state in a person or whether hope is a dynamic process that changes over time [16]. There are reasons to believe that personal qualities matter but that hope is influenced by what we encounter. This will be illuminated somewhat more in the section describing different dimensions of hope.

Kim and colleagues [16] studied the nature of hope in chronically ill people. They conducted an interview study of 12 hospitalized chronically ill patients from the United States and 16 nurses working in oncology departments. Everyone was asked to reflect on hope. Different patterns of subjective experiences of hope were described: (1) an externalism orientation, (2) a pragmatism orientation, (3) reality orientation, (4) future orientation, and lastly, (5) an internalism orientation.

Those who described an *externalism orientation* said that their sources of hope were different from themselves, such as God or significant others. They put a lot in God's hands, and they trusted family and friends to help them. Their own efforts were not important.

In a *pragmatic orientation*, the chronically ill patients stated that they found the source of hope by doing small things or enjoying things they can accomplish. Patients who fell into this pattern stated that they did not believe in the major goals as they had no belief that they could be achieved. They had accepted their illness without the prospects of getting better, and they experienced hope by having a positive attitude toward the future as well as the present.

The chronically ill with a *reality-oriented orientation* experienced hope through a sober perception of their situation. Their view of the future was thoroughly grounded in relation to the realities of their illness. They also described God as a stable and important force in life.

Patients in the *future orientation* category experienced hope by planning the future and ensuring that it contained positive opportunities. They also had a strong dependence on God. These patients do not perceive hope in relation to what other people may think but argue that everything that happens have a reason.

Patients who had an *internalism orientation* experienced hope through humor or related to advances in science. This type of hope was based on the patient's belief in what was possible in

their situation, on their own actions, on the use of humor, knowledge, or the presence of family or friends. This kind of hope was not perceived in relation to opportunities in the future or by leaving it to other people, but on the patient's own perception of the situation in question.

The researchers summarize this study by pointing out that different chronically ill patients focus on different sources of hope, and thus experience hope differently. The hope patterns described may differ due to the different characteristics of the patients. The importance of the relationship with God was highlighted in most of the different orientations. In which ways these patterns are related to health promotion and salutogenesis is not known yet.

In a literature review on hope in qualitative studies, Duggleby and colleagues summarized the characteristics of hope [9] and described two hope-processes: (1) transcendence and (2) reappraisal in re-evaluating hope when being chronically ill. Reaching inwardly and outwardly and finding meaning and purpose were sub-processes of transcendence, whereas re-evaluating hope in the context of illness and finding positive possibilities were sub-processes of positive reappraisal. These two processes are integrated. However, Duggleby and colleagues [17] concluded that hope in older persons with chronic illness involves transcendence from a difficult situation and positive reappraisal. If you cannot get rid of the chronic illness and its consequences, you can always change the way you think about your situation.

The concepts presented by Duggleby et al. [17] are central for sense of coherence and salutogenesis [18]. Still, the relationship between hope and sense of coherence is scarcely examined. In a Norwegian sample of intensive care patients 3 months after discharge from the intensive care unit, we found the correlation between hope (measured using Herth Hope Index) and sense of coherence (measured by Antonovsky's sense of coherence scale) was 0.56, meaningfulness and hope was 0.44, comprehensibility and hope was 0.45, and manageability and hope was 0.44 (unpublished data). These results suggest that hope and sense of coherence are moderately correlated in Norwegian intensive care survivors. In a study from Israel in three different cultural groups, they also concluded that hope and sense of coherence stand as separate resources even if the concepts have some overlap [19]. Møllenberg et al. showed that a stronger family sense of coherence was associated with higher hope in both persons with cancer and their family members [20]. Further research is warranted to examine the health-promoting aspects of hope.

6.2.1.1 Different Spheres and Dimensions of Hope

Dufault and Martocchio [14] stated that hope consists of two spheres. One sphere is a generalized (or general) hope and the other a particularized (or partial) hope. They defined generalized hope as a feeling that the future is uncertain but can be positive. A general feeling of hope protects the hopeful by casting a positive glow on life. A statement describing this is: "I hope for nothing special, I just hope." The other sphere of hope is the partial hope associated with a particular object that may be abstract or concrete (e.g., a new treatment).

This division of hope into spheres and dimensions was also described in Benzein's study [1] of the patients receiving palliative home care. These patients described hope as a tension between hoping for something (individualized hope) and living in hope (generalized hope). Hoping for something was related to being cured, while living in hope was a reconciliation of life and death. Which of these two spheres are dominating the palliative patient's state is seen to vary during the illness trajectory. An example of the disparity between these two spheres is that if one hopes for a treatment to succeed (individualized hope), one may not fully succumb if the treatment fails because the generalized hope can take over until one might find new particularized hopes.

The generalized hope can be a form of "fundamental" or "existential" hope [21]. A generalized hope is related to our ability to make or find meaning in our lives. A fundamental hope enables us to survive, e.g., loss of meaning.

Several definitions of hope include different dimensions or aspects of hope. Mary Nowotny

[22], based on a comprehensive literature review, has defined hope as consisting of six different dimensions:

> *a six-dimensional, dynamic attribute of the person which orients to the future, includes involvement by the individual, comes from within, is possible, relates to or involves others or a higher being, and relates to meaningful outcomes to the individual. (p. 89)*

Dufault and Martocchio [14] also described that hope has six different dimensions: an affective dimension, a cognitive dimension, a behavioral dimension, an attachment dimension, a time dimension, and a contextual dimension. Based on research using the Dufault and Martocchio hope dimensions, the next section will elaborate on these six dimensions presented by Dufault and Martocchio:

The *affective dimension* shows the emotional aspect of hope. As already shown, hope is often defined as an emotion, with many different feelings involved. Both confidence in that a positive result is possible and uncertainty about the future are central feelings in hope [23]. Travelbee emphasized both trust and courage as aspects of hope.

The *cognitive dimension* contains thoughts, ideas, goals, desires, and expectations. This dimension is related to comprehensibility in sense of coherence, which refers to the extent to which you might perceive both internal and external stimuli as being understandable in some kind of rational way [18]. An important factor here is how one assesses his or her opportunities, for example, get well or to have a good quality of life. An evaluation of the reality and hopeful factors will be central. A desire is often defined differently from hope as it may have less realism. This distinction is not easy, but hope is claimed to be based more on basic values such as experiencing community or being active. As one processes a situation, hopes and desires may become more coincidental. Still, wanting something will be part of the hope. Travelbee emphasizes both desire and having choices as important for hope.

The *behavioral dimension* of hope is related to what actions one takes, such as eating healthy food, praying, or making a decision [14]. This dimension is in accordance with m*anageability in sense of coherence and* has to do with the degree to which we might feel that there are resources at our disposal to meet demands [18]. It is pointed out that a hopeful person is better able to act than one who does not experience hope. There is energy in hope. Travelbee [11] points out that hope is linked to perseverance.

The *associational dimension* highlights the importance of good interpersonal relationships for hope [22]. These can be relationships with other people or with religion. Travelbee [11] claimed that hope is linked to dependence on others. The importance of religiosity for hope will probably differ depending on cultural differences.

The *time dimension* is fundamental for hope and implies the expectation of being able to achieve something in the future, and will in this way be time-related [14]. Travelbee [11] claims that hope is future-oriented.

Lastly, the *contextual dimension* concerns that hope is activated within a context. This dimension focuses on the specific circumstances of life that surround, influence, and challenge an individual's hopes. This dimension is the same as specific resistance resources in sense of coherence [18], which is context bounded. Hope is not regarded as a stable trait in man, but as a condition influenced by external factors such as illness and changes in life (depending on context). Consequently, it is very important how patients experience their surroundings when they are seriously ill, facing threats of their life or health. Travelbee [11] argued that nurses must prevent patients from losing their hope. Nurses can influence an individual's hope by caring behavior and the nurse–patient interaction including the way information and support are provided. We can also say that salutogenic nursing care promotes patients' hope, health, and well-being.

6.2.2 How to Measure Hope

When it comes to research on hope, the focus is often on how to identify hope using various questionnaires. Some studies have identified hope in different patient groups at different stages of illness. Furthermore, there are several qualitative studies helping to understand patients' experiences of hope [9].

Different questionnaires are developed to identify hope within health disciplines, especially by nursing researchers. Examples of such instruments are Miller Hope Scale [24], Nowotny Hope Scale [22], Stoner Hope Scale [25], Herth Hope Scale [26], and Herth Hope Index [27]. These scales are developed based on different definitions of hope. The Herth Hope Index is based on Daufalt and Martocchio's understanding of hope, which is used in several studies internationally, and found to have satisfactory psychometric properties in many countries. Herth Hope Index consists of 12 items. The answer options range on a 4-point scale from "strongly disagree" to "strongly agree." Table 6.1 shows the content of the 12 items and the scaling.

An advantage of this scale is that it is short and easy to complete [27]; therefore, it is clinically relevant. This questionnaire is currently used in patients with pain, cancer, heart failure, liver failure, cystic fibrosis, nursing home residents, and in relatives of intensive care patients. This scale has also been tested in the normal Norwegian and Swedish population [28, 29]. The instrument has the advantage that it is not specifically aimed at a specific outlook on life. Nowotny Hope Scale, which is also found in a Norwegian translation, gives religious people a higher hope than non-believers [30]. The role of religious beliefs in hope is debated, but I believe that hope will have different content for different individuals depending on one's beliefs.

Since the Herth Hope Index is short and easy to fill in, it can be used in clinical practice. There is always a danger that those patients who have the most difficulties do not contact health professionals for help. An early survey of hope using the Herth Hope Index can help to capture those who have the most difficulty. However, if using this scale in clinical practice, the results must be followed-up by adequate nursing care and actions toward the patient. If you as a health care professional, choose not to use the entire form, you may benefit from looking at the individual questions

Table 6.1 The Herth Hope Index[a] [27]

	Strongly disagree	Disagree	Agree	Strongly agree
1. I have a positive outlook toward life				
2. I have short and/or long range goals				
3. I feel all alone				
4. I can see possibilities in the midst of difficulties				
5. I have faith that gives me comfort				
6. I feel scared about my future				
7. I can recall happy/joyful times				
8. I have a deep inner strength				
9. I am able to give and receive caring/love				
10. I have a sense of direction				
11. I believe that each day has potential				
12. I fell my life has value and worth				

[a]© 1989 Kaye Herth. 1999 items 2 and 4 reworded. (Reprinted with permission of Kay Herth. Cannot be used without permission from Kaye Herth)

in the instrument and using them in conversation with the patient. Based on the patient's assessment of his or her situation, the results could be used as a starting point to talk to the patient about his/her hope and to assess whether the patient could possibly benefit from an intervention in relation to hope. Research has shown that a nurse–patient interaction including listening, acknowledging, respecting, and understanding the patient's experiences is health promoting [31] (see Chap. 10).

6.2.3 Factors That Can Facilitate or Hinder Hope

Various studies on different patient groups have examined what facilitates and what hinders hope. An Iranian study on hope and spirituality in patients with cardiovascular diseases, found a stronger hope among those being married, having higher education, good economic status and with stronger spiritual well-being [32]. This study concluded that multiple factors may influence on hope.

Another study on hope in women after cardiac surgery [33] showed that diminished hope was associated with older age, lower education, depression prior to surgery, and persistent pain at all measurement points up to 12 months after surgery. The authors concluded that e.g. promoting hope, particularly for women living alone may be important targets for interventions to improve outcomes following cardiac surgery.

Furthermore, a study examining the relationship between hope, symptoms, needs, and spirituality/religiosity in cancer patients treated in a supportive care unit [34] reported that those with less education, less symptoms, and less often had been referred to a psychologist previously to the study, as well as higher spirituality reported higher hope.

Previous studies on hope assess hope in different patient populations in various clinical and life settings as well as countries; therefore, summarizing factors that facilitate hope based on earlier research is difficult. The use of covariates to examine the impact on hope is also differing from study to study. The research on hope includes patients from different countries; hence, cultural differences might influence the results. As hope seems to be related to spiritual well-being, variations about beliefs and values might also be a disturbing factor. Furthermore, low education and many symptoms seem to negatively impact on hope.

6.2.4 Health-Promoting Interventions Strengthening Hope

Knowledge about factors that can strengthen hope in patients is important when developing interventions to impact on patients' hope. Research on factors strengthening hope is limited; however, there are reasons to believe that more research will come when instruments to assess hope are available in many countries. Caring for patients with serious illnesses and an uncertain future can be a challenge. Nurses are around patients and they are important in strengthening or maintain hope. Travelbee writes [11]:

> The job of the professional nurse is to help the sick to maintain hope and avoid hopelessness.... (p. 123)

One must be open to the fact that there are many ways of promoting hope. It can be helpful to let patients put their own words into how they look at the time they have ahead. It can be a gateway to talk about hope (see Chap. 10). As Travelbee writes, the nurse's behavior can mean a lot to patients' hopes. The fact that one dares to be present and listen to the patient is emphasized, and the patient must have confidence in the nurse.

An interview study explored critical care nurses' perceptions of hope inspiring strategies in adult patients and families [35]. The nurses told that communication was the major theme for intervention (see Chap. 10). Listening, asking questions, and educate were described. Nurses stressed to be honest and a large part of communication was getting to know the patient as a person which is an essence in nurse–patient interaction and salutogenic nursing care. They also emphasized that it was important to incorporate family into care.

The nurse–patient interaction is shown to be important for hope in cognitively intact nursing home residents [31]. Haugan et al. [36] found a direct relationship of nurse–patient interaction on hope, meaning in life and self-transcendence, and conclude that advancing caregivers' interacting and communicating skills might facilitate patients' health and global well-being and inspire professional caregivers as they perform their daily care practices.

Frankl wrote about the importance of finding hope and meaning in life, suggesting self-transcendence as the process of reaching out beyond oneself and thus discover meaning in life [37] (see Chap. 8). A way to find meaning is through the chosen attitude when faced with an unchangeable situation. Duggleby and colleagues claimed that hope is a psychosocial resource which individuals use to deal with their chronic

illness experience [9]. Finding meaning and positive reappraisals are important strategies to help older adults with chronic illnesses to maintain their hope. Ways to foster hope with older adults with chronic illness may include strategies for finding meaning and purpose which is a process of self-transcendence [9] (see Chap. 9). Strategies such as adjustment to transitions and losses, life review, reminiscence therapy, and spiritual support can help people find meaning and purpose and transcend their experience of suffering (see Chap. 8).

Ripamonti and colleagues [34] conclude that in cancer patients, hope can be encouraged by clinicians through dialog, sincerity, and reassurance, as well as assessing and considering the patients' needs (above all the psycho-emotional), symptoms, psychological frailty, and their spiritual/religious resources.

The above-presented studies describe how to strengthen hope in patients; however, they mainly focus on communication and the nurse–patient relationship and the nurse–patient interaction. This is of great importance, but it is not clear what is specific hope inspiring or what is related to other hope-related phenomena.

The effectiveness of a psychosocial supportive intervention to increase hope and quality of life was evaluated in terminally ill cancer patients 60 years and older staying at home [38]. The hope intervention termed "Living with Hope Program" (LWHP) consisted of viewing an international award-winning video on hope and a choice of one of three hope activities to work on over a 1-week period. The control group received standard care. The data were collected at the first visit in the patients' homes. Analyses showed that patients receiving the LWHP had higher hope and quality of life compared to those in the control group. They also collected qualitative data with open-ended hope questions from the treatment group. The qualitative data confirmed the findings from the statistical analyses as 62% of the patients in the treatment group reporting the LWHP increased their hope.

A recent study described smartphone delivery of a hope intervention to students [39]. The intervention was based on Snyder's theory of hope and used text messages with hope stories and pictures. Using a quasi-experimental pilot study with pretest and posttest design, the feasibility and potential impact of the mobile app were examined. The analyses showed that the participants appeared to engage with the intervention and found the experience to be user-friendly, helpful, and enjoyable. Relative to the control group, those receiving the intervention demonstrated a significantly greater increase in hope.

Research should continue to develop interventions to strengthen hope in patients. When choosing an intervention to strengthen hope, the intervention must be based on what is most important for the patient's hopes. The interventions can be individual or group-based. There is a need for studies that can further investigate how hope best can be strengthened in patients also in the specialist health service. Based on earlier research, areas like finding meaning, self-transcendence, nurse–patient interaction, and communication are important but seem not specific to hope. To secure that the interventions are related to hope one might talking with the patients about the different aspects included in the 12 items in Herth Hope Index.

A challenge in building the research on strengthening hope is that the studies presented just to a small amount are building on each other. One should base research well in what is already there. Another challenge is that hope might mean different if you are young or elderly, are very ill or in a rehabilitation phase. Further, individual's cultural and religious background impact on the content of their hope. Further research is needed about how to promote hope in different patient groups.

6.3   Conclusion

As shown in this chapter, there are many different definitions of hope. Some characteristics are included in several definitions, while other aspects vary from definition to definition. Some emphasize that hope must be realistic in order to be a hope, while others do not include this aspect at all. The degree to which hope is influenced by personal characteristics or by the surroundings is also unclear. Finally, in comparing research on hope between different international studies, the cultural differences important to hope represent a challenge. For example, when it comes to the importance of religion to hope, I expect that this will vary significantly across countries.

Given the importance of hope for patients in a variety of situations, we must continue our efforts to understand hope and to gain greater knowledge of how we can best help to strengthen patients' hope in the best possible way. There are reasons to believe that hope is a central phenomenon for health promotion and salutogenic nursing care.

Take Home Messages
- Hope is an important phenomenon for many different patient groups.
- Hope is a vital resource for health promotion in healthy as well as unhealthy people and represents a salutogenic concept.
- Hope is defined in different ways, but there is a consensus that hope is a multidimensional concept comprising both feelings and the way of thinking.
- Research on hope has been centered on how hope can be mapped to different patient groups and how hope can be strengthened in meeting patients.
- Hope can be facilitated by communication, nurse–patients interaction, and the individual's ability for self-transcendence.
- Further research is desirable and necessary to better enable the nurse to strengthen the hope of patients.

References

1. Benzein E, Norberg A, Saveman BI. The meaning of the lived experience of hope in patients with cancer in palliative home care. Palliat Med. 2001;15(2):117–26.
2. Halpern NA, Pastores SM. Critical care medicine in the United States 2000–2005: an analysis of bed numbers, occupancy rates, payer mix, and costs. Crit Care Med. 2010;38(1):65–71.
3. Maca J, Jor O, Holub M, Sklienka P, Bursa F, Burda M, Janout V, Ševčík P. Past and present ARDS mortality rates: a systematic review. Respir Care. 2017;62(1):113–22.

4. Kjærgård RS. The blink of an eye: how I died an started living. 2019 Hodder & Stoughton.

5. Folkman S. Stress, coping, and hope. Psychooncology. 2010;19(9):901–8.

6. Herth K. Enhancing hope in people with a first recurrence of cancer. J Adv Nurs. 2000;32(6):1431–41.

7. Rustøen T, Cooper BA, Miaskowski C. The importance of hope as a mediator of psychological distress and life satisfaction in a community sample of cancer patients. Cancer Nurs. 2010;33(4):258–67.

8. Fromm E. The revolution of hope, toward a humanized technology. 1st ed. New York: Harper & Row; 1968.

9. Duggleby W, Hicks D, Nekolaichuk C, Holtslander L, Williams A, Chambers T, et al. Hope, older adults, and chronic illness: a metasynthesis of qualitative research. J Adv Nurs. 2012;68(6):1211–23.

10. Lynch W. Images of hope. Notre Dame, IN: University of Notre Dame Press; 1974.

11. Travelbee J. Interpersonal aspects of nursing. Philadelphia: F. A. Davis; 1966. p. xii.

12. Snyder CR, Harris C, Anderson JR, Holleran SA, Irving LM, Sigmon ST, et al. The will and the ways: development and validation of an individual-differences measure of hope. J Pers Soc Psychol. 1991;60(4):570–85.

13. Snyder OJ. Research our great and only hope. J Am Osteopath Assoc. 2001;101(9):542–4.

14. Dufault K, Martocchio BC. Symposium on compassionate care and the dying experience. Hope: its spheres and dimensions. Nurs Clin North Am. 1985;20(2):379–91.

15. Farran CJ, Wilken C, Popovich JM. Clinical assessment of hope. Issues Ment Health Nurs. 1992;13(2):129–38.

16. Kim DS, Kim HS, Schwartz-Barcott D, Zucker D. The nature of hope in hospitalized chronically ill patients. Int J Nurs Stud. 2006;43(5):547–56.

17. Duggleby W, Bally J, Cooper D, Doell H, Thomas R. Engaging hope: the experiences of male spouses of women with breast cancer. Oncol Nurs Forum. 2012;39(4):400–6.

18. Antonovsky A. Unraveling the mystery of health: how people manage stress and stay well. 1st ed. San Francisco: Jossey-Bass; 1987.

19. Braun-Lewensohn O, Abu-Kaf S, Kalagy T. Are "sense of coherence" and "Hope" related constructs? Examining these concepts in three cultural groups in Israel. Isr J Psychiatry Relat Sci. 2017;54(2):17–23.

20. Møllerberg ML, Arestedt K, Swahnberg K, Benzein E, Sandgren A. Family sense of coherence and its associations with hope, anxiety and symptoms of depression in persons with cancer in palliative phase and their family members: a cross-sectional study. Palliat Med. 2019;33(10):1310–8.

21. Snow NA. Fundamental hope, meaning and self-transcendence. In: Frey JA, editor. Self-transcendence and virtue: perspectives from philosophy, psychology, and technology. 1st ed. New York: Taylor & Francis; 2018.

22. Nowotny ML. Assessment of hope in patients with cancer: development of an instrument. Oncol Nurs Forum. 1989;16(1):57–61.

23. Rustøen T, Hanestad BR. Nursing intervention to increase hope in cancer patients. J Clin Nurs. 1998;7(1):19–27.

24. Miller JF, Powers MJ. Development of an instrument to measure hope. Nurs Res. 1988;37(1):6–10.

25. Stoner MH, Keampfer SH. Recalled life expectancy information, phase of illness and hope in cancer patients. Res Nurs Health. 1985;8(3):269–74.

26. Herth K. Development and refinement of an instrument to measure hope. Sch Inq Nurs Pract. 1991;5(1):39–51; discussion 3–6.

27. Herth K. Abbreviated instrument to measure hope: development and psychometric evaluation. J Adv Nurs. 1992;17(10):1251–9.

28. Rustøen T, Wahl AK, Hanestad BR, Lerdal A, Miaskowski C, Moum T. Hope in the general Norwegian population, measured using the Herth Hope index. Palliat Support Care. 2003;1(4):309–18.

29. Benzein E, Berg A. The Swedish version of Herth Hope index—an instrument for palliative care. Scand J Caring Sci. 2003;17(4):409–15.

30. Rustøen T, Wiklund I. Hope in newly diagnosed patients with cancer. Cancer Nurs. 2000;23(3):214–9.

31. Haugan G, Moksnes UK, Espnes GA. Nurse-patient interaction: a resource for hope in cognitively intact nursing home patients. J Holist Nurs. 2013;31(3):152–63.

32. Yaghoobzadeh A, Soleimani MA, Allen KA, Chan YH, Herth KA. Relationship between spiritual well-being and hope in patients with cardiovascular disease. J Relig Health. 2018;57(3):938–50.

33. Bjørnnes AK, Parry M, Lie I, Falk R, Leegaard M, Rustoen T. The association between hope, marital status, depression and persistent pain in men and women following cardiac surgery. BMC Womens Health. 2018;18(1):2.

34. Ripamonti CI, Miccinesi G, Pessi MA, Di Pede P, Ferrari M. Is it possible to encourage hope in non-advanced cancer patients? We must try. Ann Oncol. 2016;27(3):513–9.

35. Fowler SB. Critical-care nurses' perceptions of hope: original qualitative research. Dimens Crit Care Nurs. 2020;39(2):110–5.

36. Haugan G. Nurse-patient interaction is a resource for hope, meaning in life and self-transcendence in nursing home patients. Scand J Caring Sci. 2014;28(1):74–88.

37. Frankl VE. The will to meaning; foundations and applications of logotherapy. New York: World Pub; 1969.

38. Duggleby WD, Degner L, Williams A, Wright K, Cooper D, Popkin D, Holtslander L. Living with hope: initial evaluation of a psychosocial hope intervention for older palliative home care patients. J Pain Symptom Manage. 2007;33(3):247–57.

39. Daugherty DA, Runyan JD, Steenbergh TA, Fratzke BJ, Fry BN, Westra E. Smartphone delivery of a hope intervention: another way to flourish. PLoS One. 2018;13(6):e0197930.

Dignity: An Essential Foundation for Promoting Health and Well-Being

Berit Sæteren and Dagfinn Nåden

Abstract

The purpose of this chapter is to illuminate different understandings of the concept of dignity and to discuss how we can make use of this knowledge to enhance human health. Dignity is viewed as a universal concept in health sciences and a feature necessary to promote health and alleviate suffering related to sickness and impending death. The ideas presented in this chapter are founded in a caring science paradigm where the human being is considered as a unique entity consisting of body, soul, and spirit. Caring science as referred to in this chapter has its scientific foundation in Gadamer's ontological hermeneutics.

Dignity is described in a historical perspective, and different meanings of dignity are clarified. Since health and dignity relate to one other, we have clarified the concept of health employing the texts of the Finnish theoretician Katie Eriksson. In order to illuminate the perspective of health promotion, we have also briefly described health in a salutogenic perspective according to the medical sociologist Aron Antonovsky. In clarifying dignity, the texts of well-known researchers from the Nordic countries and UK were employed. In reflecting on how we can make use of the knowledge of dignity and indignity to promote health, we have considered this matter in light of results of a major Scandinavian study. The main purpose of this study was to explore dignity and indignity of patients in nursing homes from the perspective of patients, family caregivers, and health personnel. The testimonies presented in this section are further interpreted employing mainly caring science and philosophical literature. Lastly, a short summary of some public policy efforts with the aim to preserve human dignity is offered.

Keywords

Dignity · Indignity · Health · Health promotion · Well-being

7.1 Introduction

The purpose of this chapter is to illuminate different understandings of the concept of dignity and to discuss how we can make use of this knowledge to enhance human health.

Dignity is a core concept in nursing science and care, as well as in other health professions that take responsibility for the health and well-being of others [1–5]. In nursing, the preservation of human dignity is often emphasized as nursing

B. Sæteren (✉) · D. Nåden
Faculty of Health Sciences, Department of Nursing and Health Promotion, Oslo Metropolitan University, Oslo, Norway
e-mail: beritsa@oslomet.no; dagfinn@oslomet.no

G. Haugan, M. Eriksson (eds.), *Health Promotion in Health Care – Vital Theories and Research*,
https://doi.org/10.1007/978-3-030-63135-2_7

is related to persons in vulnerable situations and in need of health care. The value of *protecting human dignity* is often emphasized colloquially and in professional and political settings without necessarily explaining what it really means. Consequently, no common understanding of dignity exist; thus, the health professionals are left with their individual interpretation of the meaning of dignity. Furthermore, a concept, which is used in several different context and with different meanings, is at risk of becoming meaningless. Theoretical end empirical research is therefore valuable to broaden our understanding of dignity in the health care context.

A common understanding is that human beings are unique creations with an inherent dignity and are given a specific place in the world [2–4, 6–10]. Likewise, the experience of dignity is significantly meaningful in people's lives and may be a resource for personal health and well-being. Vulnerability and dependency are basic features of human existence. As other creatures manage their own life when born, human beings have a special existential vulnerability and dependency on being seen and taken care of by others. Vulnerability is always a part of human life, actualized in situations where humans need help from their closest family members or from health care professionals [11, 12]. Vulnerability is however also a positive trait by being human, a health resource, helping persons to transform demanding experiences from life and sickness into strength and personal growth [13].

Dignity is often characterized as a complex and vague concept. Although a large amount of research related to dignity has been done in recent years, the meaning of the concept is still ambiguous. This may not be considered a problem but instead a strength, as it points to the complexity in conceptualizing a human phenomenon as complicated as dignity [14, 15].

In this chapter, the aim is to broaden the significance and meaning of the concept in a historical and professional setting based on theory and research. We do not offer a particular definition of dignity. Moreover, we emphasize the meaning and importance of dignity as a health resource in people's lives and how promoting dignity can

help persons to experience well-being and be restored to health. Tranvåg and McSherry [16] claim that nurses as well as allied health care professionals may have an intuitive understanding of dignity in their practice, but they often lack the in-depth understanding required to manifest dignity in practical situations. Indignity/violation of dignity in health care is well known and documented [5, 17]. It is therefore important that health personnel working with people in vulnerable situations seek to obtain a deeper understanding of the underlying components of dignity in order to promote health, foster humane health care, and prevent dehumanization. Buchanan [18] even emphasizes promoting dignity as the ethical dimension of health.

Dignity is viewed as a universal concept in health sciences and a feature necessary to promote health and alleviate suffering related to sickness and impending death. In this chapter, we want to call attention to the value of the concept related to experiences of health and health promotion. We understand health promotion in line with the Ottawa Charter from 1986 as "the process of enabling individuals and communities to increase control over the determinant of health and thereby improve their health." ([19], p. 15). The ideas presented in this chapter are founded in a caring science paradigm where the human being is considered as a unique entity consisting of body, soul, and spirit [2, 7, 20]. Caring science as referred to in this chapter has its scientific foundation in Hans-Georg Gadamer's [21] ontological hermeneutics. The idea of hermeneutics is to clarify terms for understanding of the human being.

7.2 Dignity in a Historical Perspective

Human dignity has held a prominent place in political discussions of human rights since the Second World War [22]. Dignity emerges as a right and a duty based on a notion of human rights that relates to inner value and objective beauty in the human being entailing strong moral implications for fellow human beings. Each person deserves respect, and because of the human being's dignity and inner value, the person holds a certain right that the world community must protect. The United Nations [23] emphasizes that all human beings have inherent dignity. Article 1 of the Universal Declaration of Human Rights [23] states:

> All human beings are born free and equal in dignity and rights. They are endowed with reason and conscience and should act towards one another in a spirit of brotherhood.

Professional codes such as the ICN Code of Ethics for Nurses [24] emphasize that the preservation of dignity is an important part of caring. *"Inherent in nursing is a respect for human rights, including cultural rights, the right to life and choice, to dignity, and to be treated with respect."*

The idea of dignity has a long history. In ancient Rome, the Latin dignitas meant "worthiness," and in a political context, "reputation" or "standing." Sensen [22] distinguishes between what he calls a contemporary and a traditional paradigm related to human dignity. The contemporary paradigm relates to human rights, and the traditional paradigm goes back to older thinkers such as Pico della Mirandola and Immanuel Kant [22]. In contrast to the contemporary paradigm related to human rights, the traditional understanding is primarily a theoretical question about the human being's place in the universe because of its rationality and freedom. Dignity is used in the traditional sense to describe the special position that human beings hold. Because of this special position, the human being has an initial dignity as well as a duty to realize it. Sensen [22] describes these two notions of dignity as "initial dignity" and "realized dignity."

In 1988 Katie Eriksson [1] (p. 22) expressed that *Human dignity is the human being's ability to constitute her life and being.* She based her thesis on the work *Praise of man's dignity* (published in 1486) by the Renaissance philosopher Giovanni Pico della Mirandola (1463–1494). According to Pico, human beings were exceptional in the *Creation*. He viewed the dignity of human beings as founded in their freedom, in their capacity to choose their own place in the chain of beings stretching from God to the lowest animals [22, 25, 26].

Later, the German philosopher Immanuel Kant (1724–1804) described dignity as an absolute inner value that all human beings possess. He refers to dignity as an elevated position, above the rest of the nature, by virtue of a certain capacity, namely freedom and reason. Kant talks about dignity mainly in relation to the duty toward oneself not to violate the prerogative one has over other creatures [22]. The historical perspectives of the meaning of dignity are still visible in the contemporary view of the concept.

7.3 Dignity and Health

Health and dignity relate to each other [4]. In traditional health and medical care the focus has been related more to illness than to health. In a health-promoting perspective, the focus is moving toward person's health resources. This perspective is clarified both in Eriksson's caring science theory [2, 7] and in Aron Antonovsky's [27, 28] salutogenic model of health. They both acknowledge suffering and disease as part of human life but find it more valuable to focus on the strength and resources, which are imparted in each human being in order to handle challenges related to illness and life. Conceptually and historically, health means wholeness and holiness [7]. Wholeness relates to a person's unseparated being as body, soul, and spirit. Holiness refers to a person's deep awareness of her uniqueness and responsibility as a fellow human being. Both health and suffering are parts of human life, and according to Eriksson [7, 8], there is an inherent dialectic between them. As human beings, we live in this dialectical movement between health as wholeness and integration and suffering as divineness and disintegration. Antonovsky [27] also described health as movement on a continuum of ease and dis-ease. According to Antonovsky [27], we are always exposed to events in life that may be considered as stressors. This can reduce health temporarily but can also make a person stronger [28]. Sense of coherence is a key concept in Antonovsky's salutogenic model. The sense of coherence points to a person's view of life and capacity to handle stressful situations. As human beings, we have the capacity to comprehend the situation we are in as comprehensive, meaningful, and manageable, thereby strengthening our sense of coherence in life [27, 28].

Eriksson [29] defines health in her earlier writings based on an analysis of the concept: *health as soundness, freshness, and well-being*. She strongly emphasizes the subjective dimension of health and health as more than the absence of illness. This is in line with Antonovsky' model. In many situations, we are not able to promote health in the sense of soundness and freshness, but in most cases, we are able to promote well-being. This will be exemplified later in this chapter.

Eriksson [7] views health in its deepest sense as an ontological concept relating to the individual's becoming and reality. She presents an ontological health model where health is a movement between three separate levels: health as doing, being, and becoming. This movement is expressed in the person's experiences of various problems, needs, or desires. At the doing level, health is related to objective external criteria; at the being level, people strive to experience a form of harmony and balance; and at the becoming level, a person is not a stranger to suffering and strives to be whole and to reconcile herself with the given circumstances. Life is movement. Human beings live in a dialectical movement between different binary opposites such as life and death, health and suffering, and dignity and indignity. To balance these opposites is the human being's responsibility and represents his personal life struggle. The direction the movement takes depends on various circumstances. These may be related to the person himself, his relationship to others, to God, or an external power, nature, or the surrounding environment [30, 31]. Among the human being's noble traits are the ability and freedom to choose the direction for this inner movement. This inner movement is not unaffected by a person's relations and circumstances, "No man is an island." This is especially true when the person's vulnerability is acute and dignity is threatened. This may happen for humans considering themselves as healthy as well as for people in obvious need of health care. The respect and confirmation of a person's strength and health resources given by health personnel are of great importance in promoting or restoring dignity when it is threatened [32, 33].

7.4 The Meaning of Dignity from Theoretical and Empirical Research

Researchers have tried to clarify dignity through theoretical and empirical studies. Investigations of the concept of dignity and its field of meanings have represented an important step in understanding the essence of dignity.

Despite ontological and empirical differences, one shared feature is the understanding of dignity as a dualistic concept [16]. This has been described in various terms. Eriksson [6], Edlund [8], and Edlund et al. [9] refer to *absolute and relative dignity*. Absolute dignity is recognized as an inherent, inviolable, and unchangeable dimension rooted in human holiness. Absolute dignity consists of values such as responsibility, freedom, duty, and service. Relative dignity comprises a bodily, external, esthetic dimension and a physical inner ethical dimension. Relative dignity is changeable and is influenced by internal and external factors.

Other theorists use the term objective dignity [3], Menneschewürde [10], and human dignity [4] to denote absolute dignity. These different terms for this dimension of dignity are rooted in human worth and human equality [23]; common features in their descriptions of dignity are dignity as inherent, universal, unchangeable, and inviolable.

Jacobson [4] describes relative dignity as social dignity and mentions two intertwined aspects of social dignity: dignity-of-self and dignity in-relation. Dignity-of-self relates to self-respect, self-confidence, autonomy, and various forms of integrity. Dignity in-relation refers to the way in which respect and worth are conveyed back to the individual through expression and recognition. Relative dignity and social dignity may be lost, or gained, threatened, violated, or promoted. Jacobson [5] claims that any human interaction may be an encounter with dignity [5] in which dignity is either promoted or violated. Also Nordenfelt [10] and Nordenfelt and Edgar [34] address the dimensions of dignity similarly, pointing to relative and social dignity through notions such as (1) dignity as merit based on formal position and rank, (2) dignity as moral stature based on personal moral values, and (3) dignity as identity based upon personal autonomy, integrity and self-respect, and also influenced by relationships and interaction with others. Relative and/or social dignity can be violated as well as supported and promoted. Relative dignity is the subjective part of dignity, and knowledge of what values are important for the individual person will always be the basis for dignity-preserving care.

As bodily changes frequently are a threat to persons in need of health care, research underscores the connection between bodily changes and dignity. Edlund [8] and Edlund et al. [9] describe the body as the bearer of relative dignity. The body often serves as a symbol for dignity when it performs actions in accordance with the culture's rules and norms for dignity. The body may also be a potential source of violation when bodily changes make it impossible to perform what both the human being and the culture of fellow humans expect. The body enables independence and freedom, but also limitations and dependency. The body generates both pride and shame and opens for vulnerability, violation, power, and powerlessness. The body is an important part of the holistic human being, a unity that must be whole to experience dignity. Bodily changes may lead to suffering and be a violation of the person's dignity [8].

It is a question as to whether it is fruitful to maintain the division between absolute and relative dignity. Research related to dignity and bodily changes in a palliative care setting questions this division. Lorentsen et al. [14, 15] emphasize patients' and relatives' need to strive for dignity in situations where patients' bodies are falling apart because of advanced cancer disease. Through the ambiguity and paradox of the body, dignity was revealed as a life-affirming will and love as healing power [15]. The relatives' confirmation of the ambivalent or rather paradoxical body was grounded in the fundamental love for the family member and an act of responsibility, both bricks in the concept of dignity. The complexity of the body lead to the question of whether the division between absolute and relative dignity was inapplicable when understanding dignity in a bodily perspective [14]. This question needs more theoretical and empirical research.

Finally, we want to shed light on an aspect of dignity related to health personnel. Gallagher [3] explored dignity as both an "another-regarding" and a "self-regarding" value: respect for the dignity of others and respect for one's own personal and professional dignity. Respect for the dignity of others is well known and the object of much attention within health professions, while respect for one's own dignity is given less attention. Other-regarding and self-regarding values appear to be inextricably linked, and Gallagher refers to Aristotle's doctrine of the mean, which enables health personnel to reflect on the appropriate degree of respect for the dignity of others and proper respect for themselves. In encounters between patients and health care personnel in our multicultural world, there may be situations of personal and cultural nature that may be challenging, and the self-respect and self-worth of the professional may be threatened.

The meaning of dignity may be summarized theoretically, as it has been a commonly shared notion among researchers that dignity has an unchangeable dimension related to just being born. The grounds of the human inherent value may differ, from a religious version, which is grounded in a belief that human beings hold an exalted place in God's creation, where life is created and given. A secular version associated with Kant is grounded in the rationality of human beings and their ability to act as moral agents as enshrined in The Universal Declaration of Human Rights (1948) [4]. Relative dignity is harder to grasp, as the subjective part of dignity will be different according to a person's own personal values, context and culture. To give an exact definition of dignity is therefore difficult because it describes the fundamental meaning of being human [4].

7.5   Making Use of the Knowledge of Dignity and Indignity to Promote Health

In the following section, we will describe and discuss from different perspectives how we can understand and make use of the knowledge of dignity and indignity to promote health, having in mind the importance of nurturing the inner strength in old people living in nursing homes [35–37]. We will consider this matter in light of the results of a major Scandinavian study called *A life in dignity*, the main purpose of which was to explore the dignity and indignity of patients in nursing homes from the perspective of patients, family caregivers, and health personnel [31, 38, 39]. The overall study had a hermeneutical design inspired by Gadamer's philosophy [21]. Individual interviews were performed with 28 residents (17 women and 11 men between 62 and 103 years), 28 family caregivers (children and spouses) and qualitative focus group interviews with health care personnel, a total of 40 staff members with five to eight participants in every interview session. The number of group sessions varied between three and four sessions, totally 20 meetings. Twelve researchers were involved, and the study was carried out in nursing homes in Norway, Sweden, and Denmark. The data material was read and interpreted by the entire research group until consensus about the results was reached. The study followed the guidelines for good scientific practice, set by the ethics committees in the Scandinavian countries [17]. Our intention in including the following presentation is not to present the study itself, but to make use of parts of the results to illustrate both dignified and undignified care in clinical practice.

7.6   Learning from the Perspective of Health Care Personnel

In the following, we present two different pictures in which dignity is preserved.

A helper's testimonies:

Some years ago, a woman with dementia was admitted to this nursing home, and she was awfully shy and scared, sitting with her purse and looking down at the floor … her hair covered her eyes. We had no contact with her; it was quite impossible. I think we tried for two hours … and then I thought … we must try something else. So, I did something no one else had done before, I think, I lay down on the floor and crawled under the table. Then I looked up at her face and smiled at her and said, "Hey there!" And then I got this beautiful smile back! And every time after that incident, she recognized me and gave me this beautiful smile, and said to me, 'Hey there!' [40]

One of our residents has serious dementia and has no family caregivers, and he loves to watch soccer; he likes Vålerenga (a well-known soccer club in Norway). Then I thought to myself, I love soccer, but I hate Vålerenga. However, I can still watch one Vålerenga match (I thought). So, I sent an e-mail to the club and told about our resident with dementia, 82 years old … And there we went. He was dressed in a dark suit and we were seated in the VIP tribune and we were treated with this and that … but what joy we shared! This was my day off duty, but we were together, both enthusiastic, and all the glances, and all the pleasant things we shared. This is what I hope my mother and father will experience in a nursing home, things they like … This is my passion! [40]

These two narratives deal with fostering dignity and promoting health, in this case in individuals who suffer from dementia living in a nursing home. The caregivers, visualized in the stories, show a deep dedication in helping human beings who suffer. We have labeled these two narratives *dignity as distinction*, meaning individuality implying respect, listening, eye contact, vocal pitch, body posture, calmness, and friendliness. Dignity is also feeling accepted as unique and complete persons [40]. Even while attending a soccer match, we experience a deep communion between the resident and the caregiver, along with togetherness, enthusiasm, and joy. The motivation for displaying this kind of attitude is aptly stated by the caregiver: *Human beings grow when they are met with dignity* [40].

Dignity is also seen as *influence and participation* through the opportunity to participate and being able to co-determine their daily activities. Through creativity, awareness and sensitivity, the health personnel had the opportunity to enhance the residents' ability to influence their own lives [40]. Nygren et al. [35] underline the importance of inner strength in being an oldest old person. The caregivers in this present study 'lived' the inner strength for those people not having the capacity possessing this quality, that nevertheless created strength and empowered the residents [40].

Both accounts relate encounters which are dimensions of caring as an art. In an investigation Nåden and Eriksson [41] concluded that the encounter is characterized by being on the same wavelength, giving oneself over, "nakedness," and of deep solidarity and closeness. One of the most human qualities is manifested in the encounter, when the person is in contact with him or herself. The encounter can be healing, life-giving, and alleviating, and the participants are first and foremost human beings. We can read these dimensions in the narratives above; the patients' wishes and needs. As one caregiver states: *One ought to be sensitive and look at facial expressions … If one does not see the other human being, then dignity is at risk* [40]. A character in a novel by Erik F. Hansen, a well-known Norwegian author, says the following about art: *I'm over sixty and I have never found out what it [art] depends on. What is it that separates the genuine from the false, the genuine from the superficial, and what is it that makes one person an artist and another a craftsman* ([42], p. 229).

For something to be called an art and not just a craft, it must be linked and connected to a foundational idea. In music it is called *cantus firmus*, the fundamental melody, which has its origin in Renaissance polyphony. In the same manner, caring and nursing become an art performance that will preserve the individual's dignity in both patients and health personnel [41]. There is an inherent obviousness in the turn to the other, where a deep ethical attitude is evident in the caregiver. It is an example of what Eriksson [2, 43] terms the mantra of caring ethics: I was there, I saw, I witnessed, and I became responsible. It is also in line with Levinas' thoughts [44–46] when he writes about the ethics of the face, becoming responsible for the other.

Levinas writes about human responsibility and freedom in context, claiming that *"I am called to a responsibility that was never contracted, inscribed on the other's face. Nothing is more passive than this accusation that precedes any freedom."* ([45], p. 100). According to Levinas [45] the ability to be affected by the vulnerability and suffering of others is a prerequisite for man to assume the responsibility that is given to us and already is there. The caregivers in the stories above possess this ability to be touched, which is why we can speak of a natural inherent obviousness in the turn to the other. Likewise, this demonstrates the very importance of Levinas' thinking in understanding the given responsibility for the other, in our case, the patients, where the caregivers lift the other so that the other can preserve his or her dignity, and experience health as becoming [2]. This is in line with the patients' wishes in Bylund-Grenklo [47] research in a palliative care context where a dignified life was about having their human value maintained by others through "coherence." Levinas emphasizes the perfection of artistic creation, the ultimate moment when the last brushstroke is made, when not a single word can be added to or subtracted from the text [45]. In light of these words, we can see the perfection of the art performance in our context, when the face and the beautiful smile were perceived by the old lady with dementia. Everything that could and should be done was done; nothing less and nothing more was needed. The last brushstroke was done with the two words: hey there! Levinas [45] claims that the artist stops because the work refuses to receive more. The artist in this narrative from clinical practice knew that at this moment, the work that these two people created together was complete. From the stories and our interpretations, we can understand, more deeply and more thoroughly, what dignity is about.

7.7 Learning from the Perspective of Family Caregivers

Brief stories from family caregivers show what dignity is for their loved one and for themselves: *Just after a short while, my mother went to concerts, bingo, church ceremonies, hobby days, digital book days and reading-aloud days. She participated in everything that was going on. She became a new human being, became healthier. Now she appreciates life* ([48], p. 513). This is consistent with Nygren et al.'s [35] research stating that *inner strength opens up the possibility of acceptance of new realities. Feeling that one is the same person even though circumstances have changed gives a feeling of stability.*

The spirit in which care is given influences the way patients and their relatives see the little extra and helps to promote the dignity of patients and thus their health: *There are some of them who do the little extra – making an omelet or doing some decoration, food and drinks, something a little extra* ([48], p. 513).

An expression of the staff's attitude from the perspective of the family caregivers reveals what it means when the patient is *really seen* as an individual with dignity. A commitment from the caregiver to look for common interests with the resident can be interpreted as creating a communion or a caring relationship [48].

Dignity as "at-home-ness" is also important for the family caregivers: *I felt warm right away, as soon as she came here, she had a value.* Another statement: *In my experience of older persons, it is more important that they feel safe than to be in a fancy surrounding, that they are cared for! When they get to a stage in life when they no longer can take care of themselves, they really have enough just trying to care for themselves* ([48], p. 512).

Family caregivers also experience situations that are the opposite of at-home-ness. They experienced situations where their dear ones became abandoned. Being deprived of dignity through physical humiliation is one kind of abandonment. One family caregiver describes feeding situations that verge on violations of law and the use of physical force [17]. In addition to hurting the residents, the caring situations were non-esthetic:

I have seen such terrible feeding situations. Totally insensitive and soulless feedings where one sits and continuously spoons food into the residents' mouths. And I, who am sitting alongside, notice that the poor human being has not swallowed any of what they just popped in his mouth. After the last ten spoonfuls, the food comes out again. The health personnel can sit and shovel food into someone at the same time as they are talking to other persons in the room or are talking on their cell phone. It makes me feel terribly sorry for the patient. This behavior is not dignified care. As a matter of fact, it has upset me very often ([17], p. 756).

From the perspective of the caregivers, one can understand the abandonment in both concrete and existential ways. In the concrete way, the residents are left alone. In the existential way, they are not met and seen when they most need it, as presented in this feeding situation [17].

To be abandoned touches deeply human sensitivities since human beings are dependent on each other. To be deprived of togetherness with other human beings or with an abstract other can abandon the individual to loneliness and despair. This experience may be perceived even worse when the individual is old, has a physical or psychological disability, or has dementia. As Nåden et al. [17] (p. 757) express: *It is especially depressing when violation occurs in a professional context where personnel are meant to care for the individual in an appropriate manner. Nursing home residences are built for individuals to let them live the last years of their lives in safe surroundings and get health care from personnel with high caring ideals as their compasses.*

The relatives also stressed the importance of the specific caregiver. Some staff members are just there for the job and are perhaps not interested in providing the little extra. If the "wrong" person gives care, the resident can be ignored. As one of the relatives noted, doing the little extra is when the residents are really seen by caregivers who are suited for their jobs and can see *the beauty in the faces of the older persons* ([48], p. 513). Levinas argues that the other's face does not expose the arbitrariness of the will, but its injustice. *Nor does the evidence of my injustice appear when I bow to facts, but when I bow to the Other* ([45], p. 53) he points out.

In this light, we can clearly see the degrading feeding situation in the above narrative. The helpers who are meant to bow to the other—in this case, those who are supposed to provide care for the persons in need, supporting them in building up their inner strength—instead turn away from them. They are prevented from seeing the other because they do not approach them. It is when approaching the other that the other's face appears to me, according to Levinas ([45], p. 53) not as a threat or an obstacle, but as something that is of importance to me.

The helpers refuse to be "the chosen ones," as Levinas [45] (p. 158), talks about. In this case this means that it is the other, the patient, that chooses me, not the opposite. To be struck by the other's face does not mean that I am set free for self-expression. On the contrary, it means that I am linked to the responsibility. The family caregivers highly value this form for responsibility from the helpers taking care of their dear ones [48].

7.8 Learning from the Perspective of Patients

What seemed to be common to almost all the residents at the nursing homes was the fact that moving into the nursing home was experienced as a threat to their dignity. The threat was related to the perception that they were becoming dependent on others, that there was a lack of time and resources on the unit, and that they were being deprived of freedom, but it was also related to the attitudes of health care personnel [49]. We present narratives of both indignity and preserved dignity.

The residents related humiliating situations in which the health care personnel were rude, impolite, and paternalistic: *Three times they have told me that they are not my slaves when I asked for help – two times when I asked for help with my ostomy, and once when I asked them if they could help me fold up my quilt. And they asked, 'Do you think this is a hotel?'* ([49], p. 44).

> I think to myself that I should be a free man, but I'm not free. If I get dressed and want to go out, I'm not allowed to go out. "You have to stay inside", they say. They say that if I want to go out, I need to have someone with me, or I can't go. That's how it is. They think I'm too weak. And I can agree that I was weak when I moved into that other place. But there is never a damned soul to take me out. Never! ([49], p. 44).

Freedom is closely linked with dignity. Freedom means that a person is free to do and use the inner strength to act or to decide for himself or herself, as well as freedom from something, such as force or paternalism. To possess autonomy implies that you construct for yourself the laws you are to follow [50]. The resident above states that he has no freedom, which is the opposite of what he had imagined. The loss of freedom can feel like a double loss for this man in that no helpers can follow him out. In this sense, the loss of physical freedom will also have consequences for the person's inner freedom. Heggestad et al. [51] found that several patients in the nursing home felt they were in captivity, like a prison without bars. In the stories above, we also experience inappropriate language from the caregivers. Rudeness, impoliteness, and paternalistic attitudes described by the residents demonstrate the asymmetric relationship between the residents and the caregivers [49]. This might be construed as abuse of power. Rundquist [52] states that power belongs to all human beings and is thus ontological—a matter of human nature. The author further states that power is given to human beings only as authority. The authoritative human being takes responsibility for his/her human office, but abandoning it means abandoning oneself and one's dignity.

The humiliating situations above are examples of misuse of power by the caregivers, a power that is not given to them by the patients in need of help. It is the opposite of ontological power that is rooted in intuitive and esthetic knowledge [53] and which does not turn the patient into a victim. Knowledge of ontological power can be linked to and is consistent with Watson's [54] statement that care necessitates a moral obligation to protect human dignity.

In line with Watson [54], Pieranunzi [53], and Rundqvist [52], Foss et al. [55] elaborate on responsibility and leadership, positing the other as the real leader. When transferred to a clinical context, the patient becomes the real leader and guiding star. This is in sharp contrast to the story told by the patient above who was deprived of his freedom, and it contrasts with the humiliation related by the family caregiver earlier in this chapter.

On the positive side, one resident explains the meaning of still being able to participate in an activity she had been part of earlier in her life: *I like to dance. I have danced for 20 years. I dance once a week, and the bus comes and picks me up. I am the only one from the nursing home. However, the nursing home organizes dancing in the afternoon for everyone. I think it's great that they arrange that, because I like it so much* ([56], p. 95). The resident feels respected and valued, when the nursing home recognized her resources and inner strength and made it possible to participate in an activity that had been a part of her previous social life and which attracted attention from others in her current life.

Two other residents are positive about their situations:

> *I'll need help to take a shower. But it is ok to be helped by others. Once a young man had to assist me. I was a little concerned about that, but when he helped me, I thought it was fine and the other ladies also liked to be assisted by him* ([56], p. 95).

> Another lady tells *I love being helped. It is not degrading. No, I am not ashamed of it. It's okay. So, I feel mostly like a baby (laughs)* ([56], p. 95).

Most residents regarded asking for help as a potential threat, and growing dependency was one of the harder adjustments they faced. Residents described these experiences in different ways. Some felt that they had been robbed of their freedom, whereas others felt valued as persons and found that the help they received improved their quality of life. In order to retain their dignity, it seemed significant to be able to make sense of the unavoidable circumstances in their lives and remain positive [56].

The quality of these meetings is of the utmost importance for those who need help to maintain their dignity. In some ways, an encounter entails going into deep water. The apprehension associated with an encounter can be altered and transformed into something greater: honesty and authenticity. On the wavelength that the encounter occurs, the person is in contact with both the self and the other. This is the profoundest level of health, where the germ and opportunity for growth are found [41]. In such a description of the encounter, the caregiver has found his place, where the potential for growth is present for both parties. In situations like this, a great responsibility is shown toward the patients. Eriksson [43] refers to Hellqvist who claims that responsibility also means a "solemn declaration." It is through a solemn declaration that we can convey the message of love that we truly desire the well-being of others. It is an assurance of the other's dignity.

7.9 Public Policy Efforts to Preserve Human Dignity

Preserving patients' dignity is not only a responsibility of the health care professional, the family, and the patient himself. It is a political responsibility. In this short section, we briefly summarize laws and regulations in the Scandinavian countries and the UK for which the aim is to preserve human dignity.

In 2011 a new national value system was implemented in the Social Services Act (2001) in Sweden [57], stipulating that elderly care shall promote a dignified life and the feeling of well-being. Local dignity guarantees are based on the national set of values for older people stipulated in the Social Services Act, which means that care of elderly people provided by social services has to focus on older people being able to live their lives in dignity and feel a sense of well-being. Similarly, The Patients' Right Act in Norway from 1999 [58] states that the provisions of the act shall help to promote a relationship of trust between the patient and the health service and safeguard respect for the life, integrity, and human dignity of each patient. In 2011, the regulation relating to "Dignity Guarantee" in elderly care entered into force in Norway [59]. The regulation aims to ensure that the care of older people is carried out in such a way that it contributes to a dignified, safe, and meaningful retirement. In 2019 Health Care Denmark presented a new white paper called "A dignified elderly care in Denmark." [60] It is stated in the foreword of this white paper that Denmark is to have a dignified elderly care system with focus on involving and empowering every citizen and an emphasis on their individual needs and preferences.

In the Health and Social Care Act (2008), United Kingdom, Regulation 2014 [61] states that service users must be treated with dignity and respect. It includes ensuring the privacy of the service user, supporting the autonomy, independence, and involvement in the community of the service user, and has any relevant protected characteristics of the Equality Act of the service user. Staff must always treat service users with dignity and respect, which means treating them in caring and compassionate ways. They must be respectful when communicating with service users, using the most suitable means of communication and respecting a person's right to engage or not to engage in their communication.

Documents like those mentioned above may contribute to a change in health care services culture in general and in nursing homes in particular, where the focus of care is on the person, not the task, as Robinson and Gallagher [62] underline, and likewise protect patients exposed to unethical acts, so that they can regain a kind of pride and dignity [63, 64]. To make a change, leaders have a crucial role to play in the promotion of dignity in care.

It is interesting to note that there is a need to enact laws and regulations on something as basic as respect for human dignity. The legislation in the examples above show the importance of supporting dignity in care, but in some of the texts of these regulations, there seems to be a lack of clarity about the meaning of the concept of dignity. A consequence of this might be that it is up to the individual reader of the text and the health personnel to understand the concept of dignity.

7.10   Conclusion

Even though there is a shared feature that dignity is important in people's life and being, and because the fact that dignity is used in political and professional settings, the meanings of dignity are seldom described. Therefore, the purpose of this chapter was to illuminate different understandings of the concept of dignity and to discuss how we can make use of this knowledge to promote and enhance human health and well-being.

Researchers have tried to clarify the concept through theoretical and empirical work. Some of these theories are presented. The theories show that there is a shared feature that dignity is a dualistic concept. One dimension is recognized as inherent dignity, which is unchangeable and rooted in human worth and equality. The other dimension is related to the subjective part of being human and dependent of a person's value system, context, and culture. This dimension can be violated as well as promoted. Hence, any human interaction may be an encounter with dignity and thereby a health promoting interaction.

Dignity is a core concept in caring, and health personnel need knowledge of the meaning of dignity in health care. There is a need of both theoretical knowledge and empirical knowledge visualized through narratives about the art of caring. In the second part of this chapter, we present testimonies from health care personnel, family caregivers, and patients. Reflections about the encounters between patients and caregivers together with knowledge about dignity may be one way to make use of the developed knowledge and the possibilities imparted in the concept of dignity in order to promote health. Both political leaders and leaders within health care have a crucial role in facilitating health care that preserves person's dignity.

Take Home Messages
- Dignity is a person's ability to constitute life and being.
- Dignity is a dualistic concept. Dignity consists of an *inherent and absolute dignity* which is universal, unchangeable, and inviolable and a *relative dignity* which is changeable and influenced by internal and external factors.
- Each human interaction may be an encounter where dignity is either promoted or violated.
- It is important to promote the inner strength of the other person to support her or him to live a life in dignity.
- Acknowledgment of and responsibility for the other person is part of performing the art of nursing care.
- Dignity is an essential foundation for promoting health and well-being.

References

1. Eriksson K. Vårdvetenskap som disciplin, forskningsområde och tillämpningsområde (Caring Science as discipline, research area and practice). Vasa: Åbo Akademi University; 1988.
2. Eriksson K. Vårdvetenskap. Vetenskap om vårdandet. Om det tidlösa i tiden. (Caring science. The science of caring. About the timeless time). Stockholm: Liber; 2018.
3. Gallagher A. Dignity and respect for dignity—two key health professional values: implications for nursing practice. Nurs Ethics. 2004;11(6):587–99.
4. Jacobson. N. Dignity and health: a review. Soc Sci Med. 2007;64:292–302.
5. Jacobson N. Dignity violation in health care. Qual Health Res. 2009;19(11):1536–47.
6. Eriksson K. Om människans värdighet (On human dignity). In: Bjerkreim T, Mathisen J, Nord R, editors. Visjon, viten og virke (Vision, knowledge and profession). Oslo: Universitetsforlaget; 1996.
7. Eriksson K. The suffering human being. Chicago: Nordic Studies Press; 2006.
8. Edlund M. Människans värdighet – ett grundbegrepp innom vårdvetenskap (Human dignity—a basic caring science concept). (Dissertation). Åbo: Åbo Akademi University Press; 2002.
9. Edlund M, Lindwall L, Von Post I, Eriksson K. Concept determination of human dignity. Nurs Ethics. 2013;20(8):851–60.
10. Nordenfelt L. The varieties of dignity. Health Care Anal. 2004;12(2):69–81.
11. Martinsen K. Care and vulnerability. Oslo: Akribe AS; 2006.
12. Martinsen K. Løgstrup og sykepleien (Løgstrup and nursing). Oslo: Akribe AS; 2012.
13. Malterud K, Solvang P. Vulnerability as a strenght: why, when, and how? Scand J Public Health. 2005;33(Suppl 66):3–6.
14. Lorentsen VB, Nåden D, Sæteren B. The paradoxical body: a glimpse of a deeper truth through relatives' stories. Nurs Ethics. 2018;26(6):1611–22. https://doi.org/10.1177/09697330118768660.
15. Lorentsen VB, Nåden D, Sæteren B. The meaning of dignity when the patients' bodies are falling apart. Nurs Open. 2019;2019.6(1):1163–70.
16. Tranvåg O, McSherry W. Understanding dignity: a complex concept of the heart of healthcare. In: Tranvåg O, Synnes O, McSherry W, editors. Stories of dignity within healthcare. Research, narratives and theories. Stuart, FL: GB, M&K Publishing; 2016.
17. Nåden D, Rehnsfeldt A, Råholm MB, Lindwall L, Caspari S, Aasgaard T, Slettebø Å, Sæteren B, Høy B, Lillestø B, Heggestad AK, Lohne V. Aspects of indignity in nursing home residences as experienced by family caregivers. Nurs Ethics. 2013;20(7):748–61. https://doi.org/10.1177/0969733012475253.
18. Buchanan DR. Promoting dignity: the ethical dimension of health. Policy Theor Soc Iss. 2016;36(2):99–104. https://doi.org/10.1177/0272684X16630885.
19. Rannestad T, Haugan G. Helsefremming i kommunehelsetjenesten (Health promotion in municipal health). In: Haugan G, Rannestad T, editors. Health promotion in municipal health. Oslo: Cappelen Damm Akademisk AS; 2014.
20. Eriksson K. Vårdandes idè (The idea of caring). Stockholm: Almqvist & Wiksell; 1987.
21. Gadamer HG. Truth and method. London: Sheed & Ward Ltd and the Continuum Publishing Group; 1989.
22. Sensen O. Human dignity in historical perspective: the contemporary and traditional paradigms. Eur J Polit Theor. 2011;10(1):71–91. https://doi.org/10.1177/1474885110386006.
23. United Nations. Universal declaration of human rights. Now York: UN; 2015. p. 1948.
24. ICN. The ICN code of ethics for nurses; 2012.
25. Pico GM. Oratio. In: Frost T, editor. Giovanni Pico della Mirandola. Lovprisning av menneskets verdighet. Om det værende og det ene (Praise og man's dignity). Latvia: Vidarforlaget; 2013.
26. Kaldestad K. Menneskets verdighet i kraft av det hellige rommet (Human dignity in virtue of the sacred space). (Dissertation). Finland: Åbo Akademi University Press; 2018.
27. Antonovsky A. Hälsans mysterium (Unraveling the mystery of health). Stockholm: Bokförlaget Natur och Kultur; 2009.
28. Eriksson M. The sense of coherence in the salutogenic model of health. In: Mittelmart MB, et al., editors. The handbook of Salutogenesis; 2017. https://doi.org/10.1007/978.3-319-04600-6_11.
29. Eriksson K. Hälsans idè (The idea of health). Stockholm: Almqvist & Wiksell; 1984.
30. Sæteren B, Lindström UÅ, Nåden D. Latching onto life: living in the area of tension between the possibility of life and the necessity of death. J Clin Nurs. 2010;20:811–8. https://doi.org/10.1111/j.1365-2702.2010.03212.x.
31. Sæteren B, Heggestad AK, Høy B, Lillestø B, Slettebø Å, Lohne V, Råholm MB, Caspari S, Rehnsfeldt A, Lindwall L, Aasgaard T, Nåden D. The dialectical movement between deprivation and preservation of a person's life space. A question of nursing home residents' dignity. Holist Nurs Pract. 2016;6(30):139–47.
32. Sæteren B. Kampen for livet I vemodets slør (Struggling for life in the veil of pensiveness). (Dissertation). Finland: Åbo Akademi University Press; 2006.
33. Sæteren B, Lindström UÅ, Nåden D. I still have so much to do – struggling for life when time is limited. Int J Hum Caring. 2015;19(1):57–62.
34. Nordenfelt L, Edgar A. The four notions of dignity. Qual Ageing. 2005;6(1):17–21.
35. Nygren B, Norberg A, Lundman B. Inner strength as disclosed in narratives of the oldest old. Qual Health Res. 2017;17(8):1060–73.
36. Lundman B, Alex L, Jonsen E, Løvheim H, Nygren B, Fischer RS, Strandberg G, Norberg A. Inner strength in relation to functional status, disease, living arrangements, and social relationships among people aged 85 years and older. Geriatr Nurs. 2012;33(3):167–76.

37. Franklin L-L, Ternestedt B-M, Nordenfelt L. Views on dignity of elderly nursing home residents. Nurs Ethics. 2006;13(8):130–46. https://doi.org/10.1191/0 969733006ne851oa.

38. Nåden D. A life in dignity. International innovation. Disseminating science, research and technology. EuroFocus: Health. 2013;2013:32–4.

39. Lindwall L, Råholm MB, Lohne V, Caspari S, Heggestad AK, Sæteren B, Slettebø Å, Høy B, Nåden D. Clinical application research through reflection, interpretation and new understanding—a hermeneutic design. Scand J Caring Sci. 2018;32:1152–67.

40. Lohne V, Høy B, Lillestø B, Sæteren B, Heggestad AKT, Aasgaard T, Caspari S, Rehnsfeldt A, Råholm MB, Slettebø Å, Lindwall L, Nåden D. Fostering dignity in the care of nursing home residents through slow caring. Nurs Ethics. 2016;24(7):778–88. Accessed 10 Feb 2020. https://doi.org/10.1177/0969733015627297.

41. Nåden D, Eriksson K. Encounter: a fundamental category of nursing as an art. Int J Hum Caring. 2002;6(1):34–9.

42. Hansen EF. Psalm at journey's end (J. Tate, Trans.). London: Secher & Warburg; 1997. Original work published 1990.

43. Eriksson K. Jag var där, jag såg, jag vittnade och jag blev ansvarig—den vårdande etikens mantra (I was there, I saw, I witnessed, and I became responsible—the mantra of caring ethics). In: Alvsvåg H, Bergland Å, Førland O, editors. Nødvendige omveier. En vitenskapelig antologi til Kari Martinsens 70-års dag. (Necessary detours. A scientific anthology to Kari Martinsen's 70 years anniversary). Oslo: Cappelen Damm Akademisk; 2013.

44. Kemp P. Emmanuel Lévinas. En introduktion (Emmauel Levinas. An introduction). Gothenburg: Daidalos; 1992.

45. Aarnes A. Emmanuel Levinas. Underveis mot den annen (Along the way towards the other). Essays av og om Levinas ved Asbjørn Aarnes. Oslo: Vidarforlaget A/S; 1998.

46. Levinas E. Den Annens Humanisme (The Humanism of the Other). Original title: Humanisme de l'autre homme (1972). Trondheim: Det Norske Akademi for Sprog og Litteratur; 2004.

47. Bylund-Grenklo T, Werkander-Harstäde V, Sandgren A, Benzein E, Östlund U. Int J Palliat Nurs. 2019;25(4):193–201.

48. Rehnsfeldt A, Lindwall L, Lohne V, Lillestø B, Slettebø Å, Heggestad AKT, Aasgaard T, Råholm MB, Caspari S, Høy B, Sæteren B, Nåden D. The meaning of dignity in nursing home care as seen by relatives. Nurs Ethics. 21(5):507–17.

49. Heggestad AKT, Høy B, Sæteren B, Slettebø Å, Lillestø B, Rehnsfeldt A, Lindwall L, Lohne V, Råholm M-B, Aasgaard T, Caspari S, Nåden D. Dignity, dependence, and relational autonomy for older people living in nursing homes. Int J Hum Caring. 2015;19(3):42–6.

50. Caspari S, Råholm M-B, Sæteren B, Rehnsfeldt A, Lillestø B, Lohne V, Slettebø Å, Heggestad AKT, Høy B, Lindwall L, Nåden D. Tension between freedom and dependence—a challenge for residents who live in nursing homes. J Clin Nurs. 2018;27:4119–27.

51. Heggestad AKT, Nortvedt P, Slettebø Å. 'Like a prison without bars': dementia and experiences of dignity. Nurs Ethics. 2013;20(8):881–92.

52. Rundqvist E. Makt som fullmakt. Et vårdvetenskapligt perspektiv (Power as authority. A caring science perspective). (Dissertation). Åbo, Finland: Åbo Akademi University Press; 2004.

53. Pieranunzi VR. The lived experience of power and powerlessness in psychiatric nursing: a Heideggerian hermeneutical analysis. Arch Psychiatr Nurs. 1997;XI(3):155–62.

54. Watson J. Nursing: human science and human care. A theory of nursing. New York: National League for Nursing Press; 1988.

55. Foss B, Nåden D, Eriksson K. Experience of events of truth in hermeneutic conversation with text: ethics and ontology. Nurs Sci Q. 2016;29(4):299–307.

56. Høy B, Lillestø B, Slettebø Å, Sæteren B, Heggestad AKT, Caspari S, Aasgaard T, Lohne V, Rehnsfeldt A, Råholm M-B, Lindwall L, Nåden D. Maintaining dignity in vulnerability: a qualitative study of the residents' perspective in nursing homes. Int J Nurs Stud. 2016;60:91–8.

57. Ministry of Health and Social Affairs, Sweden. The Social Services Act. 2001. https://ec.europa.eu/anti-trafficking/sites/antitrafficking/files/social_services_act_sweden_en_1.pdf. Accessed 1 Feb 2020.

58. The Norwegian Government. The Patients' Rights Act. 1999. https://app.uio.no/ub/ujur/oversatte-lover/data/lov-19990702-063-eng.pdf. Accessed 1 Feb 2020.

59. Ministry of Health and Care Services. Forskrift om en verdig eldreomsorg (The dignity guarantee regulation). 2011. https://lovdata.no/dokument/SF/forskrift/2010-11-12-1426?q=Verdighetsgarantien. Accessed 1 Feb 2020.

60. A dignified elderly care in Denmark. White Paper. Health Care Denmark. https://www.healthcaredenmark.dk/news/new-white-paper-a-dignified-elderly-care-in-denmark/. Accessed 2 Feb, 2019. 2020.

61. Regulation 10 of the Health and Social Care Act 2008, United Kingdom, Regulation 2014. https://app.croneri.co.uk/care-standards/cqc-fundamental-standards-england/regulation-10-dignity-and-respect. Accessed 17 Feb 2020.

62. Robinson GE, Gallagher A. Culture change impacts quality of life for nursing home residents. Top Clin Nutr. 2008;23(2):264–72.

63. Heijkenskjöld KB, Ekstedt M, Lindwall L. The patients' dignity from the nurses' perspective. Nurs Ethics. 2010;17(3):301–11.

64. Hall EOC, Høy B. Re-establishing dignity: nurses' experiences of caring for older hospital patients. Scand J Caring Sci. 2012;26:287–94.

Meaning-in-Life: A Vital Salutogenic Resource for Health

8

Gørill Haugan and Jessie Dezutter

Abstract

Based on evidence and theory, we state that facilitating and supporting people's meaning-making processes are health promoting. Hence, meaning-in-life is a salutogenic concept.

Authors from various disciplines such as nursing, medicine, psychology, philosophy, religion, and arts argue that the human search for meaning is a primary force in life and one of the most fundamental challenges an individual faces. Research demonstrates that meaning is of great importance for mental as well as physical well-being and crucial for health and quality of life. Studies have shown significant correlations between meaning-in-life and physical health measured by lower mortality for all causes of death; meaning is correlated with less cardiovascular disease,
less hypertension, better immune function, less depression, and better coping and recovery from illness. Studies have shown that cancer patients who experience a high degree of meaning have a greater ability to tolerate bodily ailments than those who do not find meaning-in-life. Those who, despite pain and fatigue, experience meaning report better quality-of-life than those with low meaning. Hence, if the individual finds meaning despite illness, ailments, and imminent death, well-being, health, and quality-of-life will increase in the current situation. However, when affected by illness and reduced functionality, finding meaning-in-life might prove more difficult. A will to search for meaning is required, as well as health professionals who help patients and their families not only to cope with illness and suffering but also to find meaning amid these experiences. Accordingly, meaning-in-life is considered a vital salutogenic resource and concept.

The psychiatrist Viktor Emil Frankl's theory of "Will to Meaning" forms the basis for modern health science research on meaning; Frankl's premise was that man has enough to live by, but too little to live for. According to Frankl, logotherapy ventures into the spiritual dimension of human life. The Greek word "logos" means not only meaning but also spirit. However, Frankl highlighted that in a logotherapeutic context, spirituality is not pri-

G. Haugan (✉)
Department of Public Health and Nursing, NTNU Norwegian University of Science and Technology, Trondheim, Norway

Faculty of Nursing and Health Science, Nord University, Levanger, Norway
e-mail: gorill.haugan@ntnu.no, gorill.haugan@nord.no

J. Dezutter
Meaning Research in Late Life Lab, Faculty of Psychology and Educational Sciences, KU Leuven, Leuven, Belgium
e-mail: jessie.dezutter@kuleuven.be

G. Haugan, M. Eriksson (eds.), *Health Promotion in Health Care – Vital Theories and Research*, https://doi.org/10.1007/978-3-030-63135-2_8

marily about religiosity—although religiosity can be a part of it—but refers to a specific human dimension that makes us human. Frankl based his theory on three concepts: meaning, freedom to choose and suffering, stating that the latter has no point. People should not look for an inherent meaning in the negative events happening to them, or in their suffering, because the meaning is not there. The meaning is in the attitude people choose while suffering from illness, crises, etc.

Keywords

Freedom to choose · Health · Human values Meaning-in-life · Meaning-making · Spiritual care · Spirituality · Suffering · Well-being Will to meaning

8.1 Meaning-in-Life: A Multi-Layered Concept

The experience of meaning is central to humans [1–3] and has become one of the core facets of the positive psychology movement [3] as well as of the health promotion field. In general, meaning has been found to be a strong individual predictor of life satisfaction [4–6] and an important psychological variable that promotes well-being [7–9] and protects individuals from negative outcomes [10, 11]. Meaning seems to serve as a mediating variable in psychological health [12–16].

In literature there is a distinction between (1) meaning-of-life and (2) meaning-in-life. The first concept pertains to the question of the significance of human existence in general. This question is discussed by a range of existential philosophers, such as Soren Kierkegaard, Albert Camus, and Friedrich Nietzsche, who wanted to explore whether and how the existence of human beings has meaning over time. The second concept refers to the individual's perceived meaning-in-life; the question is no longer focused on the more abstract and general meaning of human life but is scaled down to the question whether you experience your own individual life as meaning-

ful. This topic is more recently a focus of interest of psychologists, nurses, and health practitioners receiving increasing attention in the health literature. However, meaning-in-life is a subjective and personal phenomenon that is difficult to define.

One of the prominent scholars in the field of meaning is *psychiatrist Victor Emil Frankl*. Although he mainly refers to purpose-in-life (PIL) and not to meaning-in-life, his description of these concepts clearly overlaps. Purpose-in-life as a concept originates from Frankl's writings about the "will to meaning" as the primary motivational force for survival; he stated that meaning is a motivational and vitalizing force in humans' lives [17–19]. To find personal meaning involves understanding the nature of one's life, and to feel that life is significant, important, worthwhile, or purposeful (ibid.). In Frankl's theory, meaning is a broad construct that is conceptually and empirically related to many domains; positive associations of meaning are found in relation to constructs such as hope, faith, subjective well-being, and happiness, as well as negative associations between meaning and depression, anxiety, psychological distress, boredom, proneness, and drug/alcohol use [3, 9, 20, 21]. Frankl's theory of meaning termed logotherapy has been used as a basis for research and practice in many fields, including medicine, psychology, counseling, education, ministry, and nursing [22].

The concept of meaningfulness is also crucial in the salutogenic health theory of the *sociologist Aaron Antonovsky*, which is termed salutogenesis [23, 24]. In this model, he focused on health-promoting resources, among which sense of coherence (SOC) is a vital salutogenic resource in people's lives. Antonovsky defines SOC as a global orientation to perceive the world as comprehensible, manageable, and meaningful despite the stressful situations one encounters. Individuals with a strong SOC tend to perceive life as being manageable and believe that stressors are explicable. People with a strong SOC have confidence in their coping capacities [25]. Several studies link SOC with patient-reported and clinical outcomes such as perceived stress and coping [26], recovery from depression [25], physical and mental well-being [27], satisfying quality-of-life (QoL), and reduced mortality [28, 29]. SOC has thus been recognized as a meaningful concept for patients with different medical conditions.

Meaning-in-life is furthermore a vital aspect in the work of the *existential psychotherapist Irvin Yalom* [30]. According to Yalom, all individuals experience core anxieties or existential concerns related to their existence. He focuses on four main concerns: (1) the inevitability of death, (2) the freedom to shape our own lives, (3) our ultimate aloneness, and (4) the absence of any obvious meaning-in-life. For Yalom, meaninglessness is an existential given and cannot be solved. An individual's sudden realization of meaninglessness can be compared with an experience of total groundlessness. Yalom assumes that meaninglessness is present in everybody's life as well as in every therapy. More recently, meaning-in-life has become a topic of interest for empirical psychologists. The abstract nature of this concept, however, makes a clear conceptualization difficult, and the concept has therefore been defined in myriad ways. Steger [31], one of the leading scholars in this field, stated that people experience meaning when they comprehend who they are, what the world is like, and if they understand their unique fit in the world. Meaning is also described as an individual's sense that his/her life has value, direction and purpose, and that he/she belongs to something greater than the self, adding a sense of "belonging" [32]. In a cognitive perspective, meaning is described as a "mental representation of possible relations among things, events and relationships" [33] (p. 15), while others highlight the intuitive feeling that things make sense [34]. Some researchers have tried to disentangle meaning-in-life from purpose-in-life [35], whereas others defined purpose as part of meaning-in-life [36] or stressed that having goals or life aims are central aspects of meaning-in-life [37].

Although a comprehensive, unified framework of meaning is lacking, Martela and Steger [38] recently proposed a first theoretical step toward integrating the main aspects of meaning;

they delineate three components within the construct which capture much of the variance in the past definitions, namely (1) coherence, (2) purpose, and (3) significance (tripartite view) [38]. Looking at these components, the connection to the salutogenic health theory emphasizing comprehensibility, manageability, and meaningfulness seems clear. (1) Coherence refers to a cognitive aspect that one's life makes sense; it reflects a sense of comprehensibility in life and is situated in the domain of "understanding" [38]. (2) Purpose refers to a motivational aspect indicating that individuals have future-oriented long-term goals and feel that their lives have direction [17]. Purpose reflects the pursuit and attainment of core aims, ultimate life goals and aspirations for life [36]. (3) Significance refers to "the degree to which individuals feel that their existence is of significance and value" [39] (p. 2); that is a feeling of "existential mattering," having a life worth living. Although this tripartite view on meaning-in-life is promising in providing in-depth insight into the phenomenon of meaning in people's lives, research validating this structure of meaning is virtually absent (see George & Park, 2016 for one available study in a population of psychology students).

Since Frankl's theory of the "Will to Meaning" has been used as a basis for research and practice in many fields, including medicine, psychology, counseling, education, ministry, and nursing [22], in the next section this chapter presents Frankl's logotherapy.

8.2 Frankl's Theory: The "Will to Meaning"

Viktor Emil Frankl, psychiatrist and survivor of the Nazi concentration camps, assumed that meaning is of crucial importance to men. Based on the horror Frankl experienced in the camps, he concluded that everything can be taken away from men, from belongings and health to loved ones, but nobody can take away men's will to experience meaning. Frankl [17] described the process of "will to meaning" as a search process. He defined searching for meaning as "the primary motivational force in man" (p. 121), and a natural, healthy part of life.

Although Frankl developed his theory in the field of mental health and psychiatric diseases, the scope has been expanded and the theory is now considered relevant also to people who, for various reasons, struggle with everyday stress, disasters, losses, and crises. Today, this theory is applied not only on the individual level but also on the group level. During Frankl's working life in Europe, a set of concepts and the connection between them were referred to as a "school" and not as a theory, as we do today. As a professor of psychiatry and neurology, Frankl studied the "first Viennese school" in psychotherapy known as "The Will to Pleasure" exposed by Freud. Later, Adler developed the "second Viennese school" "The Will to Power." Frankl [19] recognized both schools, but still he believed that

> man can no longer be seen as a being whose basic concern is to satisfy drives and gratify instincts or, for that matter, to reconcile id, ego and superego; nor can the human reality be understood merely as the outcome of conditioning processes or conditioned reflexes. Here man is revealed as a being in search of meaning–a search whose futility seems to account for many of the ills of our age. (p. 17)

Thus, Frankl called his theory "The Will to Meaning," which became known as the "third Viennese school." The term "meaning" used in modern health science originates from Frankl's theory of will to meaning as the strongest driver of mental and physical survival. Experience of meaning represents a vitalization in everyday life [19], a primary force that involves understanding who one is, feeling important and valuable to oneself and others, and finding meaningful goals and purposes in one's life. In Frankl's theory, meaning is a broad concept that is theoretically and empirically related to several different dimensions; studies have shown that meaning is positively related to concepts such as hope, belief, well-being, happiness, and global QoL, while meaning is negatively related to depression, anxiety, psychological stress, boredom, and substance abuse [3, 9, 20, 21].

Frankl's logotherapy has its roots in a phenomenological understanding of human beings with existential needs, consciousness, and values [87]. Through experience from several years in Hitler's concentration camps and his many years of work as a psychoanalyst, Frankl had the following starting point for his theory: "people have enough to live by, but not enough to live for." Therefore, the individual does not tolerate stress. The key to coping with adversity and suffering lies in the fact that the individual finds meaning-in-life, day by day, year after year. Frankl claims that anyone who knows why he lives, e.g., the value of just being here, can withstand many hardships. Nonetheless, it is important to mention that Frankl was frustrated that his logotherapy was solely related to his experiences in four different concentration camps during World War II, while the ideas and essences of this theory were developed well before the war. He just had no time and opportunity to write them down. Anyway, the experience of Hitler's concentration camps became a validation of his "will to meaning."

According to Frankl [17, 19], logotherapy ventures into the spiritual dimension of human life. The Greek word "logos" means not only meaning but also spirit. Accordingly, in the early Greek language, there is a connection between spirituality and meaning. Frankl highlighted that in a logotherapeutic context, spirituality is not primarily about religiosity—although religiosity can be part of it—but refers to a specific human dimension that makes us human. The need for meaning arises from the individual's existential consciousness of mortality; one day death will come. Frankl considered an individual's conscience as the "body-of-meaning" [19]. Conscience is closely related to the individual's values, morals, responsibilities, and integrity and is an intuitive, creative, and central force in the human quest for meaning in any given situation. Conscience is thus a subjective dimension, closely linked to cultural and national values, norms, and rules that apply in the context of the individual person. It is the individual's task to decide whether to interpret his or her life's tasks based on accountability to society, to God, or to his own value system. Human beliefs, values, and integrity are crucial to what can provide meaning to the individual.

8.2.1   Three Substantial Concepts of Frankl's Theory Will to Meaning

Frankl's theory is based on three substantial concepts: (1) meaning-in-life, (2) freedom to choose, and (3) suffering. Furthermore, these three concepts are linked to three basic assumptions in humans' lives: (1) the physical body, (2) the mental mind containing emotions and thoughts, and (3) the spiritual, or what Frankl calls "noos" [17]. The physical body and mental mind can become ill, while the human spirit can become blocked and frustrated. Frankl believed that the three dimensions of body–mind–spirit are parts that act as a unified totality. That is, problems in one dimension often cause symptoms in another. For example, spiritual emptiness can be manifested as a physiological symptom such as a headache. To understand Frankl's theory, one must understand his emphasis on the human spirit, "the noos," and its vital role in the individual as an integrated unit of these three: body–mind–spirit. This corresponds well with modern nursing theory [68, 88] and recent research that indicates that people function as a unit where body–mind–spirit is fully integrated with each other and are inseparable [89]. Figure 8.1 illustrates that the body–mind–spirit levels act as parts that, through constant and infinite interaction between each other, represent an inseparable entity. The dotted circles in Fig. 8.1 illustrates the integral interaction between the body–mind–spirit parts.

8.2.1.1   Meaning-in-Life
The term meaning involves the answer to man's existential questions: "Who am I?" and "Why am I here?" The experience of purpose and meaning produces positive emotions such as satisfaction with one's place in the world. Perceived meaning-in-life relates to what the person feels dedicated to, to provide one's unique contribution to a better world bestows purpose and meaning. A purpose-in-life represents a direction of one's energy, as well as a driving force in the individual's quest for meaning; this idea is key in Frankl's theory. Meaning is discovered and determined from the uniqueness of the individual person and

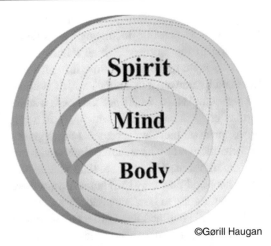

©Gørill Haugan

Fig. 8.1 The unity of body–mind–spirit in which steadily ongoing integrating processes unify the parts into one inseparable entity

his/her specific life situation. Frankl argued that meaning always changes, but never ceases to be potentially present.

Finding meaning-in-life is a subjective and unique process that takes place in the individual's mind. Meaning can neither be invented nor given as a gift. Meaning must be revealed by the individual. Thus, it is not possible for health care professionals to "tell" or "teach" the patient how to find meaning. Nor can health workers create, point to, or transfer meaning to another; finding meaning-in-life requires an inner process and active effort by the individual. Health care workers can "walk along with" the one searching for meaning, listening, asking questions, and challenging. Scholars differ in their perspectives on how meaning can be attained. Some stress that meaning needs to be discovered by the individual, implying more automatic processes, whereas other stress that the process is more deliberate and conscious, and they accordingly refer to meaning-making or meaning constructing [74]. Realizing meaning-in-life is closely related to realizing oneself. Frankl [17] argued that what people have been able to accomplish, endure, and master earlier in life represents a source of meaning here-and-now: *"All we have done, whatever great thoughts we may have had, and all we have suffered, all this is not lost, though it is past; we have brought it into being. Having been is also a* _kind of being and perhaps the surest kind"_ (p. 104). It is possible to distinguish between "meaning in the moment" which relates to the choices people make at any time in their daily lives and a "universal meaning", which is about the big picture and a confidence that there is some form of order in the universe which we are a part of. A universal meaning represents the opposite of a chaotic world where humans are victims of random impulses. The concrete thing that makes sense here-and-now may shift but is always there as an opportunity to be discovered.

Frankl [17] outlined three different sources of meaning: (1) performing good deeds or actions; to give or contribute something good or useful, or by one's creativity to create something beautiful; (2) experiencing something valuable, beautiful—experiencing goodness and loving fellowship; and (3) realizing dignified, honorable, and positive attitudes in the face of life's challenges, such as illness, suffering, and death. Hence, it seems clear that the phenomenon of self-transcendence (about self-transcendence, see Chap. 9 in this book) is closely related to purpose and meaning-in-life [17, 19, 90]. Self-transcendence refers to the ability to transcend oneself; an opening to something greater outside oneself [91]. It can be about doing a job, an effort, realizing a virtue; despite one's own life situation being demanding, painful, and difficult, to extend beyond one's self-occupation in the ego. Thus, self-transcendence implies a strategy for creating distance to oneself and one's own situation, and thereby provide a mindset without focus on one's troubles and worries. A self-transcended approach gives the opportunity to see and experience one's situation from a different perspective, and therefore an opportunity to find solutions and meaning amid the difficult and painful. For example, we have seen that parents who have lost a child in the crib have started the National Association for Unexpected Child Death to be able to help other parents in the same situation. Several similar examples exist.

Being open for other people's kindness and love does also provide an experience of meaning-in-life. Social support relates closely to the perception of meaning [49], while negative interaction with others can reduce perceived meaning-in-life [49, 92–95]. Furthermore, research has shown that positive emotions and moods appear to be a stronger source of meaning than activities toward achieving certain goals [1].

According to Frankl, the third strategy for people to create meaning-in-life is, despite any life challenges, to consciously choose their attitudes. Choosing to be positive, courageous, or optimistic despite difficult and painful events illustrates this strategy for meaning. Experience of meaning can arise from the patient voluntarily changing his attitude and consequently his perception of his current life situation.

Man's will to meaning can be frustrated, disappointed, or unfulfilled; Frankl called this "existential frustration" and "existential vacuum." When people feel despair and when they struggle to experience life as worth living, this is not an expression of mental illness, but of spiritual distress. According to Frankl, the health system often interprets and diagnoses spiritual distress as a mental illness (e.g., depression), and thus treats the condition by anesthetizing the patient's existential despair with medication. Existential vacuum is expressed by feelings such as meaninglessness, emptiness, apathy, and boredom [96] and can lead to severe neurosis. This neurosis is caused by spiritual frustration or problem, moral or ethical conflicts, existential vacuum, or frustrated will to meaning.

8.2.1.2 Freedom to Choose

Freedom to choose constitutes the second term in Frankl's logotherapy and is closely linked to the above-described sources of meaning. Many people are confronted with an undesirable fate, such as Holocaust, tsunamis, earthquakes, etc. In dealing with such life events, one can only be accepting—there is no use fighting—it is just about choosing one's attitude. Frankl [17] wrote that _"the way in which he accepts, the way in which he bears his cross, what courage he manifests in suffering, what dignity he displays in doom and disaster, is the measure of his human fulfillment"_ (p. 44). Humans can be subjected to torture and humiliation, to illness, destruction, loss and death, and yet choose to meet their destiny with courage and humanity. The sufferer's attitude is the motivating force for his actions, not the torturer. The right to choose one's attitude is regarded as human spiritual freedom and mental independence. The freedom of the will is about freedom to choose attitude regardless of external situation and circumstances. The individual cannot free himself from the conditions under which he lives. Still, he can consciously choose his attitude toward these conditions. The expression "will to meaning" indicates that meaning-in-life does not come "fleeting on a foal"; meaning does not come by itself, but requires effort, a desire and a conscious choice to actively search for meaning.

8.2.1.3 Suffering

The third concept of Frankl's theory is suffering, which represents a subjective, unique, and personal experience. Suffering is an inevitable part of humans' lives on earth. We are exposed to incidents that are undeserved, incomprehensible, and inexplicable as well as inevitable. The suffering is. It exists. At this point Frankl was quite clear; suffering has no point. There is no point in getting cancer or losing a child in an accident. Thus, people should not look for an inherent meaning in such events, because the meaning is not there. The meaning is in the attitude we choose while suffering. For example, a cancer patient chooses a positive and caring attitude toward others despite his own illness and need of care. That is, despite cancer and major losses, it is possible to realize meaning. Frankl [19] wrote about his experiences in concentration camps during World War II: *"We who lived in concentration camps can remember the men walking through the huts comforting others, giving away their last piece of bread. They may have been few in number, but they offer sufficient proof that everything can be taken from a man, but one thing: the burden of human freedoms – to choose one's attitude in any given set of circumstances, to choose one's own way"* (p. 86). Figure 8.2 illustrates the relationship between these three concepts in Frankl's Theory "Will to meaning." The individual experiences suffering in different ways; suffering is a personal and subjective experience of distress which impacts the individual as body–mind–spirit negatively. Frankl highlighted that the meaning is not in the suffering itself. Only by means of one's freedom to choose actively one's

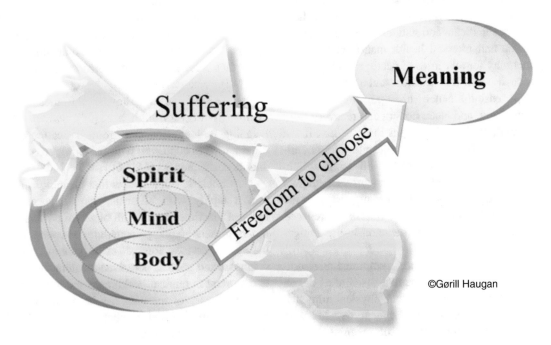

©Gørill Haugan

Fig. 8.2 Frankl's theory the "Will to meaning": Three central concepts and their relationships with each other

attitude, way of thinking, and how to approach one's life situation, meaning can be found. According to evidence and theory, we have shown that those who despite illness, crisis, suffering, etc. find meaning are better able to comprehend and manage the situation, and report better QoL and wellness.

8.3 Meaning-in-Life and (Mental) Health

Empirical studies seem to confirm that the experience of meaning is related with well-being and optimal health, representing an important resource when adjusting to or recovering from an illness [36, 40]. Accordingly, experiencing meaning-in-life is regarded as a highly desired psychological quality ("my life is meaningful") (ibid.). Positive associations between meaning-in-life and psychological well-being have been found across the lifespan, including adolescence [41], emerging adulthood [42], midlife, and older adulthood [40, 43]. The experience of meaning-in-life seems fundamental to humans [1, 2, 44] and is of significance in health and well-being particularly in later years [45–47]. Studies have shown significant correlations between meaning-in-life and physical health measured by lower mortality for all causes of death; meaning is correlated with less cardiovascular disease, less hypertension, better immune function, less depression, and better coping and recovery from illness [48–53]. This might indicate that if the individual finds meaning despite illness, ailments, and imminent death, well-being, health, and QoL will increase in the current situation. However, plausibly the relationship also goes the other way; when affected by illness and reduced functionality, finding meaning-in-life might prove more difficult [54].

Among cancer patients, symptoms related to psychological and existential discomfort are as prominent as pain and other physical ailments. Studies have shown that cancer patients who experience a high degree of meaning have a greater ability to tolerate bodily ailments than

those who do not find meaning-in-life; those who, despite pain and fatigue, experience meaning report better QoL than those with low meaning [55, 56]. Meaning is seen as a buffer that contributes to inner strength and thereby protects terminally [57] and critically ill [58, 59] patients from depression, hopelessness, and the urge to give up and desire an accelerated death. In a sample of chronic pain patients, for example, higher levels of experienced meaning-in-life predicted lower levels of depressive symptoms 1 year later [60]. Depression and hopelessness—contrary to meaning—are associated with increased mortality, dramatically higher suicide rates, and the desire for a physician-assisted death. In this context, some authors speak of a "demoralizing syndrome" [61, 62] that can occur in terminal patients when the disorder bodily-psychological-existential becomes intolerable and one's existence seems meaningless. Perceived meaning has also shown to have a strong impact on physical well-being in nursing home residents [40] and seems to moderate the relationship between illness, ailments, and functional loss on the one hand and QoL and well-being on the other.

Furthermore, research demonstrates that older people experience less meaning than other age groups [63]; on the contrary, some studies show that older people experience more meaning [42], whereas research among very old adults (85–95 years) shows that meaning declines with very high age [64]. However, meaning is suggested as a good indicator for older adults to cope well with the aging process and its consequences [65, 66].

Nevertheless, studies show that meaning correlates highly with ailments, symptoms, and reduced functionality [54]; all of which are commonly present among patients, old, or young, in the health services. Regardless of patients' age, diagnosis and gender, perceived meaning-in-life is important in clinical health care and research. Frankl's theory of meaning has been used as a basis for research and practice in many fields [22]; this chapter focuses on nursing and health science.

8.3.1 Meaning-in-Life: A Salutogenic Concept in Nursing and Health Science

Meaning-in-life is increasingly addressed in nursing and health literature [22, 67], underpinning the importance of nurses and health professionals to help patients and their families not only to cope with illness and suffering but also to find meaning in these experiences (event-related meaning) and to experience their lives as meaningful (meaning-in-life) despite the disease or illness [22, 68, 69]. Meaning seems vital in coping with severe health stressors. This is conceptualized clearly in the meaning-making model of Crystal Park [70] which proposes that people possess a global meaning system, including beliefs, goals, and a subjective sense of purpose. This global meaning system functions as an orienting system, providing individuals with a framework to interpret life experiences [71]. Stressful events impact on the meaning-making system, causing a discrepancy between the appraised situation and the global meaning system. This discrepancy creates distress, initiating a process of meaning-making. As part of the meaning-making process, both cognitive (i.e., reappraisal, rumination [72]) and emotional strategies (i.e., emotional processing [73]) can be activated. The end-products of this meaning-making process ("meaning made" [74]) can be operationalized as benefit finding (i.e., finding positive implications for a negative event) or sense-making (i.e., finding a suitable explanation for a negative event within the global meaning system). A successful resolution of the meaning-making process will then lead to better psychological functioning and better adjustment to stressful events [75].

This is in line with the salutogenic perspective of Antonovsky [76]. He described "sense of coherence" (SOC) as a measure of an individual's capacity to use various coping mechanisms and resources when faced with a stressor. Individuals with a strong SOC are assumed to effectively handle stress and maintain health, despite extremely challenging circumstances. After interviewing concentration camp survivors,

Antonovsky concluded that individuals' ability to stay healthy despite severe circumstances is related to the way they view their life and their existence [28]. He assumed that three aspects are important in this life view: the ability to understand what happens around them (comprehensibility), the ability to manage their situation (manageability), and their ability to find meaning in their situation (meaningfulness). Several studies have indeed shown that SOC is vital to coping with life's stresses such as illness, loneliness, despair, anxiety, and death [77–80].

Paying attention to meaning-in-life or to event-related meaning within care is also a focus of the bio-psycho-social-spiritual model of care as it developed by Sulmasy [81]. He argues that a person is a being in relationships and that illness involves a disruption of these relationships. Care needs to focus on restoration of the disturbed relationships. This restoration does involve not only biochemical and physiological processes (physical) but also mind–body relationships (psychological), relationships with the environment (social), and the relationship between the patient and the transcendent. This is in line with theorizing of Dossey and Keegan [68] who refer to the spiritual dimension of man as completely interwoven with the body, mind, and emotions (ibid.); that is, the human body, mind, and spirit are fully integrated with each other and constitute an indivisible whole. Bottom line, if the body is influenced, the mind and spirit will be affected at the same time. Every experience will therefore involve all dimensions of the individual: the physical, emotional-mental, social, and the spiritual-existential [82]. The holistic perspective thus emphasizes a sound integration or balance between the body–mind–spirit as crucial for health, well-being, and QoL. When discussing illness and care, Sulmasy [83] and others add the existential domain as an important fourth layer but with a focus on the transcendent (biopsychosocial *spiritual* model). A transcendental relationship with the divine is, however, not the only approach for the confrontation with meaninglessness [84]. Recent studies show that individuals, especially in West- and North-European secularized countries, also construct meaning based on secular sources such as altruism, self-actualization, family or work without the reference to spirituality or a religion [85]. Indeed, pain patients can turn toward spirituality in their search for meaningfulness, but they can also tap into other sources. A biopsychosocial *existential* model seems therefore more adequate when studying the influence of pain on all domains of life. In a Flemish study of chronic pain patients, patients reported not feeling satisfied with the attention to the social and existential life domains. Furthermore, practitioners' attention to the existential domain seems highly important for patient functioning [86]. Openness to existential concerns of pain might thus be an important aspect of care and nursing practice. The theoretical and therapeutic framework of Viktor Emil Frankl can be very useful in this vein.

8.4 To Promote Meaning Is to Promote Health

Currently, depression is the most prevalent disease worldwide [97]. This has many explanations and reasons. Frankl approached depression as a potential meaning-in-life problem and described the existential vacuum as early as in the 1960s. During the recent decades, suicides, divorces, alcoholism, intoxication, and criminality among adolescents have increased globally. Also, a growing tendency of overeating, overtraining, overworking, etc. has become evident. Frankl saw this as the result of people's attempts to cope with a lack of meaning; that is a lack of self-esteem, self-understanding, and meaningful realistic goals and purposes in life. Inspired by Frankl's logotherapy, different intervention approaches have been implemented to treat depression and anxiety [56, 98–101].

8.4.1 "Not How Your Situation Is, But How You Respond to It"

Research has so far demonstrated that people's well-being far more related with an individual's subjective perception/interpretation and evaluation of his/her objective conditions in life, than with the objective conditions per se. Consequently, personality and personal characteristics are important. Is there a personality, a gene related with greater sense of meaning-in-life? There is no doubt that personality and personality traits matter [102]. However, studies also show that therapy, cognitive, and spiritual–mental techniques such as gestalt therapy, cognitive therapy, mentalization, yoga, meditation, mindfulness, and prayer can have a positive impact on meaning-in-life and hence on mental health [40, 54, 82, 103, 104]. Being a living human comprising a unified trinity of body–mind–spirit implies steadily ongoing natural healing processes; inherent natural processes work toward homeostasis, growth, development, and healing. Humans represent inner energies that constantly integrate and heal the unity body–mind–spirit throughout life. Therefore, facilitating and supporting people's meaning-making processes represent to support and facilitate these inner processes toward healing. Hence, supporting meaning is health promoting.

8.4.2 To Facilitate and Support Patients' Search for Meaning

Health care professionals can facilitate and support patients' search for meaning by offering a relationship where the patient as a unique person can be acknowledged, welcomed, and respected [11, 105]: that is, a space of trust and confidence in which the patient feel free and relaxed, without feeling the need to care for the other. For example, the terminal husband's desire to care for and protect his wife's feelings, resulting in holding himself back keeping his innermost and heaviest thoughts and troubles by himself. Or when a child is seriously sick and dying; in care for the parents and the sick sister/brother siblings hold their feelings back, suffering silently alone, etc. The examples are many. Professionals can provide a relational spot in time and space, in which only the dying husband's or the suffering sibling's experiences and feelings are attended to. Finding meaning is about knowing who one is and why one is alive; e.g., what one lives for. Reflections on what life has been like, the individual's experiences of values and good things in life are sources of meaning and can also enhance a sense of connection. Communicational approaches in such situations may be questions such as "Are there periods in your life which you experienced particularly meaningful?" "Do you know anyone who lives a meaningful life?" "Are there people in your life who need you?" "Will you tell about an experience that made you think differently about life?" "Have you ever thought that 'I can't do this', and yet you did and experienced that you managed to do it?"

8.4.2.1 To Encounter Suffering and Negative Feelings

Often, health care professionals encounter patient's anxiety and concerns, perhaps guilt, remorse, and bad conscience, because the person feels that what he/she did in life was not good enough; it should have been better, the children should have had a better parent, etc. In such situations, health promotion is about listening with respect and acceptance to what the person tells [95, 105], without being tempted to comfort. Commonly, health care professionals tend to comfort. Instead of actively and empathically listening, they start to communicate that "Oh, you should not think like that, you should not be so harsh on yourself; do not think that way, you should rather focus on all that is good in your life," etc. By doing so, though with a good intention, health care professionals fail the person who shares his feelings and thoughts. This failure is not health promoting. Failure involves neither social nor emotional support. But listening with respect, acceptance, and attention, confirming that you acknowledge the patient's experience and recognize what really matters to him here and now, that is emotional support and health promoting [89, 94, 106]. The fact that someone is willing to be a witness, to recognize, acknowledge, endure, and pay attention, is itself health promoting [107]. When the professional does not escape but stays present, tolerates, and accepts, the patient is not left alone in the pain

and hardship. Feeling abandoned gives a feeling of loneliness, which in turn amplifies despair and pain [108].

Therefore, health professionals should develop a set of "muscles" that help to bear and endure patient's suffering; "muscles" which can withstand human's painful feelings and thoughts, which are strong enough to tolerate and accept what is expressed by the patient. Acknowledge, accept, endure, and attend to it. This is how health care professionals can contribute to meaning-in-life, by facilitating feelings of being tolerated, welcomed, and accepted. In this way, patients may experience a living space of acknowledgment, understanding, and thus connectedness, facilitating acceptance of oneself and one's life as it is [89, 105, 109]. By providing inner peace, tranquility, and releasing energy for positive aspects of life here-and-now, acceptance is healing and health promoting [105, 110, 111]. Asking questions, listening actively, supporting the patient to explain a bit more about his experiences and feelings may foster the patient's self-awareness, supporting his understanding of himself here-and-now, and what provides meaning in the present situation (about nurse-patient interaction as a salutogenic resource; see Haugan, G. (2021), Chap. 10 in this book).

The same applies in the care of terminally or critically ill patients who sometimes, in despair and exhaustion, wish to give up on life, asking for euthanasia. Health professionals need a mental "musculature" that can withstand suffering, despair, and desperation, without wanting to "fix" it, intending to change the patient focus into a more positive one. This is often framed "misunderstood comfort." In general, health professionals are trained to cure, and their main focus is therefore curing the disease. But in several situations, curing is no longer an option, and there needs to be shift to healing. Finding meaning in the event or regaining meaning despite the disease can be a pathway to healing. To support and facilitate meaning and thereby the relief of despair, it is first needed to be able to recognize and endure the patient's despair, pain, and hopelessness. From this experience, he may be able to lift his eyes looking at something brighter.

Containing other people's despair and desperation is burdensome and an intense work. To cope with this, a fit "musculature", self-understanding, and a health-promoting working culture are needed.

8.4.2.2 To Arrange for Health-Promoting Communities and Companionships

If possible, health care workers can arrange for the patient to experience health-promoting companionship, with the patient's friends, family, or peers in the ward. Many patients in hospitals are waiting for a diagnosis, feeling insecure, worrying about what might be wrong with them. Many get a serious message from the doctor about their health state: "you have cancer," "you have ALS" (amyotrophic lateral sclerosis), "you have MS" (multiple sclerosis), "your leg must be amputated," "the needed surgery is risky," etc. Diagnoses most often involve challenges and high demands on endurance and coping. Helping the patient to perceive the situation as understandable and manageable will contribute to increased meaning and a sense of coherence, both of which promoting coping and mental health [112–114]. Individually adapted and repeated information accompanied with emotional and practical support serve as a buffer of meaning in demanding life situations. Undergoing medical examinations and treatment is often a major burden for the patient; for him, this is most often new, frightening and overwhelming, while for the health care professionals, the various medical examinations and treatments might be commonplace. Therefore, it is crucial that professionals are aware of their attitudes toward various activities carried out during a working day in the hospital.

8.5 Conclusion

This chapter outlines the main ideas of the Austrian psychiatrist and neurologist Viktor Emil Frankl's theory of meaning, termed logotherapy. Research shows that meaning is essential for mental health and psychological as well as physi-

cal well-being and serves as a buffer and coping resource. This chapter demonstrates the significance of finding purpose and meaning-in-life as a resource to continue life amid great stress. However, meaning does not appear by itself; individuals need a "will to meaning," to consciously search for the unique meaning that is potentially present in any situation. Patients are often subjected to great stresses such as serious illness, painful medical examinations, and demanding treatments, as well as loss, grief, despair, and desperation. Finding meaning in these situations can be difficult. Nevertheless, studies show that patients who find meaning can tolerate symptoms, the disease, and its various outcomes better than those with low meaning. Thus, to support and facilitate patients' meaning-making processes, despite the situation, is an important health-promoting concern. Often the way to meaning goes through what the individual has managed, accomplished, contributed to, intended, and tolerated in their life ("life review")—through acceptance of who one is and one's life as it is. To integrate their lives in this way, most people need a relationship, one who listens, acknowledges, and affirms [115]. Thus, the nurse–patient relationship emerges as a significant resource for patient's meaning-in-life. Studies have shown that the nurse–patient interaction has a significant influence on nursing home resident's perceived meaning; the good "meeting" facilitating meaning is perceived as soothing and empowering [11, 93, 105, 116]. Meaning is also created by experiences of something good and beautiful, by self-transcendence, and by choosing positive and caring attitudes amid a painful and difficult situation. To facilitate and support patient's meaning-making, a relationship supported by health-promoting interaction should be provided [89, 105]. Figure 8.3 demonstrates that the three levels of body–mind–spirit interacting with each other are influenced by nurse–patient interaction: patients are affected physically, psychologically, socially, and spiritually-existentially. Health-promoting interaction impacts the patient as body–mind–spirit supporting his search for "his" meaning. However, we do not state that the nurse–patient interaction is the only way to

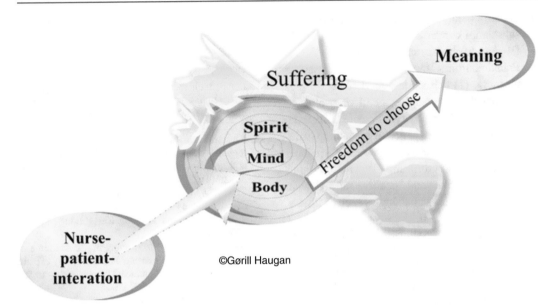

Fig. 8.3 Nurse–patient interaction affects all the three levels of body–mind–spirit and is a vital health promoting resource in facilitating patient's meaning-making processes. Nurses and health care professionals can support patients' meaningfulness in different ways. However, in the context of nursing and health care, the nurse–patient interaction has shown to be a key salutogenic resource in supporting patients' meaning-making processes

facilitate and support patients' meaning-making processes. Though, to our knowledge, the nurse–patient interaction is a key resource to support meaning in the context of health care.

Finally, health care professionals need to reflect on what gives perceived meaning in their daily work, in life, and in the face of serious illness and death. The professionals too need a conscious attention to meaning in their own life: who you are and why you are right here. This will promote health for the individual health worker, but also constitute a significant aspect of competence as professional health workers.

Take Home Messages
- Perceived meaning-in-life is essential for people's psychological functioning and is one of the core elements of positive psychology as well as health-promoting research and work.
- In the salutogenic health theory, meaning is the motivating dimension in the three-dimensional concept "sense of coherence."
- Perceived meaning-in-life is a strong individual predictor of satisfaction with life, as thus

crucial to psychological well-being; a buffer that contributes to inner strength and thereby protects the individual from depression, hopelessness, and the urge to give up.
- Positive associations between meaning-in-life and psychological well-being have been found across the lifespan, including adolescence, emerging adulthood, midlife, and older adulthood.
- Studies have shown a significant relationship between meaning-in-life and physical health measured by lower mortality for all causes of death; meaning is significantly correlated with less cardiovascular disease, less hypertension, better immune function, less depression and better coping with illness, crises and death, as well as better recovery from illness.
- Patients who find meaning despite illness, ailments, and imminent death experience more well-being and better health and quality-of-life in their life situation.
- Frankl's logotherapy emphasizes the spiritual dimension of the human life; the need for meaning arises from the existential consciousness of life and death.

- Frankl's theory of meaning is based on three substantial concepts: (1) meaning-in-life, (2) freedom to choose, and (3) suffering.
- Frankl outlines three different sources of meaning: (1) performing good deeds; to give or contribute something good or useful, or through one's creativity to create something beautiful, (2) to experience something valuable and beautiful—to experience kindness and loving fellowship, and (3) to realize dignified, honorable, and positive attitudes in meeting with life's challenges, such as illness, suffering, and death.
- Health care professionals can facilitate and support patients' search for meaning by offering a relationship where the patient's experiences, thoughts, and emotions are attended to.
- Acceptance is healing and health-promoting by providing inner peace and tranquility and thus releases energy to experience positive aspects of life here-and-now.

References

1. King LA, Hicks J, Krull J, Del Gaiso A. Positive affects and the experience of meaning in life. J Pers Soc Psychol. 2006;90:179–96.
2. Wong P, Fry P. The human quest for meaning: a handbook of psychologicasl research and clinical applications. Mahwah, NJ: Lawrence Erlbaum Associates Publishers; 1998.
3. Schulenberg SE, Hutzell R, Nassif C, Rogina J. Logotherapy for clinical practice. Psychother Theor Res Pract Train. 2009;45(4):447–63.
4. Peterson C, Park N, Seligman M. Orientations to happiness and life satisfactiom: the full life versus the empty life. J Happiness Stud. 2005; 6:25–41.
5. Morgan J, Farsides T. Measuring meaning in life. J Happiness Stud. 2009;10(2):197–214.
6. Seligman MEP. Authentic happiness. New York: Free Press; 2002.
7. Bonebright C, Clay D, Ankenmann R. The relationship of workaholism to work-life conflict, life satisfaction and purpose in life. J Couns Psychol. 2000;47:469–77.
8. Fry P. The unique contribution of key existential factors to the prediction of psychological Well-being of older adults following spousal loss. Gerontologist. 2001;41:69–81.
9. Melton A, Schulenberg S. On the measurement of meaning; Logotherapy's empirical contribu-
10. Pearson P, Sheffield B. Psychoticism and purpose in life. Personal Individ Differ. 1989;10:1321–2.
11. Haugan Hovdenes G. The nurse-patient-relationship in nursing homes: fulfillment or destruction [Pleier-pasient-relasjonen i sykehjem: virkeliggjørelse eller tilintetgjørelse]. Nord J Nurs Res Clin Stud. 2002;22(3):21–6.
12. Kleftaras G, Psarra E. Meaning in life, psychological well-being and depressive symptomatology: a comparative study. Psychol Forsch. 2012;3(4):337–45.
13. Chan DW. Orientations to happiness and subjective well-being among Chinese prospective and in-service teachers in Hong Kong. Educ Psychol. 2009;29:139–51.
14. Halama P, Dedova M. Meaning in life and hope as predictors of positive mental health: do they explain residual variance not predicted by personality traits? Stud Psychol. 2007;49:191–200.
15. Ho MY, Cheung FM, Cheung SF. The role of meaning in life and optimism in promoting well-being. Personal Individ Differ. 2010;48:658–63.
16. Holahan CK, Holahan CJ, Suzuki R. Purposiveness, physical activity, and perceived health in caridac patients. Disabil Rehabil. 2008;30:1772–8.
17. Frankl VE. Man's search for meaning. New York: Washington Square Press; 1963.
18. Frankl VE. The will to live. 1963.
19. Frankl VE. The unheard cry for meaning. New York: Simion & Scuster; 1978.
20. Melton A, Schulenberg S. On the relationship between meaning in life and boredom proneness: examining a logotherapy postulate. Psychol Rep. 2007;101:1016–22.
21. Pöhlmann K, Gruss B, Joraschky P. Structural properties of personal meaning systems: a new approach to measuring meaning in life. J Posit Psychol. 2006;1:109–17.
22. Starck PL. Theory of meaning. In: Smith MJ, Liehr PR, editors. Middel range theory for nursing. 2nd ed. New York: Springer, LLC; 2008. p. 81–104.
23. Antonovsky A. Health, stress, and coping: new perspectives on mental health and physical wellbeing. San Francisco: Jossey-Bass; 1979.
24. Antonovsky A. Unraveling the mystery of health. How people manage stress and stay well. San Fransisco: Jossey-Bass; 1987.
25. Skarsater I, Rayens M, Peden A, Hall L, Zhang M, Agren H, et al. Sense of coherence and recovery from major depression: a 4-year follow-up. Arch Psychiatr Nurs. 2009;23:119–27.
26. Zirke N, Schmid G, Mazurek B, Klapp B, Rauchfuss M. Antonovsky's Sense of Coherence in psychosomatic patients—a contribution to construct validation. GMS Psycho Soc Med. 2007;4:Doc03.
27. Pallant J, Lae L. Sense of coherence, well-being, coping and personality factors: further evaluation of

the sense of coherence scale. Personal Individ Differ. 2002;33:39–48.

28. Eriksson M, Lindstrom B. Antonovsky's sense of coherence scale and its relation with quality of life: a systematic review. J Epidemiol Community Health. 2007;61:938–44.

29. Surtees P, Wainwright N, Luben R, Khaw K, Nicholas D. Sense of coherence and mortality in men and women in the EPIC-Norfolk United Kingdom Prospective Cohort Study. Am J Epidemiol. 2003;158:1202–9.

30. Yalom I. Existential psychotherapy. New York: Basic Books; 1980.

31. Steger MF. An illustration of issues in factor extraction and indentification of dimensionality in psychological assessment data. J Pers Assess. 2006;86:263–72.

32. Roepke A, Jayawickreme E, Riffle O. Meaning and health: a systematic review. Appl Res Qual Life. 2014;9(4):1055–79.

33. Baumeister R. Meanings in life. New York: Guilford; 1991.

34. Heintzelman S, King L. (The feeling of) meaning-as-information. Pers Soc Psychol Rev. 2014;18:153–67.

35. George L, Park C. Are meaning and purpose distinct? An examination of correlates and predictors. J Posit Psychol. 2013;8:365–75.

36. Steger MF, Frazier P, Oishi S, Kaler M. The meaning in life questionnaire: assessing the presence of and search for meaning in life. J Couns Psychol. 2006;53:80–93.

37. McKnight P, Kashdan T. Purpose in life as a system that creates and sustains health and well-being: an integrative, testable theory. Rev Gen Psychol. 2009;13:242–51.

38. Martela F, Steger MF. The three meanings of meaning in life: distinguishing coherence, purpose, and significance. J Posit Psychol. 2016;11(5):531–45.

39. George L, Park C. Meaning in life as comprehension, purpose, and mattering: toward integration and new research questions. Rev Gen Psychol. 2016;20:205–20.

40. Haugan G. Meaning-in-life in nursing-home patients: a valuable approach for enhancing psychological and physical well-being? J Clin Nurs. 2014;23(13-14):1830–44.

41. Brassai L, Piko B, Steger M. Meaning in life: is it a protective factor for adolescents' psychological health? Int J Behav Med. 2011;18(1):44–51.

42. Steger MF, Oishi S, Kashdan TB. Meaning in life across the life span: levels and correlates of meaning in life from emerging adulthood to older adulthood. J Posit Psychol. 2009;4(1):43–52.

43. Zika S, Chamberlain K. On the relation between meaning in life and psychological well-being. Br J Psychol. 1992;83:133–45.

44. Schulenberg SE, Hutzell R, Nassif C, Rogina J. Logotherapy for clinical practice. Psychother Theor Res Pract Train. 2008;45:447–63.

45. Moore SL, Metcalf B, Schow E. Aging and meaning in life: examining the concept. Geriatr Nurs. 2000;21(1):27–9.

46. Sarvimäki A, Stenbock-Hult B. Quality of life in old age described as a sense of well-being, meaning and value. J Adv Nurs. 2000;32(4):1025–33.

47. Wang J-J. A structural model of the bio-psycho-socio-spiritual factors influencing the development towards gerotranscendence in a sample of institutionalized elders. J Adv Nurs. 2011;67(12):2628–36.

48. Koenig HG, George LK, Titus P, Meador KG. Religion, spirituality, and acute care hospitalization and long-term care use by older patients. Arch Intern Med. 2004;164(14):1579–85.

49. Krause N. Longitudinal study of social support and meaning in life. Psychol Aging. 2007;22(3):456–69.

50. Krause N. Meaning in life and mortality. J Gerontol B Psychol Sci Soc Sci. 2009;64B(4):517–27.

51. Starkweather A, Wiek-Janusek L, Mathews H. Applying the psychoneuroimmunology framework to nursing research. J Neurosci Nurs. 2005;37(1):56–62.

52. Vance DE, Struzick TC, Raper JL. Biopsychosocial benefits of spirituality in adults aging with HIV. J Holist Nurs. 2008;26(2):119–25.

53. Westerhof GJ, Bohlmeijer ET, van Beljouw IMJ, Pot AM. Improvement in personal meaning mediates the effects of a life review intervention on depressive symptoms in a randomized controlled trial. Gerontologist. 2010;50(4):541–9.

54. Haugan G. Meaning-in-life in nursing-home patients: a correlate to physical and emotional symptoms. J Clin Nurs. 2014;23(7-8):1030–43.

55. William B, Christopher G, Poppito Shannon R, Amy B. Psychotherapeutic interventions at the end of life: a focus on meaning and spirituality. Can J Psychiatry. 2004;49(6):366–72.

56. Breitbart W, Rosenfeld B, Gibson C, Pessin H, Poppito S, Nelson C, et al. Meaning-centered group psychotherapy for patients with advanced cancer: a pilot randomized controlled trial. Psychooncology. 2010;19(1):21–8.

57. Fitchett G, Canada AL. The role of religion/spirituality in coping with cancer: evidence, assessment, and inervention. In: Holland JC, Breitbart WS, Jacobsen PB, editors. Psychooncology. 2nd ed. New York: Oxford University Press; 2010. p. 440–6.

58. Alpers L-M, Helseth S, Bergbom I. Experiences of inner strength in critically ill patients—a hermeneutical approach. Intensive Crit Care Nurs. 2012;28(3):150–8.

59. Alexandersen I, Stjern B, Eide R, Haugdahl H, Paulsby T, Lund S, et al. "never in my mind to give up!" a qualitative study of long-term intensive care patients' inner strength and willpower-promoting and challenging aspect. J Clin Nurs. 2019;28(21-22):3991–4003.

60. Dezutter J, Luyckx K, Wachholtz A. Meaning in life in chronic pain patients over time: associations

with pain experience and psychological well-being. J Behav Med. 2015;38(2):384–96.

61. Kissane DW, Clarke DM, Street AF. Demoralization syndrome: a psychiatric diagnosis for palliative care. J Palliat Care. 2001;17(1):12–21.

62. Parker ME. Medicalizing meaning: demoralization syndrome and the desire to die. Aust N Z J Psychiatry. 2003;38(10):765–73.

63. Pinquart M. Creating and maintaining purpose in life in old age: a meta-analysis. Aging Int. 2002;27:90–104.

64. Hedberg P, Brulin C, Aléx L, Gustafson Y. Purpose in life over a five-year period: a longitudinal study in a very old population. Int Psychogeriatr. 2011;23(5):806–13.

65. Flood M. Exploring the relationships between creativity, depression, and successful aging. Activit Adapt Aging. 2007;31(1):55–71.

66. Flood M, Scharer K. Creativity enhancement: possibilities for successful aging. Issues Ment Health Nurs. 2006;27:939–59.

67. Angel S. The fight for a meaningful life [Danish]. Sygeplejersken/Danish J Nurs. 2009;109(17):48–53.

68. Dossey B, Keegan L, editors. Holistic nursing: a handbook for practice. London: Jones and Bartlett; 2009.

69. Travelbee J. Interpersonal aspects of nursing. 2nd ed. Philadelphia: F.A. Davis; 1979.

70. Park C, Folkman S. Meaning in the context of stress and coping. Rev Gen Psychol. 1997;1:115–44.

71. Reker G, Wong P. Aging as an individual process: toward a theory of personal meaning. In: Birren J, Bengston V, editors. Emergent theories of aging. New York: Springer; 1988.

72. Nolen-Hoeksema S, Davis C. Theoretical and methodological issues in the assessment and interpretation of posttraumatic growth. Psychol Inq. 2004;15:60–4.

73. Kennedy-Moore E, Watson J. How and when does emotional expression help? Rev Gen Psychol. 2001:187–212.

74. Park CL. Making sense of the meaning literature: an integrative review of meaning making and its effects on adjustment to stressful life events. Psychol Bull. 2010;136(2):257–301.

75. Janoff-Bulman R. Posttraumatic growth: three explanatory models. Psychol Inq. 2004;15(1):30–4.

76. Antonovsky A. Unraveling the mystery of health: how people manage stress and stay well. San Fransisco: Jossey-Bass; 1987.

77. Dwyer L, Nordenfelt L, Ternestedt B-M. Three nursing home residents speak about meaning at the end of life. Nurs Ethics. 2008;15(1):97–109.

78. Knestrick J, Lohri-Posey B. Spirituality and health: perceptions of older women in a rural senior high rise. J Gerontol Nurs. 2005;31(10):44–50; quiz 1-2.

79. Thomas JC, Burton M, Quinn Griffin MT, Fitzpatrick JJ. Self-transcendence, spiritual well-being, and spiritual practices of women with breast cancer. J Holist Nurs. 2010;28(2):115–22.

80. Van Orden K, Bamonti P, King D, Duberstein P. Does perceived burdensomeness erode meaning in life among older adults? Aging Ment Health. 2012;16(7):855–60.

81. Sulmasy D. A biopsychological-spiritual model for the care of patients at the end of life. Gerontologist. 2002;2002(Special Issue III):24–33.

82. Rannestad T, Hovdenes GH, Espnes GA. Hjernen er ikke alene: psykosomatikken ser kropp og sjel i sammenheng, det bør sykepleie også gjøre; Tidsskriftet Sykepleien [Norwegian Journal of Nursing], 2006. p. 52–6.

83. Astrow A, Puchalski C, Sulmasy D. Religion, spirituality, and health care: social, ethical, and practical considerations. Am J Med. 2001;110(4):283–7.

84. Moore L, Goldner-Vukov M. The existential way to recovery. Psychiatr Danub. 2009;4:453–62.

85. Silver C, Bernaud J, Pedersen H, Birkeland M, la Cour P, Schnell T. Three cultural comparisons and inferences using the Sources of Meaning and Meaning in Life Questionnaire. The biannual meeting of the International Society for Psychology of Religion; Lausanne, Switzerland; 2013.

86. Dezutter J, Offenbaecher M, Vallejo MA, Vanhooren S, Thauvoye E, Toussaint L. Chronic pain care: the importance of a biopsychosocial-existential approach. Int J Psychiatry Med. 2016;51(6):563–75.

87. Spiegelberg E. The phenomenological movement: a historical introduction. Dordrect, Boston, London: Kluwer Academic; 1994.

88. Guzzetta CE. Holistic nursing research. In: Dossey BM, Keegan L, Guzzetta CE, editors. Holistic nursing a handbook for practice. 4th ed. Boston, Toronto, London, Singapore: Jones and Bartlett; 2009. p. 211–28.

89. Haugan G. Life satisfaction in cognitively intact long-term nursing-home patients: symptom distress, well-being and nurse-patient interaction. Chapter 10 In: Sarracino F, Mikucka M, editors. Beond money: the social roots of health and well-being. New York: Nova Science; 2014. p. 165–211.

90. Haugan G, Demirci AD, Kukulu K, Aune I. Self-transcendence in individuals 65 years and older: A meta-analysis. Scand J Caring Sci. 2021. https://doi.org/10.1111/scs.12959.

91. Reed PG, Haugan G. Self-transcendence - a salutogenic resource. Chapter 9 In: Haugan G, Eriksson M, editors. Health promotion in health care—vital theories and research. London: Springer; 2021.

92. Boyraz G, Horne SG, Sayger TV. Finding meaning in loss: the mediating role of social support between personality and two construals of meaning. Death Stud. 2012;36(6):519–40.

93. Haugan G. The relationship between nurse-patient-interaction and meaning-in-life in cognitively intact nursing-home patients. J Adv Nurs. 2014;70(1):107–20.

94. Haugan G, Innstrand ST, Moksnes UK. The effect of nurse-patient-interaction on anxiety and depression

in cognitively intact nursing home patients. J Clin Nurs. 2013;22(15–16):2192–205.

95. Haugan G. Nurse-patient interaction is a resource for hope, meaning-in-life, and self-transcendence in cognitively intact nursding-home patients. Scand J Caring Sci. 2014;2014(28):74–8.

96. Frankl VE. Man's search for meaning: the classic tribute to hope from the holocaust: SD Books; 2008.

97. WHO. Depression in Europe. 2012. http://www.euro.who.int/en/health-topics/noncommunicable-diseases/mental-health/news/news/2012/10/depression-in-europe.

98. Lee V, Cohen SR, Edgar L, Laizner AM, Gagnon AJ. Meaning-making intervention during breast or colorectal cancer treatment improves self-esteem, optimism, and self-efficacy. Soc Sci Med. 2006;62(12):3133–45.

99. Lee V. The existential plight of cancer: meaning making as a concrete approach to the intangible search for meaning. Support Care Cancer. 2008;16(7):779–85.

100. Mohabbat-Bahar S, Golzari M, Moradi-Joo M, Akbari ME. Efficacy of group Logotherapy on decreasing anxiety in women with breast cancer. Iran J Cancer Prev. 2014;7(3):165–70.

101. Keall RM, Clayton JM, Butow PN. Therapeutic life review in palliative care: a systematic review of quantitative evaluations. J Pain Symptom Manage. 2015;49(4):747–61.

102. Simpson DB, Newman JL, Fuqua DR. Spirituality and personality: accumulating evidence. J Psychol Christ. 2007;26(1):33–44.

103. Haugan Hovdenes G. Troen, håpet og kjærligheten: avgjørende ressurser relatert til helse og livskvalitet. Munksgaard; 1995. p. 97-101.

104. Mwilambwe-Tshilobo L, Ge T, Chong M, Ferguson M, Misic B, Burrow A, et al. Loneliness and meaning in life are reflected in the intrinsic network architecture of the brain. Soc Cogn Affect Neurosci. 2019;14(4):423–33.

105. Haugan G. Nurse-patient interaction—a vital health promoting resource in nursing homes. Chapter 10 In: Haugan G, Eriksson M, editors. Health promotion in health care—vital theories and research. London: Springer; 2021.

106. Milberg A, Strang P. What to do when 'there is nothing more to do'? A study within a salutogenic framework of family members' experience of palliative home care staff. Psychooncology. 2007;16(8):741–51.

107. Arman M. Bearing witness: an existential position in caring. Contemp Nurse. 2007;27(1):84–93.

108. Drageset J, Eide G, Kirkevold M, Ranhoff A. Emotional loneliness is associated with mortality among mentally intact nursing home residents with and without cancer: a five-year follow-up study. J Clin Nurs. 2013;22(1-2):106–14.

109. Nåden D, Sæteren B. Cancer patients' perception of being or not being confirmed. Nurs Ethics. 2006;13(3):222–35.

110. Haugan G, Hanssen B, Rannestad T, Espnes GA. Self-transcendence and nurse-patient interaction in cognitively intact nursing-home patients. J Clin Nurs. 2012;21:3429–41.

111. Haugan G, Rannestad T, Hammervold R, Garåsen H, Espnes GA. Self-transcendence in nursing home patients—a resource for well-being. J Adv Nurs. 2013;69(5):1147–60.

112. Moksnes UK, Espnes GA, Haugan G. Stress, sense of coherence, and emotional symptoms in adolescents. Psychol Health. 2014;29(1):32–49.

113. Moksnes U, Haugan G. Validation of the orientation to Life Questionnaire in Norwegian adolescents, construct validity across samples. Soc Indic Res. 2013; https://doi.org/10.1007/s11205-013-0536-z.

114. Moksnes UK. Sense of coherence. In: Haugan G, Eriksson M, editors. Health promotion in health care—vital theories and research. London: Springer; 2021. p. 20.

115. Kagan PN. Feeling listened to: a lived experience of Humanbecoming. Nurs Sci Q. 2008;21(1):59–67.

116. Jonas-Simpson C, Mitchell GJ, Fisher A, Jones G, Linscott J. The experience of being listened to: a qualitative study of older adults in long-term care settings. J Gerontol Nurs. 2006;32(1):46–53.

Self-Transcendence: A Salutogenic Process for Well-Being

9

Pamela G. Reed and Gørill Haugan

Abstract

Self-transcendence is a concept relevant to understanding how human beings attain or maintain well-being. Not surprisingly, it is similar to other concepts that are in some way linked to human well-being. The purpose of this chapter is to discuss self-transcendence particularly for its empirical support and practical relevance in promoting well-being across the health continuum. Increasing understanding and generating new ideas about self-transcendence may also facilitate continued research into self-transcendence and identification of health-promoting interventions and practices that foster well-being, particularly in difficult life situations.

Keywords

Inherent capacity for self-organizing · Personal and contextual factors · Salutogenic resource · Self-boundaries · Self-transcendence · Vulnerability · Well-being

9.1 Theoretical Context of the Concept of Self-Transcendence

Because self-transcendence is an abstract concept, it is important to situate the concept within a theory to facilitate elaboration of its meaning and existing empirical support and how it may be assessed or measured for practical applications within a discipline. In nursing, self-transcendence is a process that promotes or supports well-being [1, 2]. The concept of self-transcendence is relevant to nursing because it is salient for well-being in health-related contexts, especially those that are particularly challenging or eventful, life-threatening, or life-changing—in other words in times of increased vulnerability.

The concept of self-transcendence is connected to vulnerability and well-being. Self-transcendence is theorized to be a resource for well-being; it is an inner resource that becomes particularly salient during events or awareness of one's vulnerability that can diminish well-being [1, 2]. A model of the theory is presented in

P. G. Reed
College of Nursing, The University of Arizona, Tucson, AZ, USA
e-mail: preed@email.arizona.edu

G. Haugan (✉)
Department of Public Health and Nursing, NTNU Norwegian University of Science and Technology, Trondheim, Norway

Faculty of Nursing and Health Science, Nord University, Levanger, Norway
e-mail: gorill.haugan@ntnu.no, gorill.haugan@nord.no

G. Haugan, M. Eriksson (eds.), *Health Promotion in Health Care – Vital Theories and Research*,
https://doi.org/10.1007/978-3-030-63135-2_9

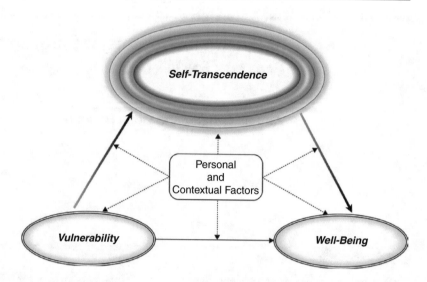

Fig. 9.1, depicting three key concepts and their relationships, including the mediating role of self-transcendence. Additional concepts in the theory are *personal and contextual factors* that can influence the relationships among vulnerability, self-transcendence, and well-being. Potential factors include age, gender, ethnicity, years of education, illness intensity, life history, social or spiritual support, and other factors concerning the person's social, cultural, and physical environment (ibid.).

9.1.1 The Main Concepts

9.1.1.1 Vulnerability
Vulnerability refers most directly to a heightened sense or awareness of one's mortality and fragility or susceptibility to be harmed in some way. A wide variety of emotional and physical human health experiences engender a sense of vulnerability, particularly those that are life-threatening or that involve loss. Examples include chronic and serious illness, disability, aging, bereavement, traumatic events, parenting and caregiving, and facing end-of-life.

9.1.1.2 Well-Being
Well-being is defined broadly as a subjective feeling of being well or healthy, based on the person's values and definition of health or being well. Well-being in this chapter is distinguished from objective health as a physical or biologically based condition, which is often described in biomedical terms or diagnoses when illness is present. Well-being refers to a subjective sense as perceived by the individuals regardless of biomedical status or diagnosis. It involves an existential judgment by the individual and is likely influenced by one's history, culture, and developmental stage in life as well as significant relationships and biophysical factors. There are various measures of subjective well-being, which indicate the diversity of perspectives on well-being in nursing and other sciences. Examples of indicators of well-being include life satisfaction, happiness, high morale in aging, meaning or purpose-in-life, as well as absence of mental health problems such as depression, anxiety, or loneliness.

9.1.1.3 Self-Transcendence
According to Reed's (e.g., [1–3]) nursing theory of self-transcendence, the concept of self-transcendence refers to perspectives and behaviors that expand (transcend) self-boundaries in multiple ways that are described, for example, *inwardly* (through intrapersonal activities and perspectives that enhance awareness of one's beliefs, values, and dreams), *outwardly* (through interpersonal connections with one's social and natural environments), *upwardly* (through per-

spectives and practices oriented beyond the ordinary or readily observable toward the transpersonal), and *temporally* (connecting perspectives of past and future to one's present) [2]. Individuals achieve these perspectives and behaviors on their own but in difficult times may also benefit from personal or professional support of others to facilitate self-transcendence. Forms of self-boundary expansion range from the mundane to the mystical, with many yet to be discovered.

9.1.2 Three Main Relationships in the Theory

Figure 9.1 depicts the three key relationships among the concepts proposed by the nursing theory of self-transcendence, each of which may be moderated by personal and contextual factors such as age, gender, cognitive ability, health status, personal beliefs, social or spiritual support, and other sociocultural factors. One relationship between vulnerability and self-transcendence posits that awareness of vulnerability may motivate an increase in self-transcendence, perhaps as a means of coping with vulnerability. A second positive relationship is proposed between self-transcendence and well-being (or an inverse relationship if the well-being outcome is a negative indicator such as depression). A third relationship proposes that self-transcendence mediates the relationship between vulnerability and well-being such that self-transcendence is the process by which an individual may attain well-being in the presence of vulnerability. The proposed relationships in this theory paint a picture not of coping but of transcending a difficult situation. Without the capacity for self-transcendence, promotion of health and well-being might not be possible in difficult situations. Self-transcendence, then, may be an underlying process that explains how well-being is possible in difficult or life-threatening situations that people endure. Accordingly, self-transcendence represents a vital resource for health and well-being and is key in health promotion.

9.2 A Nursing Theory of Self-Transcendence

Scientific theories not only provide descriptions of observable characteristics or events but also propose explanations of processes or mechanisms underlying the phenomena [4]. These explanations may be placeholders until we can learn more about what is going on behind what is readily observable. The theory of self-transcendence offers one explanation for the process of well-being. The theory draws from assumptions of two metatheories: (1) lifespan developmental psychology and the relational developmental systems perspective [4–6], which describe human development in part as a differentiation of self and changing boundaries between self and others and the environment over the lifespan; and (2) the science of unitary human beings [7–9] by which human beings are viewed as inherently open human-environment systems of changing complexity and organization.

In terms of the first assumption, differentiation of self and changing boundaries, self-transcendence involves self-boundary management as a self-organizing process that fosters well-being during significant health and life events. Change in self-boundaries is a natural developmental process according to lifespan and psychodynamic theories of human development (e.g., [10]). For example, in infancy the self-boundary between self and parent is diffuse; children and adolescents increasingly develop a self-awareness that distinguishes the self from others; adults develop a sense of interdependence between self and others; and older adults and others facing end of life may acquire more expanded and spiritual forms of self in relation to the world [11].

In terms of the second assumption, a characteristic of open systems is that they have ongoing interaction with the environment, which increases complexity. This would be chaotic without also ongoing capacity to organize complexity. The process underlying self-transcendence, then, is the broad human capacity for self-organizing the increasing complexity. The theory of self-transcendence points specifically to health-related events as bringing about increased complexity in life, and by positing that the individual's inherent self-organizing capacity—evidenced by managing personal boundaries—facilitates well-being through these events [3]. The management (or self-organizing) of complexity by expanding self-boundaries is a way to create meaning, sense of identity, and security in the face of vulnerability. In sum, self-transcendence is a "natural resource for healing that manifests the human being's capacity to self-organize for well-being at times in life when a sense of fragmentation may threaten well-being" [12].

Nursing holds deep interest and appreciation for how individuals persevere if not thrive through difficult health experiences. Translating theories about human development and complex adaptive and open systems (e.g., [13]) into nursing language means that individuals have the inherent capacity for self-organizing change that is healing and fosters well-being. Hence, this inherit capacity for self-organizing is a health-promoting resource for people's health, which [2, 14] is labeled as a "nursing" process because it is not just any self-organizing process but one that is inherent in human beings and facilitates health and well-being. Self-transcendence is one example of this self-organizing process.

Further, self-transcendence is salutogenic; it is conceptualized as an inherent resource for well-being, particularly in challenging life events such as health crises and loss. However, self-transcendence is not limited to or focused on attempts to *resist* stress as much as it is a normal, developmental outcome of co-evolving with the changing environment (and stressful life events, challenges, and other significant change) through various behaviors and mindsets or dispositions that expand self-boundaries and foster a sense of wholeness (well-being). The concept of self-transcendence covers different ways by which individuals expand their self-boundaries, which in fact is about connectedness. Thus, the core of self-transcendence is connectedness among intrapersonal, interpersonal, or transpersonal dimensions of the self. This may also include connecting to memories of one's past and anticipations about the future, drawn into one's present into a meaningful way. This connectedness involves an integration of parts of the self—such as the physical, emotional, social, and spiritual into a sense of wholeness (well-being). That is, the individual becomes healthier with stronger connections within the self, and with important others, the environment as well as one's life experiences.

Recent medical and nursing research indicates that connectedness is fundamental in well-being, health, and healing [15–18] as well as the core of people's spirituality [19–21]. Nursing and health science embrace a holistic approach to health and illness which includes a focus on interconnections between the emotional, physical, social, and spiritual. Hence, by facilitating the processes of connectedness by means of self-transcendence, the individual's inner strength, integration, and well-being are supported [22–25]. In this way, the salutogenic essence of self-transcendence seems evident. Nursing's role is to describe, explain, and facilitate these processes of connectedness promoting well-being, of which self-transcendence is one, as they occur in human beings during health experiences and events across the lifespan.

9.3 Measuring Self-Transcendence

Various instruments have been used to measure self-transcendence in research. While they share some common themes of self-transcendence such as connectedness or spirituality broadly defined, and its role in enhancing well-being, the dominant conceptualizations behind each instrument are quite distinct; for example, include religious or supernatural beliefs, intense but temporary mystical, peak, or ineffable experiences, losing or dissolution of self into a greater whole, negation of the physical world, personality temperaments or traits, and prosocial values (see [26–28] for overviews). Psychometric evaluations produce mixed results on empirical adequacy, although this can be said for most instruments measuring this complex construct of self-transcendence.

Nursing is unique in its measure of self-transcendence as expanding boundaries both inward and outward in a way that connects self to others and the environment without diminishing the individual, and not as a personality characteristic, a particular value-orientation, an ineffable experience, or belief system. Rather, and importantly, the nursing measure of self-transcendence is based upon a nursing theory by which self-transcendence involves everyday "terrestrial" experiences that individuals (and nurses and other caregivers) encounter and can readily apprehend [11, 29, 30].

In the initial and continuing research in nursing, self-transcendence is measured by the *Self-Transcendence Scale* (STS) [29]. The STS is developed as a unidimensional instrument with 15 items measured on 4-point Likert-type scaling. It originated from a psychometric study and factor analysis of a 36-item instrument, the *Developmental Resources of Later Adulthood* scale [31, 32], which generated a self-transcendence factor that described behaviors and perspectives that reflect expansion of personal boundaries. The STS has demonstrated reliability (internal consistency) and validity (content, construct) across studies of various populations and health experiences. It is brief and easy to administer either as a questionnaire or in an interview format. The STS is used widely in research and may also be used by practicing nurses to better understand areas for assessing patients. Many researchers and graduate students have used the instrument in studying self-transcendence as it relates to various health experiences and outcomes. The STS has been translated into several languages, including Spanish, Norwegian, Swedish, Turkish, Mandarin, Farsi, Japanese, and Korean.

As already described, the ST theory states that self-transcendence refers to various ways (dimensions) of transcending one's self-boundaries, for example, *outwardly* (interpersonal), *inwardly* (intrapersonal), *upwardly* (transpersonal), and *temporally* (connecting one's past and future to the present). Correspondingly, while evaluating the psychometrics of the STS one could expect four dimensions. Psychometric studies have shown that the STS is multidimensional, including at least two dimensions: an interpersonal and an intrapersonal factor [33, 34]. This differencing between the interpersonal and intrapersonal dimensions of self-transcendence is important. The outwardly dimension is an outgoing attitude and behavior, requiring a certain level of energy.

Thus, ailments such as fatigue and pain, etc., might not be a good companion for the outgoing or interpersonal way of expanding one's self-boundaries [35]. However, the inwardly dimension covers an inwardly process of self-acceptance and adaption to one's situation and functional capability, which has shown to explain the variation in quality of life/well-being better than the outgoing dimension among nursing home residents [36]. Furthermore, these two dimensions of self-transcendence seem to influence differently on other related constructs as well as the relationships between these constructs; these are perceived meaning-in-life [37], hope and nurse-patient interaction [35], depression [38], as well as physical, emotional, social, functional, and spiritual well-being [24, 25, 39]. Thus, this differentiation seems important clinically, theoretically, and scientifically.

9.4 Self-Transcendence Research

To gain a better understanding of the concept of self-transcendence as theorized here, it is helpful to review research on self-transcendence. Findings provide further insight into the breadth of vulnerable health conditions and experiences that self-transcendence is associated with or that influence human well-being in the midst of difficult life experiences. An overview of these results also suggests opportunities for developing and implementing health-promoting practices.

9.4.1 Initial Research: Depression and Cancer

Self-transcendence research in nursing was first published around the early 1990s with Reed's studies of self-transcendence as related to mental health and depression in older adults. Results consistently supported self-transcendence to be a significant correlate and sometimes predictor of depression in older adults (e.g., [11, 31, 32]). These results were repeated in subsequent research by others. For example, Klaas [40] studied self-transcendence and depression in 77 depressed and nondepressed elders, finding self-transcendence was negatively correlated with depressive feelings and positively correlated with meaning-in-life in these groups. Similarly, Haugan and Innstrand [38] found that self-transcendence significantly affected depression in 202 older nursing home residents. Moreover, self-transcendence was significantly inversely correlated with suicidal thoughts in older adults hospitalized for depression [41], and with depressive symptoms in a nursing home sample of Taiwanese older adults [42].

Doris Coward conducted several studies of self-transcendence in individuals across the trajectory of cancer, from initial diagnosis to late stage, and AIDS, and healthy individuals. She consistently found that self-transcendence was a significant correlate of various indicators of well-being involving self-esteem, hope, sense of coherence, and mental health [43–48], including especially those not considered medically healthy. Since then, self-transcendence research with individuals who have cancer has generated findings consistent with Coward's results.

9.4.2 Later Adulthood

Older adults and particularly the oldest-old (ages 80–100 years) represent a group of individuals who are very likely to be experiencing vulnerability in health conditions that they may or may not express to others. Research with them consistently reveals self-transcendence to be a key characteristic and likely contributor to their well-being [49]. For example, Reed [11] identified four patterns of self-transcendence to be more predominant in nondepressed than depressed oldest-old adults. Similarly, results from several studies by Haugan and colleagues support interpersonal and intrapersonal self-transcendence as clinically important in nurse-patient interactions to promote mental health in older adult nursing home residents [37, 38, 50, 51] and physical, emotional, social, functional, and spiritual well-being of older adults in nursing homes [24, 25, 35, 39]. Intrapersonal self-transcendence was among particularly significant health-promoting factors in long-term care residents [36]. Findings

suggested that caregivers of older adults in long-term care facilities and at home should look beyond custodial care to incorporate activities that build upon the residents' capacity for self-transcendence that can help them cope with the losses of later life.

Significant, positive, moderate size relationships were found [22] in a study of oldest-old adults between self-transcendence and indicators of well-being including resilience, sense of coherence, and purpose-in-life. In a longitudinal study by Norberg and her colleagues [52] of 190 oldest-old individuals in northern Sweden, self-transcendence was significantly related to well-being overall, but the accrual of negative life events over the 5 years effected a concerning decrease in self-transcendence. Self-transcendence is a vital but not inexhaustible psychosocial resource in older adults. For example, two different Norwegian studies among older adults in nursing homes showed that both interpersonal and intrapersonal self-transcendence were significantly influenced by the residents' perceived nurse-patient interaction [37, 51]. Walton and colleagues [53] identified a significant inverse relationship between self-transcendence and loneliness in older adults; this was supported by a recent Norwegian study among nursing home residents [54]. Hoshi [55] found that self-transcendence had a mediating effect on the relationship between vulnerability and well-being in 105 Japanese hospitalized elders. Last, self-transcendence was used to design a program to promote successful aging among older adults in the community; a series of studies generally supported the effectiveness of an intervention called the Psychoeducational Approach to Transcendence and Health (PATH) program (see [56–59]).

9.4.3 Chronic Conditions and Life-Threatening Illness

Self-care is an important aspect of health promotion in chronically ill individuals. Findings from several studies with older adults indicated that self-transcendence facilitates their engagement in instrumental activities of daily living [60, 61], and in medication adherence [62], as well as in managing stress in facing existential anxiety about the aging process [63].

Self-transcendence was found to reduce stress or enhance well-being in studies of several patient groups facing the vulnerability of serious, progressive disease including adults with multiple sclerosis and systemic lupus erythematosus [64], and in older women living with rheumatoid arthritis [65]. Results from a phenomenological study of individuals with spinal muscular atrophy indicated that self-transcendence was pivotal in maintaining a sense of integrity, hope, and meaning amidst the physical limitations experienced by this disease [66]. Similarly, individuals with amyotrophic lateral sclerosis nearing end-of-life in palliative care reported self-transcendence perspectives facilitated their sense of hope and well-being [67].

In additional research with individuals with cancer, self-transcendence was found to be an important mediator between vulnerability and well-being outcomes. Matthews and Cook [68] found that self-transcendence alone partially mediated the relationship between optimism and the outcome of emotional well-being in a sample of 93 women with breast cancer undergoing radiation treatment [68]. Farren's [69] study of 104 breast cancer survivors found self-transcendence to be a significant mediating factor in the relationship between women's participation in health care and their increased quality of life. Self-transcendence was identified as a mediator that reduced stress in men who had oral cancer [70], and in men who participated in a prostate cancer support group [71]. Finally, self-transcendence as experienced through spiritual practices promoted spiritual well-being among women with breast cancer [72].

Another group of individuals who likely experience increased vulnerability is transplant recipients. In two distinct studies of liver transplant recipients, self-transcendence was found to be positively related to quality of life and negatively related to fatigue [73] and to be a correlate and mediator of quality of life, decreasing the effects of illness distress [74]. Additionally, in a group of eight men and women who had received a stem cell transplantation 1 year prior to a phenomenology study, results suggested that effects of vulnerability on well-being were mediated by hard-won self-transcendence perspectives [75].

Homelessness presents individuals with ongoing sense of vulnerability and risks to well-being. Runquist and Reed [76] identified self-transcendence primarily, along with physical health status to be significant predictors of well-being in a sample of 61 homeless men and women, suggesting that facilitating well-being is not just a matter of providing for physical needs.

9.4.4 Nurses and Other Caregivers

Professional and family caregivers are vulnerable to diminished well-being given the nature of their challenging and stressful work and work environments. Indeed, Pask [77] elaborates on how professional nurses' self-transcendence can increase their own vulnerability without adequate support and education in their work setting. Research with family caregivers of adults with dementia starkly revealed their increased vulnerability—and thus increased risk to well-being—because of a lack of opportunities for self-transcendence within their emotional and social environment [78, 79]. On the other hand, opportunities to engage in caregiving as a self-transcendence practice facilitated personal growth and meaning among caregivers [80, 81]. Similarly, Kim et al. [82] found a significant relationship between self-transcendence and emotional well-being among family caregivers of chronically ill elders. Finally, research results also support the significance of self-transcendence for *parents* (caregivers) of children undergoing cancer treatment [83].

Self-transcendence has a role in nurse well-being. In a study sample of hospice and oncology nurses, who were vulnerable to burn out, self-transcendence was significantly inversely related to three types of burn out [84]. Palmer [85] and her colleagues found significant positive relationships between self-transcendence and vigor, dedication, and absorption in the work of 84 acute care staff registered nurses. Spiritual care intervention training resulted in increased self-transcendence as well as in spiritual well-being and positive attitudes toward work among palliative care professionals [86]. In research, using the two-factor constructs of self-transcendence by Haugan et al., [33] to create a measurement model, investigators found self-transcendence was not only significantly positively related to emotional well-being in Chinese nurses, but that self-transcendence facilitated and even "invigorated" caring behaviors [87].

9.4.5 A Value That Promotes Well-Being

Self-transcendence has been studied as one of the higher values whereby individuals feel concern for the welfare of others and interact in a way that expresses this value, for example by responding to others' needs, reaching out to marginalized individuals, being tolerant of differences, and altruism. It is conceptualized as a motivational value for growth as contrasted with the motivational value for conservation and protection. In classic work based upon a conceptual framework of values by Schwartz [88], self-transcendence was distinguished from self-enhancement values that focus on betterment of the *individual*, self-gratification, personal success, and prestige. His *Work Values Survey* continues to be used to investigate the influences of "self-transcendence" and other values. For example, a recent study in Germany by Seibert, Hillen, Pfaff, and Kuntz [89] using a *Work Values Survey* based on Schwartz's value dimensions indicated that self-transcendence as a value perspective in nurse leaders of neonatal intensive care units was significantly associated with a safer work climate, an experience considered to be highly important for nurse well-being.

Findings from another recent study of altruism indicated that self-transcendence, mediated by a multicultural perspective, was significantly related to a greater willingness to interact with People's Republic of China immigrants [90]. Altruism of self-transcendence was also evident in research by Fiske [91] who demonstrated that participating in a mission trip experience enhanced well-being.

9.5 Self-Transcendence and Applications for Health Promotion

Research findings overall support the significance of self-transcendence in contributing to health and well-being. Implications for health promotion can be drawn from the research, as well as from clinically based literature based on nurses' practice knowledge and reports of their work and the ways by which individuals expand boundaries to gain new insights for self-organizing and tackling difficult health-related situations that otherwise could fragment the individual.

Self-transcendence is a resource for well-being, regardless of health condition or diagnosis, across the lifespan from youth to end-of-life. Table 9.1 summarizes a selection of approaches, practices, or interventions that facilitate self-transcendence across individuals of various age groups and health/illness conditions.

Table 9.1 Sample of health promotion approaches to foster self-transcendence

Interventions to foster self-transcendence	References
Bereavement support groups	[92]
Peer support group	[92, 93]
Cancer support groups	[94–96]
Computer-mediated self-help intervention	[97]
Group psychotherapy	[98]
Therapeutic music video	[99, 100]
Family caregiver participation	[80]
Artmaking	[101, 102]
Memorial quilt making	[103]
Poetry writing	[104]
Expressive writing, journaling	[105]
Personal narratives	[106]
Psychoeducational Approach to Transcendence and Health (*PATH*) program	[57, 58]
Prayer and spiritual support activities	[107]
Meditation (integrative body-mind training)	[108]
Mindfulness meditation	[72, 109, 110]
Guided reminiscence intervention	[111, 112]
Life review	[113]
Nurse-patient interaction	[35, 37, 51]

9.6   Summary

As a process by which human beings may sustain well-being in times of vulnerability, self-transcendence is a salutogenic resource for expanding personal boundaries in ways that may enhance sense of well-being with broad application across the health continuum. It represents "both a human capacity and a human struggle that can be facilitated by nursing" ([30], p. 3) and specifically by the qualities embedded in the nurse-patient interaction [37, 51]. Self-transcendence theory offers an explanation as to how in the context of increased vulnerability individuals can nevertheless experience increased well-being. Achieving well-being involves intentional activity on the person's part, for example through intrapersonal reflection and interpersonal engagement that expand one's boundaries in ways that help the person find meaning in a difficult situation or gain a new sense of purpose after suffering loss. These and other behaviors that expand personal boundaries (self-transcendence) may transform loss or difficulty (increased vulnerability) into positive outcomes (well-being). Research indicates that self-transcendence is a resource for well-being, functioning either as a correlate or predictor of well-being, and as a mediator of the relationship between vulnerability and well-being across a variety of populations, particularly those experiencing serious illness or other challenging life situations. The scope of the theory has been broadened from its initial focus on later adulthood as the time of developmental maturity, to include others for whom life experiences stimulate growth and self-transcendence—individuals from adolescence on through adulthood, aging, and end-of-life who face challenging life situations that affect health and well-being. Children are another potential area for self-transcendence research. Future research and practice using self-transcendence theory may generate new discoveries about the processes by which people attain well-being.

Take Home Messages
- Self-transcendence is a salutogenic resource with broad application across the health continuum during the whole lifespan.
- Self-transcendence is a resource for well-being; it is an inner resource that becomes particularly salient during events or awareness of one's vulnerability that can diminish well-being.
- The nursing theory of self-transcendence is based on three main concepts: vulnerability, well-being, and self-transcendence. Each of these three concepts, and the relationships between them, may be moderated by personal and contextual factors such as age, gender, cognitive ability, health status, personal beliefs, social or spiritual support, other sociocultural factors and nursing interventions.
- Self-transcendence refers to perspectives and behaviors that expand (transcend) self-boundaries in multiple ways: *inwardly* (through intrapersonal activities and perspectives that enhance awareness of one's beliefs, values, and dreams), *outwardly* (through interpersonal connections with one's social and natural environments), *upwardly* (through perspectives and practices oriented beyond the ordinary or readily observable toward the transpersonal), and *temporally* (connecting perspectives of past and future to one's present).
- Without the capacity for self-transcendence, promotion of health and well-being might not be possible in difficult health situations. Self-transcendence, then, may be an underlying process that explains how well-being is possible in difficult or life-threatening situations that people endure.

References

1. Reed P. Theory of self-transcendence. In: Smith MJ, Liehr PR, editors. Middle range theory for nursing. 2nd ed. New York: Springer; 2008. p. 105–29.
2. Reed P. Theory of self-transcendence. In: Smith MJ, Liehr PR, editors. Middle range theory for nursing. 4th ed. New York: Springer; 2018. p. 119–46.
3. Reed P. Toward a nursing theory of self-transcendence: deductive reformulation using developmental theories. Adv Nurs Sci. 1991;13(4):64–77.
4. Lerner R, Hershberg R, Hilliard L, Johnson S. Concepts and theories of human development: historical and contemporary dimensions. In: Bornstein M, Lamb M, editors. Developmental science: an advanced textbook. 7th ed. New York: Psychology Press; 2015.

5. Lerner R, Lerner J. The development of a person: a relational–developmental systems perspective. In: McAdams D, Shiner R, Tackett J, editors. Handbook of personality development. New York: The Guilford Press; 2019. p. 59–75.

6. Overton W, Lerner R. Fundamental concepts and methods in developmental science: a relational perspective. Res Hum Dev. 2014;11(1):63–73.

7. Rogers M. Introduction to the theoretical basis of nursing. Philadelphia: F. A. Davis; 1970.

8. Rogers M. A science of unitary man. In: Riehl J, Roy C, editors. Conceptual modes for nursing practice. 2nd ed. New York: Appleton-Century-Crofts; 1980. p. 329–37.

9. Rogers M. Nursing: science of unitary, irreducible, human beings: update 1990. In: Barret E, editor. Visions of Rogers' science based nursing. New York: National League for Nursing Press; 1990. p. 5–12.

10. Stauffer M, Capuzzi D. Human growth and development across the lifespan. Hoboken: Wiley; 2016.

11. Reed P. Self-transcendence and mental health in oldest-old adults. Nurs Res. 1991;40:5–11.

12. Reed P, editor. The place of transcendence in nursing's science of unitary human beings: theory and research. New York: National League for Nursing Press; 1997.

13. Kauffman S. At home in the universe: the search for laws of self-organization and complexity. New York: Oxford University Press; 1995.

14. Reed P. Nursing: the ontology of the discipline. Nurs Sci Q. 1997;10(2):76–9.

15. Thauvoye E, Vanhooren S, Vandenhoeck A, Dezutter J. Spirituality among nursing home residents: a phenomenology of the experience of spirituality in late life. J Relig Spirituality Aging. 2019;32(1):88–103.

16. Burkhardt M, Nagai-Jacobson M. Spirituality: living our connectedness. New York: Delmar; 2002.

17. Jaberi A, Momennasab M, Yektatalab S, Ebadi A, Cheraghi M. Spiritual health: a concept analysis. J Relig Health. 2019;58(5):1537–60.

18. Hoseini A, Razaghi N, Panah A, Nayeri N. A concept analysis of spiritual health. J Relig Health. 2019;58(4):1025–46.

19. Nahardani S, Ahmadi F, Bigdeli S, Arabshahi K. Spirituality in medical education: a concept. Med Health Care Philos. 2019;22(2):179–89.

20. Mark G, Lyons A. Conceptualizing mind, body, spirit interconnections through, and beyond, spiritual healing practices. Explore (NY). 2014;10(5):294–9.

21. Puchalski C, Blatt B, Kogan M, Butler A. Spirituality and health: the development of a field. Acad Med. 2014;89(1):10–6.

22. Nygren B, Aléx L, Jonsén E, Gustafson Y, Norberg A, Lundman B. Resilience, sense of coherence, purpose in life and self-transcendence in relation to perceived physical and mental health among the oldest old. Aging Ment Health. 2005;9(4):354–62.

23. Nygren B, Norberg A, Lundman B. Inner strength as disclosed in narratives of the oldest old. Qual Health Res. 2007;17(8):1060–73.

24. Haugan G, Rannestad T, Hammervold R, Garåsen H, Espnes GA. Self-transcendence in nursing home patients—a resource for well-being. J Adv Nurs. 2013;69(5):1147–60.

25. Haugan G, Rannestad T, Hammervold R, Garåsen H, Espnes GA. The relationships between self-transcendence and spiritual well-being in cognitively intact nursing home patients. Int J Older People Nursing. 2014;9:65–78.

26. Akyalcin E, Greenway P, Milne L. Measuring self-transcendence: extracting core constructs. J Transpers Psychol. 2008;40(1):41–59.

27. Hanley A, Garland E. Spatial frame of reference as a phenomenological feature of self-transcendence: measurement and manipulation through mindfulness meditation. Psychol Conscious Theory Res Pract. 2019;6(4):329–45.

28. Levenson M, Jennings P, Aldwin C, Shiraishi R. Self-transcendence: conceptualization and measurement. Int J Aging Hum Dev. 2005;60(2):127–43.

29. Reed P. Demystifying self-transcendence for mental health nursing practice and research. Arch Psychiatr Nurs. 2009;23(5):397–400.

30. Reed P. Transcendence: formulating nursing perspectives. Nurs Sci Q. 1996;9(1):2–4.

31. Reed P. Developmental resources and depression in the elderly. Nurs Res. 1986;35:368–74.

32. Reed P. Mental health of older adults. West J Nurs Res. 1989;11(2):143–63.

33. Haugan G, Rannestad T, Garåsen H, Hammervold R, Espnes GA. The self-transcendence scale—an investigation of the factor structure among nursing home patients. J Holist Nurs. 2012;30(3):147–59.

34. Lundman B, Arestedt K, Norberg A, Fischer R, Norberg C, Lövheim H. Psychometric properties of the Swedish version of the self-transcendence scale among the oldest-old. J Nurs Meas. 2014;23(1):96–111.

35. Haugan G. Life satisfaction in cognitively intact long-term nursing-home patients: symptom distress, well-being and nurse-patient interaction. In: Sarracino F, Mikucka M, editors. Beyond money—the social roots of health and well-being. New York: NOVA Science Publishers, Inc; 2014. p. 165–211.

36. Haugan G, Moksnes UK, Løhre A. Intrapersonal self-transcendence, meaning-in-life and nurse-patient interaction: powerful assets for quality of life in cognitively intact nursing home patients. Scand J Caring Sci. 2016;30(4):790–801.

37. Haugan G, Kuven BM, Eide WM, Taasen SE, Rinnan E, Xi Wu V, et al. Nurse-patient interaction and self-transcendence: assets for a meaningful life in nursing home residents? BMC Geriatr. 2020;20:168. https://doi.org/10.1186/s12877-020-01555-2.

38. Haugan G, Innstrand ST. The effect of self-transcendence on depression in cognitively intact nursing home patients. ISRN Psychiatry. 2012;2012:301325.

39. Haugan G, Hanssen B, Moksnes UK. Self-transcendence, nurse-patient interaction and the outcome of multidimensional well-being in cognitively

intact nursing home patients. Scand J Caring Sci. 2013;27(4):882–93.

40. Klaas D. Testing two elements of spirituality in depressed and non-depressed elders. Int J Psychiatr Nurs Res. 1998;4(2):452–62.

41. Buchanan D, Farran C, Clark D. Suicidal thoughts and self-transcendence in older adults. J Psychosoc Nurs. 1995;33(10):31–4.

42. Hsu Y-C, Badger T, Reed P, Jones E. Factors associated with depressive symptoms in older Taiwanese adults in a long-term care community. Int Psychogeriatr. 2013;25(06):1013–21.

43. Coward DD. The lived experiences of self-transcendence in women with advanced breast cancer. Nurs Sci Q. 1990;3(4):162–9.

44. Coward DD. Self-transcendence and emotional well-being in women with advanced breast cancer. Oncol Nurs Forum. 1991;18:857–63.

45. Coward DD. The lived experience of self-transcendence in a breast cancer support group: II. Oncol Nurs Forum. 1995;30:291–300.

46. Coward DD. Self-transcendence and correlates in a healthy population. Nurs Res. 1996;45(2):116–21.

47. Coward DD, Kahn DL. Transcending breast cancer: making meaning from diagnosis and treatment. J Holist Nurs. 2005;23:264–83.

48. Coward DD, Kahn D. Resolution of spiritual disequilibrium by women newly diagnosed with breast cancer. Oncol Nurs Forum. 2004;31(2):E1–8.

49. Haugan G; Demirci, AD; Kabukcuoglu K, Aune, I. Self-transcendence among adults 65 years and older: A meta-analysis. Scand J Caring Sci. 2021. https://doi.org/10.1111/scs.12959.

50. Drageset J, Taasen S, Espehaug B, Kuven BM, Eide WM, Andre B, Rinnan E, Haugan G. Associations between nurse–patient interaction and sense of coherence among cognitively intact nursing home residents. J Holist Nurs. 2020.

51. Haugan G, Hanssen B, Rannestad T, Espnes GA. Self-transcendence and nurse-patient interaction in cognitively intact nursing-home patients. J Clin Nurs. 2012;21:3429–41.

52. Norberg A, Lundman B, Gustafson Y, Norberg C, Fischer R, Lövheim H. Self-transcendence (ST) among very old people—its associations to social and medical factors and development over five years. Arch Gerontol Geriatr. 2015;61(2):247–53.

53. Walton C, Shultz C, Beck C, Walls R. Psychological correlates of loneliness in the older adults. Arch Psychiatr Nurs. 1991;5(3):165–70.

54. Drageset J, Haugan G. The impact of nurse-patient interaction on loneliness among nursing home residents—a questionnaire survey. Geriatr Nurs. 2021 (In review).

55. Hoshi M. Self-transcendence, vulnerability, and well-being in hospitalized Japanese elders. Tucson: University of Arizona; 2008.

56. McCarthy V. A new look at successful aging: exploring a mid-range nursing theory among older adults in a low-income retirement community. J Theor Construct Test. 2011;15(1):17–23.

57. McCarthy V, Hall L, Crawford T, Connelly J. Facilitating self-transcendence: an intervention to enhance well-being in late life. West J Nurs Res. 2018;40(6):854–73.

58. McCarthy V, Jiying L, Bowland S, Hall L, Connelly J. Promoting self-transcendence and well-being in community-dwelling older adults: a pilot study of a psychoeducational intervention. Geriatr Nurs. 2015;26(6):431–7.

59. McCarthy V, Jiying L, Carini R. The role of self-transcendence: a missing variable in the pursuit of successful aging? Res Gerontol Nurs. 2013;6:178–86.

60. Upchurch S. Self-transcendence and activities of daily living: the woman with the pink slippers. J Holist Nurs. 1999;17:251–66.

61. Upchurch S, Muller WH. Spiritual influences on ability to engage in self-care activities among older African Americans. Int J Aging Hum Dev. 2005;60(1):77–94.

62. Thomas N, Dunn K. Self-transcendence and medication adherence in older adults with hypertension. J Holist Nurs. 2014;32(4):316–26.

63. Walker C. Transformative aging: how mature adults respond to growing older. J Theor Construct Test. 2002;6(2):109–16.

64. Iwamoto R, Yamawaki N, Sato T. Increased self-transcendence in patients with intractable diseases. Psychiatry Clin Neurosci. 2011;65:638–47.

65. Neill J. Transcendence and transformation in the life patterns of women living with rheumatoid arthritis. Adv Nurs Sci. 2002;24:27–47.

66. Ho H-M, Tseng Y-H, Hsin Y-M, Chou F-H, Lin W-T. Living with illness and self-transcendence: the lived experience of patients with spinal muscular atrophy. J Adv Nurs. 2016;72(11):2695–705.

67. Fanos J, Gelinas D, Foster R, Postone N, Miller R. Hope in palliative care: from narcissism to self-transcendence in amyotrophic lateral sclerosis. J Palliat Med. 2008;11(3):470–5.

68. Matthews EE, Cook PF. Relationships among optimism, well-being, self-transcendence, coping, and social support in women during treatment for breast cancer. Psycho-Oncology. 2009;18(7):716–26.

69. Farren AT. Power, uncertainty, self-transcendence, and quality of life in breast cancer survivors. Nurs Sci Q. 2010;23(1):63–71.

70. Chen H. Self-transcendence, illness perception, and depression in Taiwanese men with oral cancer. Unpublished doctoral dissertation. 2012 (in press).

71. Chin-A-Loy SS, Fernsler JI. Self-transcendence in older men attending a prostate cancer support group. Cancer Nurs. 1998;21(5):358–63.

72. Thomas JC, Burton M, Quinn Griffin MT, Fitzpatrick JJ. Self-transcendence, spiritual well-being, and spiritual practices of women with breast cancer. J Holist Nurs. 2010;28(2):115–22.

73. Wright K. Quality of life, self-transcendence, illness distress, and fatigue in liver transplant recipients. Unpublished doctoral dissertation. 2003 (in press).

74. Bean KB, Wagner K. Self-transcendence, illness distress, and quality of life among liver transplant recipients. J Theor Construct Test. 2006;10(2):47–53.

75. Williams B. Self-transcendence in stem cell transplantation recipients: a phenomenologic inquiry. Oncol Nurs Forum. 2012;39(4):E41–8.

76. Runquist JJ, Reed PG. Self-transcendence and well-being in homeless adults. J Holist Nurs. 2007;25(1):5–13.

77. Pask EJ. Self-sacrifice, self-transcendence and nurses' professional self. Nurs Philos. 2005;6(4):247–54.

78. Acton G. Self-transcendent views and behaviors: exploring growth in caregivers of adults with dementia. J Gerontol Nurs. 2002;28(12):22–30.

79. Acton G, Wright K. Self-transcendence and family caregivers of adults with dementia. J Holist Nurs. 2000;18:143–58.

80. Milberg A, Strang P. What to do when 'there is nothing more to do'? A study within a salutogenic framework of family members' experience of palliative home care staff. Psycho-Oncology. 2007;16(8):741–51.

81. Enyert G, Burman M. A qualitative study of self-transcendence in caregivers of terminally ill patients. Am J Hosp Palliat Care. 1999;16(2):455–62.

82. Kim S-S, Reed PG, Hayward RD, Kang Y, Koenig HG. Spirituality and psychological well-being: testing a theory of family interdependence among family caregivers and their elders. Res Nurs Health. 2011;34(2):103–15.

83. Bajjani-Gebara J, Reed P. Nursing theory as a guide into uncharted waters: research with parents of children undergoing cancer treatment. Appl Nurs Res. 2016;32:14–7.

84. Hunnibell LS, Reed PG, Quinn-Griffin M, Fitzpatrick JJ. Self-transcendence and burnout in hospice and oncology nurses. J Hosp Palliat Nurs. 2008;10(3):172–9.

85. Palmer B, Griffin MTQ, Reed PG, Fitzpatrick JJ. Self-transcendence and work engagement in acute care staff registered nurses. Crit Care Nurs Q. 2010;33(2):138–47.

86. Wasner M, Longaker C, Fegg M, Borasio G. Effects of a spiritual care training for palliative care professionals. Palliat Med. 2004;18:347.

87. Hwang H-L, Tu C-T, Chan H-S. Self-transcendence, caring and their associations with well-being. J Adv Nurs. 2019;75:1473–83.

88. Schwartz S. A proposal for measuring value orientations across nations. Adv Exp Soc Psychol. 1992;25:1–65.

89. Seibert M, Hillen H, Pfaff H, Kuntz L. Exploring leading nurses' work values and their association with team safety climate: results from a questionnaire survey in neonatal intensive care units. J Nurs Manag. 2020;28:112–9.

90. Michelle Y, Lim A, Pauketat J. Values predict willingness to interact with immigrants: the role of cultural ideology and multicultural acquisition. J Cross-Cult Psychol. 2020;51(1):3–24.

91. Fiske E. Self-transcendence, well-being, and vulnerability in healthcare mission participants. Nurs Sci Q. 2019;32(4):306–13.

92. Joffrion L, Douglas D. Grief resolution: facilitating self-transcendence in the bereaved. J Psychosoc Nurs. 1994;32(3):13–9.

93. Jadid M, Ashktorab T, Abed SZ, Alayi M. The impact of self-transcendence on physical health status promotion in multiple sclerosis patients attending peer support groups. Int J Nurs Pract. 2015;2(6):725–32.

94. Coward DD. Facilitation of self-transcendence in a breast cancer support group: II. Oncol Nurs Forum. 2003;30:291–300.

95. Coward DD, Reed PG. Self-transcendence: a resource for healing at the end of life. Issues Ment Health Nurs. 1996;17(3):275–88.

96. Coward DD. Facilitation of self-transcendence in a breast cancer support group. Oncol Nurs Forum. 1998;25:75–84.

97. DiNapoli J, Garcia-Dia M, Garcia-Ona L, O'Flaherty D, Siller J. A theory-based computer mediated communication intervention to promote mental health and reduce high-risk behaviors in the LGBT population. Appl Nurs Res. 2014;27(1):91–3.

98. Young C, Reed P. Elders' perceptions of the effectiveness of group psychotherapy in fostering self-transcendence. Arch Psychiatr Nurs. 1995;9:338–47.

99. Robb S, Burns D, Stegenga K, Haut P, Monahan P, Meza J, et al. Randomized clinical trial of therapeutic music video intervention for resilience outcomes in adolescents/young adults undergoing hematopoietic stem cell transplant: a report from the Children's Oncology Group. Cancer. 2014;120(6):909–17.

100. Burns D, Robb S, Haase J. Exploring the feasibility of a therapeutic music video intervention in adolescents and young adults during stem cell transplantation. Cancer Nurs. 2009;32(5):8–16.

101. Chen S, Walsh S. Effect of a creative-bonding intervention on Taiwanese nursing students' self-transcendence and attitudes toward elders. Res Nurs Health. 2009;32:204–16.

102. Walsh S, Radcliffe S, Castillo L, Kumar A, Broschard D. A pilot study to test the effect of art-making classes for family caregivers of patients with cancer. Oncol Nurs Forum. 2007;34(1):1–8.

103. Kausch K, Amer K. Self-transcendence and depression among AIDS memorial quilt panel makers. J Psychosoc Nurs. 2007;45(6):45–53.

104. Kausch KD, Amer K. Self-transcendence and depression among AIDS Memorial Quilt panel makers. J Psychosoc Nurs Ment Health Serv. 2007;45(6):44–53.

105. Kidd L, Zauszniewski J, Morris D. Benefits of a poetry writing intervention for family caregivers

of elders with dementia. Issues Ment Health Nurs. 2011;32:598–604.

106. Diener JES. Personal narrative as an intervention to enhance self-transcendence in women with chronic illness. Saint Louis: University of Missouri; 2003.

107. Haase JE, Britt T, Coward DD, Leidy NK, Penn PE. Simultaneous concept analysis of spiritual perspective, hope, acceptance and self-transcendence. Image J Nurs Sch. 1992;24(2):141–7.

108. McGee E. Alcoholics anonymous and nursing. J Holist Nurs. 2000;18(1):11–26.

109. Sharpnack PA, Benders AM, Fitzpatrick JJ. Self-transcendence and spiritual well-being in the Amish. J Holist Nurs. 2011;29(2):91–7.

110. Sharpnack P, Quinn Griffin M, Benders A, Fitzpatrick J. Spiritual and alternative healthcare practices of the Amish. Holist Nurs Pract. 2010;24:64–72.

111. Vago D, Silbersweig D. Self-awareness, self-regulation, and self-transcendence (SAR-T): a framework for understanding the neurobiological mechanisms of mindfulness. Front Hum Neurosci. 2012;6:296–316.

112. Vitale S, Shaffer C, Fenton H. Self-transcendence in Alzheimer's disease: the application of theory in practice. J Holist Nurs. 2014;23(4):347–55.

113. Stinson CK, Kirk E. Structured reminiscence: an intervention to decrease depression and increase self-transcendence in older women. J Clin Nurs. 2006;15(2):208–18.

Nurse-Patient Interaction: A Vital Salutogenic Resource in Nursing Home Care

10

Gørill Haugan

Abstract

We are now witnessing a major change in the world's population. Many people globally grow very old: 80, 90, and 100 years. Increased age is followed by an increased incidence of functional and chronic comorbidities and diverse disabilities, which for many leads to the need for long-term care in a nursing home. Quality of life and health promotive initiatives for older persons living in nursing homes will become ever more important in the years to come. Therefore, this chapter focuses on health promotion among older adults living in nursing homes. First, this chapter clarifies the concepts of health, salutogenesis, and pathogenesis, followed by knowledge about health promotion. Then insight and knowledge about the nursing home population is provided; what promotes health and well-being in nursing home residents?

Health promotion in the health services should be based on integrated knowledge of salutogenesis and pathogenesis. The saluto-genic understanding of health is holistic and considers man as a wholeness including physical, mental, social, and spiritual/existential dimensions. Research indicates that various health-promoting interventions, specifically the nurse–patient interaction, influence on older adults in nursing homes as a wholeness of body–soul–spirit, affecting the whole being. Hence, dimensions such as pain, fatigue, dyspnea, nausea, loneliness, anxiety, and depressive symptoms will be influenced through health-promoting approaches. Therefore, two separate studies on the health-promoting influences of nurse–patient interaction in nursing home residents were conducted. In total, nine hypotheses of directional influence of the nurse–patient interaction were tested, all of which finding support.

Along with competence in pain and symptom management, health-promoting nurse–patient interaction based on awareness and attentional skills is essential in nursing home care. Thus, health care workers should be given the opportunity to further develop their knowledge and relational skills, in order to "refine" their way of being present together with residents in nursing homes. Health professionals' competence involves the "*being in the doing*"; that is, both the *doing* and the way of *being* are essential in health and nursing care.

G. Haugan (✉)
Department of Public Health and Nursing, NTNU Norwegian University of Science and Technology, Trondheim, Norway

Faculty of Nursing and Health Science, Nord University, Levanger, Norway
e-mail: gorill.haugan@ntnu.no,
gorill.haugan@nord.no

G. Haugan, M. Eriksson (eds.), *Health Promotion in Health Care – Vital Theories and Research*,
https://doi.org/10.1007/978-3-030-63135-2_10

Keywords

Health promotion · Holistic health concept ·
Nursing home · Nurse–patient interaction ·
Salutogenesis and pathogenesis · Salutogenic
nursing home care · Spiritual care · The
"Being in the Doing"

10.1 Background

Currently, the world faces a shift to an older population; 125 million people are now aged 80 years
or older [1].While this shift started in high-
income countries (e.g., in Japan 30% of the population is already over 60 years old), it is now
low- and middle-income countries that are
experiencing the greatest change. Today, most
people can expect to live into their 60s and
beyond [1]. Between 2015 and 2050, the proportion of the world's population over 60 years will
nearly double from 12% to 22%; by 2050, the
world's population aged 60 years and older is
expected to total two billion, up from 900 million
in 2015 [1, 2]. Soon 30% of the world's population is 60 years and older. All countries in the
world face major challenges to ensure that their
health and social systems are ready to make the
most of this demographic shift [1].

There is, however, little evidence to suggest
that older people today are experiencing their
later years in better health than their parents. Age
is no disease. Yet, most chronically ill people
today are older adults. Increased age is followed
by an increased incidence of functional and
chronic comorbidities and diverse disabilities [3],
which for many leads to the need for long-term
care in a nursing home (NH). Accordingly, the
WHO's Global Strategy and Action Plan on
Aging and Health [1] includes the development
of systems for providing long-term care as one
among five priority areas for action. Systems of
long-term care are needed in all countries to meet
the needs of older people.

As people live longer, it is important to ensure
that the extra years of life are worth living, despite
chronic illnesses. This is important not only to
the individual elderly, but also to the families, the
local community as well as the society. Quality-
of-life (QoL) and health promotive initiatives for
older persons living in NHs will become ever
more important in the years to come. Therefore,
this chapter focuses on health promotion among
older adults living in NHs. First, this chapter clarifies the concept of health, followed by knowledge about health promotion. Then insight and
knowledge about the NH population is provided;
what is health and health promotion in the NH
context?

10.2 The Salutogenic Concept of Health

To promote health, we need knowledge of what
health is and what creates health and thus well-
being. Instead of focusing only on disease and
risk of disease (framed as pathogenesis), Aron
Antonovsky [4] focused on "What creates
health?" This question was the starting point of
the salutogenic understanding of health, which
represents a turning point in the understanding of
health research. An increasing number of
researchers have now realized that a unilateral
focus on disease and risks of getting sick (pathogenesis) does not necessarily increase or
strengthen an individual's health [5]. The human
life is multifaceted; people's health is exposed to
many different types of stress, to which the individual responds differently. Not everyone gets
sick from major stresses, risk factors, losses, crises, and illness. Who are the salutogenic ones,
those who maintain health despite stressing life
circumstances? What makes them go through
these negative life events without getting sick?
Do they just have luck? And others bad luck? Or
are there any salutogenic resources that preserve
health during difficult circumstances?

Antonovsky [4, 6] is considered the "father of
salutogenesis." The concept of salutogenesis
originates from the Greek notion of "*salus*"
which means health and the Latin term "*genesis*"
which means origin. Bottom line, salutogenesis—the salutogenic understanding of health and
the gradually evolving salutogenic concepts—
signifies knowledge about the origin of health,
that is, knowledge of what gives, facilitates, and

supports health. From a salutogenic perspective, health is a positive concept involving social and personal resources, as well as physical capacities. The concept of salutogenesis has matured since 1986 and has become a core theory of health promotion [5].

The salutogenic concept of health is holistic [4], considering man as a wholeness including a physical, mental, social, and spiritual/existential dimension. Nursing and other health professions are grounded in the holistic understanding of health, implying that human beings consist of these above-mentioned four dimensions [7]. However, by theoretically splitting the human into four, man is no longer one unit, but four "divorced" parts, which is contradictory. Health care is largely based on this fragmentation of man which causes unnecessarily suffering; often patients feel treated like a diagnosis, a case, or an object the doctor is treating and health professionals are controlling, and not as a whole living person. Figure 10.1 illustrates the entity of the human being involving a physical, emotional, social, and spiritual/existential dimension. However, this picture of a human being divided into four parts, dimensions or levels, is merely theoretical. Figure 10.1 has a red dotted line which circulates; even though we theoretically claim that there are different dimensions in the whole, it is still a

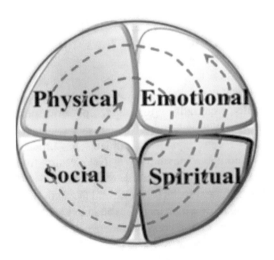

Fig. 10.1 The wholeness of man involving a physical, emotional, social, and spiritual/existential dimension, interrelated by a steady interaction between the dimensions. ©Gørill Haugan

whole because these four dimensions are integrated into each other and act like an entirely integrated wholeness, a human being. A constantly ongoing interaction integrates the dimensions or levels in the whole [8], all controlled via the brain [10]. Nothing is "just emotional" or "just physical," everything is integrated into everything. In human being, everything is interrelated and influences on everything.

Hence, man is a unique and indivisible physical-psycho-social-spiritual entity in which body, mind, and spirit are integrated and constantly interact with each other, right down to the microcellular level [9, 10]. That is, the human experiences, expectations, thoughts, and feelings are physiological states or biochemical conditions in the body, with subsequent bodily consequences impacting the whole being [11]. Research has shown and shows ever more clearly that there are connections (interaction) between the mind (our thoughts, feelings, and experiences) and the body in the development of most diseases and ailments [12]. Negative emotions and prolonged stress expose the organ systems to stress that can result in illness. Our emotions are biochemical realities in our bodies. Since they have nowhere else to be, we feel and recognize our emotions in the body [11]. Candace Pert is an internationally recognized stress researcher showing that the brain "talks" to the immune cell system by means of "messenger cells" called neuropeptides or transmitters. When the brain interprets emotions such as fear, anger, or sadness, all the immune cells are told about this interpretation. Pert [11] describes this process as "bits of the brain floating around the body." Simply put, our emotions and thoughts "float around the body," materialized as peptides (protein molecules) and a myriad of complex chemical and physiological processes. Studies on stress have claimed that feeling fear triggers more than 1400 known physical and chemical stress reactions, activating more than 30 different hormones and neurotransmitters [13]. Furthermore, the stress literature highlights that positive attitudes and expectations are not just changing moods, but biological realities in the body. Seligman [14] and Keyes [15–18] have shown that optimism and "flourishing" have a great positive impact on human health. Several studies have shown that a specific kind of white blood cells called "natural killer cells," increase during cognitive therapy, as well as by various relaxation and visualization techniques [19, 20]. Recent research implies that for example perceived meaning-in-life is important for maintaining not only mental/emotional well-being, but physical and functional well-being as well [21–23]. A novel study demonstrated humans' holistic existence showing that perceived meaning-in-life as well as loneliness affected older adults' brain function [23]. These findings advance our understanding of phenomenon such as meaning and loneliness which operate not only by emotions or experiences but represent physical states in human's brains [23]. Loneliness and meaning-in-life are reflected in the intrinsic network architecture of the brain. Thus, various health-promoting interventions, tailored to the individual and specific context, influence on the patient as body–mind–spirit impacting on the whole being. Accordingly, dimensions such as pain, fatigue, dyspnea, nausea, anxiety, and depressive symptoms will be affected through health-promoting approaches.

10.3 Health Promotion

The first international conference on health promotion was held by the World Health Organization in Ottawa, Canada, in 1986. Here, the Ottawa Charter [24] was drafted and approved, describing health promotion as "… *the process of enabling individuals and communities to increase control over the determinants of health and thereby improve their health*" [24]. Transferred to the health services, health promotion entails to develop the individual's health promotion skills by providing information, knowledge, support, guidance, care, and coping techniques. Furthermore, the goal is to reorient the health service in a health-promoting direction; the Norwegian Directorate of Health highlighted this as early as 1987 [25]. However, according to the Shanghai declaration of promoting health [26], it seems important to re-emphasize this primarily positive orientation of health promotion, as indicated in the 1986 Ottawa Charter [5, 27]. The Shanghai declaration from 2016 recognizes that health and well-being are essential to achieving sustainable development. Consequently, not only hospitals but also NHs should be developed in a health-promoting direction.

It is important to emphasize that health promotion approaches do not mean a disregard of pathogenesis. Knowledge of pathogenesis, i.e., knowledge of disease, risk, and prevention, is important in all health disciplines and of course in the health services. When people get injured or ill, whether it be heart disease, lung disease, cancer disease, mental illness, or the need for a surgical intervention, knowledge of illnesses, injuries, and trauma, as well as the treatment of them, is crucial to peoples' lives. However, the health services now need a clear and explicit synthesis of pathogenesis and salutogenesis; both paradigms are important. Instead of juxtaposing pathogenesis and salutogenesis, they should be integrated into a holistic way of understanding and working with health. Humans' health should not only be treated, but also promoted and facilitated. Health is always present, while illness and injury occur from time to time. Thus, health is the basic and the origin and should therefore be the basis, on which the health services are founded. What might health promotion look like in the NH population?

10.4 Older Adults in Nursing Homes

The NH population is characterized by high age, frailty, mortality, disability, powerlessness, dependency, vulnerability, poor general health, and a high symptom burden [3, 22, 28]. Accordingly, moving to a NH results from numerous losses, illnesses, disabilities, loss of functions and social relations, and facing the end-of-life, all of which increases an individual's vulnerability and distress. Residents in NHs have few opportunities to make personal decisions or exercise control over their lives. Many residents perceive their institutionalization as the beginning of their loss of independence and autonomy

[29–31]. Idleness and time spent in passive activities, such as doing nothing, sleeping, and waiting is commonplace among NH residents [32, 33], which leads to feelings of boredom, loneliness, and indignity [34–37]. Residents have used terms like trapped, stuck, confined, isolated, and discouraged to describe how they feel about the institutional life [29].

Consequently, the NH population is at a high risk of declined well-being and quality-of-life (QoL) [38–40]. Finding approaches to increase well-being among older adults in NHs is highly warranted. Responding to this need, the approach framed "Joy-of-Life-Nursing-Homes" (JoLNH) was developed in Norway. The JoLNH is a national strategy for promoting well-being, meaning and QoL among NH patients [41]. In accordance with recent research [37, 42–45], the JoLNH national strategy implies implementation of the "Joy-of-Life" philosophy and working approach emphasizing that spiritual and emotional needs such as perceived meaning and joy-of-life, culture, meaningful activity, connectedness, relationships, and enjoyment shall be integrated essentials of NH care. Based on the theoretical framework of salutogenesis [4, 6], well-being theory [17, 46, 47] and qualitative in-depth interviews with 29 NH residents, a conceptual structure depicting the essence of the joy-of-life phenomenon in NHs, were derived [48], and a quantitative measurement model for joy-of-life was developed and framed the Joy-of-Life Scale (JoLS) [49]. These qualitative findings revealed that positive relationships, belongingness, meaning, moments of feeling well, and acceptance conceptualized the essence of the joy-of-life phenomenon among NH residents [48].

10.4.1 Vital Salutogenic Resources in Nursing Home Care

Studies of social support in the NH population [50, 51] show significant correlations with well-being. A systematic review on well-being among older adults staying in care facilities identified four themes: (1) acceptance and adaptation, (2) attachment to others, (3) home environment, and (4) qualities in the relationship with their caregivers [52]. Moreover, a recent study among elderly in NHs showed that spiritual well-being was strongly associated with the experience of support, trust, meaning-in-life, and a perspective beyond death [53]. Experience of meaning, which is a central aspect of spiritual and emotional well-being, has also shown a clear connection with belonging/affiliation [54, 55], as well as with satisfaction [56] and dignity [37] among NH residents. Self-transcendence [57] and meaning [21, 22] are shown to explain variation in well-being, physically, emotionally, socially, functionally, and spiritually, among older adults in NHs. This means that if self-transcendence, joy-of-life, and perceived meaning-in-life increase, also the resident's well-being—physically, emotionally, socially, functionally, and spiritually—will increase. Connectedness is seen to be essential in self-transcendence, meaning, and joy-of-life.

Older people experience changes in roles, relationships, and living environments that increase their risk for experiencing social isolation and loneliness, particularly when moving to a NH. With advancing age, it is inevitable that people lose connection with their friendship networks and find it more difficult to initiate new friendships and to belong to new networks. Older adults living in NHs often experience limited opportunities for social connection despite proximity to peers [58], which has implications for mental health and QoL [59].

10.5 The Nurse–Patient Relationship: Connectedness and Well-Being

A link between well-being and connectedness is emerging in the literature [60]. Despite old age, chronical diseases, or frailty, the desire for affiliation and social bonding is an intrinsic human need, also when living in a NH. Deprivation of intimate relationships and social engagement adversely affects the physical and emotional well-being of older people. Loneliness and depression are detrimental to elderly individuals' emotional well-being [51, 61–64]. Older adults describe loneliness as "an aversive emotional state" which is associated with negative and painful feelings, "isolated from intimate relationships," "being deprived from social and external support systems," and "being abused and neglected" [65]. A lack or loss of companionship and an inability to integrate into the social environment are critical correlates of loneliness [66, 67], which is seen to associate with mortality among older adults [68–70].

A systematic review of living well in elderly care homes identified four key themes: (1) connectedness with others, (2) caring practices, (3) acceptance and adaptation, and (4) a homelike environment [52]. Moreover, studies have identified a sense of belonging (connectedness) as a core issue for well-being among NH residents [43, 48, 71–74] pointing at "feelings of support and trust," "searching for meaning and finding answers," and "a perspective beyond death" as essential to their spiritual well-being [53]. A sense of belonging and connectedness contribute to meaning-in-life [54, 55] as well as NH resident satisfaction [56] and dignity [37]. Resident's dignity was recently described related to "slow care" [75]; that is, care without rushing anything, which is seen to be particular important in care of people having dementia [76]. Accordingly, studies have shown that positive experiences in NHs can occur and are important for residents' QoL and well-being [43, 48, 52, 53, 77]. To facilitate such positive experiences, relationship-centered approaches seem required [52, 53, 78, 79].

Through the last decades, the importance of establishing the nurse–patient relationship as an integral component of nursing practice has been well documented [80–83]. International well-accepted nursing theorists describe nursing as a participatory process that transcends the boundaries between patient and nurse and can be learned and knowingly deployed to facilitate well-being [84–91]. The perspective of promoting health and well-being is fundamental in nursing and a major nursing concern in long-term care [92–94].

Communication is an important aspect of nursing; typically, a nurse's duties cannot be performed without communication with her patients.

The quality of care and the care ethics are embedded in the nurse–patient relationship. Some attributes of this relationships have been identified by older adults: in a milieu of openness and trust, the qualities of intimacy, sense of belonging, caring, empathy, respect, and reciprocity [71] appear to be health promoting, supporting resident's joy-of-life, healing, strength, and/or growth [45, 71, 95–97].

Caring nurses engage in person-to-person relationships with the NH resident as a unique person. Excellent nursing care is defined by the nurses' way of "being present" together with the older adult while performing the different nursing activities, in which attitudes and competence are inseparably connected. The competent nurse is present and respectful, sincere, friendly, sensitive, and responsive to the NH resident's feelings of vulnerability; she understands his needs, is compassionate to different sufferings, and provides emotional support and confirmation [56, 80, 81, 98, 99]. Thus, nursing care as a moral relational practice increases patients' well-being; qualitatively good nurse–patient interaction helps patients gain a sense of trust, safety, comfort, confirmation, value, dignity, and enhanced well-being (ibid). The experience of being listened to is crucial to long-term care patients, since this is how they experience feeling good, satisfied, valued, and cared about [100, 101], as a part of slow care [75]. Frustration and suffering result from the experience of not being attended to or treated with indifference [96, 102–104]. The nurse–patient interaction performs to be a fundamental health-promoting resource for older adults in NHs. Therefore, we conducted two studies investigating possible impacts of the nurse–patient interaction on well-being in the Norwegian NH population.

10.6 Nurse–Patient Interaction Is a Salutary Factor: Two Norwegian Examples

These two studies were conducted to investigate the possible influences of NH residents' perceived nurse–patient interaction on multidimen-

Fig. 10.2 Hypothesized relationships between nurse–patient interaction and variables found to be highly and significantly correlated with well-being

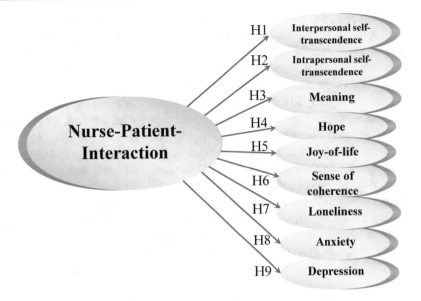

sional well-being. In order to do so, a total of nine hypotheses of direct relationships between nurse–patient interaction and interpersonal (H1) and intrapersonal (H2) self-transcendence, perceived meaning-in-life (H3), hope (H4), joy-of-life (H5), sense of coherence (H6), loneliness (H7), anxiety (H8), and depression (H9) were tested using advanced statistics such as SEM and regression analysis. Since evidence has shown that self-transcendence, meaning, hope, joy-of-life, and sense of coherence are highly positively correlated with well-being in vulnerable populations such as NH residents, these variables were included. Likewise, loneliness, anxiety and depression were selected since they are detrimental to NH residents' well-being. Figure 10.2 portrays the hypothesized directional influence of the nurse–patient interaction (H1–H9).

10.7 Methods

10.7.1 Data Collection

Study 1 collected cross-sectional data in 2008–2009 from 202 residents in 44 different Norwegian NHs; a total of nine different scales were included which totaled 130 items [94]. Study 2 was conducted in 2017–2018 and col-

lected cross-sectional data from 188 residents in 27 different NHs, including seven scales corresponding to 120 items [105]. In total, nine hypotheses of direct relationships between nurse–patient interaction and interpersonal (ST1) and intrapersonal (ST2) self-transcendence, perceived meaning-in-life, hope, joy-of-life, sense of coherence, loneliness, anxiety, and depression were tested.

Inclusion criteria were the same in both studies except residential time, which was 6 months for study 1 and 3 months for study 2: (1) local authority's decision of long-term NH care; (2) residential time 3/6 months or longer; (3) informed consent competency recognized by responsible doctor and nurse; and (4) capable of being interviewed. A nurse who knew the residents well presented them with oral and written information about their rights as participants to withdraw at any time. Each participant provided written informed consent.

Due to impaired vision, problems holding a pen, etc., this population has difficulties completing a questionnaire on their own; therefore, both studies conducted one-on-one interviews by three (study 1) and six (study 2) trained researchers in the informant's private room in the NH. Researchers with identical professional background (RN, MA, trained, and experienced in communication with elderly, as well as teaching gerontology at an advanced level) were trained to conduct the interviews as identically as possible. The questionnaires relevant for these two studies were part of a battery of nine (study 1) and seven (study 2) scales comprising 130 and 120 items, respectively. To avoid misunderstandings, the interviewers held a large-print copy of questions and possible responses in front of the participants. Approval by the Regional Committee for Medical and Health Research Ethics in Central Norway (Study1: Ref.no.4.2007.645, Study 2: Ref.nr 2014/2000/REK Central) was obtained as well as from the Management Units at the 44 (Study 1) and 27 (Study 2) NHs.

10.7.2 Participants Study 1

The sample consisted of 202 (80.8% response rate) of 250 residents who met the inclusion criteria. These 202 participants represented 44 different NHs in central Norway. Ages ranged from 65 to 104 years, with an average of 86 years (SD = 7.65). A total of 146 women (72.3%) and 56 men (27.7%) participated; the mean age was 87.3 and 82 years, for women and men, respectively. In this sample, 38 (19%) were married or cohabiting, 135 (67%) widowed, 11 (5.5%) divorced, and 18 (19%) single. The average residence time in the NH at the time of the interview was 2.6 years (range 0.5–13 years); 117 participants stayed in rural municipalities while 85 stayed in urban municipalities. Long-term NH care was defined as a 24 hours day care for 6 months or longer; short-term and rehabilitation stays along with patients diagnosed with dementia were not included. The data were collected in 2008–2009.

10.7.3 Participants Study 2

This sample consisted of 188 (92% response rate) out of 204 long-term residents who met the inclusion criteria. These 188 represented 27 different NHs in two large and two smaller urban municipalities in Norway. A total of 88 participants lived in certified joy-of-life NHs, while 100 lived in ordinary NHs. Age ranged from 63 to 104 years, with an average of 87.4 years (SD = 8.57). A total of 132 women (73.33%) and 48 men (26.67%) participated; the mean age was 88.3 years (SD = 1.80) for women and 86 years (SD = 1.16) for men. In this sample, 23 (12.2%) were married, 22 (11.7%) cohabitants, 1 (0.5%) single, 106 (56.4%) widowed, and 37 (19.7%) divorced. Long-term care in NHs was defined as 24 hours day care for 3 months or longer; short-term stays, rehabilitation stays, and residents diagnosed with dementia were not included. The data were collected during 2017–2018.

10.7.4 Measurements

The variables involved in Fig. 10.2 were measured using different scales translated into Norwegian and validated in the Norwegian NH population. Both studies involved the nurse–patient interaction scale, self-transcendence scale, the purpose-in-life test, and the hospital anxiety and depression scale. Additionally, study 1 included the Herth Hope Index, and study 2 included the joy-of-life scale, the orientation to life questionnaire and a global question assessing loneliness.

The Nurse–Patient Interaction Scale (NPIS) assessed nurse–patient interaction. The NPIS was developed in Norway to measure the NH patients' sense of well-being derived from the nurse–patient interaction [80, 96, 100, 106]. The NPIS comprises 14 items identifying essential relational qualities stressed in the nursing literature; a validation study in an NH population demonstrated good psychometric properties [97]. The NPIS is a 10-point scale from 1 (not at all) to 10 (very much); higher numbers indicate better perceived nurse–patient interaction.

The Self-Transcendence Scale (STS) developed by Reed [107, 108] was used to measure self-transcendence. The STS comprises 15 items reflecting expanded boundaries of self, identified by intrapersonal, interpersonal, transpersonal, and temporal experiences [109], all of which are characteristics of a matured view of life. Each item is rated on a 4-point Likert-type scale from 1 (not at all) to 4 (very much); higher scores indicate higher self-transcendence. The STS has been translated into Norwegian and validated in NH patients [110] showing a two-factor construct (STS1 and STS2) to be most valid and reliable among NH patients [110]. In the present studies, we applied this two-factor construct.

The Purpose-in-Life (PIL) test: Based on Viktor Frankl's [111] logotherapy, Crumbaugh and Maholick developed the PIL test [112] to assess perceived purpose and meaning-in-life. The PIL comprises 20 items worded as statements. Each statement is scored from 1 to 7; 4 represents a neutral value, whereas the numbers from 1 to 7 stretch along a continuum from one extreme feeling to the opposite kind of feeling. Higher numbers indicate stronger meaning-in-life. As part of study 1, the Norwegian version of the PIL was validated among NH residents [113], showing good psychometric properties.

The Herth Hope Index [114] assessed hope in study 1. The Herth Hope Index (HHI) comprises 12 items assessed on a 4-point Likert scale; the HHI was validated among older adults in Norwegian NHs and found to have good psychometric properties [115].

The Joy-of-life Scale (JoLS) was developed and validated for use in study 2. The JoLS includes 13 items on a 7-point scale ranging from 1 (not at all) to 7 (very much); higher number indicating stronger JOL. The JoLS demonstrated good psychometric properties in the NH population [49].

The Orientation to Life Questionnaire (OLQ) measured sense of coherence (SOC) [116]. Based in the salutogenic health theory, Antonovsky (1987) developed the original 29-item OLQ, measuring SOC. Later the 13-item short version of the OLQ was developed; the Norwegian version of the short OLQ-13 was used in the present study, rating the items on a 7-point scale providing two anchoring verbal responses, e.g., "very seldom or never" and "very often." Total score ranges from 13 to 91; higher scores indicate a stronger SOC [4, 6]. The OLQ was recently validated among nursing home residents and demonstrated satisfactory psychometric properties.

The Hospital Anxiety and Depression Scale (HADS) [117] comprising 14 items includes sub-scales for anxiety (HADS-A 7 items) and depression (HADS-D 7 items). Each item is rated from 0 to 3, where higher scores indicate more anxiety and depression. The maximum score is 21 on each subscale. The HADS has shown good to acceptable reliability and validity in the NH population [118]. The global question "Do you feel lonely?" assessed loneliness on a scale of 1–4 (1 = frequent, 2 = occasional, 3 = rare, 4 = never).

10.7.5 Analyses

Due to sample size, all paths were not tested in one complex SEM model. Thus, different SEM models of the hypothesized relations between the latent constructs of nurse–patient interaction and (1) self-transcendence (interpersonal and intrapersonal) [97], (2) meaning-in-life [55, 119], (3) hope [120], (4) anxiety and depression [45], and (5) joy-of-life [105], were tested by means of LISREL 8.8 [121] and Stata 15.1 [122], while the assoiations with sense of coherenec and loneliness were tested by regression analyses using IBM SPSS Statistics [123].

Using SEM, random measurement error is accounted for and psychometric properties of the scales in the model are more accurately derived. At the same time, the direct, indirect, and total effects throughout the model are estimated. SEM models combine measurement models (e.g., factor models) with structural models (e.g., regression); a major issue is evaluation of model fit. The conventional overall test of fit is the chi-square (χ^2); a small χ^2 and a nonsignificant p-value correspond to good fit [121]. In line with the rule of thumb given as conventional cut-off criteria [124], the following fit indices were used: The Root Mean Square Error of Approximation (RMSEA) and the Standardized Root Mean Square (SRMS) with acceptable/good fit, respectively, set to 0.08/0.05 [124, 125], the Comparative Fit Index (CFI) and the Non-Normed Fit Index (NNFI) with acceptable/good fit, respectively, 0.95/0.97, the Normed Fit Index (NFI), Tucker Lewis Index (TLI) and the Goodness-of-Fit Index (GFI) at 0.90/0.95, and the Adjusted GFI (AGFI) 0.85/0.90 (ibid.). The frequency distribution of the data was examined to assess deviation from normality; both skewness and kurtosis were statistically significant. As normality is a premise in SEM, we corrected for the non-normality by applying the Robust Maximum Likelihood (RML) estimate procedure and stated the Satorra–Bentler corrected χ^2 [126].

10.8 Findings

Study 1 (N = 202) demonstrated significant effects of residents' perceived nurse–patient interaction on anxiety and depression [45], meaning-in-life [55], interpersonal and intrapersonal self-transcendence [97], and hope [120]. Furthermore, the findings showed that the nurse–patient interaction is a resource not only for self-transcendence, hope, and meaning [79], but also for QoL [44], mental health [89], as well as physical, emotional, social, functional, and spiritual well-being [127] in the NH population. A total of 17 scientific articles have been published based on study 1, as well as a chapter in an international scientific anthology [127]. Study 2 has so far

resulted in 8 scientific publications including this chapter, showing among others a significant influence of nurse-patient interaction on sense of coherence and loneliness. Figure 10.3 summarizes the findings in study 1 and study 2: the green arrows illustrate significant direct relations, while the red tiny dotted arrows demonstrate significant mediated relations. Accordingly, Fig. 10.3 illustrates that nurse–patient interaction significantly influences on hope, joy-of-life, meaning-in-life, interpersonal and intrapersonal self-transcendence, sense of coherence, all aspects of well-being, loneliness and physical/mental symptom severity.

Furthermore, intrapersonal and interpersonal self-transcendence and meaning have shown direct and/or indirect impact on all the various dimensions of well-being, that is, physical, emotional, social, functional, and spiritual well-being. In addition, meaning revealed significant associations with symptom severity, physical, and psychological functions in the NH population [22]. Therefore, the different SEM models based on study 1 indicated significant mediated influences as illustrated by the red dotted lines in Fig. 10.3. In short, find-

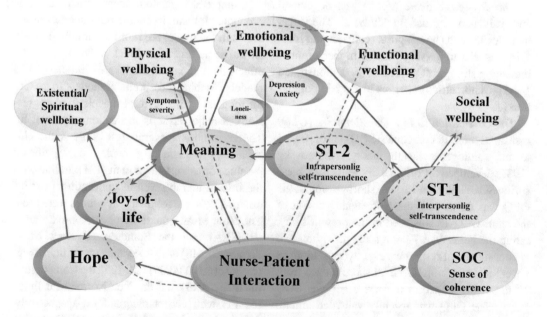

Fig. 10.3 Summary of the findings from study 1 and study 2. Relationships between nurse–patient interaction and hope, joy-of-life, meaning, intrapersonal and interpersonal self-transcendence, sense of coherence, well-being, loneli-

ness and symptom severity. *Note*: ——→ = direct relations (effects); ------→ = indirect relationships (mediated effects) © Gørill Haugan

ings from study 1 indicate that the nurse–patient interaction has significant impact on all dimensions of well-being, mediated through hope, meaning, and self-transcendence (inter and intra).

Structural equation and regression models based on data from study 2 (N = 188) indicated that the nurse–patient interaction has significant impact on joy-of-life [105], sense of coherence [128] and loneliness [...] [129]. In addition, study 2 supported the findings of study 1 showing that the nurse–patient interaction is of great importance revealing highly significant associations with both interpersonal and intrapersonal self-transcendence as well as perceived meaning-in-life [49]. Figure 10.3 illustrates the significant associations in study 1 and study 2.

10.9 Discussion

In these two studies, nine hypotheses of directional relationships of nurse–patient interaction with inter- and intrapersonal self-transcendence,

meaning-in-life, hope, joy-of-life, sense of coherence, loneliness, anxiety and depression were tested, and all of which found support. What does this mean for clinical practice? To elaborate on this, we should look at how the nurse–patient interaction was assessed. The NPIS includes 14 items, measured on a scale from 1 (not at all) to 10 (very much). The higher the score, the better is the perceived interaction with the nurses. Figure 10.4 shows in detail which aspects are included in the measurement model of nurse–patient interaction; the NPIS includes NH residents' experiences of trust, respect, feeling listened to, taken seriously and understood, acknowledged, and recognized as a unique person, as well as included in decisions regarding one's life and the experience of meaningful contact. In total, these aspects constitute the older adults' NPIS scores.

Statistical analyzes showed that residents' experience of these qualities in the nurse–patient interaction contributed to the experience of self-transcendence, meaning, hope, joy-of-life, and

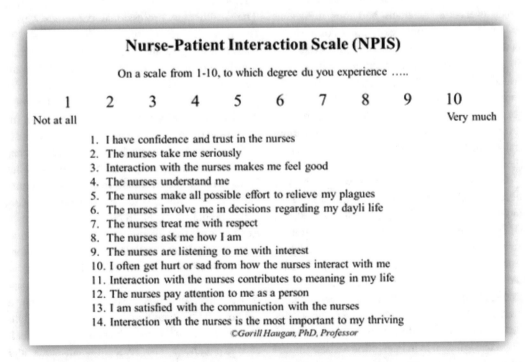

Fig. 10.4 Nurse–Patient Interaction Scale (NPIS) assesses perceived nurse–patient interaction. © Gørill Haugan

sense of coherence, and alleviation of loneliness, anxiety and depression. What is more, positively perceived nurse–patient interaction strengthens residents' joy-of-life [105], meaning-in-life, and self-transcendence [55, 97]; the latter two have shown significant impact on physical, emotional, social, functional, and spiritual well-being [21, 57, 119, 130–134]. Thus, the interaction between the nurse and the older adult can be used to promote health and well-being. By facilitating specific qualities in the interaction with their residents, nurses influence on NH residents' health and well-being. The nurse–patient interaction is a vital health-promoting resource in NH care. How can this be explained?

10.9.1 Nurse–Patient Interaction - a Salutogenic Resource

Initially, this chapter established the salutogenic understanding of health based on man being a unit of body–mind–spirit, where the physical, emotional, social, and spiritual/existential dimensions together constitute an integrated entity, in which everything interacts and thus influences everything. Accordingly, experiences of meaning as well as joy-of-life, etc. not only affect the emotional dimension. Since human being is an integrated wholeness, all experiences affect the human unity of body–mind–spirit. That is, also the body—physical well-being and symptom severity—will be affected by perceived meaning and joy-of-life. In fact, meaning and joy are biochemical states in the body [11].

Generally, NH residents have many diseases, ailments, fatigue, pain, and dyspnea [135, 136] and depend on care and help of nurses to stay well. Many are waiting for death. Missing opportunities for meaningful activities, several spend a lot of time doing nothing, sleeping, and waiting [33–37], and social contact with others outside the NH is scarce. Hence, nurses represent the most essential source of social contact as part of the nursing care. Furthermore, in this life situation, the individual might feel vulnerable in interaction and communication with others; especially in relationship with

those in power, such as the nurses and other health care professionals, who have power for both good and bad. The Danish philosopher Løgstrup [137] highlighted vulnerability related to being handed over to others, as the case is in NH care. Løgstrup [137] underlined the ethical demands arising from relationships of power, such as the nurse–patient relationship; the nurses hold some of the residents' life in their hands. Considering this, relational competence together with competent pain and symptom management is crucial for health promotion in NH care. Relational competence includes knowledge and professional skills to use the nurse–patient interaction in health-promoting ways, that is, to carefully observe and competently influence the older adults, so that health and well-being increase.

10.9.1.1 Practical Implications: Professionals' Attention and Influencing Skills

Relational competence involves both attentional and influencing skills [138]. Nurse's attention is the leading "tool." Therefore, health-promoting interaction is based on attention-related skills. The health care professional consciously uses and regulates one's attention; that is, what one sees, hears, feels, smells, senses, and thinks during the interaction with the residents. What are you paying attention to? Or where do you direct your attention? Health-promoting interaction requires awareness skills that are based on an active and openly receiving presence. By a sensitive presence [88], the professional nurse uses her senses and presence to perceive and receive what is important to the resident, in order to welcome and attend to what the older adults expresses, verbally and non-verbally. In this way, nurses create trust; a sense of being taken seriously, being acknowledged and attended to as a real person. This promotes health and well-being in vulnerable older individuals in NHs. However, nurse–patient interaction is also about fostering a common understanding of what is at stake right here-and-now; what does the resident think, feel, and experience? The resident's emotions and experiences should be given attention and understood by the health care professional. This is how nurses let the older NH resident become a person, which is highly health promoting.

Attention skills include being sensitive to the NH resident's choice of words, volume, tone, and power in the voice, as well as rhythm of expression (staccato), tempo (fast-slow, pauses), nonverbal expressions such as a sigh, breath, gaze, facial expressions, skin color, posture, congruence, authenticity. There is a wealth of information in such cues [138, 139], which are vital in achieving health-promoting nurse–patient interaction. The instrument of your attention is yourself and what you see, hear, feel, and sense. Therefore, health care professionals need to stay well connected with one's inner self. Still, any focus of attention will always include something and consequently exclude something else. Therefore, it is important to notice whether undue attention is paid or if there is any lack of attention to something that should be attended to. An example illustrating this point is a resident who dares to open up and tell about her loneliness. She is crying. What are you as a health care professional paying attention to? The fact told about her loneliness? Or the emotional expression of crying? What are you doing? Are you listening? Do you explore what this is about? Or do you start to comfort? There is no facet. But, taking time to listen and explore, allowing the resident room and space to become clear to herself, would be health promoting and even more soothing than any well-intentioned comfort. In some cases, health professionals' attempts to comfort become more of a strategy that maintains the problem, rather than helping to solve it. For example, focusing on what this old lady is saying about being lonely instead of focusing on her crying can, paradoxically, cause this lady to feel overlooked, rejected, and thus feel even more lonely. Attention to the matter and a cognitive understanding of its content is usually not enough. Attention to emotional expressions is usually fundamental. This is especially important while caring for older adults having dementia.

Health-promoting interaction rests on health professionals' listening techniques and their ability to create rapport, i.e., to identify and care for the true essence of the resident's experience. In every health professional nurse–patient relationship, professionals are dependent on their attention skills. Nurses need attention to get a clear picture of what is at stake, so they can competently and ethically influence the resident's health and well-being. Not least, this applies to various physical signs such as pain, urinary infection, and pneumonia, or when caring for a wound. Nurses are aware of several small hints that give valuable information.

Health-promoting interaction is about competent influence, sustaining the boundaries between the two, so respect and dignity are maintained. Empathic listening providing unconditional acceptance, recognition, and empathy creates experiences of acceptance and respect and can lead to positive changes and thereby health and well-being. Nevertheless, attentional skills represent impact and thus signify a use of power [138]; such power is part of all relationships between health professionals and their patients. Openly or hidden, power, influence, and authority are always integrated aspects of any relationship between people [88, 137]. Thus, nurse–patient interaction requires that health care professionals are perceptive of one's power and how they use it. The consideration is not about *if or whether* power is being used, but *how* it is used. Wanting the resident well, unconditional acceptance, authenticity, and warmth are always the foundation on which health-promoting interaction is based.

10.9.2 Competent Health-Promoting Nurse–Patient Interaction

The focus of this chapter is nurse–patient interaction as a health-promoting resource in NH care; the relational qualities of the nurse–patient interaction signify essential influences on residents' well-being physically, emotionally, socially, functionally, and spiritually. Being attentive, communicating, and interacting respectfully and empathically while making all possible effort to relieve the old persons' infirmities are relational qualities fostering dignity, wellbeing and confidence in the nurses [140], as well as encouraging personal goals, values, and comprehensibility. In light of limited staffing, taking time for "slow care" as well as emphatical listening might sometimes prove difficult. Nevertheless, because this includes the way professionals use their eyes, face, voice, hands, and their body which is not time-consuming by itself, an accepting and attending way of being present is not necessarily more time-consuming than an indifferent presence. Moreover, a relationship requires two partakers. That is, the NH resident does also have to contribute to the interaction. However, the professionals should be responsible for at least 75% of the contact qualities in the nurse–patient interaction, aiming at facilitating joy-of-life, sense of coherence, meaning-in-life, hope, self-transcendence and thereby well-being. Professional nursing care is determined by nurses' use of their knowledge, attitudes, behavior, and communication skills to appreciate the uniqueness of the person being cared for [141], which is fundamental for dignity [134], meaning-in-life [55], self-transcendence and well-being [44, 97], loneliness [129], anxiety and depression [45]. Frustration, suffering, hopelessness, meaninglessness, and loneliness result from the experience of not being attended to or treated with indifference [96, 102].

Consequently, health care professionals need knowledge and skills in health-promoting interaction; they should utilize their attentional and influencing skills competently and ethically as part of any caring situation. Moreover, an explicit and clear integration of the pathogenesis and salutogenesis into the health services is needed. Therefore, this chapter proposes a competence triangle where salutogenesis and pathogenesis constitute the sides, while the foundation of the triangle is relational competence, which usually determines how far health professionals can reach in their health-promotion work. Figure 10.5 illustrates the competence triangle, indicating that all three kinds of knowledge (relational, salutogenesis, pathogenesis) are essential parts of competence in NH care.

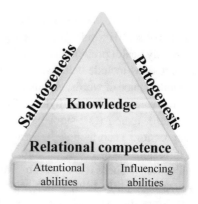

Fig. 10.5 The triangle of competence: salutogenesis and pathogenesis based upon the basis of relational competence. © Gørill Haugan

Professor Baldacchino [142] emphasized the *"being in the doing."* Health professionals' way of being present while performing various tasks in collaboration with the NH resident determines the older adult's experience of care quality. Studies have shown that the perceived qualities in the nurse–patient interaction significantly influence on NH residents' loneliness, anxiety, depression, hope, meaning, and self-transcendence, as well as joy-of-life and sense of coherence. This means that by means of awareness, tenderness, and attentional skills, nurse–patient interaction can be used to positively influence on patients' health, QoL, and well-being, physically, emotionally, socially, and spiritually/existentially. Figure 10.6 illustrates a tentative theory of how the salutogenic and pathogenic knowledge together with relational competence, the *"being in the doing,"* can influence on NH residents.

Health promotion in NHs should be based on integrated knowledge of salutogenesis and pathogenesis. Competence in pain and symptom management is central in NH care, together with relational knowhow based on awareness and influencing skills. Health workers, not only in NHs but in the entire health services, should be given the opportunity to further develop their knowledge, relational competence, and interactional skills, in order to "refine" their way of being present together with their patients and residents. Health professionals' competence

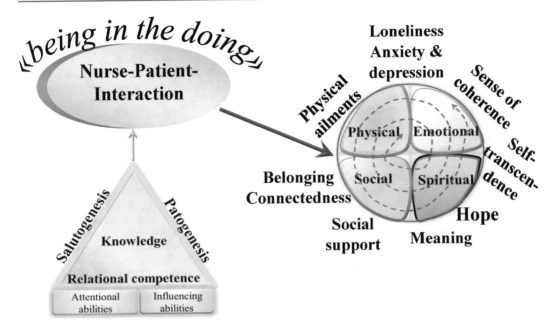

Fig. 10.6 Tentative theory of health promotion interaction in nursing. © Gørill Haugan

should include both the doing and the way of being in NHs and the health services.

Take Home Messages
- Salutogenesis represents the origin of health, while pathogenesis covers knowledge of disease, risk, and prevention. Salutogenesis and pathogenesis need to be integrated in a holistic understanding of human health and well-being.
- The importance of establishing the nurse–patient relationship as an integral component of nursing practice has been well documented. The nurse–patient interaction embodies the foundation of the nurse–patient relationship.
- Nurse–patient interaction has shown to influence on nursing home residents' perceived meaning-in-life, hope, inter- and intrapersonal self-transcendence, joy-of-life, sense of coherence, as well as loneliness, anxiety and depression.
- Accordingly, the nurse–patient interaction is a resource for health, quality-of-life, and well-being in nursing homes; by means of ethical and competent nurse–patient interaction, health professionals influence on older adults'

well-being, physically, emotionally, socially, functionally, and spiritually.
- Empathic listening, awareness, tenderness, and attentional skills are key assets to positively influence on NH residents' health, quality-of-life, and well-being.
- Nevertheless, empathic listening, awareness, tenderness, and attentional skills also signify a use of power; thus, nurse–patient interaction requires that health care professionals are perceptive of their power and how they use it. The issue is not about if or whether power is being used, but how it is used, which is specified by the *"being in the doing."*

References

1. WHO. Ageing and health. World Health Organization; 2018. https://www.who.int/newsroom/fact-sheets/detail/ageing-and-health. Accessed 5 Feb 2018.
2. Kinsella K, He W. An Aging World: 2008. Washington, DC: U.S. Department of Health and Human Services National Institutes of Health National Institute on Aging, U.S. Department of Commerce Economics and Statistics; 2009. Contract no.: report no.: P95/09-1.

3. WHO. Global status report on non-communicable diseases. 2010. http://www.who.int/chp/ncd_global_status_report/en/index.html. Accessed 23 Aug 2012.
4. Antonovsky A. Unraveling the mystery of health. How people manage stress and stay well. San Francisco: Jossey-Bass; 1987.
5. Mittelmark MB, Sagy S, Eriksson M, Bauer GF, Pelikan JM, Lindström B, et al., editors. The handbook of Salutogenesis. New York: Springer; 2017.
6. Antonovsky A. Health, stress, and coping: new perspectives on mental health and physical wellbeing. San Francisco: Jossey-Bass; 1979.
7. Dossey B, Keegan L, editors. Holistic nursing: a handbook for practice. London: Jones and Bartlett; 2009.
8. Guzzetta CE. Holistic nursing research. In: Dossey BM, Keegan L, Guzzetta CE, editors. Holistic nursing a handbook for practice. 4th ed. Boston, Toronto, London, Singapore: Jones and Bartlett; 2009. p. 211–28.
9. Kiecolt-Glaser J, McGuire L, Robles T, Glaser R. Emotions, morbidity, and mortality: new perspectives from psychoneuroimmunology. Annu Rev Psychol. 2002;53:83–107.
10. Starkweather A, Wiek-Janusek L, Mathews H. Applying the psychoneuroimmunology framework to nursing research. J Neurosci Nurs. 2005;37(1):56–62.
11. Pert CB. Molecules of emotion—why you feel the way you feel. New York: Simon and Schuster.; 1999.
12. Ehlert U, Gaab J, Heinrichs M. Psychoneuroendocrinological contributions to the etiology of depression, posttraumatic stress disorder, and stress-related bodily disorders: the role of the hypothalamus-pituitary-adrenal axis. Biol Psychol. 2001;57(1–3):141–52.
13. Haugan G. Helsefremmende interaksjon [health promoting interaction]. In: Haugan G, Rannestad T, editors. Helsefremming i kommunehelsetjenesten [health promotion in the municipality health services]. Oslo: Cappelen Damm Akademiske; 2014.
14. Seligman MEP. Learned optimism: how to change your mind and your life. New York: Vintage Books; 2006.
15. Seligman MEP. Flourish: a visionary new understanding of happiness and well-being. New York: Simon and Schuster; 2012.
16. Keyes CL. Promoting and protecting mental health as flourishing: a complementary strategy for improving national mental health. Am Psychol. 2007;62(2):95–108.
17. Keyes CL. Mental health as a complete state: how the salutogenic perspective completes the picture. In: Bauer GF, Hämmig O, editors. Bridging occupational, organizational and public health. Dordrecht: Springer; 2014. p. 179–92.
18. Keyes CL. The mental health continuum: from languishing to flourishing in life. J Health Soc Behav. 2002;43(2):207–22.
19. Haugan Hovdenes G. Troen, håpet og kjærligheten: avgjørende ressurser relatert til helse og livskvalitet. 1995.
20. Rannestad T, Haugan Hovdenes G, Espnes GA. Hjernen er ikke alene : psykosomatikken ser kropp og sjel i sammenheng, det bør sykepleie også gjøre; 2006. p. 52–6.
21. Haugan G. Meaning-in-life in nursing-home patients: a valuable approach for enhancing psychological and physical well-being? J Clin Nurs. 2014;23(13-14):1830–44.
22. Haugan G. Meaning-in-life in nursing-home patients: a correlate to physical and emotional symptoms. J Clin Nurs. 2014;23(7-8):1030–43.
23. Mwilambwe-Tshilobo L, Ge T, Chong M, Ferguson M, Misic B, Burrow A, et al. Loneliness and meaning in life are reflected in the intrinsic network architecture of the brain. Soc Cogn Affect Neurosci. 2019;14(4):423–33.
24. WHO. The Ottawa Charter for health promotion. 1986. http://www.who.int/healthpromotion/conferences/previous/ottawa/en/.
25. Helsedirektoratet. Helsefremmende arbeid www.forebygging.no/en/Ordbok/F-K/Helsefremmende-arbeid. Helsedirektoratet; 1987.
26. WHO. Shanghai Declaration on promoting health in the 2030 Agenda for sustainable development: 9th global conference on health promotion, Shanghai 2016; 2016.
27. Eriksson M, Lindström B. A Salutogenic interpretation of the Ottawa charter. Health Promot Int. 2008;23(2):190–9.
28. Barca ML, Selbæk G, Laks J, Engedal K. Factors associated with depression in Norwegian nursing homes. Int J Geriatr Psychiatry. 2009;24(4):417–25.
29. Choi N, Ransom S, Wyllie R. Depression in older nursing home residents: the influence of nursing home environmental stressors, coping, and acceptance of group and individual therapy. Aging Ment Health. 2008;12(5):536–47.
30. Otsuka S, Hamahata A, Komatsu M, et al. Prospects for introducing the Eden Alternative to Japan. J Gerontol Nurs. 2010;36(3):47–55.
31. Tuckett A. The meaning of nursing-home: 'waiting to go up to St. Peter, OK! Waiting house, sad but true': an Australian perspective. J Aging Stud. 2007;21(2):119–33.
32. Björk S, Lindkvist M, Wimo A, Juthberg C, Bergland Å, Edvardsson D. Residents' engagement in everyday activities and its association with thriving in nursing homes. J Adv Nurs. 2017;73(8):1884–95.
33. Harper IG. Daily life in a nursing home—has it changed in 25 years? J Aging Stud. 2002;16:345–59.
34. Brownie S, Horstmanshof L. Creating the conditions for self-fulfilment for aged care residents. Nurs Ethics. 2012:1–10.

35. Grönstedt H, Frändin K, Bergland A, Helbostad J, Granbo R, Puggaard L, et al. Effects of individually tailored physical and daily activities in nursing home residents on activities of daily living, physical performance and physical activity level: a randomized controlled trial. Gerontology. 2013;59(3):220–9.

36. Haugland BØ. Meningsfulle aktiviteter på sykehjemmet [Meaningful activities in nurisng homes]. Sykepleien Forskning. 2012;7(1):42–9.

37. Slettebo A, Saeteren B, Caspari S, Lohne V, Rehnsfeldt AW, Heggestad AKT, et al. The significance of meaningful and enjoyable activities for nursing home resident's experiences of dignity. Scand J Caring Sci. 2017;31(4):718–26.

38. Drageset J, Eide G, Corbett A. Health-related quality of life among cognitively intact nursing home residents with and without cancer—a 6-year longitudinal study. Patient Relat Outcome Meas. 2017;27(8):63–9.

39. Drageset J, Eide GE, Ranhoff A. Anxiety and depression among nursing hoeme residents without cognitive impairment. Scand J Caring Sci. 2013;27(4):872–81.

40. Sanderson WC, Scherbov S. Demography. Remeasuring aging. Science. 2010;329(5997):1287–8.

41. Ministry of Health Care Services. Morgendagens omsorg [Tomorrows' Care]. In: Services MoHC, editor. www.regjeringen.no. Fagbokforlaget, Bergen, Norway; 2012–2013. p. 141.

42. Ververda J, Hauge S. Implementing active care through (cultural) activities of daily living: a person-centred approach to achieve flourishing. Nurs Open. 2019;6(2):583–90.

43. Drageset J, Haugan G, Tranvåg O. Crucial aspects promoting meaning and purpose in life: perceptions of nursing home residents. BMC Geriatr. 2017;17(1):254.

44. Haugan G, Moksnes UK, Løhre A. Intra-personal self-transcendence, meaning-in-life and nurse-patient interaction: powerful assets for quality of life in cognitively intact nursing home patients. Scand J Caring Sci. 2016;30(4):790–801.

45. Haugan G, Innstrand ST, Moksnes UK. The effect of nurse-patient-interaction on anxiety and depression in cognitively intact nursing home patients. J Clin Nurs. 2013;22(15-16):2192–205.

46. Seligman MEP. Authentic happiness. New York: Free Press; 2002.

47. Seligman MEP. Flourish. North Sydney, NSW: Random House; 2011.

48. Rinnan E, Andrè B, Drageset J, Garåsen H, Espnes GA, Haugan G. Joy of life in nursing homes: a qualitative study of what constitutes the essence of joy of life in elderly individuals living in Norwegian nursing homes. Scand J Caring Sci. 2018;32(4):1468–76.

49. Haugan G, Rinnan E, Espnes GA, Drageset J, Rannestad T, André B. Development and psychometric properties of the Joy-of-Life Scale among cognitively intact nursing home patients. Scand J Caring Sci. 2019;33(4):801–14.

50. Drageset J, Eide G, Nygaard H. The impact of social support and sense of coherence on health-related quality of life among nursing home residents: a questionnaire survey in Bergen, Norway. Int J Nurs Stud. 2009;46(1):66–76.

51. Drageset J, Espehaug B, Kirkevold M. The impact of depression and sense of coherence on emotional and social loneliness among nursing home residents without cognitive impairment—a questionnaire survey. J Clin Nurs. 2012;21(7-8):965–74.

52. Bradshaw SA, Playford ED, Riazi A. Living well in care homes: a systematic review of qualitative studies. Age Ageing. 2012;41(4):429–40.

53. Thauvoye E, Vanhooren S, Vandenhoeck A, Dezutter J. Spirituality among nursing home residents: a phenomenology of the experience of spirituality in late life. J Religion Spirit Aging. 2019.

54. Stavrova O, Luhmann M. Social connectedness as a source and consequence of meaning in life. J Posit Psychol. 2016;11(5):470–9.

55. Haugan. G. The relationship between nurse-patient-interaction and meaning-in-life in cognitively intact nursing-home patients. J Adv Nurs. 2014;70(1):107–20.

56. Tejero L, Marie S. The mediating role of the nurse-patient dyad bonding in bringing about patient satisfaction. J Adv Nurs. 2012;68(5):994–1002.

57. Haugan G, Rannestad T, Hammervold R, Garåsen H, Espnes GA. Self-transcendence in nursing home patients—a resource for well-being. J Adv Nurs. 2013;69(5):1147–60.

58. Bergland A, Kirkevold M. Thriving in nursing homes in Norway: contributing aspects described by residents. Int J Nurs Stud. 2006;43(6):681–91.

59. Annear M, Elliott K, Tierney L, Lea E, Robinson A. "Bringing the outside world in": enriching social connection through health student placements in a teaching aged care facility. Health Expect. 2017;20(5):1154–62.

60. Cooney A, Dowling M, Gannon M, Dempsey L, Murphy K. Exploration of the meaning of connectedness for older people in long-term care in context of their quality of life: a review and commentary. Int J Older People Nurs. 2014;9(3):192–9.

61. Routasalo P, Savikko N, Tilvis R, Strandberg T, Pitkälä K. Social contacts and their relationship to loneliness among aged people—a population-base study. Gerontology. 2006;52:181–7.

62. Savikko N. Loneliness of older people and elements of an intervention for its alleviation. Doctoral dissertation. Annales Universitatis Turkuensis Turku: University of Turku, Finland; 2008.

63. Drageset J, Eide G, Ranhoff A. Depression is associated with poor functioning in activities of daily living among nursing home residents without cognitive impairment. J Clin Nurs. 2011;20(21-22):3111–8.

64. Drageset J, Eide G, Ranhoff A. Anxiety and depression among nursing home residents without cogni-

tive impairment. Scand J Caring Sci. 2013;27(4): 872–81.

65. Heravi-Karimooi MMMMTE. Understanding loneliness in the lived experiences of Iranian elders. Scand J Caring Sci. 2010;24(2):274–80.

66. Duppen D, Machielse A, Verté D, Dury S, De Donder L, Consortium D-S. Meaning in life for socially frail older adults. J Community Health Nurs. 2019;36(2):65–77.

67. Brownie S, Horstmanshof L. The management of loneliness in aged care residents: an important therapeutic target for gerontological nursing. Geriatr Nurs. 2011;32(5):318–25.

68. Drageset J, Eide G, Kirkevold M, Ranhoff A. Emotional loneliness is associated with mortality among mentally intact nursing home residents with and without cancer: a five-year follow-up study. J Clin Nurs. 2013;22(1–2):106–14.

69. Holt-Lunstad J, Smith TB, Layton JB. Social relationships and mortality risk: a meta-analytic review. PLoS Med. 2010;7(7):1–19.

70. Cacioppo JT, Hawkley LC, Crawford E, et al. Loneliness and health: potential mechanisms. Psychosom Med. 2002;64:407–17.

71. Phillips-Salimi CR, Haase JE, Kooken WC. Connectedness in the context of patient-provider relationships: a concept analysis. J Adv Nurs. 2012;68(1):230–45.

72. Welsh D, Moore SL, Getslaf BA. Meaning in life: the perspective of long-term care residents. Res Gerontol Nurs. 2012;5(3):185–94.

73. Prieto-Flores M, Fernandez-Mayoralas G, Forjaz M, Rojo-Perez F, Martinez-Martin P. Residential satisfaction, sense of belonging and loneliness among older adults living in the community and in care facilities. Health Place. 2011 Nov;17(6):1183–90.

74. Prieto-Flores M, Forjaz M, Fernandez-Mayoralas G, Rojo-Perez F, Martinez-Martin P. Factors associated with loneliness of noninstitutionalized and institutionalized older adults. J Aging Health. 2011;23(1):177–94.

75. Lohne V, Høy B, Lillestø B, Sæteren B, Heggestad A, Aasgaard T, et al. Fostering dignity in the care of nursing home residents through slow caring. Nurs Ethics. 2017;24(7):778–88.

76. Lillekroken D, Hauge S, Slettebø Å. The meaning of slow nursing in dementia care. Dementia (London). 2017;16(7):930–47.

77. Van der Heyden K, Dezutter J, Beyers W. Meaning in life and depressive symptoms: a person-oriented approach in residential and community-dwelling older adults. Aging Ment Health. 2015;19(12): 1063–70.

78. Bernard M, Strasser F, Gamondi C, Braunschweig G, Forster M, Kaspers-Elekes K, et al. Relationship between spirituality, meaning in life, psychological distress, wish for hastened death, and their influence on quality of life in palliative care patients. J Pain Symptom Manage. 2017;54:514–22.

79. Haugan G. Nurse-patient interaction is a resource for hope, meaning-in-life, and self-transcendence in cognitively intact nursing-home patients. Scand J Caring Sci. 2014;2014(28):74–8.

80. Rchaidia L, Dierckx de Casterlé B, De Blaeser L, Gastmans C. Cancer patients' perceptions of the good nurse: a literature review. Nurs Ethics. 2009;16(5):528–42.

81. Nåden D, Eriksson K. Understanding the importance of values and moral attitudes in nursing care in preserving human dignity. Nurs Sci Q. 2004;17(1):86–91.

82. Nåden D, Sæteren B. Cancer patients' perception of being or not being confirmed. Nurs Ethics. 2006;13(3):222–35.

83. Appleton C. The art of nursing: the experience of patients and nurses. J Adv Nurs. 1993;1993(18):892–9.

84. Watson J. Postmodernism and knowledge development in nursing. Nurs Sci Q. 1995;8:60–4.

85. Watson J. Nursing: human science and human care. A theory of nursing. New York: National League for Nursing; 1988.

86. Eriksson K, editor. Mot en Caritativ Vårdetik (towards a Caritative caring ethics). Åbo: Åbo Akademi; 1995.

87. Eriksson K. Det Lidende Menneske (The Suffering Human Being). Otta: TANO AS; 1995.

88. Martinsen K. Fra Marx til Løgstrup. Om etikk og sanselighet i sykepleien (from Marx to Løgstrup. About ethics and awareness in nursing). Otta: TANO AS; 1993.

89. Neuman B, editor. The Neuman systems model. 3rd ed. Norwalk, CT: Appleton & Lange; 1995.

90. Reed PG. Nursing: the ontology of the discipline. In: Reed PG, Shearer NBC, editors. Perspectives on nursing theory. 5th ed. Philadelphia, Baltimore, New York, London, Buenos Aires, Hong Kong, Sydney, Tokyo: Wolters Kluwer, Lippincott Williams & Wilikns; 2009. p. 615–20.

91. Eriksson K. Vårdvetenskap som akademisk disiplin [caring science as academic discipline]. Vasa, Finland: Department of Caring Science, Åbo Akademi University; 2001.

92. Drageset J. Health-related quality of life among nursing home residents. Bergen: University of Bergen; 2009.

93. Nakrem S, Vinsnes AG, Seim A. Residents' experiences of interpersonal factors in nursing home care: A qualitative study. Int J Nurs Stud. 2011;48(11):1357–66.

94. Haugan G. Self-transcendence, well-being and nurse-patient interaction in cognitively intact nursing home patients [PhD]. Trondheim, Norway: Norwegian University of Science and Technology; 2013.

95. Miner-Williams D. Connectedness in the nurse-patient relationship. San Antonio: University of Texas Health Science Center; 2005.

96. Haugan HG. The Nurse-patient-relationship in nursing homes: fulfillment or destruction [Pleier-pasient-relasjonen i sykehjem: virkeliggjørelse eller tilintetgjørelse]. Nord J Nurs Res Clin Stud. 2002;22(3):21–6.

97. Haugan G, Hanssen B, Rannestad T, Espnes GA. Self-transcendence and nurse-patient interaction in cognitively intact nursing-home patients. J Clin Nurs. 2012;21:3429–41.

98. Moss B. Communication skills in health and social care. 4th ed. London: Sage; 2017.

99. Cartter M. Trust, power, and vulnerability: a discourse on helping in nursing. J Clin Nurs. 2009;44(4):393–405.

100. Finch LP. Patients' communication with nurses: relational communication and preferred nurse behaviors. Int J Hum Caring. 2006;10(4):14–22.

101. Finch LP. Nurses' communication with patients: examining relational communication dimensions and relationship satisfaction. Int J Hum Caring. 2005;9(4):14–23.

102. Jonas-Simpson C, Mitchell GJ, Fisher A, Jones G, Linscott J. The experience of being listened to: a qualitative study of older adults in long-term care settings. J Gerontol Nurs. 2006;32(1):46–53.

103. Braaten K, Malmedal W. Preventing physical abuse of nursing home residents—as seen from the nursing staff's perspective. Nurs Open. 2017;4(4):274–81.

104. Malmedal W, Ingebrigtsen O, Saveman B. Inadequate care in Norwegian nursing homes—as reported by nursing staff. Scand J Caring Sci. 2009;23(2):231–42.

105. Haugan G, Eide WM, Taasen S, Rinnan E, Kuven BM, Xi WV, et al. The relationships between nurse-patient interaction and joy-of-life in cognitively intact nursing home patients. Scand J Caring Sci. 2020 Mar 22. https://doi.org/10.1111/scs.12836

106. Hollinger-Samson N, Pearson JL. The relationships between staff empathy and depressive symptoms in nursing home residents. Aging Ment Health. 2000;4(1):56–65.

107. Reed PG. Spirituality and well-being in terminally ill hospitalized adults. Res Nurs Health. 1987;10(5):335–44.

108. Reed PG. An emerging paradigm for the investigation of spirituality in nursing. Res Nurs Health. 1992;15(5):349–57.

109. Reed PG. Demystifying self-transcendence for mental health nursing practice and research. Arch Psychiatr Nurs. 2009;23(5):397–400.

110. Haugan G, Rannestad T, Garåsen H, Hammervold R, Espnes GA. The self-transcendence scale—an investigation of the factor structure among nursing home patients. J Holist Nurs. 2012;30(3):147–59.

111. Frankl VE. Man's search for meaning. New York: Washington Square Press; 1963.

112. Crumbaugh JC, Maholick LT. An experimental study in existentialism: the psychometric approach to Frankl's concept of noogenic neurosis. J Clin Psychol. 1964;20(2):200–7.

113. Haugan G, Moksnes UK. Meaning-in-life in nursing-home patients: a validation study of the purpose-in-life test. J Nurs Meas. 2013;21(2):296–319.

114. Herth K. Abbreviated instrument to measure hope: development and psychometric evaluation. J Adv Nurs. 1992;17(10):1251–9.

115. Haugan G, Utvær BKS, Moksnes UK. The Herth Hope index—a psychometric study among cognitively intact nursing-home patients. J Nurs Meas. 2013;21(3):378–400.

116. Antonovsky A. The structure and properties of the sense of coherence scale. Soc Sci Med. 1993;36:969–81.

117. Snaith R, Zigmond A. The hospital anxiety and depression scale manual. Windsor: NEFER-Nelson; 1994.

118. Haugan G, Drageset J. The hospital anxiety and depression scale—dimensionality, reliability and construct validity among cognitively intact nursing home patients. J Affect Disord. 2014.

119. Haugan G, Kuven BM, Eide WM, Taasen S, Rinnan E, Wu Xi V, Drageset J, André B. Nurse-patient interaction and self-transcendence: assets for meaning-in-life among nursing home residents? BMC Geriatrics. 2020;20:168. https://doi.org/10.1186/s12877-020-01555-2.

120. Haugan G, Moksnes UK, Espnes GA. Nurse-patient-interaction: a resource for hope among cognitively intact nursing home patients. J Holist Nurs. 2013;31(3):152–63.

121. Jøreskog K, Sørbom D. LISREL 8: structural equation modeling with the SIMPLIS command language. Chicago: Scientific Software International; 1995.

122. StataCorp Stata 15 Base Reference Manual 2017. StataCorp; 2017.

123. IBM Corp. Released 2020. IBM SPSS Statistics for Windows, Version 27.0. Armonk, NY: IBM Corp.

124. Schermelleh-Engel K, Moosbrugger H, Muller H. Evaluating the fit of structural equation models: tests of significance and descriptive goodness-of-fit measures. Meth Psychol Res. 2003;8(2):23–74.

125. Hu L, Bentler P. Fit indices in covariance structure modeling: sensitivity to underparametrized model misspesification. Psychol Methods. 1998;3(4):424–53.

126. Satorra A, Bentler P. Corrections to test statistics and standard errors in covariance structure analysis. In: Von Eye A, Cloggs C, editors. Latent variables analysis: applications for developmental research. Thousand Oaks, CA: Sage; 1994. p. 399–419.

127. Haugan G. Life satisfaction in cognitively intact long-term nursing-home patients: symptom distress, well-being and nurse-patient interaction. In: Sarracino F, Mikucka M, editors. Beyond money—the social roots of health and well-being. New York: NOVA Science; 2014. p. 165–211.

128. Drageset J, Taasen S, Espehaug B, Kuven BM, Eide WM, Andre B, et al. The relationships between

nurse-patient interaction and sense of coherence in cognitively intact nursing home patients. J Clin Nurs. 2019; in review.

129. Drageset J, Haugan G. The impact of Nurse-Patient Interaction on loneliness among nursing home residents-a questionnaire survey. Geriatric Nursing. 2021. In review.

130. Haugan G, Rannestad T, Hammervold R, Garåsen H, Espnes GA. The relationships between self-transcendence and spiritual well-being in cognitively intact nursing home patients. Int J Older People Nurs. 2014;9:65–78.

131. Farren AT. Power, uncertainty, self-transcendence, and quality of life in breast cancer survivors. Nurs Sci Q. 2010;23(1):63–71.

132. Runquist JJ, Reed PG. Self-transcendence and well-being in homeless adults. J Holist Nurs. 2007;25(1):5–13.

133. Bauer-Wu S, Farran CJ. Meaning in life and psychospiritual functioning: a comparison of breast cancer survivors. J Holist Nurs. 2005;23(2):172–90.

134. Burack OR, Weiner AS, Reinhardt JP, Annunziato RA. What matters most to nursing home elders: quality of life in the nursing home. J Am Med Dir Assoc. 2012;13(1):48–53.

135. Haugan G. Meaning-in-life in nursing-home patients: a correlate with physical and emotional symptoms. J Clin Nurs. 2014;23(7-8):1030–43.

136. Drageset J, Natvig GK, Eide GE, Bondevik M, Nortvedt MW, Nygaard HA. Health-related quality of life among old residents of nursing homes in Norway. Int J Nurs Pract. 2009;15(5):455–66.

137. Løgstrup KE. Den etiske fordring. Klim: København; 1956/2010.

138. Kvalsund R. Oppmerksomhet og påvirkning i hjelperelasjoner [attention and influence in professional helping relationships]. Trondheim: Tapir Academic Publisher; 2007.

139. Tveiten S. Veiledning—mer enn Ord [Counselling—more than words]. Bergen: Fagbokforlaget; 2013.

140. Carter M. Trust, power, and vulnerability: a discourse on helping in nursing. Nurs Clin North Am. 2009;44(4):393–405.

141. Warelow P, Edward KL, Vinek J. Care: what nurses say and what nurses do. Holist Nurs Pract. 2008;22(3):146–53.

142. Baldacchino D. Spiritual care: being in doing. Malta: Preca Library; 2010.

Social Support

11

Jorunn Drageset

Abstract

Social support by our social network proves to be important for our health. The opposite of good social support is loneliness. First and foremost, it seems that social support includes emotional support, belonging in a social community, being valued, practical help, and information and guidance. Social support represents a vital salutogenic resource for individuals' mental health.

This chapter explains the concept of social support in relation with other concepts of specific relevance, such as coping and quality of life. In a health-promoting perspective, this chapter presents the concept of social support and its theoretical basis. A brief description of questionnaires assessing social support is provided, as well as a brief summary of evidence demonstrating the salutogenic potential of social support, both as a preventive and a health-promoting resource.

Keywords

Social support · Social relationships · Health promotion · Sense of coherence · Older people · Social networks

11.1 Introduction

The concept of social support is multidimensional and can be incorporated into a larger context termed social capital, where social support and social networks are parts [1]. Social support and social networks are described in different ways; mainly these can be presented as (1) structurally and functionally and (2) formally and informally [2]. Nursing care can, for example, be a formal support to people who have no close friends.

The *structural aspect of social support* refers to the existence and size of a social network, and the extent to which the person is connected within a social network, like the number of social ties (quantity of the relationships) and the characteristics of the social exchanges between individuals (e.g., social support activities, frequency of interactions). Relationships with family, friends, and members in organizations might contribute to social integration [2, 3]. The *functionally/qualitative aspect of social support* refers to a person's appraisals of the social support he or she experience, or how integrated a person is within his or

J. Drageset (✉)
Western Norway of Applied Sciences, Bergen, Norge

University of Bergen, Bergen, Norway
e-mail: jorunn.drageset@hvl.no,
jorunn.drageset@uib.no

G. Haugan, M. Eriksson (eds.), *Health Promotion in Health Care – Vital Theories and Research*,
https://doi.org/10.1007/978-3-030-63135-2_11

her social network; that is, the quality or depth of the relationships [2, 3]. Furthermore, the specific functions that members in a social network can provide such as emotional (i.e., reassurance of worth, empathy, affection), instrumental (i.e., material aid), and informational (i.e., advice, guidance, feedback) [2, 4, 5] are also vital aspects of social support. Thus, social support refers to the cognitive/functional qualitative aspects of human relationships, such as the content and availability of relationships with significant others, whereas social network refers to the quantitative and structural aspects of these relationships [2, 5].

Social support occurs in the presence of a social network [2, 6]; the concept is often used in a broad sense, referring to any process through which social relationships might provide health and well-being [2, 7]. Reviewing the literature reveals that social support is understood from a subjective viewpoint, including emotional support, esteem support, social integration or network support, provision of information and feedback and tangible assistance [2, 4, 5]. Measures that reflect each dimension of social support are therefore needed [4].

Researchers have commonly made a distinction between perceived and received support [2, 3, 8]. Perceived support refers to a person's subjective judgment that will give help or have given help during times of need. Received support refers to specific support (e.g., advice) that is given if needed, actually provided to the person [2, 5, 8]. The different, specific types of social support that an individual may experience include emotional support (listening support, comfort, and security), informational support (advice and guidance), esteem support (increasing the person's sense of competence), and tangible support (concrete assistance such as providing transportation or financial assistance). These different, specific types of social support have shown different correlations with health and personal relationships; only perceived support is consistently linked to better mental health, whereas received support and social integration are not found to relate with health [9]. Accordingly, there is an agreement in the literature that the only aspect of social support that is linked to health outcomes is perceived support, or the belief that help is avail-

able if needed, rather than the help and support that is actually received [2, 5, 8, 9].

Based on the relationships between social support, stressful life events, and physical and mental health, the literature of social support proposes two models: (1) "buffering support" and (2) "main support" [2, 10–12]. The first model reflects the fact that social support is beneficial only under conditions of high stress, that is, the buffering effect. This means that individuals with a high level of perceived social support will have fewer negative health effects following stressful events than those with a low level of perceived social support. The second model states that social support is beneficial regardless of an individual's level of life stress and predicts positive influences of social support on physical and mental health, independently of the presence and the absence of stressful events [2, 10–12].

In his salutogenic theory of health, Antonovsky [13] introduced the concept of "sense of coherence" (SOC) as a global life orientation of viewing the world and one's environment as comprehensible, manageable, and meaningful. Antonovsky (1987) claimed that the way people view their life influences on their health. These three elements, comprehensibility, manageability, and meaningfulness, formed the concept of SOC. Another salutogenic concept is general resistance resources (GRR), involving aspects such as knowledge, intelligence, coping strategy, and social support. The GRRs are characterized by consistency, participation in shaping one's outcome, and a balance between underload and overload. These resistance resources are shaped by life experiences and reinforce the SOC. Social support is a GRR that builds up a strong SOC which in turn has proven to have a buffering and key effect on health [12].

11.2 Theoretical Approaches to the Concept of Social Support

11.2.1 Social Capital

Putnam, Leonardi, and Nanetti [14] make a distinction between two kinds of social capital: bonding capital and bridging capital. Bonding capital occurs when you are socializing with people who are alike you: same age, same religion, and so on (interconnecting dimensions). Bridging is what you do when you make friends with people who are not like you (e.g., between generations). These two kinds of social capital, bonding and bridging, do strengthen each other.

Coleman [15] describes social capital as a support that facilitates an individual's or a collective's action generated by networks of relationships through reciprocity, trust, and social norms, depending entirely on the individuals. That means that an individual can use these embedded resources whenever needed. Social capital is thereby inherent in the structure of relations between individuals [1, 15].

11.2.2 Social Relationships and Social Provisions Theory

Weiss's [16] theory of social relationships incorporates six major elements/provisions of the most current conceptualizations of social support which are (1) attachment, (2) social integration, (3) opportunity for nurturance, (4) reassurance of worth, (5) guidance, and (6) reliable alliance proposed by theorists in this area. Hence, Weiss theory compares the six social provisions with the dimensions of social support that have been described by other authors [4, 5, 17]. The theory of social relationships by Weiss focuses on the person's need to interact with others. The theory differentiates between primary and secondary relationships. The former comprises close, warm, and frequent relationships and is obtained from family and friends. The latter includes working relationships of less emotional importance than the primary ones, although it has great influence [16, 18]. Weiss [16] describes six different social relationships/provisions that must be obtained through relationships with other people, and all provisions are needed for an individual to feel adequate support. Each of the six provisions is usually obtained from a specific kind of relationship, but several may be obtained from the same person. Different provisions may be critical at different stages of the life cycle.

Weiss' concept of social provisions includes the functioning of social networks; that certain types of relationships usually provide each of the social provisions (attachment, social integration, opportunity for nurturance, reassurance of worth, guidance, and reliable alliance). Deficits in the specific provisions might lead to loneliness, boredom, low self-esteem, and anxiety. As older people experience changes in close relationships, failing health, or death of a spouse or friends, Weiss' concept of social provisions appears to be appropriate for understanding the relationships between social interaction and psychological well-being among older adults [19]. To the extent that deficits in social provisions affect health, social support may affect health-related quality of life directly through the dimensions of emotional support, network support, and esteem support. The six provisions are described as follows:

1. Attachment
    (a sense of emotional closeness and security often provided by a spouse or romantic partner).
2. Social integration
    (a sense of belonging to a group that shares common interests and activity, often provided by friends).
3. Opportunity for nurturance
    (a sense of responsibility for the well-being of another person, often obtained from children).
4. Reassurance of worth
    (acknowledgement of one's competence and skill, usually obtain from co-workers).
5. Guidance
    (advice and information, usually obtained from teachers, mentors and parents).
6. Reliable alliance (the assurance that one can count on people for assistance under any circumstances, usually obtained from close family member).

11.3   The Measurement of Social Support

So far, this chapter has shown that social support is important for both mental and physical health. Therefore, regardless of illness and age, the evaluation of social support is often part of interview surveys about health in the general population and among patients. The questionnaires assessing social support cover subjective experiences of social support. The Social Support Scale (OSS-3) (WHO Regional Office for Europe: EUROHIS, 2003) is a three-question form commonly used in the general population. This scale contains questions about "number of close people," "interest from others," and "help from neighbors." The responses are grouped into weak, medium, and good social support according to the scores on each of the three questions in the OSS-3 [20].

Another form is the Social Provisions Scale (SPS) which is often used in clinical settings, across diagnosis and ages [4]. This form builds on Weiss' theory of social relationships and the six provisions of social support (reliable alliance, guidance, affiliation, social integration, self-esteem affirmation, and the opportunity to mean something to others/provide care). This scale has 24 questions, four for each of the six sub-dimensions. The 24 questions are presented in the form of statements rated from "Strongly Disagree," "Disagree," "Agree," and "Strongly Agree." The SPS also exists in a shorter version including 16 questions covering "affiliation," "social integration," "affirmation of self-worth," and "opportunity to mean something to others/care." This 16-item short version is most often used among older people. The 16-item version scale has proven to be a valid and reliable instrument when used among older people living in the community [21, 22] and in nursing homes [22, 23].

11.4 Social Support and Health Promotion

Social support has proven to be health promoting by strengthening individual's coping abilities, health, and quality of life while facing stress; these associations have been seen in many different populations of both healthy and sick people [13, 24, 25]. The salutogenic nursing approach focuses on identifying the individual's health resources and actions to promote the person's health processes toward the positive side of the disease/ease-continuum [13].

Antonovsky introduced the salutogenic concept Sense of Coherence (SOC) [13, 24]. The salutogenic health theory was founded on the basic idea of what creates health; the concepts of SOC and generalized resistance resources (GRRs) represent the central ideas of Antonovsky's salutogenesis [13, 24]. These concepts harmonize well with the philosophy of the Ottawa Charter in 1986 [25, 26] stating health as a process enabling people to develop health through their assets and thus having the opportunity to lead a good life. The way people view the world affects their ability to manage tension and stress. The outcome (health) depends on perceived SOC and the GRRs available, i.e., material, ego identity, and social support [27]. The SOC consists of three dimensions: comprehensibility, manageability, and meaningfulness, reflecting the interaction between the individual and the environment. Evidence shows that SOC is strongly associated with perceived health, especially mental health [12, 27]. Furthermore, SOC has demonstrated a main, moderating, or mediating role in the explanation and prediction of health among adult in Swedish and Finnish population [12, 27].

Social support is a vital generalized resistance resource and thereby seen as a salutogenic concept [28]. Close supportive relations is according to Antonovsky [13], a prerequisite for developing a strong SOC. The importance of the different aspects of supportive relations or dimensions of social support can vary among different populations. A systematic review showed that social support from spouse, friends, and health professionals was an important factor in establishing and maintaining healthy habits for nutrition and lifestyle in people diagnosed with diabetes [29]. Social support from close friends has also shown a positive effect on mental health problems in older people (aged 65 years or older) and is described as a "buffer" between mental disorders and physical impairments such as hearing impairment. In the same study, social support was significant independently associated with psychological distress [30]. Wang, Mann, Lloyd-Evans, Ma, and Johnson [31] found substantial evidence from prospective studies that people with depression who perceive their social support as poorer have worse outcomes in terms of depressive symptoms, recovery, and social functioning. Further, studies show that social support perceived as emotional support, and reassurance of one's worth, is important for quality of life and loneliness among older nursing home patients with and without cancer as well as in home-dwelling older adults [23, 32, 33]. Kvale and Synnes [34] found that, by providing good care, health care personnel performed to be a vital resource strengthening cancer patients' general resistance resources in a stressful life situation. Nurses, doctors, family, and friends functioned as vital resources at these individuals' disposal when needed; thus, nursing care can be a specific resistance resource buffering stress [34]. The studies listed above signify the significance of having one special person in one's life to be confident in and feel appreciated by. This special relationship involves being listened to so that the person feels understood, seen, accepted, acknowledged, and confirmed. This kind of emotional support creates a sense of security and well-being and thus acts as a health promotion resource.

Social support and the quantity of close relationships are of great importance for mortality risk. A group of older adults ($N = 2.347$) who were examined about close friends/family, marital status, and mortality three times over 10 years disclosed that widowed older adults who had fewer than 4–6 close relationships had a significantly increased risk of death 10 years later compared to their married counterparts [35]. Clearly, the social relationships serve a critical role in overall health and well-being.

Furthermore, research shows that social support is important for the burden of care among older people giving care to a partner with dementia. A cross-sectional observation study of 97 individuals, ≥65 years old living with a partner having symptoms of dementia, showed that lower level of burden of care was significantly related with higher level of attachment and higher level of SOC [36]. Similarly, the findings from a study of cognitively intact nursing home residents (mean age 85 years) showed a strong positive correlation of nurse–patient interaction with anx-

iety, depression, hope, meaning, and self-transcendence [37–40]. These studies indicate that the relational qualities embedded in the nurse–patient interaction have a health-promoting influence.

Lämås and colleagues [41] conducted a cross-sectional study of 136 participants (mean 82 years) showing that participation in social relations and the experience of self-determination in activities in and around the house are significantly associated with thriving. Moreover, the experience of social support has been found to be health-promoting among people 75 years or older living at home; the frequency of home nursing was important for health promotion [21]. People with higher education who experienced good social support reported less need for home care than those who did not experience good support [21]. This indicate that besides higher education, support from social network is health promotion.

In summary, based on this literature review, social support has shown to significantly impact on psychological distress, quality of life, loneliness, burden of care, as well as anxiety, depression, hope, meaning, self-transcendence, and mortality risk. Social support has also shown to be a "buffer" between mental disorders and physical impairments. Thus, based on the existing evidence, social support shows to act as a vital health promotion resource representing a salutogenic concept.

11.5 How Can the Health Service Contribute to Social Support of Older Persons and Relatives?

11.5.1 Clinical Implications

The quality of social support from family and friends as well from caregivers is a vital resource in health promotion for older people. Consequently, knowledge about social support is important for health care workers providing care and treatment in all ages. This knowledge should be included in different health educations as well as to health care leaders.

Quality of care for the elderly requires good competence and knowledge of the importance of psychosocial care for health and well-being. Attention should be made to the importance of facilitating the opportunity to maintain contact with family (i.e., spouse, children) and close friends. Emotional support from significant others has proven to be important for health and well-being, embodying a salutogenic health resource. Health care professionals should facilitate, safeguard, or improve social support and, if necessary, provide social support. The starting point must be based on each person's needs, ensuring that the patient's autonomy and integrity are respected.

The different, specific types of social support (attachment, social integration, opportunity for nurturance, reassurance of worth, guidance, and reliable alliance) have certain types of relationships that are usually provided to each of the social provisions.

Appropriate strategies to ensure emotional support (the need for love and friendship) can be to ask the person if he/she has one or more confidants and then facilitate social contact based on the needs and wishes. Spend time and meeting the patient where he/she is based on the care needs. The emotional support creates a sense of security and well-being and thus acts as a health promotion resource. To ensure network support (need for affiliation) could be to facilitate social contact with friends and significant others, with patients and other residents (for those living in nursing homes), and motivate the patient to take the initiative and participate in social contexts. Further, being valued (support when it comes to self-esteem), nursing care personnel should be aware of the importance to help and support the person's self-esteem in their daily contact, i.e., the care should be based on the people's needs and not on what care personnel believe they need, because the person's autonomy and integrity should be respected.

Concrete support (practical help) could be done by identifying the person's previous strengths and the internal and external resources that are currently available and helping and moti-

vating the person to use these available resources despite any limitations.

Regarding instrumental support (information and guidance), professionals should provide health care information to the person in a way that is easy for them to understand.

The evidence shows both a "main" and "buffer" effect of social support as important health-promoting resource in maintaining health and well-being. What type of support that has "main" or "buffering" effect can vary among situations and different persons and population. The most important is that the only aspect of social support that is linked to health outcomes is perceived support, or the belief that help is available if needed, rather than the help and support that is received.

11.6 Conclusion

Social support involves that you experience security and closeness, can have the opportunity to care for others, that you belong to a social network, feel respected and valued, and participate in a community with mutual obligations. The opposite of social support is loneliness. Our social network has an impact on our health. First and foremost, it seems that social support includes emotional support, belonging in a social community, being valued, practical help and information, and guidance which are the health-promoting factors.

Take Home Messages
- The concept of social support is multidimensional and can be incorporated into larger context termed social capital, where social support and social networks are parts.
- Social support can be categorized and measured in several different ways, where emotional support, belonging in a social community, being valued, practical help, and information and guidance are the common functions.
- According to the salutogenic health theory, social support is a general resistant resource which can influence on people's sense of coherence.

- Social support is a predictor of physical and mental health, and a buffer that protects (or "buffers") people from the bad effects of stressful life events (e.g., death of a spouse, relocation).
- Positive associations between social support and individual's coping abilities, health and quality of life while facing stress, have been found in many different populations of both healthy and sick people.
- Social support has shown to significantly impact on psychological distress, quality of life, loneliness, burden of care, as well as anxiety, depression, hope, meaning, self-transcendence, and mortality risk.

References

1. Rostila M. The facets of social capital. J Theory Soc Behav. 2011;41(3):308–26.
2. Kent de Grey R, Uchino B, Trettevik R, Cronan S, Hogan J. Social support. Oxford Bibliogr Pscychol. 2018.
3. Taylor SE. Social support: a review. In: IMSF, editor. The handbook of health psychology. New York: Oxford University Press; 2011. p. 189–214.
4. Cutrona CE, Russel DW. The provisions of social relationships and adaptation to stress. In: Jones WH, Perlman D, editors. Advances in personal relationships a research annual I. Greenwich, CT: Jai Press; 1987. p. 37–67.
5. Sarason BR, Sarason IG, Pierce GR. Social support: an interactional view. A Wiley-interscience publication. Hoboken, NJ: Wiley; 1990.
6. Langford CP, Bowsher J, Maloney JP, Lillis PP. Social support: a conceptual analysis. J Adv Nurs. 1997;25(1):95–100.
7. Cohen S, Lynn U, Gottlieb B. Social support measurement and intervention: a guide for health and social scientists. Oxford: Oxford University Press; 2000.
8. Beauchamp M, Eys M. Coping, social support, and emotion regulation in teams. In: Eys MRBMA, editor. Group dynamics in exercise and sport psychology: contemporary themes. London: Routledge; 2014. p. 222–39.
9. Uchino BN. Understanding the links between social support and physical health: a life-span perspective with emphasis on the Separability of perceived and received support. Perspect Psychol Sci. 2009;4(3):236–55.
10. Cutrona C, Russell D, Rose J. Social support and adaptation to stress by the elderly. Psychol Aging. 1987;1(1):47–54.
11. Cohen S. Social relationships and health. Am Psychol. 2004;59(8):676–84.
12. Eriksson M, Lindstrom B. Antonovsky's sense of coherence scale and the relation with health: a systematic review. J Epidemiol Community Health. 2006;60(5):376–81.
13. Antonovsky A. Unraveling the mystery of health: how people manage stress and stay well. San Fransisco: Jossey-Bass; 1987.
14. Putnam RD, Leonardi R, Nanetti RY. Making democracy work: civic traditions in modern Italy. Princeton, NJ: Princeton University Press; 1994.
15. Coleman JS. Social capital in the creation of human capital. In: Networks in the knowledge economy; 2003. p. 57–81.
16. Weiss RS. The provisions of social relationships. In: Rubin Z, editor. Doing unto others. Englewood Cliffs, NJ: Prentice Hall; 1974. p. 17–26.
17. Cohen S, Syme SLE. Social support and health. New York: Academic Press; 1985.
18. Weiss RS. Loneliness. The experience of emotional and social isolation. Cambridge, MA: The Massachusetts Institute of Technology; 1973.
19. Mancini JA, Blieszner R. Social provisions in adulthood: concept and measurement in close relationships. J Gerontol. 1992;47(1):P14–20.
20. Abiola T, Udofia O, Zakari M. Psychometric properties of the 3-item Oslo social support scale among clinical students of Bayero university Kano. Niger Malay J Psychiatry. 2013;22(2):32–41.
21. Saevareid HI, Thygesen E, Lindstrom TC, Nygaard HA. Association between self-reported care needs and the allocation of care in Norwegian home nursing care recipients. Int J Older People Nurs. 2012;7(1):20–8.
22. Bondevik M, Skogstad A. Loneliness among the oldest old, a comparison between residents living in nursing homes and residents living in the community. Int J Aging Hum Dev. 1996;43(3):181–97.
23. Drageset J, Kirkevold M, Espehaug B. Loneliness and social support among nursing home residents without cognitive impairment: a questionnaire survey. Int J Nurs Stud. 2010;48(5):611–9.
24. Antonovsky A. Health, stress and coping: new perspective on mental and physical well-being. San Fransisco: Jossey-Bass; 1979.
25. Eriksson M, Lindstrom B. A salutogenic interpretation of the Ottawa charter. Health Promot Int. 2008;23(2):190–9.
26. World Health Organization, WHO. Ottawa charter for health promotion: an international conference on health promotion, the move towards a new public health. Ottawa, Geneva: WHO; 1986a.
27. Eriksson M, Lindstrom B. Antonovsky's sense of coherence scale and its relation with quality of life: a systematic review. J Epidemiol Community Health. 2007;61(11):938–44.
28. Eriksson M. Unravelling the mystery of Salutogenesis. The evidence base of the salutogenic research as measured by Antonovsky's sense of coherence scale; 2007.

29. Mohebi S, Sharifirad G, Feizi A, Botlani S, Hozori M, Azadbakht L. Can health promotion model constructs predict nutritional behavior among diabetic patients? J Res Med Sci. 2013;18(4):346–59.

30. Boen H, Dalgard OS, Bjertness E. The importance of social support in the associations between psychological distress and somatic health problems and socioeconomic factors among older adults living at home: a cross sectional study. BMC Geriatr. 2012;12:27.

31. Wang J, Mann F, Lloyd-Evans B, Ma R, Johnson S. Associations between loneliness and perceived social support and outcomes of mental health problems: a systematic review. BMC Psychiatry. 2018;18(1):156.

32. Elovainio M, Kivimake M. Sense of coherence and social support—resources for subjective well-being and health of the aged in Finland. Int J Soc Welfare. 2000;9:128–35.

33. Drageset J, Eide GE, Dysvik E, Furnes B, Hauge S. Loneliness, loss, and social support among cognitively intact older people with cancer, living in nursing homes--a mixed-methods study. Clin Interv Aging. 2015;10:1529–36.

34. Kvale K, Synnes O. Understanding cancer patients' reflections on good nursing care in light of Antonovsky's theory. Eur J Oncol Nurs. 2013;17(6):814–9.

35. Manvelian A, Sbarra DA. Marital status, close relationships, and all-cause mortality: results from a 10-year study of nationally representative older adults. Psychosom Med. 2020;82:384.

36. Stensletten K, Bruvik F, Espehaug B, Drageset J. Burden of care, social support, and sense of coherence in elderly caregivers living with individuals with symptoms of dementia. Dementia. 2016;15(6):1422–35.

37. Haugan G. The relationship between nurse-patient interaction and meaning-in-life in cognitively intact nursing home patients. J Adv Nurs. 2014;70(1):107–20.

38. Haugan G. Nurse–patient interaction is a resource for hope, meaning in life and selftranscendence in nursing home patients. Scand J Caring Sci. 2014;28(1):74–88.

39. Haugan G, Moksnes UK, Lohre A. Intrapersonal self-transcendence, meaning-in-life and nurse-patient interaction: powerful assets for quality of life in cognitively intact nursing home patients. Scand J Caring Sci. 2016;30:790.

40. Haugan G, Innstrand ST, Moksnes UK. The effect of nurse-patient interaction on anxiety and depression in cognitively intact nursing home patients. J Clin Nurs. 2013;22(15–16):2192–205.

41. Lamas K, Bolenius K, Sandman PO, Bergland A, Lindkvist M, Edvardsson D. Thriving among older people living at home with home care services—a cross-sectional study. J Adv Nurs. 2020;76(4):999–1008.

Self-Efficacy in a Nursing Context

12

Shefaly Shorey and Violeta Lopez

Abstract

Self-efficacy is one of the most ubiquitous term found in social, psychological, counselling, education, clinical and health literatures. The purpose of this chapter is to describe and evaluate self-efficacy theory and the studies most relevant to the nursing context. This chapter provides an overview of the development of self-efficacy theory, its five components and the role of self-efficacy in promoting emotional and behavioural changes in a person's life with health problems. This chapter also discusses the role of self-efficacy in nursing interventions by providing examples of studies conducted in health promotion in patients and academic performance of nursing students.

Keywords

Self-efficacy · Nursing · Health promotion

12.1 Introduction

Albert Bandura derived the concept of self-efficacy from his psychological research [1]. Based on Bandura' self-efficacy theory [2] which was later renamed social cognitive theory, self-efficacy was defined as the individual's perception of one's ability to perform particular behaviours through four processes [3] including cognitive, motivational, affective and selection processes. The stronger their cognitive perception of self-efficacy, the higher they set their goals and commitment to achieve these goals [4]. Through cognitive comparisons of one's own standard and knowledge of their performance level, people will choose what challenges they have to meet and how much effort is needed to undertake or overcome those challenges. Motivation based on goals leads to perseverance to accomplish their goals. Perceived self-efficacy determines their level of motivation [5]. People's affective processes influence how they control and manage threats such as stress and depression in life and thus a strong source of incentive motivation. It has been reported that affective processes have dual motivating roles. The more self-satisfaction people have, the more motivated they are in accomplishing their goals. On the other hand, the more self-dissatisfied people are, the more heightened efforts they will do to accomplish their set goals [6]. Thus, in social cognitive theory, Bandura [3] believes that self-

S. Shorey (✉)
Alice Lee Centre for Nursing Studies, National University of Singapore, Singapore, Singapore
e-mail: nurssh@nus.edu.sg

V. Lopez
School of Nursing, Hubei University of Medicine, Shiyan, China

© The Author(s) 2021
G. Haugan, M. Eriksson (eds.), *Health Promotion in Health Care – Vital Theories and Research*,
https://doi.org/10.1007/978-3-030-63135-2_12

efficacy plays a major role in self-regulation in appraising and exercising control over potential threats. Through the selection process, people can select beneficial social environments and exercise control over them as they can judge their capability of handling challenging activities [7].

12.2 Self-Efficacy Theory and Other Psychological Theories

Self-efficacy theory has been compared to other theoretical models mostly among psychological theories on explaining human behaviour so as to place self-efficacy in a larger context. Self-efficacy relates to how a person perceives his or her ability to feel, think, motivate and act upon to change particular behaviour. The person processes, weighs and integrates diverse sources of information concerning his or her capability and integrates choice behaviour and effort expenditure accordingly [1]. Expectations concerning mastery and efficacy their ability to perform such activities are related to how they see themselves in terms of self-concept and self-esteem. Self-concept is a term used to describe the person's attitudes and beliefs about the self and what he or she is capable to doing well. On the other hand, self-esteem is one's evaluation of their beliefs and assessment of their value as a person. If a person's assessment of their self-concept and self-esteem is high, the more they will be able or competent enough to change their behaviour.

Self-efficacy is also compared to *locus of control* which refers to a person's belief that one is capable of controlling outcomes through one's own behaviour [8]. People's locus of control can either be affected by external or internal forces. Self-efficacy focuses on the person's belief in the ability to perform a specific task, and having a feeling of success and accomplishment is a form of reinforcement to effect behavioural change and an example of internal locus of control [9, 10]. Bandura [7, 11] argued that locus of control is a kind of outcome expectancy as it is concerned about whether a person's behaviour can control outcomes. Self-efficacy expectancy refers to perceived subjective judgement on the effective execution of a course of action.

Self-efficacy theory has also been linked to intrinsic motivation theory [12]. Bandura [7, 11] purported that people must serve as agents of their own motivation and action. Self-motivation relies on goal setting and evaluation of one's own behaviour which operate through internal comparison processes [13]. Motivation predicts performance outcomes as it is concerned with what task people want or need to accomplish and successfully achieving it to have incentive value that is satisfying and pleasurable [9].

12.3 Sources of Self-Efficacy

Bandura [14] emphasised the four major sources of self-efficacy. First is through mastery experiences in overcoming obstacles. Mastery experiences build coping skills and exercise control over potential threats. Second is through various experiences provided by social models and seeing people similar to themselves who are successfully performing similar behaviours. These experiences are considered as the most influencing source of efficacy. Third is their own belief that they have what it takes to succeed. Fourth is altering their negative emotions and misinterpreting their physiological states. Physiological state can affect the level of self-efficacy when they interpret their somatic symptoms based on aversive arousal [7, 15]. People who believe they can manage these threats tend to be less disturbed by them [16].

12.4 Concept Analyses of Self-Efficacy

Concept development is an important process to generate nursing knowledge which ultimately be used to build evidence-based practice [10]. Self-efficacy has been identified as a middle-range theory, that is recognised as a predictor of health behaviour change and health maintenance [17]. There are many publications in nursing literature regarding the broad concept of self-efficacy. In general, and as used across disciplines, the concept of self-efficacy has been described as self-regulation, self-care, self-monitoring, self-management and self-monitoring [18]. The concept of self-efficacy has been analysed extensively in different nursing and education disciplines to provide an in-depth understanding of the theory's applicability. A number of methods such as Rodgers, Walker and Avant [19] and Wilson [20] have been used to conduct concept analysis of self-efficacy in terms of its defining attributes, antecedents and references. Below are some of the examples of concept analyses in nursing.

Liu [21] analysed the concept of self-efficacy and its relationship with self-management among elderly patients with type 2 diabetes in China using Walker's and Avant [19] method. The analysis found that the defining attributes of self-efficacy among this population were "cognitive recognition of requisite specific techniques and skills, perceived expectations of outcomes of self-management, sufficient confidence in their ability to perform the self-management, and sustained efforts in diabetes management" (p. 230). Liu [21] found that the consequences of self-efficacy among the Chinese elderly with type 2 diabetes were adherence to the prescribed regimen and successful management of the disease which were influenced by having relevant knowledge about diabetes, family support and learning from other similar cases with diabetes.

White et al. [22] analysed the concept of self-efficacy in relation to symptom management in patients with cancer. If cancer patients are not able to manage their symptom, the outcomes would be increased symptom distress, poor prognosis, decreased quality of life (QoL) and survival [23]. White et al. [22] also used Walker's and Avant [19] concept analysis method to determine the antecedents, defining attributes and consequences. For the patients with cancer, the attributes of self-efficacy are cognitive, affective processes, motivation, confidence, competence and awareness of how they perceive and evaluate the symptoms. Symptom awareness and management decisions are affected by the patients' emotions and distress. Motivation, confidence and

competence must all be present for symptom management. White et al. [22] reported that the consequences of having low self-efficacy in patients with cancer leads to increased distress, depression and anxiety, interference with treatment and potential for untreated malignancies. As self-efficacy for managing cancer symptoms is influenced positively or negatively, utilising individual care plans based on the attributes, antecedents and consequences of self-efficacy concept among these patients is needed.

Sims and Skarbek [24] conducted concept analysis of self-efficacy to examine if the levels of parental self-efficacy are correlated with nursing care delivery and developmental outcomes for parents and their infants. As with White et al. [22], confidence (the ability to trust oneself) and competence (the ability to perform in a given situation) emerged as the most prominent defining attributes of parental self-efficacy. Previous experiences with infants and observational learning were found to be antecedents of parental self-efficacy, and the consequences included "parental satisfaction in parenting role, parental well-being, positive parenting skills and beneficial health outcomes for children" (p. 11). They recommended further research to survey objective parents' level of confidence with parenting and level of comfort in their role.

Using Rogers' [25] concept analysis method, Voskuil and Robbins [26] examined the concept of youth physical activity self-efficacy due to the decline in physical activity from childhood to adolescents. They defined physical activity as "complex, multi-dimensional behaviour that involves bodily movement produced by the contraction of skeletal muscle with resultant increases in physiological attributes, including energy expenditure above the basal metabolic rate and physical fitness" (p. 2004). They found that youth self-efficacy involves self-appraisal process in their belief and action about their capability for physical activity. The antecedents include prior and current physical activity experiences, modelling of physical activity by other youths and strong social support networks. There are of course positive and negative consequences of physical activity self-efficacy in youth. For example, physiological state in children with cardiac defect can lower self-efficacy while mastery and satisfactory experiences from participating in sport result in higher self-efficacy. The authors suggested that examination of the development of physical activity self-efficacy is needed as well as developing theory-based interventions designed to increase the sources of self-efficacy and physical activity self-efficacy to promote physical activity among youth.

Self-efficacy is also a concept used in nursing education to bridge the theory–practice gap [27], acquisition of clinical skills, critical thinking and overall academic success [28, 29]. Robb [30] conducted a concept analysis of self-efficacy to identify behaviours needed for students' goal attainment. It was noted that clinical simulations, cooperative learning and personalised classroom structure influence students' level of self-efficacy. Students utilised Bandura's [2] concept of vicarious experiences by relying on theory learned from the classroom, clinical experiences and by observing other nurses and their teachers perform certain procedures successfully. Verbal persuasion from teachers is often the sources of self-efficacy in nursing education. Robb [30] found that students' low level of self-efficacy requires emotional and academic support and suggested that nurse educators should be aware of the strategies used by millennial students to gain information and how they provide feedback about students' performance.

12.5 Self-Efficacy in Nursing Research

Self-efficacy theory has been receiving much attention as a predictor of behavioural change and self-care management in health-related and educational research. This may be partially attributed to the shift in the health care paradigm from a disease-centred (pathogenic) to a health-centred (salutogenic) orientation. The salutogenic orientation emphasises personal well-being and an ideal state of health as the ultimate goals and works towards achieving these, as opposed to the pathogenic approach, which is primarily based

on identifying problems or diseases and only attempting to solve them [31, 32]. One of the major concepts of the salutogenic theory is the sense of coherence, which refers to an individual's ability to adopt existing and potential resources to counter stress and promote health. It is measured based on one's perceived value of the outcome of the behaviour (meaningfulness), one's belief that the behaviour will actually lead to that outcome (comprehensibility), and one's capability of successfully performing the behaviour (manageability), of which Antonovsky [32] drew analogous comparison to the three conditions for self-efficacious behaviour: self-efficacy beliefs, behavioural efficacy beliefs and the value of anticipated outcomes [33]. The salutogenic approach has much in common with Bandura's self-efficacy theory [1] that highlighted perceived self-efficacy's crucial influence on choice of behavioural settings. Antonovsky [32] drew reference to it stating how an individual with a strong sense of coherence would more likely choose to enter situations without evaluating it as stressful, or in stressful situations, would appraise a stressor as benign. Under the salutogenic umbrella, self-efficacy is one of the key components that drive health-promoting practices, behaviour and self-care management [34–37]. In a recent study, self-efficacy is found to be positively related to sense of coherence, with this association being the strongest among people with low sense of coherence [38]. Additionally, self-efficacy was found to have either a significant direct effect on behaviours [39–41] or it becomes a mediator between other psychological factors and health behaviour [42, 43].

An electronic search was conducted on four databases (PsycInfo, PubMed, Embase and Cinahl) for English language articles that were published from each database's inception up to December 2019. Keywords used revolved around the concept of self-efficacy in nursing and health care, such as "self-efficacy", "chronic disease", "nursing education", and "patients". The search generated a repertoire of studies, which primarily involved patients with chronic illnesses, parents during the perinatal period, nursing or medical students, and the youth or elderly population.

12.5.1 Use of Self-Efficacy in Health Promotion Among Patients with Chronic Illness

For patients with chronic medical conditions (e.g. sickle cell disease, asthma, cardiovascular disease (CVD), inflammatory bowel disease, cancer), higher levels of self-efficacy to manage their own chronic conditions are related to higher health-related QoL [44–48], reduced perceived stress [49–51], lesser anxiety and depressive symptoms [47, 48, 52] and lower symptom severity [48, 53] and also predict symptom resolution [49]. Similar results were found in mental illness studies examining unipolar and bipolar disorders, where higher self-efficacy was positively related to mental and physical health-related QoL [54, 55]. Conversely, a study on multi-morbid primary care patients reported that lower self-efficacy and higher disease burden leads to lower QoL [56]. The notable two-way relationship between certain predictors and outcomes highlights the complexity of addressing patient self-efficacy.

Given the rise in the ageing population and an increasing prevalence of chronic diseases [57], patient empowerment is imperative to reduce health care burden. Community and individual empowerment are one of the key health promotion principles stated in the Ottawa Charter for health promotion that focuses on enabling people to exercise more control over their health, environment and health choices [58]. Besides, an intervention study using an empowering self-management model that focused on self-awareness, goal setting, planning, adjusting physical, psychological and social structures, and evaluation was found to improve self-efficacy and sense of coherence among elderlies with chronic diseases [59]. In particular, self-efficacy is strongly related to the competence component of the empowerment concept, and it plays a critical role in the initiation and maintenance of positive behaviour change and is a vital mechanism for effective self-management [39, 60, 61]. Higher self-efficacy results in better self-management, which leads to improved health outcomes that not only reduce health care service burdens but also health care utilisation [36, 62, 63].

In terms of patient self-care and management, there is substantial evidence confirming the relationship between self-efficacy (both general and specific, e.g. pain self-efficacy) and self-management behaviours. Studies have identified a positive relationship between self-efficacy and opioid or medication adherence [61, 64–67], increased communication, partnership, self-care [37, 65] and positive patient-centred communication [68, 69]. A diabetes study reported diabetes management self-efficacy as the only predictor of diabetes control [70]. Higher education level and receiving health education were shown to boost management self-efficacy that was associated with self-care activities (i.e. nutrition, medication, physical exercise) and glycaemic control [70]. This also holds true for cancer patients, where self-efficacy and social support directly and indirectly affected self-management behaviours, specifically, patient communication (e.g. communicating concerns, asking questions, expressing treatment expectations), exercise and information seeking [71]. Pertaining to patients with physical disabilities, social functioning, stronger resilience and less pain and fatigue were strongly associated with disability management self-efficacy [72], which is crucial for increasing odds of employment among disabled youths [73].

Studies have identified a few predictors of self-efficacy among patients with chronic diseases such as duration of diagnosis, severity of disease symptoms, age, availability of social support and health education, and absence of complications and depression [74–77]. Of these variables, availability of social support and healthy literacy can easily be manipulated through intervention programs. Most studies have found a positive relationship between self-efficacy and health literacy, especially functional health literacy [77–81], but there are a few that found no significant associations between self-efficacy and health literacy [75, 82]. In addition, social support is a major factor affecting patients' self-efficacy and self-management behaviours. Apart from boosting self-efficacy and self-management [71, 83, 84], higher social support was shown to reduce difficulties in medical inter-actions among breast cancer patients [85] and enhance well-being among diabetes patients [84]. Therefore, it is necessary for health care and educational interventions to include components of social support, health education when target-ing patients' management self-efficacy.

According to a recent review by Allegrante et al. [62], much of the empirical research and reviews that have been conducted on the effec-tiveness of interventions to support behavioural self-management of chronic diseases have demonstrated small to moderate effects for changes in health behaviours, health status, and health care utilisation for certain chronic condi-tions. Such interventions that targeted or exam-ined self-efficacy as an outcome included web-based, mobile app-based and face-to-face educational training or programs. In Chao et al.'s [86] study, a cloud-based mobile health platform and mobile app service for diabetic patients to self-monitor progress and goals set was found to increase self-efficacy, improve health knowledge and increase behaviour compliance rate, espe-cially in women. Ali and colleagues [87] reported higher pharmaceutical knowledge, patient satis-faction and self-efficacy among cardiovascular disease patients who were qualified to self-administer medication, as compared to those who were just provided educational brochures by nurses. In another study [88], an 8-week Patient and Partner Education Programme for Pituitary disease (PPEP-Pituitary) was found to increase patient and partner's self-efficacy. Self-care behaviour and self-efficacy of asthma patients also improved after attending a self-efficacy intervention constituting educational videos, resources, social support group and phone-based medical follow-up [89]. Other interventions focused on caregivers' self-efficacy by providing caregiver trainings and stress management train-ings, which were effective in improving caregiv-ers' self-efficacy in managing patients' symptoms, reducing caregiver stress and increas-ing preparedness in caregiving [90, 91]. The effectiveness of these interventions in improving self-efficacy suggests the importance of educa-tion, progress monitoring, information resources,

social support, and patient–provider trust and communication in self-management behaviour, promoting interventions for patients with chronic diseases and their caregivers.

12.5.2 Role of Self-Efficacy in Parental Outcomes in the Perinatal Period

The emergence of self-efficacy studies on new parents or parents during the perinatal period has revealed the association of self-efficacy with childbirth and psychological well-being and childbirth outcomes. During pregnancy, maternal childbirth self-efficacy is positively correlated with vigour, sense of coherence, maternal sup-port and childbirth knowledge, and negatively correlated with history of mental illnesses [92–94]. Moreover, maternal childbirth self-efficacy affects maternal well-being during pregnancy in terms of negative mood, anxiety, depressive symptoms and fear of childbirth [93–96]. The level of maternal self-efficacy also influences birth choices, with elective caesarean and higher dosage of analgesic epidural during childbirth being more common among mothers with lower childbirth self-efficacy [92–94, 97]. In order to better prepare mothers for childbirth, few studies have adopted a blended approach of antenatal mindfulness practice and skill-based education programs, which was effective in improving childbirth self-efficacy, mindfulness, reducing fear of childbirth, stress, antenatal depression, and opioid analgesic use [98–100]. The mindful-ness programs also saw a reduction in postnatal depression, anxiety, and stress [98, 99]. Other studies that implemented antenatal psychoeduca-tion programs also report increase in childbirth self-efficacy among mothers and reduction in fear of childbirth [101, 102].

After childbirth, receiving informal social support is essential for maternal parenting self-efficacy, which helps to reduce risk of postnatal depression [103]. A study by Salonen et al. [104] comparing parenting self-efficacy levels between mothers and fathers revealed that mothers tend to score higher than fathers on parenting self-efficacy. Age, multiparity, presence of depressive symptoms, perception of infant's health and contentment, and quality of partner relationship were shown to be significant predictors of parenting self-efficacy in mothers and fathers [94, 104, 105]. Parenting self-efficacy not only is crucial for personal health and well-being but also contributes to healthy marital relations, family functioning and child development [106]. Therefore, various educational and technology-based interventions have been developed in hopes of boosting parental self-efficacy in the postpartum period. A postnatal psychoeducation program designed for the first-time mothers, consisting of a face-to-face educational session during a home visit, an educational booklet and three follow-up telephone calls was found to be effective at enhancing maternal self-efficacy, reducing postnatal depression, and increasing perceived social support [107]. A more recent technology-based Supportive Educational Parenting Program (SEPP) targeting both parents, comprised of two telephone-based educational sessions and 1 month follow-up via an educational mobile health app [108]. As compared to routine postpartum care, the SEPP was effective in promoting parenting self-efficacy, parenting satisfaction, parental bonding, better perceived social support and reducing postnatal depression in both mothers and fathers [108].

Self-efficacy in the postpartum period also includes breastfeeding. Dennis [109] reported significant predictors of breastfeeding self-efficacy as maternal education, support from other mothers, type of delivery, satisfaction with labour pain relief, satisfaction with postpartum care, perceptions of breastfeeding progress, infant feeding method as planned and maternal anxiety [109]. A study conducted among Japanese women found that breastfeeding self-efficacy is also associated with maternal perceptions of insufficient milk, leading to discontinuation of breastfeeding during the immediate postpartum period [110]. Breastfeeding is highly encouraged by health care professionals due to its nutritional value, benefits to the infant's development and potential mother–child bonding; therefore, stud-

ies seek to develop educational or support programs to promote breastfeeding. During pregnancy, antenatal educational interventions using breastfeeding workbook or videos and demonstrations have shown to be effective in increasing mothers' breastfeeding self-efficacy at 4 weeks postpartum [111, 112]. During the postpartum period, peer-support interventions for breastfeeding are more common [113]. Combined with professional support, peer-support breastfeeding programs are effective in boosting breastfeeding self-efficacy [113].

Despite the heavy focus on maternal self-efficacy during and after pregnancy, there has also been an increase in health care research on fathers' involvement during the perinatal period, as early paternal involvement during and after pregnancy was found to positively influence maternal well-being and benefit the biopsychosocial development of infants 14 months and below [114–116]. A recent study by Shorey et al. [117] found that high paternal self-efficacy is one of the main factors of high paternal involvement during infancy, especially among first-time fathers. Higher paternal self-efficacy also leads to increase in parenting satisfaction over the first 6 months postpartum [118]. According to a review on informational interventions aiming to improve paternal outcomes [117], there were only three interventions (via online dissemination of information or self-modelled videotaped interaction and feedback) that reported on paternal self-efficacy [119–121], but only Hudson et al.'s [119] study found an intervention effect on parenting self-efficacy and parenting satisfaction in fathers. In addition to informational interventions, educational interventions are also useful and important in boosting paternal self-efficacy and other paternal outcomes [108, 122].

Overall, in order to effectively enhance parental self-efficacy across these various aspects (i.e. childbirth, parenting, breastfeeding) during the perinatal period, it is necessary for interventions to incorporate and target at least a component of the self-efficacy theory (mastery experiences, vicarious experiences, verbal persuasion, and emotional and physiological arousal).

12.5.3 Role of Self-Efficacy in Nursing Education

Another application of self-efficacy in the health care setting is with regard to nursing education and training. Effective clinical trainings should establish a sense of self-efficacy among nursing students, which is a key component for acting independently and competently in the nursing profession [123–125]. Students' clinical performance, course completion and achievement motivations are also dependent on individual perceived self-efficacy [125–127]. According to Bandura [128], students with low self-efficacy will tend to avoid situations that led to past failures; therefore, strong sense of self-efficacy and job satisfaction is crucial in reducing attrition in the nursing profession [126, 129]. Lastly, as a future health care practitioner, clinical self-efficacy and competence are essential for providing quality health care and ensuring patient safety [125].

Evidence has suggested that older age, being married, more working experience in the nursing field, individual interest and willingness to work in a nursing unit contributes to high nursing self-efficacy in students [127, 130, 131], which is also an important factor in creating clinical confidence [132]. Clinical environments, nursing colleagues, and clinical educator's capabilities can influence the creation of clinical self-efficacy in nursing students [123]. A weak relationship between faculty and hospitals, lack of staff and training facilities, and unprofessional trainers could adversely influence self-efficacy [133, 134]. More specifically, students have reported that using logbooks, having more authentic clinical simulations, working alone, more ward time, being under the guidance of one instructor, and receiving constant verbal validation, positive feedback and support can increase one's own sense of self-efficacy [123, 135, 136]. These corresponds with components of the self-efficacy theory [128] in terms of mastery experiences, vicarious experiences and verbal persuasion.

Numerous education and clinical training curriculums are being developed and constantly revised to target promotion of self-efficacy in specific clinical skills among nursing students. Sabeti and colleagues [137] found that students' self-efficacy ranges from weak to excellent across different skills, with high self-efficacy in medication administration and nursing procedures, and low self-efficacy in care before, during and after diagnostic procedures. In Pike et al.'s study [136], despite undergoing a clinical simulation program aimed to improve learning self-efficacy, students still reported low self-efficacy in communication skills. However, in another study, a blended learning pedagogy was used to redesign a nursing communication module from didactic lectures to an online and face-to-face interactive classroom sessions, which resulted in increased communication self-efficacy and better learning attitudes among nursing students [138]. In nursing education, clinical simulations are widely used to create authentic scenarios and training environments and were often the most effective method in boosting students' self-efficacy. A study comparing the effectiveness of a peritoneal dialysis simulation with watching videos reported higher psychomotor skills score and self-efficacy among students who underwent the simulation than those who just watched videos of the procedure [139]. Similarly, a Diverse Standardised Patient Simulation was also seen to improve students' transcultural self-efficacy perceptions [140]. Notably, simulation exercises were more effective at improving students' self-efficacy and critical thinking skills when conducted after a role-play than after a lecture [141]. Overall, nursing curriculum and clinical simulations play a vital role in mastery experiences, and the integration of positive feedback (verbal persuasion) and observation of clinical educators in ward settings (vicarious experiences) would present an ideal method of enhancing self-efficacy among nursing students.

12.6 Conclusion

The self-efficacy theory is in itself linked with other psychological theories to influence health-promoting behavioural changes in various life situations. The applications of self-efficacy in various nursing contexts ultimately boil down to health promotion and improvement of the quality of health care and patient safety. The concept of self-efficacy has played a significant role in not only predicting individual physical and psychological wellbeing, competencies, and self-care management, but also often serve as a theoretical framework for existing clinical and educational interventions. Despite its well-established literature base, emerging evidence on self-efficacy's positive relationship with sense of coherence and the gradual shift of the health care paradigm to a salutogenic orientation indicate a need for subsequent nursing research to continue to tailor and refine ways to enhance self-efficacy in specific population groups.

Take Home Messages
- Self-efficacy is an individual's perception of their own ability to perform a particular behaviour through cognitive, motivational, affective and selection processes.
- Self-efficacy is derived from mastery experiences, vicarious experiences, verbal persuasion and individual emotional and physiological state.
- Self-efficacy theory is commonly compared to other psychological behaviour theories such as locus of control, self-esteem and intrinsic motivation theory.
- The self-efficacy theory is analogous to Antonovsky's salutogenic theory where self-efficacy is also discovered to be positively associated with sense of coherence.
- The concept of self-efficacy is applied in self-regulation, self-care, self-monitoring and self-management in the nursing context.
- Self-efficacy promotes patients' competence that is vital for self-care and management and is associated with better physical and psychological health among chronically ill patients.
- High maternal self-efficacy is crucial for positive childbirth and breastfeeding experiences, and better psychological well-being during and after pregnancy.
- High paternal self-efficacy increases paternal involvement during infancy and parenting satisfaction.

- In nursing education, self-efficacy plays a vital role in enhancing students' competence, motivation and clinical performance, which influences job satisfaction and quality of patient care provided.
- Education and social support through informational, emotional, formal and informal means are the primary contributors to self-efficacy.
- Overall, self-efficacy is a key health-promoting component among patients with chronic illnesses, parents during the perinatal period, youth and the elderly.

References

1. Bandura A. Self-efficacy: toward a unifying theory of behavioral change. Psychol Rev. 1977;84(2):191–215.
2. Bandura A, Walters RH. Social learning theory. Englewood Cliffs, NJ: Prentice-Hall; 1977.
3. Bandura A. Self-efficacy mechanism in physiological activation and health-promoting behavior. New York: Raven; 1989.
4. Bandura A. Recycling misconceptions of perceived self-efficacy. Cognit Ther Res. 1984;8(3):231–55.
5. Bandura A. Human agency in social cognitive theory. Am Psychol. 1989;44(9):1175.
6. Schwarzer R. Self-efficacy: thought control of action. Hoboken, NJ: Taylor & Francis; 2014.
7. Bandura A. Social foundations of thought and action: a social cognitive theory. Englewood Cliffs, NJ: Prentice-Hall; 1986.
8. Rotter JB. Generalized expectancies for internal versus external control of reinforcement. Psychol Monogr Gen Appl. 1966;80(1):1.
9. Maddux JE, Rogers RW. Protection motivation and self-efficacy: a revised theory of fear appeals and attitude change. J Exp Soc Psychol. 1983;19(5):469–79.
10. Zulkosky K, editor. Self-efficacy: a concept analysis. Nursing forum: Wiley Online Library; 2009.
11. Bandura A. Self-efficacy: the exercise of control. New York: W. H. Freeman; 1997.
12. Deci EL. SpringerLink. Intrinsic motivation. Boston, MA: Springer US; 1975.
13. Bandura A, Schunk DH. Cultivating competence, self-efficacy, and intrinsic interest through proximal self-motivation. J Pers Soc Psychol. 1981;41(3):586–98.
14. Bandura A. Self-efficacy. In: Ramachaudran VS, editor. Encyclopedia of human behaviour. New York: Academic Press; 1994. p. 71–81.
15. Bandura A. Self-efficacy mechanism in human agency. Am Psychol. 1982;37(2):122.

16. Bandura A. Self-efficacy in changing societies. Cambridge: Cambridge University Press; 1995.

17. Carpenito LJ. Nursing diagnosis: application to clinical practice. Philadelphia: Wolters Kluwer Health; 2009.

18. Novak M, Costantini L, Schneider S, Beanlands H, editors. Approaches to self-management in chronic illness. Seminars in dialysis, vol. 26: Wiley Online Library; 2013. p. 188.

19. Walker LO, Avant KC. Strategies for theory construction in nursing. Norwalk: Appleton & Lange; 2005.

20. Wilson J. Thinking with concepts. Cambridge: Cambridge University Press; 1969.

21. Liu T. A concept analysis of self-efficacy among Chinese elderly with diabetes mellitus. Nurs Forum. 2012;47(4):226–35.

22. White LL, Cohen MZ, Berger AM, Kupzyk KA, Swore-Fletcher BA, Bierman PJ. Perceived self-efficacy: a concept analysis for symptom management in patients with cancer. Clin J Oncol Nurs. 2017;21(6):E272–e9.

23. Gapstur RL. Symptom burden: a concept analysis and implications for oncology nurses. Oncol Nurs Forum. 2007;34(3):673–80.

24. Sims DC, Skarbek AJ. Parental Self-efficacy: a concept analysis related to teen parenting and implications for school nurses. J Sch Nurs. 2019;35(1):8–14.

25. Rodgers BL, Knafl K. Concept analysis: an evolutionary view, concept development in nursing: foundations. Tech Appl. 2000:77–102.

26. Voskuil VR, Robbins LB. Youth physical activity self-efficacy: a concept analysis. J Adv Nurs. 2015;71(9):2002–19.

27. Kuiper R, Pesut D, Kautz D. Promoting the self-regulation of clinical reasoning skills in nursing students. Open Nurs J. 2009;3:76–85.

28. Bambini D, Washburn J, Perkins R. Outcomes of clinical simulation for novice nursing students: communication, confidence, clinical judgment. Nurs Educ Perspect. 2009;30(2):79–82.

29. Blackman I, Hall M, Darmawan IJIEJ. Undergraduate nurse variables that predict academic achievement and clinical competence in. Nursing. 2007;8(2):222–36.

30. Robb M. Self-efficacy with application to nursing education: a concept analysis. Nurs Forum. 2012;47(3):166–72.

31. Antonovsky A. Health, stress, and coping. London: Jossey-Bass; 1979.

32. Antonovsky A. Unraveling the mystery of health: how people manage stress and stay well. London: Jossey-Bass; 1987.

33. Saltzer EB. The relationship of personal efficacy beliefs to behaviour. Br J Soc Psychol. 1982;21(3):213–21.

34. Eriksson M, Mittelmark MB. The sense of coherence and its measurement. In: Mittelmark MB, Sagy S, Eriksson M, Bauer GF, Pelikan JM, Lindstrom B,

et al., editors. The handbook of Salutogenesis, vol. 2017. Cham: Springer. p. 97–106.

35. Lindström B, Eriksson M. The Hitchhiker's guide to salutogenesis: Salutogenic pathways to health promotion: Folkhälsan Research Center, Health Promotion Research; 2010.

36. Lorig KR, Ritter P, Stewart AL, Sobel DS, Brown BW, Bandura A, et al. Chronic disease self-management program: 2-year health status and health care utilization outcomes. Med Care. 2001;39(11):1217–23.

37. Sarkar U, Fisher L, Schillinger D. Is self-efficacy associated with diabetes self-management across race/ethnicity and health literacy? Diabetes Care. 2006;29(4):823–9.

38. Trap R, Rejkjaer L, Hansen EH. Empirical relations between sense of coherence and self-efficacy, National Danish Survey. Health Promot Int. 2016;31(3):635–43.

39. Baldwin AS, Rothman AJ, Hertel AW, Linde JA, Jeffery RW, Finch EA, et al. Specifying the determinants of the initiation and maintenance of behavior change: an examination of self-efficacy, satisfaction, and smoking cessation. Health Psychol. 2006;25(5):626–34.

40. Hendriksen ES, Pettifor A, Lee S-J, Coates TJ, Rees HV. Predictors of condom use among young adults in South Africa: the reproductive health and HIV research unit National Youth Survey. Am J Public Health. 2007;97(7):1241–8.

41. Scholz U, Sniehotta FF, Schwarzer R. Predicting physical exercise in cardiac rehabilitation: the role of phase-specific self-efficacy beliefs. J Sport Exerc Psychol. 2005;27(2):135–51.

42. Darker CD, French DP, Eves FF, Sniehotta FF. An intervention to promote walking amongst the general population based on an 'extended' theory of planned behaviour: a waiting list randomised controlled trial. Psychol Health. 2010;25(1):71–88.

43. Motl RW, Dishman RK, Saunders RP, Dowda M, Felton G, Ward DS, et al. Examining social-cognitive determinants of intention and physical activity among black and White adolescent girls using structural equation modeling. Health Psychol. 2002;21(5):459–67.

44. Adegbola M. Spirituality, self-efficacy, and quality of life among adults with sickle cell disease. South Online J Nurs Res. 2011;11(1):5.

45. Akin S, Kas Guner C. Investigation of the relationship among fatigue, self-efficacy and quality of life during chemotherapy in patients with breast, lung or gastrointestinal cancer. Eur J Cancer Care (Engl). 2019;28(1):e12898.

46. Börsbo B, Gerdle B, Peolsson M. 988 impact of the interaction between self efficacy, symptoms, and catastrophizing on disability, quality of life, and health in chronic pain patients. Eur J Pain. 2009;13(S1):S277–S8.

47. Chao CY, Lemieux C, Restellini S, Afif W, Bitton A, Lakatos PL, et al. Maladaptive coping, low

self-efficacy and disease activity are associated with poorer patient-reported outcomes in inflammatory bowel disease. Saudi J Gastroenterol. 2019;25(3):159–66.

48. Omran S, Symptom Severity MMS. Anxiety, depression, self-efficacy and quality of life in patients with Cancer. Asian Pac J Cancer Prev. 2018;19(2):365–74.

49. Byma EA, Given BA, Given CW, You M. The effects of mastery on pain and fatigue resolution. Oncol Nurs Forum. 2009;36(5):544–52.

50. Fleming G, McKenna M, Murchison V, Wood Y, Nixon JO, Rogers T, et al. Using self-efficacy as a client-centred outcome measure. Nurs Stand. 2003;17(34):33–6.

51. Hoffman AJ, von Eye A, Gift AG, Given BA, Given CW, Rothert M. Testing a theoretical model of perceived self-efficacy for cancer-related fatigue self-management and optimal physical functional status. Nurs Res. 2009;58(1):32–41.

52. Sympa P, Vlachou E, Kazakos K, Govina O, Stamatiou G, Lavdaniti M. Depression and self-efficacy in patients with type 2 diabetes in northern Greece. Endocr Metab Immune Disord Drug Targets. 2018;18(4):371–8.

53. Kurtz ME, Kurtz JC, Stommel M, Given CW, Given B. Physical functioning and depression among older persons with cancer. Cancer Pract. 2001;9(1):11–8.

54. Abraham KM, Miller CJ, Birgenheir DG, Lai Z, Kilbourne AM. Self-efficacy and quality of life among people with bipolar disorder. J Nerv Ment Dis. 2014;202(8):583–8.

55. Houle J, Gascon-Depatie M, Bélanger-Dumontier G, Cardinal C. Depression self-management support: a systematic review. Patient Educ Couns. 2013;91(3):271–9.

56. Peters M, Potter CM, Kelly L, Fitzpatrick R. Self-efficacy and health-related quality of life: a cross-sectional study of primary care patients with multi-morbidity. Health Qual Life Outcomes. 2019;17(1):37.

57. WHO. The world health report 2002: reducing risks, promoting healthy life. Geneva: World Health Organization; 2002.

58. WHO. The Ottawa charter for health promotion. Geneva: World Health Organization; 1986.

59. Hourzad A, Pouladi S, Ostovar A, Ravanipour M. The effects of an empowering self-management model on self-efficacy and sense of coherence among retired elderly with chronic diseases: a randomized controlled trial. Clin Interv Aging. 2018;13:2215–24.

60. Lorig KR, Holman HR. Self-management education: history, definition, outcomes, and mechanisms. Ann Behav Med. 2003;26(1):1–7.

61. Nafradi L, Nakamoto K, Schulz PJ. Is patient empowerment the key to promote adherence? A systematic review of the relationship between self-efficacy, health locus of control and medication adherence. PLoS One. 2017;12(10):e0186458.

62. Allegrante JP, Wells MT, Peterson JC. Interventions to support behavioral self-management of chronic diseases. Annu Rev Public Health. 2019;40(1):127–46.

63. Marks R, Allegrante JP. A review and synthesis of research evidence for self-efficacy-enhancing interventions for reducing chronic disability: implications for health education practice (part II). Health Promot Pract. 2005;6(2):148–56.

64. Archiopoli A, Ginossar T, Wilcox B, Avila M, Hill R, Oetzel J. Factors of interpersonal communication and behavioral health on medication self-efficacy and medication adherence. AIDS Care. 2016;28(12):1607–14.

65. Curtin RB, Walters BAJ, Schatell D, Pennell P, Wise M, Klicko K. Self-efficacy and self-management behaviors in patients with chronic kidney disease. Adv Chronic Kidney Dis. 2008;15(2):191–205.

66. Liang SY, Yates P, Edwards H, Tsay SL. Factors influencing opioid-taking self-efficacy and analgesic adherence in Taiwanese outpatients with cancer. Psychooncology. 2008;17(11):1100–7.

67. McCann TV, Clark E, Lu S. The self-efficacy model of medication adherence in chronic mental illness. J Clin Nurs. 2008;17(11c):329–40.

68. Austin JD, Robertson MC, Shay LA, Balasubramanian BA. Implications for patient-provider communication and health self-efficacy among cancer survivors with multiple chronic conditions: results from the health information National Trends Survey. J Cancer Surviv. 2019;13(5):663–72.

69. Finney Rutten LJ, Hesse BW, St Sauver JL, Wilson P, Chawla N, Hartigan DB, et al. Health Self-efficacy among populations with multiple chronic conditions: the value of patient-centered communication. Adv Ther. 2016;33(8):1440–51.

70. Amer FA, Mohamed MS, Elbur AI, Abdelaziz SI, Elrayah ZA. Influence of self-efficacy management on adherence to self-care activities and treatment outcome among diabetes mellitus type 2. Pharm Pract (Granada). 2018;16(4):1274.

71. Geng Z, Ogbolu Y, Wang J, Hinds PS, Qian H, Yuan C. Gauging the effects of Self-efficacy, social support, and coping style on self-management behaviors in Chinese cancer survivors. Cancer Nurs. 2018;41(5):E1–E10.

72. Amtmann D, Bamer AM, Nery-Hurwit MB, Liljenquist KS, Yorkston K. Factors associated with disease self-efficacy in individuals aging with a disability. Psychol Health Med. 2019;24(10):1171–81.

73. Andersén Å, Larsson K, Pingel R, Kristiansson P, Anderzén I. The relationship between self-efficacy and transition to work or studies in young adults with disabilities. Scand J Public Health. 2018;46(2):272–8.

74. Kang Y, Yang IS. Cardiac self-efficacy and its predictors in patients with coronary artery diseases. J Clin Nurs. 2013;22(17–18):2465–73.

75. Lee H, Lim Y, Kim S, Park HK, Ahn JJ, Kim Y, et al. Predictors of low levels of self-efficacy among

patients with chronic obstructive pulmonary disease in South Korea. Nurs Health Sci. 2014;16(1):78–83.

76. Sanchez AI, Martinez MP, Miro E, Medina A. Predictors of the pain perception and self-efficacy for pain control in patients with fibromyalgia. Span J Psychol. 2011;14(1):366–73.

77. Xu XY, Leung AYM, Chau PH. Health literacy, self-efficacy, and associated factors among patients with diabetes. Health Literacy Res Pract. 2018;2(2):e67–77.

78. Bohanny W, Wu SFV, Liu CY, Yeh SH, Tsay SL, Wang TJ. Health literacy, self-efficacy, and self-care behaviors in patients with type 2 diabetes mellitus. J Am Assoc Nurse Pract. 2013;25(9):495–502.

79. Inoue M, Takahashi M, Kai I. Impact of communicative and critical health literacy on understanding of diabetes care and self-efficacy in diabetes management: a cross-sectional study of primary care in Japan. BMC Fam Pract. 2013;14(1):40.

80. Reisi M, Tavassoli E, Mahaki B, Sharifirad G, Javadzade H, Mostafavi F. Impact of health literacy, self-efficacy and outcome expectations on adherence to self-care behaviors in Iranians with type 2 diabetes. Oman Med J. 2016;31(1):52–9.

81. Zuercher E, Diatta ID, Burnand B, Peytremann-Bridevaux I. Health literacy and quality of care of patients with diabetes: a cross-sectional analysis. Prim Care Diabetes. 2017;11(3):233–40.

82. Murphy DA, Lam P, Naar-King S, Harris DR, Parsons JT, Muenz LR. Health literacy and antiretroviral adherence among HIV-infected adolescents. Patient Educ Couns. 2010;79(1):25–9.

83. Lee YH, Wang RH. Helplessness, social support and self-care behaviors among long-term hemodialysis patients. Nurs Res. 2001;9(2):147.

84. Schiotz ML, Bogelund M, Almdal T, Jensen BB, Willaing I. Social support and self-management behaviour among patients with type 2 diabetes. Diabet Med. 2012;29(5):654–61.

85. Collie K, Wong P, Tilston J, Butler LD, Turner-Cobb J, Kreshka MA, et al. Self-efficacy, coping, and difficulties interacting with health care professionals among women living with breast cancer in rural communities. Psychooncology. 2005;14(10):901–12.

86. Chao DY, Lin TM, Ma W-Y. Enhanced self-efficacy and behavioral changes among patients with diabetes: cloud-based mobile health platform and Mobile App Service. JMIR Diabetes. 2019;4(2):e11017.

87. Ali Beigloo RH, Mohajer S, Eshraghi A, Mazlom SR. Self-administered medications in cardiovascular ward: a study on patients' self-efficacy, knowledge and satisfaction. J Evid Based Care. 2019;9(1):16–25.

88. Andela CD, Repping-Wuts H, Stikkelbroeck N, Pronk MC, Tiemensma J, Hermus AR, et al. Enhanced self-efficacy after a self-management programme in pituitary disease: a randomized controlled trial. Eur J Endocrinol. 2017;177(1):59–72.

89. Chen SY, Sheu S, Chang CS, Wang TH, Huang MS. The effects of the self-efficacy method on adult asthmatic patient self-care behavior. J Nurs Res. 2010;18(4):266–74.

90. Havyer RD, Havyer RD, van Ryn M, van Ryn M, Wilson PM, Wilson PM, et al. The effect of routine training on the self-efficacy of informal caregivers of colorectal cancer patients. Support Care Cancer. 2017;25(4):1071–7.

91. Hendrix CC, Hendrix CC, Bailey DE Jr, Bailey DE Jr, Steinhauser KE, Steinhauser KE, et al. Effects of enhanced caregiver training program on cancer caregiver's self-efficacy, preparedness, and psychological well-being. Support Care Cancer. 2016;24(1):327–36.

92. Berentson-Shaw J, Scott KM, Jose PE. Do self-efficacy beliefs predict the primiparous labour and birth experience? A longitudinal study. J Reprod Infant Psychol. 2009;27(4):357–73.

93. Carlsson I-M, Ziegert K, Nissen E, Hälsofrämjande P, Centrum för forskning om välfärd hoi, Akademin för hälsa och v, et al. The relationship between childbirth self-efficacy and aspects of well-being, birth interventions and birth outcomes. Midwifery. 2015;31(10):1000–7.

94. Schwartz L, Toohill J, Creedy DK, Baird K, Gamble J, Fenwick J. Factors associated with childbirth self-efficacy in Australian childbearing women. BMC Pregnancy Childbirth. 2015;15:29.

95. Salomonsson B, Gullberg MT, Alehagen S, Wijma K. Self-efficacy beliefs and fear of childbirth in nulliparous women. J Psychosom Obstet Gynaecol. 2013;34(3):116–21.

96. Sieber S, Germann N, Barbir A, Ehlert U. Emotional well-being and predictors of birth-anxiety, self-efficacy, and psychosocial adaptation in healthy pregnant women. Acta Obstet Gynecol Scand. 2006;85(10):1200–7.

97. Dilks FM, Beal JA. Role of self-efficacy in birth choice. J Perinat Neonatal Nurs. 1997;11(1):1–9.

98. Byrne J, Hauck Y, Fisher C, Bayes S, Schutze R. Effectiveness of a mindfulness-based childbirth education pilot study on maternal self-efficacy and fear of childbirth. J Midwifery Womens Health. 2014;59(2):192–7.

99. Duncan LG, Cohn MA, Chao MT, Cook JG, Riccobono J, Bardacke N. Benefits of preparing for childbirth with mindfulness training: a randomized controlled trial with active comparison. BMC Pregnancy Childbirth. 2017;17(1):140–11.

100. Pan W-L, Chang C-W, Chen S-M, Gau M-L. Assessing the effectiveness of mindfulness-based programs on mental health during pregnancy and early motherhood—a randomized control trial. BMC Pregnancy Childbirth. 2019;19(1):346.

101. Sercekus P, Baskale H. Effects of antenatal education on fear of childbirth, maternal self-efficacy and parental attachment. Midwifery. 2016;34:166–72.

102. Toohill J, Fenwick J, Gamble J, Creedy DK, Buist A, Turkstra E, et al. A randomized controlled trial of a psycho-education intervention by midwives in

reducing childbirth fear in pregnant women. Birth. 2014;41(4):384–94.

103. Leahy-Warren P, McCarthy G, Corcoran P. First-time mothers: social support, maternal parental self-efficacy and postnatal depression. J Clin Nurs. 2012;21(3–4):388–97.

104. Salonen AH, Kaunonen M, Åstedt-Kurki P, Järvenpää AL, Isoaho H, Tarkka MT. Parenting self-efficacy after childbirth. J Adv Nurs. 2009;65(11):2324–36.

105. Bryanton J, Gagnon AJ, Hatem M, Johnston C. Predictors of early parenting self-efficacy: results of a prospective cohort study. Nurs Res. 2008;57(4):252–9.

106. Albanese AM, Russo GR, Geller PA. The role of parental self-efficacy in parent and child well-being: a systematic review of associated outcomes. Child Care Health Dev. 2019;45(3):333–63.

107. Shorey S, Chan SWC, Chong YS, He HG. A randomized controlled trial of the effectiveness of a postnatal psychoeducation programme on self-efficacy, social support and postnatal depression among primiparas. J Adv Nurs. 2015;71(6):1260–73.

108. Shorey S, Ng YPM, Ng ED, Siew AL, Mörelius E, Yoong J, et al. Effectiveness of a technology-based supportive educational parenting program on parental outcomes (part 1): randomized controlled trial. J Med Internet Res. 2019;21(2):e10816.

109. Dennis CLE. Identifying predictors of breastfeeding self-efficacy in the immediate postpartum period. Res Nurs Health. 2006;29(4):256–68.

110. Otsuka K, Dennis C-L, Tatsuoka H, Jimba M. The relationship between breastfeeding self-efficacy and perceived insufficient milk among Japanese mothers. J Obstet Gynecol Neonatal Nurs. 2008;37(5):546–55.

111. Mizrak B, Ozerdogan N, Colak E. The effect of antenatal education on breastfeeding self-efficacy: primiparous women in Turkey. Int J Caring Sci. 2017;10(1):503–10.

112. Otsuka K, Taguri M, Dennis C-L, Wakutani K, Awano M, Yamaguchi T, et al. Effectiveness of a breastfeeding self-efficacy intervention: do hospital practices make a difference? Matern Child Health J. 2014;18(1):296–306.

113. Kaunonen M, Hannula L, Tarkka MT. A systematic review of peer support interventions for breastfeeding. J Clin Nurs. 2012;21(13–14):1943–54.

114. Bronte-Tinkew J, Carrano J, Horowitz A, Kinukawa A. Involvement among resident fathers and links to infant cognitive outcomes. J Fam Issues. 2008;29(9):1211–44.

115. Shorey S, He H-G, Morelius E. Skin-to-skin contact by fathers and the impact on infant and paternal outcomes: an integrative review. Midwifery. 2016;40:207–17.

116. Stapleton LRT, Schetter CD, Westling E, Rini C, Glynn LM, Hobel CJ, et al. Perceived partner support in pregnancy predicts lower maternal and infant distress. J Fam Psychol. 2012;26(3):453–63.

117. Shorey S, Ang L, Tam WWS. Informational interventions on paternal outcomes during the perinatal period: a systematic review. Women Birth. 2019;32(2):e145–e58.

118. Shorey S, Ang L, Goh ECL, Gandhi M. Factors influencing paternal involvement during infancy: a prospective longitudinal study. J Adv Nurs. 2019;75(2):357–67.

119. Hudson DB, Campbell-Grossman C, Ofe Fleck M, Elek SM, Shipman AMY. Effects of the new fathers network on first-time fathers' parenting self-efficacy and parenting satisfaction during the transition to parenthood. Issues Compr Pediatr Nurs. 2003;26(4):217–29.

120. Magill-Evans J, Harrison M, Benzies K, Gierl M, Kimak C. Effects of parenting education on first-time fathers' skills in interactions with their infants. Fathering. 2007;5(1):42–57.

121. Salonen AH, Kaunonen M, Åstedt-Kurki P, Järvenpää A-L, Isoaho H, Tarkka M-T. Effectiveness of an internet-based intervention enhancing Finnish parents' parenting satisfaction and parenting self-efficacy during the postpartum period. Midwifery. 2011;27(6):832–41.

122. Shorey S, Lau YY, Dennis CL, Chan YS, Tam WWS, Chan YH. A randomized-controlled trial to examine the effectiveness of the 'home-but not alone' mobile-health application educational programme on parental outcomes. J Adv Nurs. 2017;73(9):2103–17.

123. Abdal M, Masoudi Alavi N, Adib-Hajbaghery M. Clinical self-efficacy in senior nursing students: a mixed-methods study. Nurs Midwif Stud. 2015;4(3):e29143.

124. Dearnley CA, Meddings FS. Student self-assessment and its impact on learning—a pilot study. Nurse Educ Today. 2007;27(4):333–40.

125. Mohamadirizi S, Kohan S, Shafei F, Mohamadirizi S. The relationship between clinical competence and clinical self-efficacy among nursing and midwifery students. Int J Pediatr. 2015;3(6.2):1117–23.

126. McLaughlin K, Moutray M, Muldoon OT. The role of personality and self-efficacy in the selection and retention of successful nursing students: a longitudinal study. J Adv Nurs. 2008;61(2):211–21.

127. Zhang Z-J, Zhang C-L, Zhang X-G, Liu X-M, Zhang H, Wang J, et al. Relationship between self-efficacy beliefs and achievement motivation in student nurses. Chin Nurs Res. 2015;2(2):67–70.

128. Bandura A. Perceived self-efficacy in cognitive development and functioning. Educ Psychol. 1993;28(2):117–48.

129. Lee TW, Ko YK. Effects of self-efficacy, affectivity and collective efficacy on nursing performance of hospital nurses. J Adv Nurs. 2010;66(4):839–48.

130. Reid C, Jones L, Hurst C, Anderson D. Examining relationships between socio-demographics and self-efficacy among registered nurses in Australia. Collegian. 2018;25(1):57–63.

131. Soudagar S, Rambod M, Beheshtipour N. Factors associated with nurses' self-efficacy in clinical setting in Iran, 2013. Iran J Nurs Midwifery Res. 2015;20(2):226–31.

132. Boi S. Nurses' experiences in caring for patients from different cultural backgrounds. NT Res. 2000;5(5):382–9.

133. Ekstedt M, Lindblad M, Löfmark A. Nursing students' perception of the clinical learning environment and supervision in relation to two different supervision models—a comparative cross-sectional study. BMC Nurs. 2019;18(1):49.

134. Nabolsi M, Zumot A, Wardam L, Abu-Moghli F. The experience of Jordanian nursing students in their clinical practice. Procedia Soc Behav Sci. 2012;46:5849–57.

135. Gibbons C. Stress, coping and burn-out in nursing students. Int J Nurs Stud. 2010;47(10):1299–309.

136. Pike T, O'Donnell V. The impact of clinical simulation on learner self-efficacy in pre-registration nursing education. Nurse Educ Today. 2010;30(5):405–10.

137. Sabeti F, Akbari-nassaji N, Haghighy-zadeh MH. Nursing students' self-assessment regarding clinical skills achievement in Ahvaz Jundishapur University of Medical Sciences (2009). IJME. 2011;11(5):506–15.

138. Shorey S, Kowitlawakul Y, Devi MK, Chen HC, Soong SKA, Ang E. Blended learning pedagogy designed for communication module among undergraduate nursing students: a quasi-experimental study. Nurse Educ Today. 2018;61:120–6.

139. Topbas E, Terzi B, Gorgen O, Bingol G. Effects of different education methods in peritoneal dialysis application training on psychomotor skills and self-efficacy of nursing students. Technol Health Care. 2019;27(2):175–82.

140. Ozkara SE. Effect of the diverse standardized patient simulation (DSPS) cultural competence education strategy on nursing students' transcultural self-efficacy perceptions. J Transcult Nurs. 2019;30(3):291–302.

141. Kim E. Effect of simulation-based emergency cardiac arrest education on nursing students' self-efficacy and critical thinking skills: role play versus lecture. Nurs Educ Today. 2018;61:258–63.

Empowerment and Health Promotion in Hospitals

13

Sidsel Tveiten

Abstract

Health promotion in hospitals may be an unusual concept to many—experience seems to show that public health and health promotion are considered to be the remit of the local authority. However, hospitals also have responsibility for health promotion. This chapter enlightens empowerment as a concept, a process and an outcome and relates empowerment to health and health promotion in hospitals. Supervision as an empowerment-based intervention is described. The central principles of empowerment can be connected with the central elements of the theory of salutogenesis, recognising patients' self-consciousness and participation as described at the end of the chapter.

Keywords

Empowerment · Empowerment interventions · Health promotion · Hospitals · Participation

S. Tveiten (✉)
Department of Nursing and Health Promotion, Section of Health Science, Oslo Metropolitan University, Oslo, Norway
e-mail: stveiten@oslomet.no

13.1 Empowerment as a Concept

From a scientific perspective, "empowerment" is an immature concept. In other words, it is a broad, vague term that lacks a consensual definition [1]. Consensus means agreement within an academic or professional community around the internal content of a concept. An overview of literature showed that related to health, psychology and pedagogics, there exist 17 definitions of empowerment [2]. In the interest of validity, therefore, it is important to look at some definitions and possible interpretations of empowerment before applying this concept to the hospital context.

The term is a broad one and has connections to many different fields such as occupational psychology, management, health science, pedagogics, social science, politics and democratisation processes. Online searches for the term in scientific databases in 2019 resulted in hundreds of thousands of hits. Both qualitative and quantitative research methods are used in research connected to empowerment.

An immature concept is broadly defined, described and characterised. Immature concepts are easily misused and misunderstood [3–5]. This is confirmed in an academic article that documents and attempts to correct myths and misunderstandings connected to empowerment [6]. Including immature concepts in the production of scientific knowledge implicates the risk of weak-

G. Haugan, M. Eriksson (eds.), *Health Promotion in Health Care – Vital Theories and Research*,
https://doi.org/10.1007/978-3-030-63135-2_13

ening validity because there is uncertainty as to whether one is actually studying what one thinks one is studying. The concept appears in administrative letters from the 1700s [7]. From around 1970, the concept is found in scientific literature connected to the civil rights movement in the USA and other democratisation processes [8, 9].

The New International Webster's Comprehensive Dictionary of the English Language [10] defines "empower" as (to) "give authority to", "delegate authority to", "commission" or "permit". Illustrated Oxford Dictionary [11] defines empowerment as "to authorise", "give permission to", "give power to" or "put in working order". These definitions may seem paternalistic, which in itself is incompatible with what is implied by the term, namely democratisation. To *give* someone authority or to *delegate* authority implies that someone is in possession of that authority and consequently passes it on or delegates it further. One may wonder whether there are conditions attached to this delegation.

13.2 Empowerment and Health

The Ottawa Conference in 1986 represents kind of a shift in paradigm regarding health, from paternalistic to democratic [12]. The World Health Organization (WHO) declared that it was necessary to pay *more attention to health promotion* within the health care services, arguing that people had to take more responsibility for their own health [12]. The main idea was to redistribute power, from the health professionals to the patients, and the term "The *new* public health" was introduced by the WHO, underlining this increased attention.

Within the health (and social) care fields, the concept of empowerment is linked to individuals and groups who are/have been in a situation of powerlessness and how they can emerge from that powerlessness [9]. Illness and symptoms such as severe pain, nausea and discomfort, or fear and exhaustion can easily contribute to feelings of powerlessness.

A frequently used definition in health contexts describes empowerment as giving someone the authority or power to do something, "...to make someone stronger and more confident, especially in controlling their life and claiming their rights" [13]. However, this definition too, may be perceived as paternalistic.

A concept analysis of empowerment within an health care context published in 2014 showed that empowerment is characterised by active participation, informed change (change that one undertakes after attaining relevant knowledge, e.g. about the significance of a better diet and physical activity), knowledge to problem solve, self-care responsibility, sense of control, awareness, development of personal abilities, autonomy and coping [14].

Another concept analysis concludes that individual patient empowerment is a process that enables patients to exert more influence over their individual health by increasing their capacities to gain more control over issues they themselves define as important. The authors combine patient empowerment with patient participation and patient centredness and state that patient participation might lead to patient centredness that at last can lead to patient empowerment [15].

A study of the principles of empowerment in a psychiatric context showed that the patients found it difficult to understand every decision in relation to what was "allowed and not allowed" and to understand the reasons given by the staff for implementing measures within the department. Similarly, they found it difficult to be perceived as experts on themselves [16]. Another study on the perception of empowerment among elderly people with diabetes indicated the same challenges [14]. A literature review and a concept analysis of empowerment in critical care showed that the common attributes of empowerment were a mutual and supportive relationship, skills, power within oneself and self-determination. The author concludes that even if empowerment is sparsely used in relation to critical care, it appears to be a very useful concept in this context [17].

Rapaport [18] once claimed that it is easier to define the opposite of empowerment: powerlessness or learned helplessness, alienation and the perception of not having control over one's own life. This is a particularly interesting observation for our context. The health service and hospitals in particular can easily be perceived as paternalistic, and it can be difficult to participate and be acknowledged as an expert on oneself as a patient. It is easy to fall into the traditional role of patient and leave decisions to the professionals, to be taught helplessness and feel powerless.

The concept of empowerment is of particular interest to the health professions [8]. This is because the concept underscores the importance of supporting people who find themselves in a vulnerable situation and because the concept per se emphasises the importance of seeing people as actors in their own lives who "know best where the shoe pinches" [19, 20]. It is precisely this, supporting someone in a vulnerable position, while not taking over but helping the person to take as much control as possible that is challenging in relation to empowerment in hospitals. Most patients may be able to participate *a little* in some areas.

13.2.1 Empowerment as a Process

The empowerment process can be described as a social and a helping process, as well as a dynamic and interactive process [14, 17, 21, 22]. Describe how the empowerment process in elderly care claims that the health professionals surrender control. To surrender control might be easier said than done to the health professionals [23, 24]. The health professionals themselves often define the needs of the patients and even how to meet those needs.

Askheim [9] claims that empowerment is characterised by a positive view of the individual and by the individual as active and acting in their best interests where the right conditions are in place. Empowerment is further characterised as a concept that has an emotional dimension [9]. The individual is not always rational, and situations that may involve, e.g. shame and dejectedness or enthusiasm, and the joy of mastery may influence the empowerment process.

When studied from the perspective of the individual, empowerment is called "psychological empowerment". Empowerment may also be studied from a group, organisation or societal perspective. Further, empowerment can be studied from a

systemic perspective, e.g. structural empowerment. All levels of empowerment are connected. The system holds major significance for psychological or individual empowerment [25].

Psychological empowerment is based on social psychology theory and developmental psychology and builds on the assumption that empowerment centres around internal, psychological processes such as perceptions of self-determination, impact, competence and meaning [7, 26, 27]. Individual or psychological empowerment is about the individual's ability to make decisions and have control over his/her own life [28] and about self-control, belief in and opportunities for one's own efficacy (efficacy expectation or self-efficacy) [29].

Structural empowerment deals with a person's power with regard to his/her position within the organisation. Kanter [30] describes four empowerment structures: opportunity, information, support and resources. Structural empowerment may be understood as the structures in which the patient is a part representing opportunities for or obstacles to empowerment. Specifically, systems that provide opportunities for participation, such as joint meetings in mental health care settings where the patient is able to influence conditions within the department, represent an example of structural empowerment, along with procedures or systems gathering information about patients' experiences, views and needs during conversations. A study of patients' perceived opportunities for participation at an outpatient pain clinic showed that the patients perceived that their participation was obstructed by an inability to understand their treatment plan. The patients also had very limited knowledge about their rights in relation to participation [25].

Gibson [31] defines empowerment as a social process that contributes to recognising, promoting and enhancing people's abilities to meet their own needs, solve their own problems and mobilise the necessary resources in order to feel in control of their own lives or the factors which affect their health. The definition is still used in scientific articles despite the year of publication, so long ago. This definition emphasises the social process between health professional and patient. Being a partner in an empowerment process requires the health professional to adopt a different role than that of traditional assistant who solves problems for the patient: the health professional takes on a supervisory role [32]. In this context, the affective dimension is significant. The affective dimension deals with the way the health professional relates to the patient, whether she communicates respect, empathy or understanding, for example, or conveys that she is short on time, appears impatient or is inattentive to the patient. According to Askheim and Starrin [8], it is precisely this emotional dimension between helper and helpee (here: patient) that is important in empowerment.

13.2.2 Public Health and Health Promotion

What is public health and what does it have to do with hospitals? In 1920, public health was defined as: *"The science and art of preventing disease, prolonging life and promoting health through the organized efforts and informed choices of society, organizations, public and private, communities and individuals"*. This definition is still used ([33], pp. 17–18). Public health can be understood as society's responsibility for the health of the people, or society's duty to protect, promote and strengthen people's health. Public health can also be understood as the duty of medicine to protect and improve the health of the nation [34].

Public health work may further be understood as the collective effort of society to strengthen factors promoting health, to reduce factors that result in increased health risks and to protect against external threats to health and as the practical means by which information about the science of public health is applied for the purpose of promoting health [35]. Health promotion and disease prevention are forms of intervention in public health work. The Ottawa Charter provides guidelines for substantially strengthening health promotion work [12]. Health promotion and preventing disease are strategies that overlap to a certain degree.

13.2.3 Health

Views on health hold significance for health promotion work. WHO's definition of health from 1948 [36] was somewhat expanded in 1986 [12], and emphasis was placed on the significance of well-being and quality of life [37]. In the 1946 definition [38], health was understood as more than just absence of disease and as complete physical, mental and social well-being. WHO later modified the definition and describes health as the ability to live an economically and socially productive life [39]. Hjorth [40] describes health as the ability to cope and function in one's current context and with the challenges one may face at any time. Health is understood as a resource that gives people the strength and resilience to endure stresses and strains [39].

Views of health reflect ideology, value-based priorities and cultural and social relations. In recent times, the term "health" has to some extent been replaced by "quality of life" [39]. Fugelli and Ingstad [41] describe health as an ephemeral phenomenon that shifts between time and space and is both individual and general. Health professionals are supposed to contribute to health promotion, prevent disease, alleviate suffering and restore health. Health promotion work centres around how one lays the groundwork for the individual to feel more in control over his/her life and health. Health promotion work focuses on empowerment principles (redistribution of power, participation and acknowledging) and building capacity within the individual and the local community. Participation through involving people in decisions about their lives and health is one part of this work [42].

13.2.4 Empowerment and Health Promotion

Since the 1970s, empowerment has been defined as a central concept in health promotion work, and Andrews and Rootman et al. [43, 44] state that empowerment represents a framework for health promotion. The Brazilian educator Paulo Freire [45] focused his pedagogical efforts on the poor of Brazil in the 1960s and was particularly interested in how the situation these people found themselves contributes to oppression. Freire believed that what was most important for the poor and oppressed was to become *conscious* of why they were oppressed, because this awareness could help them change their behaviour and thereby create a new situation for themselves. *Consciousness raising* is therefore important to be able to take control of one's own life. According to Freire, the central method of this liberation was *dialogue* [45]. Dialogue as a method of health promotion will be discussed later in this chapter.

Empowerment may be a social, cultural, psychological or political process through which individuals and social groups are able to express their needs, present their concerns, devise strategies for involvement in decision-making and achieve political, social and cultural action to meet those needs. Through such a process, people see a closer correspondence between their goals in life and a sense of how to achieve them and a relationship between their efforts and life outcomes. Health promotion not only encompasses actions directed at strengthening the basic life skills and capacities of individuals, but also at influencing underlying social and economic conditions and physical environments which impact upon health. In this sense health promotion directs creating conditions facilitating a relationship between the efforts of individuals and groups, and subsequent health outcomes in the way described above.

A distinction is made between individual and community empowerment. Individual empowerment refers primarily to the individuals' ability to make decisions and have control over their personal life. Community empowerment involves individuals acting collectively to gain greater influence and control over the *determinants of health* and the *quality of life* in their *community* and is an important goal in *community action for health*. In health promotion, enabling involves taking action in *partnership* with individuals or groups to empower them, through the mobilisation of human and material resources, which are important to promote and protect their *health*.

The World Health Organisation ([46], p. 11) provides the following description of empowerment: "Patient and consumer empowerment has emerged in the last decades as a proactive partnership and patient self-care strategy to improve health outcomes and quality of life". In this description, empowerment is thus linked to health and quality of life.

One may wonder whether the philosophy of empowerment is universally appropriate. What about the seriously ill and children? What about people who are unconscious? It is the most seriously ill who are admitted to hospital. This issue touches on the central principles of empowerment. What does participation entail? Participation can be ranked and seen in the context of the patient's capacity level at any time. One can participate a little; for example, one can participate in relation to what one would like to drink, whether one wants to sit up or lie down in bed. It is easy to make such choices on behalf of the patient. To find anything out about the patient's capacity, the health professional must be attentive, aware of his/her interactions and acknowledge the patient's competence at all times. In this context, affective competence is of particular importance. In encounters with unconscious patients, who has not whispered into the patient's ear that he/she must squeeze your hand if they can hear what you are saying? This is an example of acknowledging the patient's personal competence and inviting him/her to participate. This involves a kind of redistribution of power. In this context, it is also appropriate to see the patient and his/her next of kin as one unit.

13.3 Empowerment and Health Promotion in Hospitals

Our context is empowerment in connection with health promotion in hospitals. The guidelines in the Ottawa Charter place greater emphasis than before on health promotion and described health promoting strategies as "the *new* public health". The guidelines centre around giving special priority in health promotion work to *the redistribution of power from professional to patient or user,* participation and acknowledgement of the patient's [12]. WHO further states that empowerment means:

> "...the process of increasing capacity of individuals or groups to make choices and to transform those choices into desired actions and outcomes" to "build individual and collective assets, and to improve the efficiency and fairness of the organizational and institutional context which govern the use of these assets" and the "expansion of assets and capabilities of poor people to participate in, negotiate in, negotiate with, influence, control, and hold accountable institutions that affect their lives" ([12], p. 17).

Health promotion in hospitals has to do with the interaction between patients and health professionals and the hospital as the system within which this interaction takes place. Health promotion is about helping the patient to participate in his/her own treatment and care, acknowledging the patient's self-competence and redistributing power. Health promotion is about everything we do to enable the patient to develop or improve competence in relation to sustaining health and quality of life. You may be forgiven for thinking that such interactions take too much time in hospitals and that seriously and/or acutely ill people do not need or have the energy to participate. Of course, this may be the case, but health professionals cannot take it for granted. In interactions with the patient, health professionals can identify the patient's needs in relation to participation. Expressing that one does not wish to participate is in itself a form of participation. Again, it is important to be aware that one can participate a little and in certain areas. Acknowledgement may also be expressed in many ways. A seriously ill patient may for example feel acknowledged by the health professional communicating empathy and respect. WHO has provided guidelines for the recognition of Health Promoting Hospitals and has set up a network for these hospitals [47]. All health trusts and organisations interested in public health and willing to follow the WHO concept of Health Promoting Hospitals can become members. Membership in the network can be seen as an aspect of empowerment at the system level.

There are several examples of health promotion in hospitals. For example, some hospitals have "**patient schools**" for patients with heart disease, diabetes, stomas or breast cancer. These patient schools offer for example teaching and supervision that is intended to help patients cope with their symptoms and treatment. However, studies emphasise that competence in health education is crucial for ensuring that patients and service users derive benefit from the patients' schools or programs [48].

13.4 Empowerment-Based Interventions

As we have seen, the central principles of empowerment are *power redistribution, participation and being acknowledged as an expert on oneself*. These principles are connected; one is virtually a natural consequence of the other. The principles will be preserved through *the interaction* between health care professionals and patients [12]. The strategies for this interaction can be described as empowerment "interventions". These are interventions that aim to develop competence and coping skills or that help patients cope as well as possible with health challenges and their attendant consequences [49–51]. The empowerment interventions must be commensurate with the patient's competence, for example, the patient's resources, needs and opportunities to participate.

> *Empowerment-based interventions include both a process and an outcome component. The process component occurs when the true purpose of the intervention is to increase the patient's capacity to think critically and make autonomous, informed decisions. The outcome component occurs when there is a measurable increase in the patient's ability to make autonomous, informed decisions* ([6], p. 278)

The result of empowerment may be described as coping [49]. Coping may be understood as ever-changing cognitive and behavioural efforts to manage specific external and/or internal challenges that are perceived as burdensome or that adversely affect the resources one has at one's disposal [52, 53]. Coping can also be understood as attempts by the individual to manage challenge or stressful situations. Vifladt and Hopen [54] define coping as "the perception of having the resources to face challenges and a sense of having control over one's own life. Active and effective coping helps you to adapt to new realities and enables you to see the difference between the things you have to live with and the things you can play a part in changing" ([54], p. 61, translated by the author).

The concept of *compliance* is interesting in this context. Traditionally, the term denotes manageability or assent, or the patient's ability to follow the doctor's advice. According to Fielding and Duff [55], "compliance" can have a deeper meaning; the ability to take control of the factors that affect your health. In other words, not just following advice, but playing an active role, responding actively to advice, speaking up when advice is not perceived as beneficial, for example. "Compliance" can also be understood as an active, intentional and responsible process [56]. In concrete terms, this means the ability to understand and act in relation to changing symptoms and to understand and act when treatment perhaps does not work the way it was supposed to. Another interpretation of "compliance" leads to empowerment. "Compliance" is influenced by age, socio-economic circumstances, how one copes with having an illness and by psychological stress. "Compliance" may be strengthened by education, reflection, emotional processing and skills training [55].

Patient education is recognised as an important part of the nurse's role and includes patient teaching, advice and information-giving as well as supervision. The purpose of patient and eventually next of kin education is to contribute to improving health and quality of life and help patients and next of kin cope with illness and/or functional impairment. Further, education can lead to patients being able to make informed choices together with their health care providers. The hospitals must also contribute to health-promoting processes through interaction with the individual patient and his/her next of kin and groups of patients and next of kin. Patient and next of kin education can therefore be seen as health-promoting work at the hospital [20, 51].

Supervision is an empowerment-based intervention. The concept of supervision might seem unusual regarding patients and next of kin, since the concept usually is related to health professionals or students [57]. Supervision may be defined as: *A formal, relational and pedagogical process that enables, and that aims to strengthen personal mastery competence through a dialogue based on knowledge and humanistic values* [32, 58]. This definition emphasises the relationship between health professional and patient. It is through this relationship that the health professional gains insight into the patient's thoughts, perceptions and needs. The affective aspect of the interaction centres around laying the foundations for trust and meeting the patient where he/she is. Health-promoting measures can thus be customised.

Dialogue requires the health professional to be a skilled listener. The dialogue entails reflection, in the sense of *exchange*. The health professional must listen to the patient and tell the patient his/her perception of what the patient is saying and of the situation the patient is in. Thus, exchange and reflection take place. This creates an enhanced mutual understanding of the patient's situation, and further health-promoting measures are implemented in line with the patient's needs.

The purpose of supervision is to strengthen **coping competence.** What to be overcome is individual, situational and contextual. Coping competence includes knowledge, abilities and attitudes. All these aspects are important in the supervision dialogue. A patient in hospital may be in an acute state of illness or injury and may be dealing with pain, fear or reduced consciousness. The dialogue with the patient must be informed by the patient's condition. It would be easy to think that the most seriously ill patients have no need for dialogue. However, assessment of the patient's competence must be ongoing. A dialogue with a patient may, for example, involve investigating what the patient knows about the illness and treatment options, and conveying to the patient the information that he/she needs in order to understand, actively participate and make choices. Dialogue entails helping the patient to gain a deeper understanding.

An example from a hospital, as told by the patient's next of kin:

An 80-year-old man with stomach pains was an emergency admission to the hospital. He was lucid and oriented and was lying in bed when his next of kin arrived. A nurse arrived at the same time and asked if the man would like something to drink. The man answered "Yes please..." and a glass of fruit cordial was placed on the bedside table. The next of kin asked if the man would like to sit up to make it easier for him to drink the cordial. The man answered that he was unsure whether he was allowed to sit up. The next of kin left the room, located the nurse and asked if it was OK for the man to sit up in bed. The nurse replied that of course it was OK, he could even get out of bed if he wanted to. The patient later said that he had been lying on his back in bed since he was admitted two days ago, no-one had informed him that he was free to move around, and he had not asked any questions.

This is an example of a patient feeling powerless and presenting learned helplessness, but it is also an example of the importance of providing supervision to patients to enable them to start using their own resources. Knowing that one can safely get out of bed and move around is of major significance in terms of health. Being bed-bound may in itself cause complications due to inactivity. This is also an example of when a dialogue with the patient may have had a health-promoting effect. The purpose of the dialogue is to produce an enhanced understanding of what the dialogue is about. It is of major importance in terms of coping that patients understand and can appropriately relate to the information they are given, e.g. about medicines and treatment. This is known as "health literacy" [59].

Health literacy concerns the knowledge and competences of persons to meet the complex demands of health in modern society and can be defined as "people's knowledge, motivation and competence to access, understand, appraise, and apply health information in order to make judgements and take decisions in everyday life con-

cerning health care, disease prevention and health promotion to maintain or improve quality of life during the life course" ([60], p. 3). Health literacy may also be defined as the use of medical terminology that may for example prevent a patient from understanding. The patient's health literacy is an important factor in empowerment and health promotion work [61].

There are many ways to provide supervision and dialogue: solution-focused guidance, change-focused guidance or counselling, empathic communication, health coaching, shared decision-making, or motivational interview, to name just a few [20]. Patients in hospital may be facing multiple choices in relation to treatment, lifestyle and follow-up. Actively participating in choices requires, among other things, awareness, understanding, knowledge and skills. In this context, supervision is a relevant method.

To fulfil their health-promoting duty, health professionals need pedagogical competence or competence related to **health pedagogics.** Health pedagogics may be understood as everything that is connected to development, learning, teaching and supervision in a health-related setting [20, 62]. The purpose of health pedagogics is to encourage the patient to change his/her relationship to his/her own health and lifestyle [63]. The concept of *health competence* is recently used to describe the result of health education and is in Norway defined as a consensus concept connected to health literacy [64]. Health pedagogics is the general term we use to denote everything we do as health professionals (e.g. empowerment interventions, training and supervision) to strengthen the patient's and next of kin's ability to cope with health-related challenges and to achieve health competence.

13.5   Some Empirical Studies

In an intervention study, the purpose of which was to look at the empowerment process in the rehabilitation of women with breast cancer, Stang and Mittelmark [65] found that self-help groups as intervention resulted in consciousness raising.

Knowledge building, community learning and discovering new perspectives contributed to the consciousness raising. Consciousness raising, as we saw earlier, is a prerequisite for empowerment [45].

Anderson and Funnell's [6] study shows that implementing empowerment interventions entails a type of paradigm shift that can be complex because the education received by health professionals taught more traditional types of intervention. Empowerment interventions may involve new and different ways of relating to patients and require the ability of self-reflection. Ruud Knutsen and Foss [66] studied understandings of and strategies for empowerment in lifestyle change courses at one hospital's Learning and Mastery Centre. The analysis showed that when health professionals develop empowerment interventions, it is essential to be aware of the power dynamic that will always be present in relation to patients in this context. Power can lie within systems.

Communication between health professionals and patients is an important factor in interactions. Cegala et al. [67] concluded in their study that when the parents of sick children are active communicators, the surgeon will provide more information. When parents are more active, this may lead to them receiving clarification on what they were unsure about. This promotes empowerment. In a systematic literature review, Pearson [68] showed that involving patients in goal-setting processes for lifestyle change may be useful. In addition, a questionnaire conducted by Rosenlund et al. [69] shows that patients value communication when they themselves are active. When the patient is active, empowerment is promoted. A quantitative study of patients' experiences with the empowerment process concludes that it is of importance regarding quality of life and health outcomes that health professionals actively ask for the patients' experiences of the process or how it felt to participate and being acknowledged [70]. Stiffler et al. [71] conclude in a qualitative study that the interaction between the patient and the health professionals was more important to the patient than medical control regarding the disease.

Studies of health education interventions are often related to specific diagnoses. For example, one study of patient experiences connected to diagnosis-specific health education interventions showed limited effects [72]. Perhaps it would be more useful to carry out training irrespective of diagnosis and based on the needs of the individual. The need for a scientific basis for the development of strategies for health education is confirmed by Smith et al. [73], who concluded that much of the material being used in this context is outdated. However, one may argue that the patient's perspective and participation challenge equality in the relationship between the patient and the health professionals due to the fact that the health professionals themselves often define the patient's needs and goals [24]. The health professionals need health education competence or health pedagogy competence in order to practice in line with the empowerment principles. Research regarding this area sparsely exists. Therefore, qualitative as well as quantitative studies are of high importance in the future, and there is a need of further developing health-promoting strategies and education of health professionals within health pedagogy [48].

13.5.1 Empowerment and Salutogenesis

As we have seen in this chapter, central principles of empowerment are distribution of power from the health professionals to the patients, patient participation and acknowledging the patient as an expert regarding herself/himself. Antonovsky's theory of salutogenesis [74] emphasises positive aspects of health and well-being. A key component in the theory is "sense of coherence" (SOC). This component has a particular relevance to health promotion, since it represents characteristics that contribute to help individuals gain control:

> The sense of coherence is…a global orientation that expresses the extent to which one has a pervasive, enduring though dynamic feeling of confidence that one's internal and external environments are predictable and that there is a high probability

that things will work out as well as can reasonably be expected. ([74], p. 122)

The elements of coherence are *comprehensibility*, which means that the world is ordered consistent, structured and clear and that the future is predictable rather than noisy, chaotic, disordered, random, accidental and unpredictable. Further, *manageability*, which means that individuals believe that they have the resources at their disposal which can help them to manage their lives. *Meaningfulness* means that life make sense emotionally, that people are committed and that they invest energy in worthwhile goals [74, 75]. The elements of SOC can be viewed as interrelated with the principles of empowerment, to take control in one's life and to obtain power *within* oneself claims self-consciousness and participation. SOC claims self-consciousness and participation as well.

Take Home Messages

- Empowerment can be understood as a concept, a process and an outcome.
- Empowerment can be a health promotion strategy (empowerment-based interventions) in hospitals.
- Acting or interacting in line with the principles of empowerment philosophy, power redistribution, participation and acknowledgement of the patient's competence is complex.
- Health promotion and empowerment-based interventions (e.g. supervision) require health education skills.
- Knowledge-based practice is a goal for the health service. There is a great need for scientific knowledge related to empowerment-based interventions in hospitals.
- The principles of empowerment connect with the central elements of the salutogenic theory.

References

1. Istomina N, Suominen T, Razbadauskas A, Martikenas A, Kuokkanen L. Lithuanian nurses' assessment of their empowerment. Scand J Caring Sci. 2011;26:3. https://doi.org/10.1111/j.1471-6712.2011.00894.x.
2. Cerezo PG, Juvè-Udina ME, Delgado-Hito P. Concepts and measures of patient empowerment: a comprehensive review. Rev Esc Enferm USP. 2016;50(4):664–71.
3. Morse JM. Exploring the theoretical basis of nursing using advanced techniques of concept analysis. Adv Nurs Sci. 1995;17(3):31–46.
4. Morse JM, Mitcham C, Hupcey JE, Cerdas Tason M. Criteria for concept evaluation. J Adv Nurs. 1996a;24:385–90.
5. Morse JM, Hupcey C, Lenz ER. Concept analysis in nursing research: a critical appraisal. Sch Inq Nurs Pract. 1996b;10(3):253–77.
6. Anderson RM, Funnell M. Patient empowerment: myths and misconceptions. Patient Educ Couns. 2010;79:277–82.
7. Kuokkanen L, Leino-Kilpi H. Power and empowerment in nursing: three theoretical approaches. J Adv Nurs. 2000;31:235–41.
8. Askheim OP, Starrin B. Empowerment i teori og praksis [empowerment in theory and practice]. Oslo: Gyldendal Academic; 2007.
9. Askheim OP. Empowerment i helse- og sosialfaglig arbeid: floskel, styringsverktøy eller frigjøringsstrategi? [Empowerment in health and social work: meaningless jargon, management tool or strategy for liberation?]. Oslo: Gyldendal Academic; 2012.
10. Wbster's Comprehensive Dictionary of the English language. 1996.
11. Illustrated Oxford Dictionary. Oslo: Teknologisk forlag; 1998.
12. World Health Organization. The Ottawa charter for health promotion. Geneva: WHO; 1986.
13. Pearsall J, editor. The new Oxford dictionary of English. Oxford: Clarendon Press; 1998.
14. Fotoukian Z, Shahboulaghi FM, Khoshknab MF, Mohammadi E. Concept analysis of empowerment in old people with chronic diseases using a hybrid model. Asian Nurs Res. 2014;8:118–27.
15. Castro EM, Van Regenmortel T, Vanhaecht K, Sermeus W, Van Hecke A. Patient empowerment, participation and patient-centeredness in hospital care: a concept analysis based on literature review. Patient Educ Couns. 2016;99:1923–39.
16. Tveiten S, Haukland M, Onstad RF. The patient's voice—empowerment in a psychiatric context. Nord J Nurs Res. 2011;101(31):20–4.
17. Wåhlin I. Empowerment in critical care—a concept analysis. Scand J Caring Sci. 2016;31:164–76. https://doi.org/10.1111/scs.12331.
18. Rapaport J. Studies in empowerment: introduction to the issue. Prev Hum Serv. 1984;3:1–7.
19. Tveiten S. Den vet best hvor skoen trykker…om veiledning I empowermentprosessen. [the wearer knows best where the shoe pinches... On supervision in the empowerment process]. Bergen: Fagbokforlaget; 2007.
20. Tveiten S. Helsepedagogikk (Health Pedagogics). Bergen: Fagbokforlaget; 2016.
21. McCarthy V, Holbrook Freeman L. A multidisciplinary concept analysis of empowerment:

implications for nursing. J Theor Construct Test. 2008;12(2):68–74.

22. Bennett L, Bergin M, Wells SG. The social space of empowerment within epilepsy services: the map is not the terrain. Epilepsy Behav. 2016;56:139–48.

23. Tveiten S, Meyer IS. «Easier said than done»—empowering dialogues with patients at the pain clinic. J Nurs Manag. 2009;17:804–12.

24. Tveiten S, Onstad RF, Haukland M. Refleksjon over praksis i lys av empowerment—en fokusgruppeundersøkelse (Reflections on practice in the light of empowerment—a focus group study). Nord J Nurs Res. 2015;35:136–43.

25. Tveiten S, Ruud Knutsen I. Empowering dialogues—the patients' perspective. Nord Coll Caring Sci. 2010. https://doi.org/10.1111/j.1471-6712.2010.00831.x.

26. Spreitzer GM. Psychological empowerment in the workplace: dimensions, measurement, and validation. Acad Manage J. 1995;38(5):1442–65. https://doi.org/10.2307/256865.

27. Knol J, van Linge R. Innovative behaviour: the effect of structural and psychological empowerment in nurses. J Adv Nurs. 2009;65(2):359–70.

28. Israel BA, Checkoway B, Schulz A, Zimmerman M. Health education and community empowerment: conceptualization and measuring perceptions of individual, organizational and community control. Health Educ Q. 1994;21(2):149–70.

29. Wallerstein N. Power between evaluator and community relationships with New Mexico's healthier communities. Soc Sci Med. 1999;49(1):39–53.

30. Kanter RM. Men and women of the corporation. New York: Basic Books; 1993.

31. Gibson CH. A concept analysis of empowerment. J Adv Nurs. 1991;16:354–61.

32. Tveiten S. The public health nurses' client supervision. Doctoral thesis. University of Oslo; 2006.

33. Småland Goth U, editor. Folkehelse i et norsk perspektiv [public health from a Norwegian perspective]. Oslo: Gyldendal Academic; 2014.

34. Last JM. A dictionary of epidemiology. New York: Oxford University Press; 1995.

35. Dreyer Fredriksen ST. The enigmatic knowledge of intensive care patients—experience and interpretation based knowledge in intensive care tutoring. Doctoral thesis. Nordic College for Public Health and Harstad University College; 2011.

36. United Nations Department of Public Information. The universal declaration of human rights. 1948. https://www.un.org/en/universal-declaration-human-rights/.

37. Sletteland N, Donovan RM. Helsefremmende lokalsamfunn. [the health-promoting community]. Oslo: Gyldendal Academic; 2012.

38. World Health Organisation. Constitution. 1946. www.who.int/about/who-we-are/constitution.

39. Mæland JG. Forebyggende helsearbeid i teori og praksis [Preventive health work in theory and practice]. Oslo: Universitetsforlaget; 2016.

40. Hjorth PF. "Om samsykdommene" [On psycho-social disease]. I: Hjorth, P. F. Helse for alle! [Health for Everyone!] Foredrag og artikler [Essays and articles] 1974–1993. Investigation report no. U1–1994. Oslo: The Norwegian Institute of Public Health, Section for Health Services Research; 1994.

41. Fugelli P, Ingstad B. Helse på norsk [Norwegian perspectives on health]. Oslo: Ad Notam Gyldendal; 2009.

42. Mittelmark M, Kickbusch I, Rootman I, Scriven A, Tones K. Helsefremmende arbeid – ideologier og begreper [Health promotion work—ideologies and concepts]. In: Gammersvik Å, Larsen T, editors. Helsefremmende sykepleie [Health promotion in nursing]. Bergen: Fagbokforlaget; 2012.

43. Andrews T. "New" ideological basis for preventive health work. A discussion on views of power and change. Norwegian J Welfare Res. 2003;6(1):30–42.

44. Rootman I, Goodstadt M, Potvin L, Springett J. A framework for health promotion. WHO Regional Publication European Series, vol. 92; 2001. p. 7–38.

45. Freire P. Pedagogy of the oppressed. Oslo: Ad Notam Gyldendal; 1999.

46. World Health Organization. What is the evidence of effectiveness of empowerment to improve health? Geneva: WHO; 2006.

47. Johnson A, Baum F. Health promoting hospitals: a typology of different organizational approaches to health promotion. Health Promot Int. 2001;16(3):281–7.

48. Vågan A, Eika K, Skirbekk H. Helsepedagogisk kompetanse, læring og mestring (Health pedagogic competence, learning and coping). Sykepleien.no/ Forskning; 2018. https://doi.org/10.4220/sykepeleienf.2006.59702s.

49. Espnes GA, Smedslund G. Helsepsykologi [Health Psychology]. Oslo: Gyldendal Academic; 2009.

50. Lerdal A, Fagermoen MS. Learning and mastery—a health promotion perspective in practice and research. Oslo: Gyldendal Academic; 2011.

51. Crawford T, Roger P, Candlin S. The interactional consequences of "empowering discourse" in intercultural patient education. Patient Educ Couns. 2017;100:495–500.

52. Lazarus RS, Folkman S. Stress, appraisal and coping. New York: Springer; 1984.

53. Folkman S, Lazarus BS. The relationship between coping and emotion: implications for theory and research. Soc Sci Med. 1988;26:309–17.

54. Vifladt E, Hopen L. Helsepedagogikk—Samhandling om læring og mestring [health education—interaction in learning and mastery]. Oslo: Norwegian National Advisory Unit on Learning and Mastery in Health; 2004.

55. Fielding D, Duff A. Compliance with treatment protocols: intervention for children with chronic illness. Arch Dis Child. 1999;80:196–200.

56. Kyngäs H. A theoretical model of compliance in young diabetics. J Clin Nurs. 1999;8(1):73–80.

57. Tveiten S. Evaluation of the concept of supervision related to public health nurses I Norway. J Nurs Manag. 2005;13:13–21.

58. Tveiten S. Veiledning, mer enn ord…(Supervision, more than words…). Bergen: Fagbokforlaget; 2019.

59. Carolan M. Health literacy and the information needs and dilemmas of first-time mothers over 35 years. J Clin Nurs. 2007;16:1162–72.

60. Sørensen K, Van den Broucke S, Fullam J, et al. Health literacy and public health: a systematic review and integration of definitions and models. BMC Public Health. 2012;12:80. http://www.biomedcentral.com/1471-2458/12/80.

61. Sand-Jecklin K, Coyle S. Efficiently assessing patient health care literacy: the BHLS instrument. Clin Nurs Res. 2014;23:581. https://doi.org/10.1177/1054773813488417.

62. Tveiten S. Empowerment og veiledning—sykepleierens pedagogiske funksjon i helsefremmende arbeid [Empowerment and supervision—the pedagogical role of the nurse in health promotion work]. In: Gammersvik Å, Larsen T, editors. Helsefremmende sykepleie [Health promotion in nursing]. Bergen: Fagbokforlaget; 2012.

63. Holman HR, Lorig KR. Patient education: essentials in good health care for patients with chronic arthritis. Rheumatology. 1997;40(8):1371–3.

64. The Health and Caring Department, Norway. Strategy to develop the health of the population. 2019.

65. Stang I, Mittelmark M. Learning as an empowerment process in breast cancer self-help groups. J Clin Nurs. 2008;18:2049–57.

66. Ruud Knutsen I, Foss C. Caught between conduct and free choice—a field study of an empowering programme in lifestyle change for obese patients. Scand J Caring Sci. 2010. https://doi.org/10.1111/j.1471-6712.2010.00801.x.

67. Cegala DJ, Chisolm DJ, Nwomeh BC. Further examination of the impact of patient participation on physicians' communication style. Patient Educ Couns. 2012;89:25–30.

68. Pearson ES. Goal setting as a health behavior change strategy in overweight and obese adults: a systematic literature review examining intervention components. Patient Educ Couns. 2011;87:32–42.

69. Rosenlund Lau S, Christensen ST, Andersen JT. Patients' preferences for patient-centered communication: a survey from an outpatient department in rural Sierra Leone. Patient Educ Couns. 2014;93:312–8.

70. Chen M-F, Tsai CT, Hsu S-M, Tu S-Y, Kao P-L, Chen S-L. Patient perceptions of empowerment processes, health outcomes and related factors in living with diabetes in Taiwan: a cross-sectional survey. J Community Health Nurs. 2013;30:201–15.

71. Stiffler D, Cullen D, Luna G. Diabetes barriers and self-care management: the patient perspective. Clin Nurs Res. 2013;23(6):601–26.

72. Hamilton Larsen M, Hagen KB, Krogstad A-L, Aas E, Klopstad Wahl A. Limited evidence of the effects of patient education and self-management interventions in psoriasis patients: a systematic review. Patient Educ Couns. 2014;94:158–69.

73. Smith F, Carlsson E, Kokkinakis D, Forsberg M, Kodeda K, Sawatzky R, Friberg F, Öhlén J. Readability, suitability and comprehensibility in patient education materials for Swedish patients with colorectal cancer undergoing elective surgery: a mixed method design. Patient Educ Couns. 2014;94:202–9.

74. Antonovsky A. The sense of coherence as a determinant of health. In: Matarazzo JD, Weiss SM, Herd JA, et al., editors. Behavioral health. New York: Wiley; 1984. p. 114–29.

75. Mittelmark MB, Sagy S, Eriksson M, Bauer GF, Pelikan JM, Lindström B, Espnes GA, editors. The handbook of Salutogenesis. Berlin: Springer; 2017. https://doi.org/10.1007/978-3-319-04600-6.

Part III

Empirical Research on Health Promotion in the Health Care

Health Promotion Among Families Having a Newborn Baby

14

Shefaly Shorey

Abstract

Pregnancy, childbirth, and the postpartum period are the stressful transition periods to parenthood. With medicalization of perinatal period, parents feel left out and less confident in their parenthood journey, which may pose serious threats to the family dynamics. Salutogenesis theory offers the potential to influence a shift away from negative health outlooks and outcomes, medicalization of childbirth, toward health promotion and positive well-being focus for maternity care services design and delivery in the future.

Keywords

Salutogenesis · Health promotion · Perinatal period

14.1 Introduction

This chapter describes the need of health promotion strategies among families having a newborn baby. The focus of the utilization of the Salutogenesis theory in health promotion and future directions in health promotion research has

S. Shorey (✉)
Alice Lee Centre for Nursing Studies, National University of Singapore, Singapore, Singapore
e-mail: nurssh@nus.edu.sg

been discussed. The following discussions are based on the research on perinatal mental health, trends in childbirth, health promotion, and, particularly, the integration of the Salutogenesis theory in health promotion during the perinatal period. The extensive discussions constitute a basis for development of future policies or initiatives to promote health promotion among families having a newborn that meet the standards for health care education and research.

14.2 Perinatal Mental Health

The perinatal period spans from the start of one's pregnancy to the first 12 months after childbirth [1]. This period is a stressful and remarkably dynamic period of growth that poses significant challenges for both pregnant women and their partners [2]. Right from pregnancy till after child birth, the perinatal period is a complex phenomenon that consists of a myriad of adjustments to physical, social, and emotional lifestyles, that influence the overall well-being of the parents [3].

There is increasing research on parental perinatal mental health, in which systematic reviews revealed that 6.5% to 12.9% of pregnant and postpartum mothers experienced depression and anxiety [4, 5]. Likewise, depression and anxiety have been reported to be the most common mental health issues faced by fathers during the perinatal period [6, 7]. Existing meta-analyses

G. Haugan, M. Eriksson (eds.), *Health Promotion in Health Care – Vital Theories and Research*,
https://doi.org/10.1007/978-3-030-63135-2_14

have reported that the prevalence rate for paternal depression during the perinatal period was approximately 8.4% [8] and the prevalence of anxiety in fathers ranged between 3.4% and 25% during the prenatal period, to 2.4% and 51% during the postnatal period [9]. The striking prevalence of mental health issues among both mothers and fathers urge the need for a focus shift toward familial health promotion throughout the perinatal period.

In recent years, the experiences and needs of both mothers and fathers during the perinatal period have been explored. During pregnancy, mothers reported that it was an emotional roller-coaster ride that made them feel overwhelmed with the evolving pregnancy needs [10]. During postpartum, mothers felt varied emotional issues and many of them felt neglected to seek any help [10]. Mothers also experienced unpreparedness, anxiety, stress over infant care, breast-feeding concerns, and physical discomfort [11]. Existing barriers such as stigma, shame, and the lack of time and interactions with health care professionals prevented mothers from disclosing their feelings and needs [10, 12]. Hence, mothers expressed their need for (1) continuity of care, (2) mental health enquiries to include less common disorders on top of depression and anxiety, (3) culturally appropriate postnatal practices in infant care and upbringing, and (4) professional support needs, i.e. more information with regard to health care services [10, 11, 13]. Similarly, fathers exhibited negative feelings and psychological difficulties during the perinatal period. They expressed feelings of insecurity and inadequacy, felt isolated and excluded from the events that happened throughout the perinatal period [14–18]. Fathers also expressed stress, anxiety, depression, and role strain and conflict while they tried to cope with other role demands such as their jobs, parental stress from their children (e.g., fear of developmental problems), and conflict with in-laws and partners [14, 19, 20]. Therefore, fathers reported their needs: (1) including more educational information about pregnancy and parenting (during antenatal classes), (2) engaging them with other experienced fathers through small groups and focused group discussions [14, 17,

18], (3) having topics of discussion beyond the infant and partner care such as to include mental health topics [14, 20], (4) ensuring continuity of care after hospital discharge after the childbirth to seek timely help from health care professionals, and (5) incorporating technology (e.g., mobile health applications) to receive information covering mental health [21]. These evidences highlight the need to explore health promotion strategies among parents with a newborn to ensure smooth transition to parenthood and overall well-being of new parents and eventually their entire families.

14.3 Trends in Childbirth

Before the twentieth century, childbirth was considered a natural, normal, female-centred event, and hospital birth was uncommon [22, 23]. Female midwives predominantly helped with the childbirth, whereas men were rarely involved, and if they did, it was mainly during difficult deliveries [22]. In the nineteenth and twentieth centuries, medical influence on childbirth exaggerated with the development of medical procedures such as anesthesia and caesarean section [22]. Presently, the increased use of ultrasounds, fetal heart monitors, and increasing caesarean delivery rates illustrate multiple ways that women's pregnancy and childbirth experiences have been heavily medicalized [22–24].

14.3.1 Medicalization of Childbirth

Medicalization is defined as the tendency to pathologize normal bodily processes and states, resulting in unnecessary medical management [25]. Some factors influencing childbirth medicalization include the complexity of maternal health care, culture of medical dominance, submissive culture in nursing and midwifery [26], technological advancement (e.g. emergence of biomedicine) [27, 28], and focus on risks involved with natural childbirth [29]. Childbirth medicalization is apparent in the widespread and increasing rates of medical interventions (i.e. caesarean and instrumental deliveries). In Western countries (e.g. the United States, Italy, and the United Kingdom), caesarean births account for approximately 20% of childbirth procedures [22, 30]. In Spain, the extent of medicalization is demonstrated in some of the highest caesarean delivery rates in Europe (e.g. 40% increase of the procedure in Catalonia over 5 years) and obstetricians are held accountable for not allowing women to be involved in childbirth decision-making [22, 31]. Furthermore, Eastern countries such as China and Singapore have one of the highest caesarean delivery rates in the world and South East Asia, respectively [32, 33]. In China, caesarean rates in the 90s rose from below 5% to above 10%, with urban rates as high as 20% by 1996. In 2010, of the 16 million babies born in China, approximately 50% were born by caesarean delivery [32]. In Singapore, the overall caesarean delivery rate increased from 32.2% (Year 2005) to 37.4% in year 2014 [34]. Some contributing factors to the alarming rates of caesarean delivery in China and Singapore include the obstetric care system (i.e. urbanization, medicalization of childbirth, and financial incentives), provider factors (i.e. obstetric training and staffing), and patient factors (i.e. parity where primiparas prefer caesarean delivery as it is deemed as more effective, and education level where university-educated women prefer caesarean births) [32].

The potential impacts of medicalization of childbirth and pregnancy include (1) dependence on medicine and the medical field [35], (2) hampering the embodiment process that neglects the body as somato-psychic [36, 37], and (3) hindering the gift dynamic at play during natural childbirth [38]. The medicalization of childbirth, at times can be a life-saving and effective procedure, but if done unnecessarily it may put women and their babies at increased susceptibility to mortality and morbidity and has aversive effects on maternal health and pregnancy outcomes [39, 40]. Hence, it should be limited to instances of medical emergencies. Finally, the medicalization of childbirth and pregnancy is coupled with a negative connotation, in which natural pregnancy and childbirth are now conceptualized as illnesses or diseases that require medical technologies and interventions [23, 41].

14.3.2 Latest Move Toward Natural Physiological Birth

In response to the increasing rates of medical intervention and medicalization of childbirth and pregnancy, there has been increasing efforts in promoting natural childbirth [42]. The World Health Organization (1997) highlighted the need to eliminate unnecessary medical interventions in childbirth [43] and countries have passed policies, initiatives, and guidelines to promote and protect natural childbirth. In Australia, the current maternity care reform (*National Maternity Services Plan*) is grounded on the underlying philosophy of childbirth as a natural physiological process [44]. Guidelines to protect, promote, and support natural childbirth were established and published in Queensland [45]. A policy in New South Wales (*Towards Normal Birth in New South Wales*) required all birthing facilities and institutions in the Australian state to have a written policy for natural childbirth by 2015 [46]. In the United Kingdom (UK), the Royal College of Midwives established the *Campaign for Normal Birth* that is now integrated as part of the *Better Births Initiative* [47]. Health care providers in Canada published a *Joint Policy Statement on Normal Birth* to protect the practice of natural birth [48]. In the Netherlands, the maternity care system is grounded on the principle that childbirth and pregnancy are natural physiological processes and community-based midwifery continue to play an important role [49] facilitating natural birth and continuity of care after childbirth. Hence, home birth remains a widely accepted and well-integrated part of the health care system [50].

Researchers have explored the role of midwives in encouraging natural birth as midwifery-led models of care are associated with the reduced use of medical interventions and mothers' increased satisfaction with the natural birthing experience [51]. Thompson et al.'s (2016) qualitative study explored Dutch midwives' attitudes and motivations toward the promotion of natural childbirth, and identified factors associated with these attitudes and motivations [52]. Findings revealed that midwives perceive the safeguarding and promotion of natural physiological childbirth as the focus of their role, and hospital culture is deemed as a barrier to practices that promote natural childbirth [52]. To overcome this barrier, midwives expressed the need to be aware of factors that inhibit and encourage natural childbirth practices, and to employ strategies that promote natural childbirth in home and hospital settings [52]. A recent UK evaluation study examined the effectiveness of an educational training package designed for midwives and maternity support workers [53]. The training package included a core workshop entitled "Keeping Birth Normal" (KBM), workshops that focused on antenatal education, communication skills, and baby massage [53]. Findings revealed that midwives were appreciative of the educational materials (e.g. videos and lectures) and expressed that small group discussions helped to facilitate learning [53]. They described two barriers to the implementation of training: (1) cultural focus on risk and (2) hospital culture of low prioritization of natural childbirth [29, 52, 53]. Despite the barriers, the training provided opportunities (1) to build a community of practice around natural childbirth that helped in overcoming the existing risk-focused culture and (2) created awareness within the midwifery unit that the promotion of natural physiological childbirth is central to their role [53]. These evidences urge the need for future midwifery education and research to focus on developing and testing strategies that support midwives in delivery health-promoting care and services [52, 53].

Moreover, a recent qualitative study that aimed to clarify how primiparous women in Turkey experience childbirth and intrapartum care revealed that the women wanted a natural birth without interventions [54]. Grounded theory guided interviews with 12 women were conducted and they reported wanting vaginal birth without interventions, which required empowerment and social support from others (i.e. health care professionals, family, and friends) [54]. Also, they expressed that routine medical interventions during the birth process cause their anxiety and frustration [54]. These interventions become obstructions to women's natural posi-

tion during birth, interrupt the birth process, and compromise their dignity and sense of autonomy [54]. This is an exceptionally important finding as Turkey has one of the highest caesarean rates, in which care during labor often entails the overuse of medicalized interventions such as episiotomy (i.e. experienced by 93.3% of primiparous women in Turkey) and augmentation with oxytocin and caesarean section [55]. With women who voiced their "want" for natural birth without interventions due to the negative consequences of medicalized interventions, it is a "need" to work toward a less- or non-medicalized childbirth process through positive health promotion.

With the progression toward less-medicalized models of birth through promotion of natural childbirth, existing barriers such as hospital and risk-focused culture are still apparent in many parts of the health care system. Therefore, it is imperative to adopt an appropriate approach of health promotion that will provide the necessary shift of focus from the risks and complications associated with childbirth to one that provides a positive and health-promoting experience for families with a newborn [56].

14.4   Health Promotion: Use of Salutogenesis Theory

Health promotion is purported to enable individuals with increased control over their own health [57]. One such approach is to integrate the Salutogenesis theory that was coined by the medical sociologist Antonovsky (1979) who focused on the origin of good health rather than the origin of illness [58]. Salutogenesis illustrates that the state of health lies on a spectrum—from complete absence of health to absolute state of health on the other extreme [58]. This theory implies that one has the ability and control to move toward better health with available resources around them. Salutogenesis consists of two: (1) *generalized resistance resources (GRR)*, i.e. characteristics of an individual, family, or community that are resources to aid the individual in coping with stressors and (2) *sense of coherence (SOC)*, i.e. one's ability to use available resources

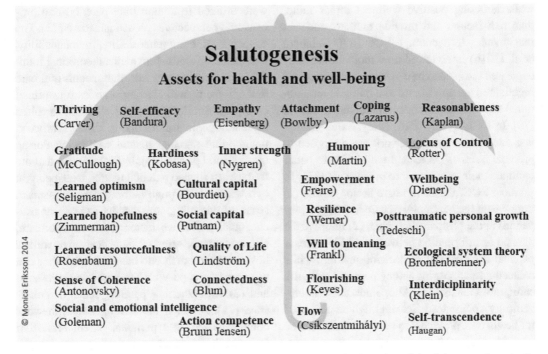

Fig. 14.1 Salutogenesis Umbrella (Reproduced with permission from Folkhälsan Research Center, Lindstrom & Eriksson, 2010) [65] According to Monica Eriksson, there is a revised version of the Salutogenesis umbrella which is used now)

for stress-coping and health promotion ([59]. In recent years, the salutogenic framework has been explored and expanded, in which more concepts were included within the framework. It is known as the Salutogenesis umbrella (Fig. 14.1) that constitutes concepts (e.g. *Gratitude, Self-efficacy, Connectedness, Coping,* and *Well-Being* [60–64] with the positive view of health as a resource for life and executing behaviors to restore and maintain good health even when one is not ill [65]. Hence, Salutogenesis is a potential school of thought that urges health care professionals to adopt positive and health-promoting care to assist families during the perinatal period.

Presently, there is an increasing trend in the utility of Salutogenesis for guiding health promotion under various disciplines. For instance, García-Moya and Morgan (2016) assessed the theoretical status of Salutogenesis and the utility of SOC to advance health promotion practices for young people's well-being [66]. SOC has been shown to be associated with well-being, in which it can be an asset that operates by increas-

ing one's ability to mobilize both internal and external resources for well-being [66, 67]. More recently, Johansson et al. (2018) developed and implemented a salutogenic treatment model in a clinical setting of emergency child and adolescent psychiatry in Sweden [68]. Eight GRRs (e.g. clear language, daily information, and participation in decision-making) were developed and implemented in the emergency unit, and parents reported increased satisfaction with the treatment and care provided [68]. Mental health of children improved during their stay at the hospital, and results revealed reduced treatment length and readmission rates [68]. Therefore, the salutogenic framework can be applied as a strong and effective theoretical basis to direct the development and implementation of health care services.

Multiple studies have adopted the salutogenic framework to highlight important qualities of health care providers and areas of improvements to promote SOC in new mothers [69–71]. Findings revealed that midwives should stay calm in tight time-constraint environments while targeting positive wellness topics rather than risk factors and provide mothers constant reassurances to encourage SOC [69]. Dahlberg et al. (2016) interviewed new mothers and they expressed the need to be cared for exclusively and highlighted the importance of a midwife for emotional support, coaching, and parenting guidance [70]. In Kelly et al. (2016) study, Salutogenesis was adopted, and a framework was proposed to promote families' SOC and well-being to better facilitate their transition into parenthood [71]. To promote SOC, the health care sector should (1) improve on the continuity of care and support for parents in the postpartum period, (2) improve the method of information delivery, and (3) increase parental involvement in decision-making, while balancing relationships among parents and health care professionals [71]. Altogether, these salutogenically focused studies highlighted the need for health care providers to possess more humane qualities (i.e. midwives to stay calm and provide emotional support), as opposed to just the delivery of tangible materials (e.g. provision of educational booklets) to provide positive and health-promoting services.

14.4.1 Salutogenesis Theory in Perinatal Health Care

The salutogenic framework has been applied in perinatal health care, specifically for families having a newborn. Existing salutogenically focused studies addressed several phenomena across the perinatal period. Greer et al. (2014) explored mothers' fear of childbirth and its impact on birth choices among women and their partners through interviews carried out within the SOC theoretical framework [72]. The findings (i.e. riskiness, ways of coping, and being a good parent) were related to the three dimensions of SOC (i.e. comprehensibility, manageability, and meaningfulness) [72]. For instance, pregnant couples feared the repercussions of natural childbirth and preferred medical interventions over natural childbirth to cope with uncertainties and to ensure a smooth and safe transition to parenthood [72]. The three dimensions of SOC

were utilized to demonstrate parental and professional perspectives on neonatal care [73]. The concepts of comprehensibility, manageability, and meaningfulness provided a theoretical foundation to develop and integrate meaningful care that complemented existing services for optimal care [73]. Similarly, Kelly et al. (2016) applied the salutogenic framework to discuss ways in maintaining parental mental well-being during the perinatal period [71]. It was reported that the framework shaped parental mental well-being in two ways: (1) through helping parents to make sense of parenting stressors by examining psychosocial protective factors such as optimism, self-esteem, and stressor identification as well as how these factors fit into their lives, and they can use them to cope with the parenting stressors, and (2) strengthening parents' sense of coherence [71]. As such the salutogenic framework could be used as a perinatal parent education framework to promote overall parental well-being during the perinatal period [71]. There are only two existing reviews that consolidated existing studies that examined Salutogenesis in perinatal health care. Smith et al. (2014) identified salutogenically focused outcomes ($n = 16$; e.g. maternal satisfaction and breastfeeding) and non-salutogenically focused outcomes ($n = 49$; e.g. measures of neonatal morbidity) during the intrapartum period (Smith et al. 2014). The review implied a lack of salutogenically focused outcomes reported in intrapartum intervention-based research [74]. Perez-Botella et al. (2015) examined how the Salutogenesis theory can be utilized to address several parenting outcomes across the perinatal period, and implied that the theory is rarely used in maternity care research and urged future research to measure salutogenitcally oriented outcomes to provide a balance in maternity care design [75]. Though there are increasing but limited perinatal studies that adopted the salutogenic framework with majority of studies focussing on only SOC, there is a crucial need to expand the utilization of the salutogenic framework and concepts in the salutogenic umbrella (other than SOC) to ensure a holistic application of the theory to encourage health promotion during the perinatal period.

14.4.2 Managing the Perinatal Period with Physical Activity: A Salutogenic Approach

Women during pregnancy are generally sedentary and could gain excessive weight due to physical limitations, increased appetite, and tiredness [76, 77]. As a result, majority of the pregnant women fail to meet the recommended level of physical activity and this increases their risk of negative pregnancy conditions such as gestational diabetes and pregnancy-induced hypertension [77, 78]. Also, the children of obese women during pregnancy are more likely to become obese adults [79]. Therefore, there is a need for health care professionals to inform pregnant couples about healthy lifestyle choices such as the engagement in physical activity for health promotion during the perinatal period [78]. Physical activity is recommended as a health promoting approach that aid pregnant couples to cope with the bodily changes throughout the perinatal period [80]. Also, physical activity has been found to be associated with increased overall well-being during pregnancy, self-esteem, shorter duration of labor, fewer depressive symptoms, higher prevalence of natural childbirth [77], and reduced occurrence of gestational diabetes [81] and pregnancy-induced hypertension [82].

The Salutogenesis theory has been found useful in directing families to engage in physical activity as a mean to cope with potential negative pregnancy conditions during the perinatal period [83]. Frequent physical activity has been shown to be associated with strong SOC [83]. In Hassmen et al.'s (2000) population study significant correlations were found between individuals, both men and women, who exercised more frequently with higher SOC than those who exercise less frequently [84]. Another study from the Netherlands revealed that individuals with a strong SOC engaged in sports more frequently and have better health outcomes such as lower average blood pressure [85]. The individuals with increased physical activity not only found to have stronger SOC but also higher self-esteem, stronger control over bad habits, and more positive attitudes toward changes in life [86]. A review conducted by Eriksson and Lindström (2006) synthesized empirical findings on SOC and reported that stronger SOC is linked to better health outcomes [87]. Stronger SOC was found to be associated with lower mortality risk [85], delay onset of cancer [88], and lower rates of diabetes [89].

During the perinatal period, one of the main contributing factor that lead to physical inactivity is lack of social support [76, 78]. Women reported that due to lack of support from their partners to run errands at home and to care for older children, they often have limited time and tend to neglect their physical exercise. To promote a strong social support and to increase physical activity, the salutogenic framework can pave the path in encouraging families to engage in physical activities together. On top of the two main components (i.e. GRR and SOC) of the salutogenic theory, the other concepts from the salutogenic umbrella such as connectedness [61], coping [63], and well-being [62], can be included to form a conceptual framework in the development of family-focused interventions catered for the pregnant couples. For instance, during prenatal care, health care professionals (i.e. doctors and midwives) have the unique opportunity to inform pregnant couples about the benefits of healthy lifestyle choices such as walking and swimming and to recommend individualized exercise routines and nutritional plans for couples to follow through. At this stage, pregnant couples can be motivated to have a shared physical activity plan to enhance their connectedness [61] and thus supporting each other for a shared activity that will eventually benefit them both physically and mentally. These individualized couple-based exercise routines and nutritional plans can be then enhanced with other shared physical and mental changes with the addition of the newborn during the postpartum period.

During postpartum, shared physical activities and nutritional plans could continue to direct couples and their newborn through connecting and benefitting the overall familial well-being. Hence, health care professionals who recommend physical activities and nutritional plans (Coping) help to provide a common ground for both mothers and fathers (GRR) with a newborn (Connectedness) to manage the likelihood of negative pregnancy conditions. The adherence to exercise routines and nutritional plans could aid in parental overall physical and mental well-being (Well-being; SOC), improving their physical and mental health. With connectedness and appropriate coping to stressors throughout the perinatal period, the overall familial well-being and SOC could be maintained using the available resources, and thus, result in positive perinatal health outlooks and outcomes. Therefore, additional concepts in the salutogenic umbrella can be included on top of GRR and SOC in directing the development of family-focused services.

14.5 Literature Gaps, Implications, and Future Research

With rising prevalence rates of negative parental mental health during the perinatal period, mothers and fathers reported negative feelings and expressed needs to assist them during this period. The medicalization of childbirth resulted in aversive effects on maternal health and pregnancy outcomes and is coupled with a negative connotation that pregnancy and childbirth are conceptualized as illnesses or diseases. Despite the increasing efforts to promote natural physiological childbirth, hospital and risk-focused cultures continue to pose as strong barriers to normalizing natural childbirth. Therefore, these pose as existing gaps in the literature that imply a necessary shift of focus to one that provides a positive and health-promoting experience for families with a newborn. To bridge these gaps, health promotion that integrates the Salutogenesis theory forms a foundational basis that directs health care professionals and providers to design and deliver well-being focused interventions and care services for the pregnant couples and the new parents. Existing salutogenically focused studies that adopted quantitative (i.e. correlational studies and randomized controlled trials) and/or qualitative approaches (i.e. in-depth interviews and grounded-theory studies), implied that the saluto-

genic framework is a potential school of thought that urges health care professionals to adopt in providing positive and health-promoting services and care to assist families during the perinatal period. Also, salutogenically focused qualitative studies that interviewed pregnant women and midwives during the perinatal period highlighted the need for health care providers to possess more humane qualities (e.g. emotional support) to deliver positive and health-promoting care. This implies the need to train health care professionals such as midwives to be prepared and proactive in delivering optimal positive perinatal care. Future research can consider the salutogenic framework in designing midwifery education that focuses on developing and testing strategies to support midwives in this endeavour. The salutogenic framework is well-positioned as a perinatal parent education framework and future research can aim to design salutogenically focused interventions (e.g. support groups and perinatal classes) to promote parental well-being during the perinatal period.

Existing quantitative and correlational studies have shown the benefits of being physically active during the perinatal period, but the majority remains physically inactive. This implies the need for health care professionals to inform pregnant couples about healthy lifestyle choices for health promotion and prevention of negative pregnancy conditions during the perinatal period. Future research can aim to adopt the salutogenic framework in developing family-focused care services (i.e. exercise routines and nutritional plans) catered to pregnant couples during the perinatal period. It is also important to conduct further research on pregnant couples and factors that promote physical activity.

14.6 Conclusion

There are increasing but limited perinatal studies that adopted the salutogenic framework, especially elements of SOC in isolation. Future research could expand the utilization of the framework and concepts in the salutogenic umbrella beyond SOC to ensure a holistic application of the theory to encourage health promoting outcomes during the perinatal period. As majority of the existing studies are from the West, more studies from geographically diverse backgrounds such as the Middle East and Asia are required to explore and garner a holistic view of salutogenic framework and health promotion across the perinatal period. In summary, salutogenic theory offers the potential to influence a shift away from negative health outlooks and outcomes, medicalization of childbirth, toward health promotion and positive well-being focus for maternity care services design and delivery in the future.

Take-Home Messages

- It is imperative to enhance quality of care for families having a newborn to ensure optimal parental mental health and newborn health.
- A fundamental step is to recognize and acknowledge the problem of medicalization interventions during the perinatal period, and to adopt an appropriate approach of health promotion that will provide a shift of focus from the risks and complications associated with childbirth to one that is positive and health-promoting for families with a newborn.
- It is timely to evaluate and implement the up-and-coming salutogenic framework in health care services that focuses on positive well-being and health promotion, especially with its increasing but limited application in perinatal health care. The framework serves as a guide for health care professionals in developing health-promoting services to families with a newborn.
- There is a crucial need to expand and integrate the salutogenic framework in promoting the engagement in physical activities as families tend to become sedentary during the perinatal period. The framework serves as a common ground for health care professionals and families to discuss individualized activity plans that can optimize their experience and positive well-being during the perinatal period.
- Theory-based research is the way to describe and evaluate evidence-based quality care to families with a newborn. Health care professionals need to be equipped with relevant

skills in conducting quality research that work toward the expansion of the framework and concepts in the salutogenic umbrella beyond SOC to ensure a holistic application of the theory to encourage health promoting outcomes during the perinatal period.

References

1. Leach LS, Poyser C, Cooklin AR, Giallo R. Prevalence and course of anxiety disorders (and symptom levels) in men across the perinatal period: a systematic review. J Affect Disord. 2016;190:675–86.
2. Duncan LG, Bardacke N. Mindfulness-based childbirth and parenting education: promoting family mindfulness during the perinatal period. J Child Fam Stud. 2010;19(2):190–202.
3. Buultjens M, Murphy G, Robinson P, Milgrom J. The perinatal period: a literature review from the biopsychosocial perspective. Clin Nurs Stud. 2013;1(3):19–31.
4. Gavin NI, Gaynes BN, Lohr KN, Meltzer-Brody S, Gartlehner G, Swinson T. Perinatal depression: a systematic review of prevalence and incidence. Obstet Gynecol. 2005;106(5 Pt 1):1071–83.
5. Leach LS, Poyser C, Fairweather-Schmidt K. Maternal perinatal anxiety: a review of prevalence and correlates. Clin Psychol. 2017;21(1):4–19.
6. Gao L, Chan SW, Mao Q. Depression, perceived stress, and social support among first-time Chinese mothers and fathers in the postpartum period. Res Nurs Health. 2009;32(1):50–8.
7. Paulson JF, Bazemore SD. Prenatal and postpartum depression in fathers and its association with maternal depression: a meta-analysis. JAMA. 2010;303(19):1961–9.
8. Cameron EE, Sedov ID, Tomfohr-Madsen LM. Prevalence of paternal depression in pregnancy and the postpartum: an updated meta-analysis. J Affect Disord. 2016;206:189–203.
9. Philpott LF, Savage E, FitzGerald S, Leahy-Warren P. Anxiety in fathers in the perinatal period: a systematic review. Midwifery. 2019;76:54–101.
10. Nagle U, Farrelly M. Women's views and experiences of having their mental health needs considered in the perinatal period. Midwifery. 2018;66:79–87.
11. Ong SF, Chan W-CS, Shorey S, Chong YS, Klainin-Yobas P, He H-G. Postnatal experiences and support needs of first-time mothers in Singapore: a descriptive qualitative study. Midwifery. 2014;30(6):772–8.
12. Edwards E, Timmons S. A qualitative study of stigma among women suffering postnatal illness. J Ment Health. 2005;14(5):471–81.
13. Slade P, Morrell CJ, Rigby A, Ricci K, Spittlehouse J, Brugha TS. Postnatal women's experiences of man-

agement of depressive symptoms: a qualitative study. Br J Gen Pract. 2010;60(580):e440–e8.

14. Darwin Z, Galdas P, Hinchliff S, Littlewood E, McMillan D, McGowan L, et al. Fathers' views and experiences of their own mental health during pregnancy and the first postnatal year: a qualitative interview study of men participating in the UK Born and Bred in Yorkshire (BaBY) cohort. BMC Pregnancy Childbirth. 2017;17(1):45.

15. Finnbogadóttir H, Crang Svalenius E, Persson E. Expectant first-time fathers' experiences of pregnancy. Midwifery. 2003;19(2):96–105.

16. Iwata H. Experiences of Japanese men during the transition to fatherhood. J Transcult Nurs. 2014;25(2):159–66.

17. Poh HL, Koh SSL, Seow HCL, He H-G. First-time fathers' experiences and needs during pregnancy and childbirth: a descriptive qualitative study. Midwifery. 2014;30(6):779–87.

18. Rowe HJ, Holton S, Fisher JRW. Postpartum emotional support: a qualitative study of women's and men's anticipated needs and preferred sources. Aust J Prim Health. 2013;19(1):46.

19. Edhborg M, Carlberg M, Simon F, Lindberg L. Waiting for better times: experiences in the first postpartum year by Swedish fathers with depressive symptoms. Am J Mens Health. 2016;10(5): 428–39.

20. Pålsson P, Persson EK, Ekelin M, Kristensson Hallström I, Kvist LJ. First-time fathers experiences of their prenatal preparation in relation to challenges met in the early parenthood period: implications for early parenthood preparation. Midwifery. 2017;50:86–92.

21. Shorey S, Dennis CL, Bridge S, Chong YS, Holroyd E, He HG. First-time fathers' postnatal experiences and support needs: a descriptive qualitative study. J Adv Nurs. 2017;73(12):2987–96.

22. Johanson R, Newburn M, Macfarlane A. Has the medicalisation of childbirth gone too far? BMJ. 2002;324(7342):892–5.

23. Parry DC. "We wanted a birth experience, not a medical experience": exploring Canadian Women's use of midwifery. Health Care Women Int. 2008;29(8–9):784–806.

24. Mitchell LM. Baby's first picture: ultrasound and the politics of fetal subjects. Toronto: University of Toronto Press; 2001.

25. Inhorn MC. Defining Women's Health: a dozen messages from more than 150 ethnographies. Med Anthropol Q. 2006;20(3):345–78.

26. Clesse C, Lighezzolo-Alnot J, de Lavergne S, Hamlin S, Scheffler M. The evolution of birth medicalisation: a systematic review. Midwifery. 2018;66:161–7.

27. Nye RA. The evolution of the concept of medicalization in the late twentieth century. J Hist Behav Sci. 2003;39(2):115–29.

28. Saintôt B. More managing for pregnancy and childbirth? [In French: Gérer toujours plus la grossesseet l'accouchement ?]. Laennec. 2015;63(4):6–15.

29. Parry DC. Women's lived experiences with pregnancy and midwifery in a Medicalized and Fetocentric context: six short stories. Qual Inq. 2006;12(3):459–71.

30. Thomas J, Paranjothy S. The national sentinel caesarean section audit report. National Sentinel Caesarean Section Audit Report. 2001.

31. Topçu S, Brown P. The impact of technology on pregnancy and childbirth: creating and managing obstetrical risk in different cultural and socio-economic contexts. Health Risk Soc. 2019;21(3–4):89–99.

32. Hellerstein S, Feldman S, Duan T. China's 50% caesarean delivery rate: is it too high? BJOG. 2015;122(2):160–4.

33. Hou L, Hellerstein S, Vitonis A, Zou L, Ruan Y, Wang X, et al. Cross sectional study of mode of delivery and maternal and perinatal outcomes in mainland China. PLoS One. 2017;12(2):e0171779.

34. Chi C, Pang D, Aris IM, Teo WT, Li SW, Biswas A, et al. Trends and predictors of cesarean birth in Singapore, 2005–2014: a population-based cohort study. Birth. 2018;45(4):399–408.

35. Chanial P. The fugitive moment in which society takes: the gift, the game and the whole. [in French: L'instant fugitif où la société prend. Le don, la partie et le tout.]. Revue du MAUSS semestrielle. 2010;36:521–38.

36. Davis-Floyd R. The technocratic, humanistic, and holistic paradigms of childbirth. Int J Gynecol Obstet. 2001;75:S5–S23.

37. Shabot SC. Making loud bodies "feminine": a feminist-phenomenological analysis of obstetric violence. Hum Stud. 2016;39(2):231–47.

38. Azcue M, Tardif J. Begetting in the perspective of gift: what it means to give birth in our modern health care system. Revue du MAUSS. 2012;39(1):163–79.

39. Rosen T. Placenta accreta and cesarean scar pregnancy: overlooked costs of the rising cesarean section rate. Clin Perinatol. 2008;35(3):519–29. x

40. Silver RM, Landon MB, Rouse DJ, Leveno KJ, Spong CY, Thom EA, et al. Maternal morbidity associated with multiple repeat cesarean deliveries. Obstet Gynecol. 2006;107(6):1226–32.

41. Walters V. Women's perceptions regarding health and illness. In: Bolaria BS, Dickinson HD, editors. Health, illness and health care in Canada. Toronto: Hartcourt Brace; 1994. p. 307–25.

42. Prosser SJ, Barnett AG, Miller YD. Factors promoting or inhibiting normal birth. BMC Pregnancy Childbirth. 2018;18(1):241–10.

43. Technical Working Group WHO. Care in Normal Birth: a practical guide. Birth. 1997;24(2):121–3.

44. Conference AHM. National maternity services plan 2010. 2010.

45. Program QMaNCG. Normal birth. 2012.

46. Health NSW. Towards normal birth in NSW. 2010.

47. Midwives TRCo. Better birth initiative. 2018.

48. Joint Policy Statement on Normal Childbirth. J Obstet Gynaecol. 2008;30(12):1163–5.

49. De Vries R, Press AU. Pleasing birth: midwives and maternity care in the Netherlands. Amsterdam: Amsterdam University Press; 2005.

50. Christiaens W, Nieuwenhuijze MJ, de Vries R. Trends in the medicalisation of childbirth in Flanders and the Netherlands. Midwifery. 2013;29(1):e1–8.

51. Sandall J, Soltani H, Gates S, Shennan A, Devane D, Sandall J. Midwife-led continuity models versus other models of care for childbearing women. Cochrane Database Syst Rev. 2016;2016(4):CD004667.

52. Thompson SM, Nieuwenhuijze MJ, Low LK, de Vries R. Exploring Dutch midwives' attitudes to promoting physiological childbirth: a qualitative study. Midwifery. 2016;42:67–73.

53. Walker S, Batinelli L, Rocca-Ihenacho L, McCourt C. 'Keeping birth normal': exploratory evaluation of a training package for midwives in an inner-city, alongside midwifery unit. Midwifery. 2018;60:1–8.

54. Deliktas Demirci A, Kabukcuglu K, Haugan G, Aune I. "I want a birth without interventions": women's childbirth experiences from Turkey. Women Birth. 2019;32(6):e515.

55. Kartal B, Kızılırmak A, Calpbinici P, Demir G. Retrospective analysis of episiotomy prevalence. J Turk German Gynecol Assoc. 2017;18(4):190–4.

56. Sinclair M, Stockdale J. Achieving optimal birth using salutogenesis in routine antenatal education. Evid Based Midwif. 2011;9(3):75.

57. WHO. What is health promotion. 2016.

58. Antonovsky A. Health, stress, and coping. London: Jossey-Bass; 1979.

59. Antonovsky A. The salutogenic model as a theory to guide health promotion. Health Promot Int. 1996;11(1):11–8.

60. Bandura A. Self-efficacy: the exercise of control. New York: W.H. Freeman; 1997.

61. Blum RJMCI. School connectedness: improving students' lives; 2005. p. 1–18.

62. Diener E. The science of well-being: the collected works of Ed Diener. 1. Aufl.;1; ed. Dordrecht: Springer; 2009.

63. Folkman S, Lazarus RS. Coping as a mediator of emotion. J Pers Soc Psychol. 1988;54(3):466–75.

64. McCullough ME, Emmons RA, Tsang J-A. The grateful disposition: a conceptual and empirical topography. J Pers Soc Psychol. 2002;82(1):112–27.

65. Lindström B, Eriksson M. The hitchhiker's guide to salutogenesis: Salutogenic pathways to health promotion. Folkhälsan Research Center, Health Promotion Research; 2010.

66. Garcia-Moya I, Morgan A. The utility of salutogenesis for guiding health promotion: the case for young people's well-being. Health Promot Int. 2017;32(4):723–33.

67. Morgan A, Hernán M. Promoting health and well-being through the asset model. Revista Española de Sanidad Penitenciaria. 2013;15(3):78–86.

68. Johansson BA, Pettersson K, Tydesten K, Lindgren A, Andersson C. Utvecklingsrelaterade störningar asoåib-ou, et al. implementing a salutogenic treatment model in a clinical setting of emergency child and adolescent psychiatry in Sweden. J Child Adolesc Psychiatr Nurs. 2018;31(2–3):79–86.

69. Browne J, O'Brien M, Taylor J, Bowman R, Davis D. 'You've got it within you': the political act of keeping a wellness focus in the antenatal time. Midwifery. 2014;30(4):420–6.

70. Dahlberg U, Persen J, Skogas AK, Selboe ST, Torvik HM, Aune I. How can midwives promote a normal birth and a positive birth experience? The experience of first-time Norwegian mothers. Sex Reprod Healthc. 2016;7:2–7.

71. Kelly RG, Hauck Y, Thomas S. Salutogenesis: a framework for perinatal mental wellbeing. Aust J Child Fam Health Nurs. 2016;13(2):4.

72. Greer J, Lazenbatt A, Dunne L. 'Fear of childbirth' and ways of coping for pregnant women and their partners during the birthing process: a salutogenic analysis. Evid Based Midwif. 2014;12:95–100.

73. Thomson G, Moran VH, Axelin A, Dykes F, Flacking R, Högskolan D, et al. Integrating a sense of coherence into the neonatal environment. BMC Pediatr. 2013;13(1):84.

74. Smith V, Daly D, Lundgren I, Eri T, Benstoem C, Devane D, et al. Salutogenically focused outcomes in systematic reviews of intrapartum interventions: a systematic review of systematic reviews. Midwifery. 2014;30(4):e151–e6.

75. Perez-Botella M, Downe S, Meier Magistretti C, Lindstrom B, Berg M, Sahlgrenska A, et al. The use of salutogenesis theory in empirical studies of maternity care for healthy mothers and babies. Sex Reprod Healthc. 2014;6(1):33–9.

76. Gaston A, Cramp A. Exercise during pregnancy: a review of patterns and determinants. J Sci Med Sport. 2011;14(4):299–305.

77. Gjestland K, Bø K, Owe K, Eberhard-Gran M. Do pregnant women follow exercise guidelines? Prevalence data among 3482 women, and prediction of low-back pain, pelvic girdle pain and depression. Br J Sports Med. 2012;47:515–20.

78. Birkheim SL. Association between sense of coherence and participation in a free offer of exercise for pregnant women. 2015.

79. de Jersey SJ, Nicholson JM, Callaway LK, Daniels LA. An observational study of nutrition and physical activity behaviours, knowledge, and advice in pregnancy. BMC Pregnancy Childbirth. 2013;13:115.

80. Cioffi J, Schmied V, Dahlen H, Mills A, Thornton C, Duff M, et al. Physical activity in pregnancy: women's perceptions, practices, and influencing factors. J Midwifery Womens Health. 2010;55(5):455–61.

81. Dempsey JC, Sorensen TK, Williams MA, Lee IM, Miller RS, Dashow EE, et al. Prospective study of gestational diabetes mellitus risk in relation to maternal recreational physical activity before and during pregnancy. Am J Epidemiol. 2004;159(7):663–70.

82. Sorensen TK, Williams MA, Lee IM, Dashow EE, Thompson ML, Luthy DA. Recreational physical activity during pregnancy and risk of preeclampsia. Hypertension. 2003;41(6):1273–80.

83. Kuuppelomäki M, Utriainen P. A 3 year follow-up study of health care students' sense of coherence and

related smoking, drinking and physical exercise factors. Int J Nurs Stud. 2003;40(4):383–8.

84. Hassmen P, Koivula N, Uutela A. Physical exercise and psychological well-being: a population study in Finland. Prev Med. 2000;30(1):17–25.

85. Super S, Verschuren WMM, Zantinge EM, Wagemakers MAE, Picavet HSJ. A weak sense of coherence is associated with a higher mortality risk. J Epidemiol Community Health. 2014;68(5):411–7.

86. Pallant JF, Lae L. Sense of coherence, well-being, coping and personality factors: further evaluation of the sense of coherence scale. Personal Individ Differ. 2002;33(1):39–48.

87. Eriksson M, Lindström B, Högskolan V, Institutionen för omvårdnad hok, Avd för hälsa och k. Validity of Antonovsky's sense of coherence scale: a systematic review. J Epidemiol Community Health. 2005;59(6):460–6.

88. Poppius E, Virkkunen H, Hakama M, Tenkanen L. The sense of coherence and incidence of cancer—role of follow-up time and age at baseline. J Psychosom Res. 2006;61(2):205–11.

89. Kouvonen AM, Väänänen A, Woods SA, Heponiemi T, Koskinen A, Toppinen-Tanner S. Sense of coherence and diabetes: a prospective occupational cohort study. BMC Public Health. 2008;8(1):46.

Salutogenic-Oriented Mental Health Nursing: Strengthening Mental Health Among Adults with Mental Illness

15

Nina Helen Mjøsund and Monica Eriksson

Abstract

This chapter focuses on mental health promotion with a salutogenic understanding of mental health as an individual's subjective well-being encompassing both feelings and functioning. Mental health is an ever-present aspect of life, relevant for everybody; thus, to promote mental health is a universal ambition. Our chapter is written with adults with mental illness in need of mental health nursing in mind. To understand the present and make suggestions for the future, knowledge of the past is needed. We elaborate on historical trends of nursing, nursing models, and the hospital setting to support our statement; persons with mental illness need a more complete mental health nursing care, including salutogenic mental health promotion. In the last part of the chapter, we introduce the salutogenic-oriented mental health nursing, and further showing how salutogenesis can be integrated in nursing care for persons with mental illness. As well as elaborating on the features of salutogenic-oriented mental health nursing, and briefly present the Act-Belong-Commit framework for mental health promotion as an example of salutogenesis in nursing practice.

Keywords

Act-Belong-Commit · Mental health · Mental illness · Mental health nursing · Mental health promotion · Nursing models · Psychiatric nursing · Salutogenic-oriented mental health nursing · Salutogenesis

15.1 Introduction

We aim to use our own experiences to guide the presentation in this chapter. For me, Nina, the first author of this chapter, the occupational and professional life has been a journey of transformation from a nurse educated in psychiatric nursing, mental disorders, symptoms, and risk factors to find my identity as a *mental health nurse*. Today I am intrigued by the constitutional characteristic of resources and strengths in human beings, which of course also applies to persons with mental illness. These values, beliefs, and my respect for persons struggling with mental disorders are grounded in experiences acquired

N. H. Mjøsund (✉)
Division of Mental Health and Addiction, Department of Mental Health Research and Development, Vestre Viken Hospital Trust, Drammen, Norway
e-mail: nina.helen.mjosund@vestreviken.no

M. Eriksson
Department of Health Sciences, University West, Trollhattan, Sweden
e-mail: monica.eriksson@hv.se

at wards in hospital settings. The majority of my training gave prominence to the traditional role of caring for the sick. The opportunity to be educated in public health and health promotion was a turning point to embrace an expanded role as a "mental health nurse." In this journey, Monica has been an excellent guide into the theoretical landscape of salutogenesis.

For me, Monica, the second author, salutogenesis has been my research interest from the very beginning and up to date, more than 30 years of education and research. As a former social worker at a hospital and with work experiences among disabled people, my focus has always been on peoples' resources and their ability to overcome difficulties. Aaron Antonovsky and his salutogenic theory and model of health gave me the knowledge and prerequisites to immerse myself in what leads to health instead of the causes of illness.

Together we, Nina and Monica, share the desire to enhance the prerequisite for strengthening mental health of persons in need of hospitalization in mental health care. Salutogenesis has become the air we breathe. We possess extensive experiences from close collaboration with persons living with severe mental disorders in projects, both in health research and in clinical quality enhancement projects. We pay tribute to service user involvement. Thereby, this chapter emphasizes an insider perspective on how mental health promotion is perceived grounded in patients' lived experiences.

An elaboration of the salutogenic orientation applied on health and mental health clarifies the main theoretical underpinning in this chapter. Until we have arrived at explaining the content and application of salutogenic-oriented mental health nursing, we start with our understanding of health in general and mental health in particular. We continue to explain what we mean by salutogenic mental health promotion. The difference between interventions aiming for health promotion and the prevention of disorders will further be elaborated.

The promotion of mental health for people with mental illnesses is an issue for the nursing workforce all over the world. People who live with mental disorders deserve support to cope and recover from their illness as well as support to strengthen their general health. We claim that the population with mental disorders is in great need of *health promotion* interventions including the improvement of physical, social, spiritual, and mental health, due to 15–20 years shorter life expectancy compared with the general population [1]. However, the focus in this chapter is on salutogenic *mental health promotion*.

To understand the present and the future, knowledge about the past is needed. Thus, we highlight elements from some widely used nursing theories, which several decades ago brought health promotion and health maintenance into nursing science. Building on nursing theories, salutogenesis, and knowledge of the essence of health in general and mental health in particular, we end up with a proposal for a more holistic and coherent nursing care, including both *salutogenic-oriented nursing,* and *pathogenic-oriented nursing*. In order to emphasize the significance of salutogenic mental health promotion in nursing practice, we describe features of the salutogenic-oriented mental health nursing, and its application in clinical practice in mental health services.

15.1.1 Methods

The choice of theoretical perspectives, models, interventions, and evaluations presented in this chapter have been influenced by the usefulness for performance of clinical nursing and health care in the specialized health care services. Further, this chapter emphasizes an insider perspective on how mental health promotion is perceived grounded in patients' lived experiences. The chapter is inspired from our own empirical research [2–7], as well as extensive theoretical analysis and review reports [8–14]. The literature we build on is mainly grounded in qualitative research. More common in the field of public health as well as in medicine dominated hospital settings are the observational data and quantitative research.

Theoretically we rely on two salutogenic health theories, the salutogenic theory by Antonovsky [9, 15, 16] and mental health as flourishing by Keyes [17–20]. Additionally, the presentation was substantiated with a literature search including the words health care, health promotion, mental health promotion, mental health care, mental illness, mental disorders, nursing, salutogenesis, and service user involvement. The examples in this chapter are drawn from the context of the Nordic countries, as this is where we, the authors, are educated, have our work experience, and are living.

15.2 Health in Salutogenic Theoretical Framework

Salutogenesis offers a resource-oriented and strength-based perspective on health, and we will therefore especially emphasize some aspects of the existing knowledge base.

15.2.1 Health

Everyone's health gets affected. Health is a fundamental part of human beings. However, what constitutes the quality of health might be perceived differently. The authors of this chapter share a common understanding of the concept of health, i.e. health is always something positive, something we want more of, and want to promote and protect. A salutogenic approach to the study of health focuses on the genesis or sources of health, as well as circumstances promoting or undermining health. A salutogenic orientation includes a broad focus on resources, assets, and strengths leading to positive outcomes, which is different from the more limited focus in Antonovsky's [16] *Model of health.* Antonovsky

(1979) explained health as a movement along a continuum between ease and dis/ease,[1] and rejected the dualism of the health–disease dichotomy. Health promotion is about the movement towards health, with emphasis on assets, actions, and interventions that aim to promote health as a positive outcome. Adult lay people in Norway conceptualized health by six essential elements: well-being, function, nature, a sense of humour, coping, and energy [21]. In the same study, health was characterized by three qualities; *Wholeness*: health is a holistic phenomenon. Health is related to all aspects of life and society. *Pragmatism*: health is a relative phenomenon. Health is experienced and evaluated according to what people find reasonable to expect, given their age, medical condition, and social situation. *Individualism*: health is a personal phenomenon. Every human being is unique, and health and strategies for health must be individualized [21]. It has also been shown that nurses in mental health services perceived health as more than the absence of disorder [22].

15.2.2 Mental Health

No health without mental health—indicating a discourse including mental health in a positive sense [23]. Antonovsky [24] described mental health as a continuum. A person's location on a mental health continuum included the presence of a positive aspect, a sense of psychological well-being. Antonovsky defined mental health as more than the absence of something negative:

> Mental health, as I conceive it, refers to the location, at any point in the life cycle, of a person on a *continuum* which ranges from excruciating emotional pain and total psychological malfunctioning at one extreme to a full, vibrant sense of psychological wellbeing at the other [24], p. 274].

---

[1] In Antonovsky's original writings he consequently used a hyphen between dis and ease describing the health continuum as ease–dis-ease; however, according to programs that automatically correct misspelled words the hyphen often disappears, therefore, in this chapter we will use a slash; ease-dis/ease).

A salutogenic orientation focuses on the achievement of a successful coping, which facilitates movement towards that part of the mental health continuum that is a vibrant sense of psychological well-being. Mittelmark and Bull [25] show passages by Antonovsky indicating that his understanding of health was an aspect of the broader construct of well-being.

Inspired by salutogenesis, the research of Corey Keyes [17] focuses on subjective experiences of mental health. Keyes views mental health as the presence of positive states of human capacities and functioning in cognition, affect, and behavior. In line with Antonovsky, Keyes also questioned the commonly accepted definition of mental health as the absence of psychopathology. As elaborated in Chap. 5, Keyes describes mental health as the presence of psychological and functional well-being, thus a positive experience, not the absence of infirmity. He labels a continuum and uses the term *flourishing* to describe high quality of mental health or the most appealing position on the mental health continuum. The opposite position is labeled languishing, with moderate mental health in-between. Keyes [26] argues that it is not enough to see how people react. We also need to know how they feel and how they perceive their world. Mentally healthy people are described as being content with who they are and what they have, they feel socially and mentally competent, and emotionally stable [26]. Further, mentally healthy people experience to be generally happy, enthusiastic, and energetic most of the time, as well as being able to cope with problems and crisis in life [27].

Mjøsund et al. [6] used the salutogenic framework as the theoretical foundation for studying how persons with severe mental illness perceived their world of mental health. The study participants were not talking about absence of illness or disorder symptoms in their descriptions; they claimed mental health was an aspect of being, that was always present and experienced in everyday life as a sense of energy. Health was not perceived as changeless, but as a fluctuating and dynamic phenomenon. The participants perceived mental health as a movement, like walking up or down a spiral staircase, equivalent to a continuum [6], as illustrated in Fig. 5.2 in Chap. 5.

15.2.3 Mental Health Promotion

In the field of mental health promotion, it is essential to reflect on the understanding of health and mental health, as well as how promotion relates. WHO [28] states that mental health promotion involves actions that improve psychological well-being. Mental health promotion is a contested term and might be enlightened from multiple perspectives [29, 30]. Salutogenic health promotion is an endeavor to promote health by actively and consciously focusing on strength and resources in people. Mental health promotion can be explained as activities to sustain, restore, and enhance mental health. Mental health promotion might be applied on a policy and societal level, as well as on an individual, family, group, and community level. Salutogenic mental health promotion is directed towards improving, strengthening, or increasing the well-being of all people regardless of mental illness or not. Interventions designed to enhance mental health and well-being by increasing the coping capacities of communities and individuals and by improving environments that affect mental health are also described as mental health promotion [27]. The goal for health promotion in society and on a population level should be to make health promoting behaviors easier and more likely, and simultaneously make health-depleting actions more difficult. In this chapter, salutogenic mental health promotion is explored by focusing on strength and resources at an individual level in mental health care settings.

15.2.4 The Salutogenic Model of Health

Aron Antonovsky (1923–1994) challenged the conventional paradigm of pathogenesis and its dichotomous classification of persons as being either healthy or diseased [16]. He coined the concept of salutogenesis, which means the origin of health. Antonovsky saw health as a movement along a continuum on a horizontal axis between health/ease and dis/ease (see Fig. 15.1) [10]. He saw the relationship between the two orientations—pathogenesis and salutogenesis—as complementary [15].

This model of health within the salutogenic framework is resource-oriented focusing on peoples' ability to manage stress and still stay healthy. Salutogenesis is a way of thinking, being, acting, and meeting people in a health promotion manner [10]. It is not a personal trait or a special personality, but a life orientation or a way of viewing life as comprehensible, manageable, and meaningful [31]. More generally, salutogenesis refers to a scholarly orientation focusing attention to the origins of health and assets for health, contra the origins of disease and risk factors [32]. The core resources to counteract stressors are the sense of coherence (SOC) and generalized and specific resistance resources (GRRs/SRRs) and deficits (GRDs/SRDs) [15, 31, 33, 34]. SOC is defined as:

"a global orientation that expresses the extent to which one has a pervasive, enduring though dynamic feeling of confidence that: (a) the stimuli from one's internal and external environments in the course of living are structured, predictable and explicable; (b) the resources are available to one to meet the demands posed by these stimuli; and (c) these demands are challenges, worthy of investment and engagement" [15 , p. 19]

SOC includes three core dimensions: (a) comprehensibility, which refers to the extent to which one perceives the stimuli that confront one as consistent, structured, and clear; (b) manageability, which is the extent to which one perceives that the resources at one's disposal are adequate to meet life's demands; and (c) meaningfulness, which refers to the extent to which one feels that life makes sense emotionally ([15], p. 16–18). How the core dimensions interact and together influence SOC is illustrated in Fig. 15.2. The cognitive dimension comprehensibility is illustrated with a thought bubble over the face to draw attention to a capacity to judge the reality, to understand what is happening. The hand illustrated under manageability draws attention to the instrumental or behavioral dimension, a practical capacity to manage the situation. The heart

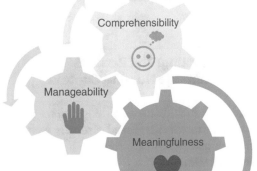

Fig. 15.2 The dimensions of the sense of coherence

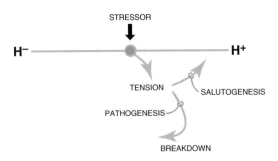

Fig. 15.1 The health continuum "ease/dis-ease" (Published with permission from Folkhälsan Research Center, Helsinki, Lindström & Eriksson [3])

under meaningfulness draws attention to which one feels that life makes sense emotionally, that the challenges in life are worth investing energy in, and are worth our commitment and engagement. The arrows around the dimensions help us to remember that these dimensions are involved when individuals are in interaction with the environment as they constantly go through challenging situations.

GRRs provide a person with sets of resources to promote meaningful and coherent life experiences. GRRs are found in people and bound to their person and capacity, but also to their immediate and distant environment [15, 33]. SRRs are context and situation bounded. Through SOC the GRRs enable one to recognize, pick up, and use SRRs in ways that keep tension from turning into debilitating stress [34]. Salutogenic nursing interventions aim to aid the patients to be aware, and use their GRRs/SRRs.

The Global Working Group on Salutogenesis (GWG-Sal) has identified key avenues for future development of the concept of salutogenesis to create a sound scientific base of health promotion [35]. There is a need to advance the original salutogenic model of health by adding an additional positive health continuum operating independently of stressors, as well development of alternative approaches to the conceptualization and measurement of the SOC [35].

15.3 Setting: The Patients' and the Nursing Context

The population discussed in this chapter is persons diagnosed with mental disorders receiving nursing and health care services in specialized mental health care.

15.3.1 Persons with Mental Disorders

People experiencing mental disorders are just as different as anyone else is. The understand-

ing of mental disorders are influenced by time and culture, and the use of terminology associated with disease is complicated and contested [36–38]. Dominant diagnostic systems in the field of psychiatry use different terminologies, the ICD-10 [39] uses classification of diseases and the DSM-5 [40] uses classifications of disorders. Severe conditions of mental disorders often broadly include disorders in the bipolar and schizophrenia spectrums, and complex comorbid conditions with substance abuse disorders, as well as life-threatening depressions. Severe conditions often persist over time and contribute to serious difficulties in personal and social functioning, thereby reducing the affected person's quality of life [41].

The experiences of mental distress, problems, and mental disorders are common and often underreported. According to an EU survey, one third of Europeans suffers from mental, neurological or substance abuse diagnoses (prevalence) [42]. Nordic patients with mental disorders seem to have 15–20 years shorter life expectancy than the general population largely due to lifestyle-related noncommunicable diseases [43]. A systematic review and meta-analysis [44] showed that people with schizophrenia are associated with at least 14 years potential life lost. To reduce this mortality gap, the situation requires urgent development and implementation of interventions.

We do not underestimate the fact that persons with mental disorders are in great need of lifestyle interventions targeting behavior to prevent somatic illnesses and to improve their physical health. However, less attention seems to be on behavior related to strengthening mental health. We realize that in clinical practice, it is difficult, nor desirable, to separate initiatives to promote physical, social, spiritual, or mental health. However, theoretically, in publications and in compilation of knowledge it can be relevant to shed light on certain parts of a larger context. Here, we aim to elaborate on one part of a larger picture, which is salutogenic mental health promotion for persons with mental disorders.

To avoid confusion with Antonovsky's ease-dis/ease terminology we avoid the use of the word disease. To denote a diagnosed condition we use the term *mental disorder*. When focusing on the individual experiences of struggling with mental problems or living with a diagnosed condition we use the term *mental illness*.

15.3.2 Nursing in the Context of Mental Health Care

Traditionally, mental health nursing and health care in hospitals have been directed towards persons diagnosed with a mental disorder or a suspected mental disorder. The main issue for nursing is the consequences of the disorder and coping in daily life. Hospitalized patients are often individuals with severe, multiple, and complex needs and long-term conditions. The impairment of self-care and disturbance of daily activities, as altered sleep pattern, bad nutrition, inactivity, strained relationships, and use of drugs in combination with increased intensity of symptoms of the disorders might require hospitalization. Patients affected with a severe mental disorder might be in great need of nursing; acute episodes might require total and lifesaving care. Nurses must apply their comprehensive knowledge about mental disorders to assist the patients to cope with consequences of the individual illness in daily life. User-led qualitative research revealed that individuals with complex needs appreciate trusting relationships with professionals, within a positive framework that fosters self-belief and which is focused on salutogenesis rather than pathogenesis [45].

A large part of the global nursing workforce, practices within primary and secondary health care settings in a rehabilitation, residential, or community setting. This workforce is claimed to be a sleeping giant in health promotion [46]. Promotion and maintenance of mental health, beyond the responsibility to provide curative services for adults with severe mental illnesses,

do not get the attention they deserve by nurses and other health professionals in the health care sector. Nurses are in a unique position for health promotion due to their presence in services across society, their continual attendance with patients night and day, and the close relationships they often develop with patients and next of kin. Nurses constitute a powerful group when wanting to reach and impact a large part of the population.

Besides somatic treatment and psychotherapeutic interventions, treatment for patients with severe mental illness should also include psychosocial interventions [41]. Berg and Sarvimäki [47] introduced a holistic-existential approach to health promotion in nursing. They defined health promoting nursing as "planned nursing actions designed to meet the needs of individuals, families and communities in their efforts to deal or cope with health challenges that they presently encounter in daily life or that might appear in the future... The aim of nursing is to support human beings in their need of knowledge and to offer practical assistance in order to cope with illness experiences and suffering and, thus, to stimulate healthy living" ([47], p. 390).

15.3.3 Health Promotion in the Specialized Mental Health Care Services

Despite launching the Ottawa charter nearly four decades ago [48], and the messages reinforced in the New Haven recommendations [49], hospitals all over the world are still characterized mostly by a pathogenic and biomedical approach. Psychiatric treatment and care of patients in mental health care hospitals are dominated by diagnosing, treating, and caring for persons with severe episodes of mental disorders, as well as acute and lifesaving interventions. Both nursing and medical interventions are often introduced with rather acute and short-sighted perspectives, putting the long-term focus of health promotion and quality of life in the shadow. A reorientation of the health care services is stated to be the least systematically developed, implemented, and evaluated key action area outlined in the Ottawa Charter [50], and new ways to reorient the health services towards the promotion of health are requested [51, 52]. The reorientation of the health care system is also requested by patients with mental disorders [3]. The timing for health promotion seems to be good during hospitalization when the awareness of health is heightened [53]. Former inpatients have described the hospital admission as a *window of opportunity* for choosing a healthier way of living, with the help of all the (human) resources available under hospitalization [5].

The role of nurses in the hospital is undergoing transitions, including redefining aspects of professional work, more complex and complicated conditions and acute crises as well as changing reimbursement systems [54, 55]. The scene has changed and other health care providers such as psychologists, social educators, social workers, psychiatrists, and counselors overlap with the nurses in mental health care hospital settings. This situation might cause controversies and role confusion in everyday life at the workplace. To define the scope of nursing as well as the other professions and to promote distinct roles of mental health nurses and other professions will be important for future development of these services.

15.3.4 Towards a More Complete Mental Health Nursing

We want to argue for a development towards a mental health nursing science and practice that more explicitly includes knowledge from salutogenesis. We do not claim this is a new approach, as many years ago, the salutogenic model was claimed to be suitable for adaptation in nursing milieu [56, 57]. Salutogenic-oriented mental health nursing is rather a conscious application of health promotion, based on beliefs about the human potential, intertwined in interventions to increase coping, competences, good feelings, and well-being. Our aim is to promote a nursing practice based in salutogenic thinking, feeling, and acting. Antonovsky saw early the potential in nursing to become an important profession to promote a salutogenic orientation. In the preface of his second book he said: *In writing this book, I have also had another group in mind: nurses, going through the fascinating throes of formulating a new professional identity, are perhaps more open to my ideas and ways of thinking than almost anyone else* ([15], p. xiv).

Our vision is to contribute to a more complete mental health nursing practice, where an illness and disorder-oriented approach are complemented with a health-oriented approach based on salutogenesis. For the understanding of salutogenic-oriented mental health nursing, we want to clarify the distinction between a salutogenic versus a pathogenic orientation. We explain the different meanings of treatment and *prevention* of disorders and disability, on to *protect and maintain* mental health, as well as the understanding of *promotion* of health, including physical, social, spiritual, and mental health. There are differences between these concepts, which have significance for how to work in different contexts. Our suggestion is explicitly to include salutogenic mental health promotion in nursing practice. Nurses should utilize salutogenic knowledge to emphasize the persons' level of mental health and initiate health promoting interventions, alongside a focus on the status of mental illness in planning these nursing interventions. We claim that nursing in mental health care services should include two complementary purposes in their portfolio; a health-oriented and an illness-oriented approach, as illustrated in Fig. 15.3.

Figure 15.3 illustrates the combination of knowledge from both salutogenesis and pathogenesis, as the base for promotion and protection of health, as well as the treatment and prevention of disorders. The knowledge base of salutogenesis in partnership with the knowledge base of pathogenesis complements each other, as well as contrasts each other by different area of interest

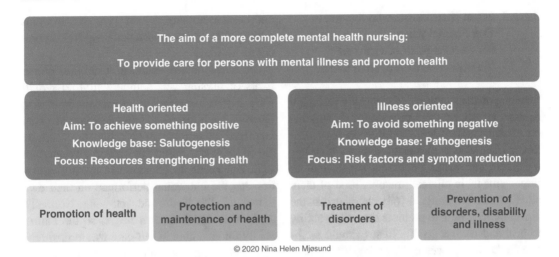

Fig. 15.3 Aims, knowledge base, and focus of a more holistic mental health nursing

[8, 58–60]. Our message is underlined by Becker and Rhynders' [61] use of mathematic analogy: "Pathogenesis is about subtraction and how to take away bad conditions, risk factors, or threats. Salutogenesis, on the other hand, is about addition and how to add positive actions, opportunities, conditions, and outcomes" [61, p. 2.].

Antonovsky [62] described similarities and differences between the two paradigms and argued for salutogenesis as a more powerful guide for health promotion research and practice than the pathogenesis. A pathogenic orientation embraces a dichotomous classification of disease or absence of disease. Pathogenesis assumes that if nothing causes mental illness, good mental health will be manifest. Antonovsky [16] followed a continuum line of thought in his salutogenic model of health. The health continuum contains an end of ease where you aim to stay and to protect your position, as well as an adverse end of dis/ease from which you want to leave. Both paradigms have a focus on factors; salutogenesis on salutary factors that promote health and pathogenesis on risk factors that might cause disorders. Taking a point of departure in salutogenesis helps nurses relate to all aspects of a person using a holistic approach. Within the pathogenic paradigm, a more reductionist approach leads to a focus on a particular diagnostic category [62].

Moreover, the desired positive outcomes are different in these two paradigms. Within a salutogenic way of working, the anticipated outcome is to have more health and well-being. Inspired by salutogenesis, the aim is to create progress towards desired improvements and gains and protect against something that may cause regression of health. This is the realm of promotion. In contrast, to be working within a paradigm of pathogenesis where the anticipated outcome is no disease, the emphasis will be on a problem. The best possible outcome from a problem is the lack of a problem, i.e. no symptoms of a mental disorder. A more complete mental health nursing practice requires knowledge from both paradigms.

To understand the present and the future, we need to understand the past. Thus, after giving the theoretical contextualization of mental health nursing we proceed forward to explain the work of influential nursing theorists. In the next section, we highlight some nursing theories, which have contributed substantially to the nursing science of today. Their work might help us to a) differentiate the role of nurses from other health care professionals by delineating the unique focus of nursing, and b) facilitate a reorientation of the nursing practice to include an explicit focus on salutogenic mental health promotion.

15.3.5 From Nightingale to Keyes: The Foundation for Salutogenic-Oriented Mental Health Nursing Care

Standing on the shoulders of giants is a metaphor to draw attention to the importance of building on existing knowledge. Standing on a foundation of knowledge makes us able to visualize the future and make theoretical suggestions to improvements in clinical practice. First of them all, Florence Nightingale [63] claimed that the aim of nursing were to promote the body's ability to heal and recover itself. Nurses should facilitate the healing processes by caring for a proper selection and administration of a diet, fresh air, light, warmth, cleanliness, and hygienic conditions, and reduce unnecessary emotional stress as well as carefully observe the patient's condition. Nightingale [63] believed that the patient in their environment was the main focus for nurses. Nightingale claimed that nursing was to care for the basic needs of human beings and promote health and well-being. Inspired by a salutogenic approach, we argue that Nightingale was the first health promoter in nursing science with her focus on promoting health and well-being of her patients.

Another influential nursing theorist for mental health nursing was Virginia Henderson. In her book "the Nature of Nursing" [64], she defined the unique function of nursing as to assist the person in performing activities contributing to health or recovery that the individual could have performed themselves if they had the strength, the will and knowledge, and always with the aim to help them gain independence as rapidly as possible [64]. Both Nightingale and Henderson saw nursing acts as assisting or doing on behalf of the patient, but never doing more than the patient can do independently or by supervision. This tuning towards the patient's mental and physical condition and environmental situation was the essence of the art of nursing. It was crucial to empower the patient to self-care as soon as possible. Seeing the patients as part of a greater society, always in interaction with their environment contributed to a broader view and holistic nursing, which were what persons with mental disorders also demanded and appreciated [2, 6].

Dorothea Orem claimed that the proper focus of nursing was self-care [65]. Her *Self-Care Deficit Nursing Theory* has similarities to those of Nightingale and Henderson, but Orem increased the emphasize on achieving health by the individual's ability to care for themselves [65]. According to Orem, self-care was activities that the individual performed on their own to maintain life, health and well-being. Normally, adults care for their own needs, so the human ability for engaging in self-care was termed self-care agency. Infants, children, the aged, the ill or the disabled required nursing in form of complete care or assistance with self-care activities in their day-to-day living [65]. Self-care contributed to human functioning and development based on self-care requisites in three categories: (a) universal, (b) developmental, and (c) conditions of illness, disorder, or injury [65]. The category of universal self-care requisite includes resources vital to the continuation of life, to growth and development, as such as air, food, water, elimination processes, activity and rest, social interaction and solitude, as well as human well-being. The developmental requisite comprised conditions to support life processes and needs related to various stages of development in the life course. The last category of requisite was related to situations of disorders or injury. There was a need to seek appropriate medical assistance for conditions of human pathology and carry out medical prescribed treatments, caring for side effects of the treatment, as well altering one's life-style to promote personal development while living with the side effects of pathology and medical treatments such as medicine.

The self-care deficits delineated when nursing was needed, and a nurse–patient relationship was required. Where the nursing relationship was not limited to just one individual, but the receiver of nursing care could be a family, a group or communities. The roles of the nurse and the patient were complementary in that a certain behavior of the patient elicited a certain response in the nurse, and vice versa. A self-care deficit requires nursing activities. The self-care concept facilitates an involvement of the patient in the nursing planning, prescribing, providing and evaluating. A model of practice termed *Treating Self-Care Deficits Related to Mental Health Functioning* has been developed as part of a mental health nurse practitioner master's program grounded in Orem's model [66].

Katie Eriksson's theory of *caritative caring* has been influential in nursing and other caring professions in the Nordic countries [67]. In her philosophical theory of caring, Eriksson claimed that the basic motive, the substance and the distinctive character for caring were caritas, which was by nature unconditioned love. In a health promotion context, it is appropriate to highlight her concept analysis of health [68]. She defined health to be constituted by two dimensions; the objective dimension of soundness and freshness and the subjective dimension of well-being. Health was seen as more than the absence of illness, and was conceived as movement and integration, *a becoming*. Eriksson [68] illustrated the health dimensions in a crosshair which included a vertical line representing the subjective dimension of well-being, and a horizontal line which represented objective dysfunctional attributes.

15.3.6 Towards a Distinct Understanding of Mental Health in Mental Health Nursing

In the nursing science we see traces on health promotion already in Nightingale's work [63] when she claimed long ago that nursing is to promote health and well-being for the patients. Also Henderson [64] argued that the aim of nursing was to contribute to health and Eriksson [65] claimed health to be more than the absence of illness. As one of many nursing theories we judge the conceptual framework of Orem [65] to be highly compatible with a salutogenic orientation. We want to inspire mental health nurses and other health professionals working with persons with mental disorders to build on

former nursing giants to apply health promotion more explicit in their clinical practice. The reason for this is based on knowledge we possess about contemporary clinical practices, the population in focus, and international guidelines as the Ottawa charter [69], as well as the fact that persons with mental disorder demand more health promotion [3].

To be able to develop, implement and measure the outcome of mental health promotion initiatives, we need to make overt the applied definition of mental health. Rather than arriving to a consensus on a definition of health for the use in the total field of health promotion, Mittelmark and Bull [25] argue for a pragmatic approach where scientist and health promoters make overt which definition they use in different project and settings.

Antonovsky's [15, 16, 62] work on salutogenesis and health promotion is essential for nursing and health promotion. However, we claim that his definition of health as a continuum between ease and dis/ease is not sufficient. A close reading of Antonovsky's writings gives no indication that he separated health from disease. Further, several passages of his writing might be understood as he included disorders and similar conditions in the dis/ease pole of the health continuum. Antonovsky [15] defined the positive end of the continuum in a negative way by the focus on the absence of pain, functional limitations, acute or chronic prognosis and health-related action implications [35]. See also discussion in the Handbook of Salutogenesis, chap. 49 [70].

Katie Eriksson [68] gave an important contribution to the understanding of health through her concept analysis. She included by her health definition an objective dimension representing symptoms of disorder or objective dysfunctional attributes, together with a subjective dimension of well-being. Later, and even more specific, we again can find a subjective dimension of well-being in a mental health definition. Keyes [20] defines mental health as an individual's subjective well-being, in term of their affective state and their psychological and social functioning, and good mental health is described by the metaphor flourishing (see Chap. 5 for a thoroughly elaboration of Keyes work). Besides Keyes' work on a definition of mental health [20], he has also given important contribution to the field by his two continua model of mental health and mental illness in the same context or picture (see Fig. 5.4). This complete picture is helpful for nurses and health promoters working with adults living with a mental disorder by making it possible to hold both of these phenomena in mind at the same time. In the setting of mental health nursing, based on the elaboration and assessment of the theoretical models and conceptual frameworks presented in this chapter, we suggest applying a distinct definition of mental health encompassing both feelings and functioning, based on Keyes' model of mental health (see Chap. 5).

Inspired by the work of Keyes, we see the potential in combining elements of theoretical framework from different times, cultures, disciplines and sciences to underpinning the today's art of nursing. Fig. 15.4 illustrates essential elements and areas of knowledge to make up a more complete mental health nursing practice.

In Fig. 15.4 the salutogenic orientation is of equal value as the pathogenic orientation. We do not claim this collection to be complete;

rather we challenge health professionals to put in elements to adapt the theoretical foundation to their actual setting. The main issue for us is to complement the pathogenic orientation with a salutogenic orientation to promote mental health for everybody and in the context of this chapter especially for adults with mental disorders. Further, we want to elaborate on one of the elements in Fig. 15.4, namely the salutogenic orientation as one important ingredient in the art of nursing.

15.4   Implementing Salutogenesis in Mental Health Nursing Practice

The time is ripe. Nurses have the knowledge to design evidence-based nursing aiming actively to promote patients' mental health, i.e. salutogenic mental health promotion. In the context of this book we want to give a more comprehensive elaboration of some features of the salutogenic-oriented mental health nursing, including some practical examples. We will continue with a presentation of some features of salutogenic-oriented mental health nursing as illustrated in the highlighted chart pie in Fig.15.5.

First, we give attention to the holistic approach to the person in need of care, including the person's environment. The second feature is attention to the person's strength and resources and to the persons own experiences of coping and adaption in life. The third feature we want to elaborate on is saluseducation, a concept first used by Mjøsund [3, 8]. When the nurses teach and supervise persons about salutogenic mental health promotion, they conduct saluseducation. The fourth prerequisite for salutogenic-oriented mental health nursing is to get access to the patients' experiences, which demands an active involvement of the patient in planning and implementation of nursing. We also want to emphasize the need to bring the patient perspective into this knowledge production; the service user involvement in research. Nursing research should involve patients and other service users actively in studies.

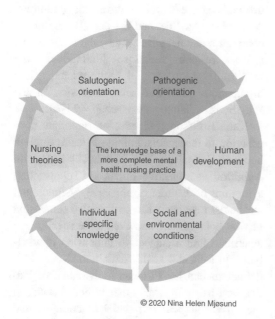

© 2020 Nina Helen Mjøsund

Fig. 15.4 The knowledge base of a more complete mental health nursing practice

Fig. 15.5 Features of salutogenic-oriented mental health nursing – as part of a more complete mental health nursing practice

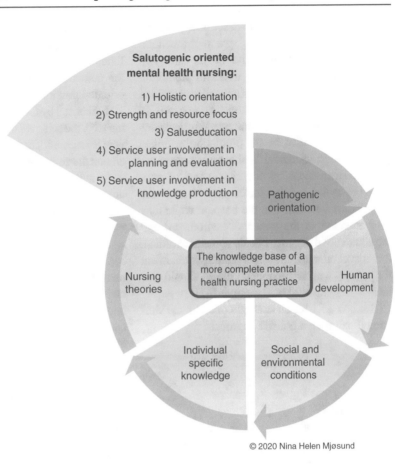

Salutogenic oriented
mental health nursing:

1) Holistic orientation
2) Strength and resource focus
3) Saluseducation
4) Service user involvement in planning and evaluation
5) Service user involvement in knowledge production

Pathogenic orientation

Nursing theories

The knowledge base of a more complete mental health nursing practice

Human development

Individual specific knowledge

Social and environmental conditions

© 2020 Nina Helen Mjøsund

15.4.1 A Holistic Orientation to the Patient with Mental Illness

Salutogenic-oriented mental health nursing includes a view of human beings as whole persons (mind, body and spirit) who are inseparable from their environment. In a holistic approach, the nurse includes a broader perspective and considers the patient as part of a larger context. The history of a person is significant beyond the illness history, or the person's single symptom of illness [71]. The patient's socio-economic status and social network, such as family or next of kin, friends, and professional relationships, are significant sources in the nursing assessment. They might contribute to understand more of the individual's daily life, as well as being sources of GRRs and potential stressors in the patients' environment. A nurse trained in salutogenic-

oriented nursing will always expect to find some assets and resources in every human being, which make the patients able to cope with simple or difficult tasks that can promote a feeling of mastery, even in the most acute situation.

A salutogenic approach to nursing in mental health care services might balance the dominant emphasis on disorder symptoms and risks, as well as the common language that reinforces a focus on disorder. Acquiring new concepts from salutogenic theory will contribute to more comprehensive and holistic knowledge. One example is given by Langeland [72]; she claims using the word person and not patient consistently will help us be aware that it is the whole person we are focusing on and not just the diagnosis. Antonovsky [15] was occupied with a holistic view on human beings, focusing on the history of the person more than the symptoms, risk factors, and the organ dysfunction.

Different labels are used to describe approaches similar to salutogenic nursing; we might mention holistic nursing and integrative health care [73]. A review of the nurses' role in health promotion practice shows that their activities were guided by an individualistic and holistic approach to help patients and families make health decisions and support them in health promotion activities [74]. Salutogenic mental health promotion nursing is characterized by targeting issues of coping in everyday living. Nurses need to mind the here-and-now situation in the hospital while they give attention to the patients' environment and the context of daily life. Beside somatic treatment and psychotherapeutic interventions, treatment for patients with severe mental illness should also include psychosocial interventions [41].

See box 15.1 for an example of a clinical situation illustrating a holistic approach.

> **Box 15.1 Example of a Clincial Situation Focusing on a Holistiv Approach**
> *Nursing situation*: Afternoon shift in an open inpatient unit. A man in his 50s is troubling with psychosis symptoms and do not want to take a shower.
> *Nurse*: Can you remember taking a footbath from your childhood?
> *Patient*: … hmm, I remember taking footbath at my grandmother's place.
> *Nurse*: I can arrange it for you now, your feet need some care. You deserve some wellness by hot water and a softening soap. I can cut your nails and apply some cream to your feet as well.
> *Assessment*: This situation facilitated a dialog about the patient's situation at home and the troublesome relationship to his brother. He had not talked to him for 5 years. The story ended with a telephone call to his brother, assisted by the nurse.

15.4.2 A Strength- and Resource-Focused Approach

Salutogenesis leads us to consider the human resources to strengthen health. Sharing positive expectations of what the patient can manage and achieve currently, and increasingly more in the future, creates hope and optimism. An explicit focus on salutogenic mental health nursing has the potential to strengthen a holistic and health-oriented nursing practice [57].

Influenced by Orem's conceptual model of nursing [65], the self-care agency of the patient here and now is assessed. The nurse need to take into consideration the ability of the patient to act independently, or by supervision, to satisfy self-care requisites of universal, developmental, or disorder-related conditions. Mental health nurses applying salutogenic mental health nursing emphasize the opportunities, resources and coping methods, as well as creating confidence for the patient that growth and development are possible. Building qualitatively good relations based on subject-to-subject relationships is an important foundation of the salutogenic approach, and nursing planning conducted in an atmosphere of partnership and equality with the patient is essential. A nurse–patient relationship should be established based on the recognition that each hold expertise in different fields. Where the patient is the expert in their life, with a range of experiences living with a mental disorder, and the trained nurse brings experiences from a large range of patient-meetings. Together these perspectives form the base for nursing interventions, and finding the right "fit" between the patient and the nurse.

A nursing planning process includes an assessment of the patient's resources and strengths. Significant knowledge is part of the patient's actual GRRs/SRRs, as well as the ability to use the resources. An explicit focus on coping and manageability based on utilization of GRRs/SRRs or getting access to new or extended GRRs/SRRs might bring important hope, energy and optimism. This is a counterpart to the more common focus on symptoms, risk assessment, and what is wrong.

See box 15.2 for an example of a clinical situation illustrating a strength- and resource-focused approach.

> **Box 15.2 Example of a Clinical Situation Focusing on a Strength- and Resource-Focused Approach**
> *Nursing situation:* A primary nurse approaches a patient with psychosis who

just started antipsychotic medicine. The nurse intends to become better acquainted with her patient's daily life and her family situation. They are together working with the nursing plan for the next 2 weeks.

Nurse: Now when you are on antipsychotic medication I know it is important to take a notice on your eating habits and your relationship to food.

Patient: I like to cook, and I like new recipes.

Nurse: Wow, your interest in cooking is positive, and a resource you possess. Do you know how to find out what the ingredients contain of calories, fat, sugar and proteins?

Patient: Yes, I think so, but I'm not sure. …

Nurse: Should we go to a grocery shop together on Wednesday to discuss some shopping and possible ingredients to make healthy meals?

15.4.3 Saluseducation: Learning Processes in Mental Health Promotion

An important area of the nurse profession' is the education, supervision, and guidance intentions of nursing. Nurses should use their broad knowledge to educate patients and families in the realm of mental health promotion to increase coping and empowerment. Patient education is mandatory for specialized health care services in Norway [75]. One of the first traces of an educational function in nursing is found in Nightingale's writings [63], when she claimed that nurses' role was not only to care for the sick, but also to teach proper caring for those who care for the health of others. The purpose of the book "Notes on Nursing" was to write a guide to women on how to care for their family's health, not a manual on nursing [63]. Nightingale's messages translated into current mental health care practice of today: the role of nurses includes educational and training activities for the patients themselves, as well as for those who care for their relatives or family members.

Potential opportunities associated with coping in daily life after hospitalization is requested in recovery and health promotion processes for persons with mental disorder [76]. A talk-therapy-group intervention based on Antonovsky's model of health for persons with mental disorders promoted SOC, coping, and mental health [76]. Talk-therapy based on salutogenesis treatment principles might be helpful in increasing coping among people with mental disorders [77]. Psychosocial interventions aimed at families are among the interventions supported by available evidence for individuals with severe mental disorders [41, 78, 79]. The health benefits rising from patient and family interventions aiming to increase health literacy, social and practical skills are relevant for mental health promoting nursing. Family intervention is a structured method for involving the patient and the patient's family members in treatment and rehabilitation, including family psychoeducation and skills training. Family interventions helps patients and families to cope through providing knowledge about the disorder and its symptoms, signs, crisis management, emotional support, and training in communication and problem solving in every-day life [41]. The broad and various elements in these interventions inspired from mental disorder knowledge, as well as a solution orientation to increase coping and mastery, make psychoeducation compatible with a salutogenic mental health promotion approach.

Psychoeducational interventions are associated with improved individual and social functioning and decreased relapse rates [41], therefore might educational activity be a GRR that enhances the patients' SOC. Many years ago, Landsverk and Kane [80] proposed that one of the processes through which psychoeducation works is in maintaining and enhancing an individual's SOC. The relationship between GRRs/SRRs and SOC seems to be a feedback loop: GRRs/SRRs provide experiences that lead to coping and enhanced SOC, and enables the patient to mobilize and use available resources [80].

Persons with severe mental health disorders express an appetite for learning [3], both about their disorder as well as their health in general. They requested *saluseducation* complementing a psychoeducational focus [3]. The saluseducation represents learning processes about health and health promotion, including knowledge and skills relevant for everybody—to increase health and well-being. Saluseducation is not delineated to people with some illnesses, although saluseducation should be tailored to each person's individual situation. Saluseducation in groups might have a synergetic effect as persons with mental disorders emphasize the positive impact of spending time with others with the same mental disorder [3].

Empowerment represents a corner stone in the field of health promotion. Nurses have the responsibility to provide care to promote empowerment by the means of emancipation, self-efficacy, and self-management of patients with long-term mental illness [81]. Empowerment was rated as the most important intervention in health promotion in a study on attitudes towards aspects of health promotion interventions, and the patients rated alliance and educational support significantly higher than the staff did [82]. Empowerment might be reached by customizing learning processes, that takes into account the person's individual situation, and sharing knowledge in a health promoting manner.

The participants in a study by Mjøsund et al. [6], described the importance of being of significance to each other and being able to support or assist others were perceived as health promoting. Langeland, Gjengedal, and Vinje [83] investigated salutogenic talk-therapy groups; receiving constructive feedback from other participants in the group was significant in order to develop good relationships and a participatory competence, resulting in stronger identity, useful advices and tips as well as seeing things in new ways. Persons in the group built salutogenic capacity based on a sense of community and from the opportunities to discuss and reflect together with other group participants who were perceived as like-minded [83].

Clinical experiences from psychoeducational treatment groups involving persons with bipolar disorders [84] and family groups for persons with schizophrenia spectrum disorders [85] have been an important inspiration to coin and introduce the term *saluseducation*. Persons with mental disorders and their families embrace knowledge they can apply immediately, without any assessment, diagnosing, or remedies, just to help themselves to live healthy lives with better mental health and well-being. Saluseducation together with psychoeducation provides opportunities to satisfy the knowledge appetite that persons with severe mental disorders have articulated [3].

See box 15.3 for an example of a clinical situation illustrating saluseducation.

Box 15.3 Example of a Clinical Situation Focusing on Saluseducation

Nursing situation: The nurse is holding an evening educational session for three patients with bipolar disorder and their next of kin at an inpatient ward.

Nurse: Some of my patients are curious about what to do for themselves to achieve better quality of life in their everyday activities. One of the things we all might be conscious about is our sleeping pattern. How long we sleep; when; sleeping hygiene like lower temperature in the sleeping room; open window for fresh air; what the bed should be reserved for; and regularities through the week and weekend. Now you might write down some questions coming up and we discuss some of them in a minute.

A father: I wonder about this afternoon nap. Could that be something that could help when you are a bit manic?

Nurse: I put the question at the board.

A young girl newly diagnose with bipolar disorder: When I visit my sister at weekends, we stay awake until early morning—that is probably not wise, or? Is it an explanation why? …

15.4.4 Service User Involvement in Planning and Evaluation of Nursing

We argue that it is essential to involve the perspectives of patients and their relatives to secure a patient relevant focus in knowledge development and practice. Service user involvement is a prerequisite for salutogenic mental health nursing. Persons with mental disorders should be empowered and involved in mental health advocacy, policy, planning, legislation, service provision, monitoring, research, and evaluation according to WHO [86]. The message to nurses is that it should be mandatory and naturally for patients to be brought into the decision-making processes. Crucial in recovery processes and in promotion of health is that patients and their families should be given the opportunity to participate actively in partnership to promote shared decisions about care and treatments. A recent systematic review concludes that family interventions are effective for reducing relapse rates, duration of hospitalization, and psychotic symptoms, and for increasing functionality in patients with a first episode of psychosis [87].

In collaboration with the main person and their next of kin the intents for nursing interventions and activities beyond life-saving care, must be agreed on. The relationship between the patient and the nurse has been described, also by patients with serious mental disorders, as essential to achieve successful outcomes of health promotion programs [88]. However, a recent study by Terry and Coffey [89] showed that service user involvement did not form an important part of mental health nursing processes. Service user involvement was seldom mentioned by nurses themselves and nursing work was rather described as task-focused, with limited collaboration with the patients in areas like care planning [89].

Patient-centered care involves the patient in planning, delivering, and evaluation of the nursing care [90]. Patient-centeredness secures a focus on the needs of the user as opposed to the needs of the hospital or the nurse. Applying patient-centered care, the focus is on the patient's needs, values, and preferences. Only by actively taking the individual's specific situation as a starting point can sustainable lifestyle changes that promote health occur.

See box 15.4 for an example of a clinical situation illustrating involvement of the patient in planning and evaluation of nursing.

Box 15.4 Example of a Clinical Situation Focusing on Involvement of the Patient in Planning and Evaluation of Nursing

Nursing situation: A primary nurse is walking in the park with a young patient Ann, who was admitted a few days prior with her first episode of psychosis. That afternoon, a meeting is scheduled to plan the treatment and care for the next week. The psychiatrist and the social worker will be there together with the nurse. Ann is invited; however, she is unsure if she will be there.

Nurse: I know you have experiences and information important for the planning of your treatment and care. For you, what is most important?

Ann: I don't know… I am not going to that meeting—and my cat has been alone since Thursday and I cannot give her food being here.

Nurse: I see… So the wellbeing of your cat is important? This is exactly what we need to know. I want to facilitate the information exchange between you and your team. We can do it in different ways. You and I can write down three important things for you, I bring it into the team and come back to you after the meeting. Alternatively, you come with me and I tell the others what you and I have been talking about. You have also another option. You might bring with you somebody you trust. And you can of course leave whenever you want.

Patient: I do not want my father to be there, neither my mother… I called my aunt Ellen yesterday…

Nurse: Your aunt Ellen, do you trust her? Maybe she is someone you can invite to be together with you when we discuss how to facilitate your treatment and care… and what we can do to take care of your cat.

15.4.5 Salutogenic Service User Involvement in Knowledge Production and Research

Experiential knowledge is an essential ingredient in the knowledge base of salutogenic-oriented mental health nursing. Lived experiences of receiving nursing and other treatments in health care are valuable for the development and improvement of the health care services. The field of mental health research has a long history of engagement with service users [91]. In research and knowledge production, the perspective of service users should be included, not only as informants but also in the research teams. Involvement takes place when research is carried out "with" or "by" patients rather than "to," "about" or "for" them [92]. The involvement of service users in the research process should be conducted in the salutogenic way, as claimed by Mjøsund et al. [2]. An advisory team was included in the research team; the five members were different persons from the participants interviewed in the project. Either the research advisors were diagnosed with a severe mental disorder or had family members with a severe mental disorder. They articulated features of the collaboration process and labeled it a *salutogenic service user involvement* [2]. Six features of the collaboration process which encouraged and empowered the advisors to make significant contribution to the research process and the outcome were articulated; leadership, meeting structure, role clarification, being members of a team, a focus on possibilities, and being seen and treated as holistic individuals. These features were perceived to constitute a salutogenic and mental health promotive involvement [2].

Service user involvement is also essential in clinical quality improvement projects. Evidence-based knowledge always need to be adapted to a local setting and environment, then service users with experiences from the same context possess important knowledge to be included in improvement processes. Service user involvement also has the potential to enhance the research quality [4].

See box 15.5 for an example of a clinical situation illustrating the recruitment of a service user to a research project.

> **Box 15.5 Example of a Clinical Situation Focusing on Service User Involvement in Knowledge Production and Research**
> *Nursing situation*: Under a discharge conversation between the nurse and her primary patient, the nurse wants to recruit her patient to become a service user in a project they plan at the ward. The project aim is to implement a national guideline for the involvement of family or next of kin, when persons with severe mental disorder are admitted to the hospital.
>
> *Nurse*: I know you want to actively use your experiences from receiving treatment from this ward over years. We need two persons with patient experience to join the project team, together with three persons being family members to someone being admitted to our section. Could you be interest?
>
> Patient: hmm… What am I supposed to do? And where are the meetings? It is a long bus ride for me to come here. Who else is in the team?
>
> Nurse: I have an information flyer here. Besides the persons I mentioned, three nurses from the section, including me and a nurse researcher are supposed to be in the team. How the involvement is designed will be developed in collaboration with the researcher. Is it ok if I contact you in a couple of days, then I probably know more about those practical things? …

15.5 Act-Belong-Commit: A Framework for Exemplifying Salutogenesis in Mental Health Nursing

The use of body- and movement-related actions for the prevention and healing of illnesses has a long tradition. Apart from the various physical benefits, psychological changes have been postulated [41]. The Act-Belong-Commit (ABC) mental health promotion campaign is assessed to be a comprehensive, population-wide program with a strong evidence base, demonstrating success in implementation and comprises universal principles of mental health and well-being [93]. The ABC campaign aims to target people in communities to engage in activities that enhanced their mental health. ABC might be used in different settings, both on a population level, in specified setting, and on an individual level [27].

The ABC-framework encourages individuals to engage in mentally healthy activities, and it appears to empower people with mental illness to take steps of their own to enhance their mental health [94]. The ABC-framework adapted in a health care and nursing context provides nurses and other health professionals with a practical framework for actually doing mental health promotion activities together with the patients. A population-based study of Irish older adults showed that the increase in the number of ABC-activities inversely predicted the onset of depression, anxiety, and cognitive impairment [95].

Mental health as well as physical and social health are related to lifestyle and cultivated by practice and what we do; *we become mentally healthy by engaging in mentally healthy activities* [27]. The ABC framework offers a structural approach to specific subpopulations in clinical settings. The ABC campaign is about keeping mentally healthy by keeping active, keeping up friendships and make connections with others, as well as engaging in activities that provide meaning and purpose in life [96].

- Act: Keep alert and engaged by keeping mentally, socially, spiritually, and physically active.
- Belong: Develop a strong sense of belonging by keeping up friendships, joining groups, and participating in community activities.
- Commit: Do things that provide meaning and purpose in life like taking up challenges, volunteering, learning new skills, and helping others.

Additionally, the ABC framework might be interpreted in three ways by which nurses and other health professionals in charge can enhance the mental health of those in their care. It is to: **A**ctively involve (those in your care), **B**uild (their) skills, and **C**elebrate (their) achievements [97]. The situation in Box 15.6 illustrates how the ABC-principles might be turned into action. The nurse invites the patient to an activity (**Act**) they are going to do together (**Belong**) in the future (**Commit**), based on the patient's interest in nature (**Commit**).

Box 15.6 Example of a Clinical Situation Focusing on ABC Activities

Nursing situation: Morning shift at a closed acute inpatient unit. The patient has been staying mostly in bed not talking for a couple of days.

Nurse: Good morning, my friend! I brought some flowers from my garden to you. I remember you were looking at the picture of some spring flowers in the newspaper yesterday.

Patient: ...Hmm.

Nurse: I'm on duty the day after tomorrow. Do you agree to come with me to the park by the main road to look at the trees over there – the leafs are in thousands of colors. ...

15.6 Conclusion

Mental health promotion is important to all of us, no matter if we are young or old and healthy or diseased. Salutogenic mental health promotion provides a resource and strength-based approach to promote mental health. Nurses in mental health care services are in an excellent position to include health promotion in their daily work with their continuous presence with the patients. In mental health care services, we claim that nurses need to provide a more complete mental health nursing to persons with mental disorders based in knowledge from both the paradigms of salutogenesis and pathogenesis. To emphasize the importance of salutogenesis in nursing care, we introduce the term salutogenic-oriented mental health nursing practice. Features of the salutogenic-oriented mental health nursing are the holistic orientation, with emphasize on strengths and resources, facilitating learning processes in health promotion, saluseducation, and the involvement of patients and next of kin in salutogenic nursing practices as well as in research.

Take-Home Messages
- Everybody could benefit from being involved in interventions aiming to promote mental health the salutogenic way.
- In mental health care services, the patients should receive a more complete nursing, based on knowledge from both the paradigms of salutogenesis and pathogenesis.
- Salutogenic-oriented mental health nursing is aiming to promote mental health as subjective well-being, understood in terms of the emotional state and psychological and social functioning of the patients.
- Salutogenic-oriented mental health nursing in mental health care services will be holistically oriented. Where patients are viewed as whole persons, body and mind, and part of a social environment and larger context.
- Salutogenic-oriented mental health nursing emphasizes the patients' capabilities, resources and ability to cope, and where personal growth and development are possible.
- The prerequisites for salutogenic-oriented mental health nursing is to put the patient at the center of shared decisions and evaluation of treatment and care.
- Salutogenic-oriented mental health nursing includes educational intervention to promote learning processes about mental health and how to promote, maintain, or protect good mental health.
- Salutogenic-oriented mental health nursing is evidence-based embedded in research including experiential knowledge and service user involvements.
- The Act-Belong-Commit framework for mental health promotion is an example of how to apply salutogenesis in mental health nursing practice.

Acknowledgement The authors would like to thank Vestre Viken Hospital Trust, Department of Mental Health Research and Development and University West, Department of Health Sciences for making it possible to write this chapter. Magnus Lien Mjøsund, thank you for reviewing the language and for assisting in fine-tuning of the figures.

References

1. The Norwegian Directorate of Health. National guideline about somatic health and lifestyle for persons with mental illness or additions. . In: Services MoHaC, editor. Oslo: The Norwegian Directorate of Health; 2018.
2. Mjøsund NH, Eriksson M, Haaland-Øverby M, Jensen SL, Kjus S, Norheim I, et al. Salutogenic service user involvement in nursing research: a case study. J Adv Nurs. 2018;74(9):2145–56. https://doi.org/10.1111/jan.13708.
3. Mjøsund NH, Eriksson M, Espnes GA, Vinje HF. Reorienting Norwegian mental healthcare services: listen to patients' learning appetite. Health Promot Int. 2018;34:541–51. https://doi.org/10.1093/heapro/day012.
4. Mjøsund NH, Eriksson M, Espnes GA, Haaland-Øverby M, Jensen SL, Norheim I, et al. Service user involvement enhanced the research quality in a study using interpretative phenomenological analysis: the power of multiple perspectives. J Adv Nurs. 2017;73(1):265–78. https://doi.org/10.1111/jan.13093.
5. Mjøsund NH. Positive mental health—from what to how. A study in the specialized mental healthcare service. Trondheim: Norwegian University of Science and Technology, Faculty of Medicine and Health Sciences, Department of Public Health and Nursing; 2017.
6. Mjøsund NH, Eriksson M, Norheim I, Keyes CLM, Espnes GA, Vinje HF. Mental health as perceived by persons with mental disorders—an interpretative phenomenological study. Int J Ment Health Promot. 2015;17(4):215–33. https://doi.org/10.1080/1462373 0.2015.1039329.
7. Mjøsund NH. Health promotion nursing in mental health care—patients' dream hospital. Norwegian J Clin Nurs. 2020. https://doi.org/10.4220/Sykepleienf.2020.80478.
8. Mjøsund NH. Helsefremming for personer med psykisk lidelse innlagt i sykehus [health promotion for persons with severe mental illness in hospital]. In: Haugan G, Rannestad T, editors. Helsefremming i spesialisthelsetjenesten [health promotion in specialized health care services]. Oslo: Cappelen Damm Akademisk; 2016. p. 236–54.
9. Mittelmark MB, Sagy S, Eriksson M, Bauer GF, Pelikan JM, Lindström B, et al. The handbook of Salutogenesis. Cham: Springer International Publishing AG; 2017.

10. Lindström B, Eriksson M. The Hitchhiker's guide to salutogenesis: salutogenic pathways to health promotion. Helsinki: Folkhälsan; 2010.

11. Eriksson M, Lindström B. A salutogenic interpretation of the Ottawa charter. Health Promot Int. 2008;23(2):190–9.

12. Eriksson M, Lindström B. Antonovsky's sense of coherence scale and its relation with quality of life: a systematic review. J Epidemiol Community Health. 2007;61(11):938–44.

13. Eriksson M, Lindström B. Antonovsky's sense of coherence scale and the relation with health: a systematic review. J Epidemiol Community Health. 2006;60(5):376–81. https://doi.org/10.1136/jech.2005.041616.

14. Eriksson M, Kerekes N, Brink P, Pennbrant S, Nunstedt H. The level of sense of coherence among Swedish nursing staff. J Adv Nurs. 2019;75(11):2766–72. https://doi.org/10.1111/jan.14137.

15. Antonovsky A. Unraveling the mystery of health: how people manage stress and stay well. San Francisco: Jossey-Bass; 1987.

16. Antonovsky A. Health, stress, and coping. San Francisco: Jossey-Bass; 1979.

17. Keyes CLM. Mental health as a complete state: how the Salutogenic perspective completes the picture. In: Bauer GF, Hämmig O, editors. Bridging occupational, organizational and public health: a transdisciplinary approach. London: Springer; 2014. p. 179–92.

18. Keyes CLM. Towards a mentally flourishing society: mental health promotion, not cure. J Public Ment Health. 2007;6(2):4–7. https://doi.org/10.1108/17465729200700009.

19. Keyes CLM, Haidt J. Flourishing: Positive psychology and the life well-lived. Washington, DC: American Psychological Association; 2003.

20. Keyes CLM. The mental health continuum: from languishing to flourishing in life. J Health Soc Behav. 2002;43(2):207–22.

21. Fugelli P, Ingstad B. Helse—slik folk ser det. Tidsskrift for Den norske legeforening. 2001;(Årg. 121, nr 30):3600–4.

22. Jormfeldt H, Svedberg P, Fridlund B, Arvidsson B. Perceptions of the concept of health among nurses working in mental health services: a phenomenographic study. Int J Ment Health Nurs. 2007;16(1):50–6. https://doi.org/10.1111/j.1447-0349.2006.00444.x.

23. Herrman H, Saxena S, Moodie R. Promoting mental health: concepts, emerging evidence, practice : a report of the World Health Organization, Department of Mental Health and Substance Abuse in collaboration with the Victorian Health Promotion Foundation and the University of Melbourne. Geneva: World Health Organization; 2005.

24. Antonovsky A. The life cycle, mental health and the sense of coherence. Isr J Psychiatry Relat Sci. 1985;22(4):273–80.

25. Mittelmark MB, Bull T. The salutogenic model of health in health promotion research. Glob Health Promot. 2013;20(2):30–8. https://doi.org/10.1177/1757975913486684.

26. Keyes CLM. Promoting and Protecting positive mental health: early and often throughout the lifespan. In: Keyes CLM, editor. Mental well-being: international contributions to the study of positive mental health. Dordrecht: Springer; 2013. p. 3–28.

27. Donovan RJ, Anwar-McHenry J. Act-belong-commit: lifestyle medicine for keeping mentally healthy. Am J Lifestyle Med. 2014;10(3):193–9. https://doi.org/10.1177/1559827614536846.

28. WHO. Mental health: strengthening our response. 2018. Accessed 18 Dec 2019.

29. Barry MM, Jenkins R. Implementing mental health promotion. Edinburgh: Churchill Livingstone; 2007.

30. Cattan M, Tilford S. Mental health promotion: a lifespan approach. Maidenhead: Open University Press, Mc Graw-Hill; 2006.

31. Eriksson M. The sense of coherence in the Saltogenic model of health. In: Mittelmark MB, Sagy S, Eriksson M, Bauer GF, Pelikan JM, Lindström B, et al., editors. The handbook of Salutogenesis. Cham: Springer International Publishing AG; 2017. p. 91–6.

32. Mittelmark MB, Bauer GF. The meanings of Salutogenesis. In: Mittelmark MB, Sagy S, Eriksson M, Bauer GF, Pelikan JM, Lindström B, et al., editors. The handbook of Salutogenesis. Cham: Springer International Publishing AG; 2017. p. 7–13.

33. Idan O, Eriksson M, Al-Yagon M. The Salutogenic model: the role of generalized resistance resources. In: Mittelmark MB, Sagy S, Eriksson M, Bauer GF, Pelikan JM, Lindström B, et al., editors. The handbook of Salutogenesis. Cham: Springer International Publishing AG; 2017. p. 57–70.

34. Mittelmark MB, Bull T, Daniel M, Urke H. Specific resistance resources in the Salutogenic model of health. In: Mittelmark MB, Sagy S, Eriksson M, Bauer GF, Pelikan JM, Lindström B, et al., editors. The handbook of Salutogenesis. Cham: Springer International Publishing AG; 2017. p. 71–6.

35. Bauer GF, Roy M, Bakibinga P, Contu P, Downe S, Eriksson M, et al. Future directions for the concept of salutogenesis: a position article. Health Promot Int. 2019;35:187. https://doi.org/10.1093/heapro/daz057.

36. Schramme T. On the autonomy of the concept of disease in psychiatry. Front Psychol. 2013;4:457. https://doi.org/10.3389/fpsyg.2013.00457.

37. Zachar P, Kendler KS. Psychiatric disorders: a conceptual taxonomy. Am J Psychiatry. 2007;164(4):557–65.

38. Hofmann B, Wilkinson S. Mange betegnelser for sykdom (Several terms for disease). Tidsskrift for den norske legeforening. 2016;136(12/13):1125–6. https://doi.org/10.4045/tidsskr.16.0316.

39. WHO. ICD-10: International statistical classification of diseases and related health problems. Geneva: World Health Organization; 2009.

40. American Psychiatric Association. Diagnostic and statistical manual of mental disorders: DSM-5. 5th ed. Washington, DC: American Psychiatric Association; 2013.

41. Gühne U, Weinmann S, Arnold K, Becker T, Riedel-Heller SG. S3 guideline on psychosocial therapies in severe mental illness: evidence and recommendations. Eur Arch Psychiatry Clin Neurosci. 2015;265(3):173–88. https://doi.org/10.1007/s00406-014-0558-9.

42. Wittchen HU, Jacobi F, Rehm J, Gustavsson A, Svensson M, Jönsson B, et al. The size and burden of mental disorders and other disorders of the brain in Europe 2010. Eur Neuropsychopharmacol. 2011;21(9):655–79. https://doi.org/10.1016/j.euroneuro.2011.07.018.

43. Wahlbeck K, Westman J, Nordentoft M, Gissler M, Laursen TM. Outcomes of Nordic mental health systems: life expectancy of patients with mental disorders. Br J Psychiatry. 2011;199(6):453–8. https://doi.org/10.1192/bjp.bp.110.085100.

44. Hjorthøj C, Stürup AE, McGrath JJ, Nordentoft M. Years of potential life lost and life expectancy in schizophrenia: a systematic review and meta-analysis. Lancet Psychiatry. 2017;4(4):295–301. https://doi.org/10.1016/S2215-0366(17)30078-0.

45. Woodall J, Cross R, Kinsella K, Bunyan A-M. Using peer research processes to understand strategies to support those with severe, multiple and complex health needs. Health Educ J. 2019;78(2):176–88. https://doi.org/10.1177/0017896918796044.

46. Whitehead D, Irvine F. Ottawa 25+—'All aboard the Dazzling Bandwagon'—developing personal skills: what remains for the future? Health Promot Int. 2011;26(suppl 2):ii245–i52. https://doi.org/10.1093/heapro/dar072.

47. Berg GV, Sarvimäki A. A holistic-existential approach to health promotion. Scand J Caring Sci. 2003;17(4):384–91. https://doi.org/10.1046/j.0283-9318.2003.00240.x.

48. WHO. In: Promotion FICoH, editor. Ottawa Charter for health promotion. Ottawa: WHO; 1986. p. 5.

49. International Health Promotion Hospitals and Health Services. The New Haven recommendations on partnering with patients, families and citizens to enhance performance and quality in health promoting hospitals and health services. Clin Health Promot. 2016;6(1):1–15.

50. Wise M, Nutbeam D. Enabling health systems transformation: what progress has been made in re-orienting health services? Promot Educ. 2007;45(Suppl 2):23–7.

51. de Leeuw E. Have the health services reoriented at all? Health Promot Int. 2009;24(2):105–7.

52. Catford J. Turn, turn, turn: time to reorient health services. Health Promot Int. 2014;29(1):1–4. https://doi.org/10.1093/heapro/dat097.

53. Latter S. The potential for health promotion in hospital nursing practice. In: Scriven A, Orme J, editors. Health promotion: professional perspectives. 2nd ed. New York: Palgrave; 2001.

54. Whitehead D. Exploring health promotion and health education in nursing. Nurs Standard. 2018;33(8). https://doi.org/10.7748/ns.2018.e11220.

55. Hudson K. Salutogenesis: the origin of health. Nurs Manage. 2013;44(11):12–3. https://doi.org/10.1097/01.numa.0000436369.45139.81.

56. Langius A, Björvell H. Salutogenic model and utilization of the KASAM form (sense of coherence) in nursing research—a methodological report. Vård i Norden. 1996;16(1):28–32. https://doi.org/10.1177/010740839601600106.

57. Sullivan GC. Evaluating Antonovsky's Salutogenic model for its adaptability to nursing. J Adv Nurs. 1989;14(4):336–42.

58. Haugan G, Rannestad T. Helsefremmende helsearbeid -patogenese og salutogenese [health promotion in health care work—pathogensis and salutogensis]. In: Haugan G, Rannestad T, editors. Helsefremming i spesialisthelsetjenesten [health promotion in specialized health care services]. Oslo: Cappelen Damm Akademisk; 2016. p. 34–58.

59. Haugan G. Helsefremmende sykepleie i spesialist- og kommunehelsetjenesten [health promotion in nursing the specialized and municipality health care services]. In: Larsen TB, Gammersvik Å, editors. Helsefremmende sykepleie—i teori og praksis [health promotion in nursing—in theory and practice]. Oslo: Fagbokforlaget; 2018.

60. Haugan G. Helsefremming i kommunehelsetjenesten [Health promotion in the municipality health care services]. In: Ingstad K, Hedlund M, Moe A, editors. Kunnskap i praksis—fellesskap og kommunal omsorg [Knowledge for practice—community and municipality care]. In review: Universitetsforlaget 2020.

61. Becker CM, Rhynders P. It's time to make the profession of health about health. Scand J Public Health. 2013;41(1):1–3. https://doi.org/10.1177/1403494812467506.

62. Antonovsky A. The salutogenic model as a theory to guide health promotion. Health Promot Int. 1996;11(1):11–8.

63. Nightingale F. Notes on nursing: what is nursing and what is not. New York: Dover; 1860.

64. Henderson V. The nature of nursing: a definition and its implications for practice, research, and education. Third printing, 1969 ed. New York: Macmillan; 1966.

65. Orem DE. Nursing: concepts of practice. 6th ed. St. Louis, MO: Mosby; 2001.

66. Grando VT. A self-care deficit nursing theory practice model for advanced practice psychiatric/mental health nursing. SelfCare Depend Care Nurs. 2005;13(1):4–8.

67. Lindström UÅ, Lindholm L, Zetterlund JE. Theory of Caritative caring. In: Alligood MR, editor. Nursing theorists and their work. 8th ed. Greenville, NC: Elsevier; 2014. p. 171–202.

68. Eriksson K. Hälsans idé (the idea of health). 2. Uppl. Ed. Vårdserie. Stockholm: Almqvist & Wiksell; 1984.

69. WHO. Ottawa charter for health promotion. Can J Public Health. 1986;77(6):425–30.

70. Espnes GA. Salutogenesis: the Book's editors discuss possible futures. In: Mittelmark MB, Sagy S, Eriksson M, Bauer GF, Pelikan JM, Lindström B, et al., editors. The handbook of Salutogenesis. Cham: Springer International Publishing AG; 2016.

71. Vinje HF, Langeland E, Bull T. Aaron Antonovsky's development of Salutogenesis, 1979 to 1994. In: Mittelmark MB, Sagy S, Eriksson M, Bauer GF, Pelikan JM, Lindström B, et al., editors. The handbook of Salutogenesis. Cham: Springer International Publishing AG; 2017.

72. Langeland E. Sense of coherence and life satisfaction in people suffering from mental health problems: an intervention study in talk-therapy groups with focus on salutogenesis [PhD]. The University of Bergen; 2007.

73. Frisch NC, Rabinowitsch D. What's in a definition? Holistic nursing, integrative health care, and integrative nursing: report of an integrated literature review. J Holist Nurs. 2019;37(3):260–72. https://doi.org/10.1177/0898010119860685.

74. Kemppainen V, Tossavainen K, Turunen H. Nurses' roles in health promotion practice: an integrative review. Health Promot Int. 2013;28(4):490–501. https://doi.org/10.1093/heapro/das034.

75. Specialized Health Services Act. Act 1999-07-02-61. Act relating to specialized health services. 1999.

76. Langeland E, Wahl AK, Kristoffersen K, Hanestad BR. Promoting coping: salutogenesis among people with mental health problems. Issues Ment Health Nurs. 2007;28(3):275–95. https://doi.org/10.1080/01612840601172627.

77. Langeland E, Riise T, Hanestad BR, Nortvedt MW, Kristoffersen K, Wahl AK. The effect of salutogenic treatment principles on coping with mental health problems a randomised controlled trial. Patient Educ Couns. 2006;62(2):212–9. https://doi.org/10.1016/j.pec.2005.07.004.

78. Pharoah F, Mari JJ, Rathbone J, Wong W. Family intervention for schizophrenia. Cochrane Libr. 2010. https://doi.org/10.1002/14651858.CD000088.pub3.

79. Dixon LB, Dickerson F, Bellack AS, Bennett M, Dickinson D, Goldberg RW, et al. The 2009 schizophrenia PORT psychosocial treatment recommendations and summary statements. Schizophr Bull. 2009;36(1):48–70. https://doi.org/10.1093/schbul/sbp115.

80. Landsverk SS, Kane CF. Antonovsky's sense of coherence: theoretical basis of psychoeducation in schizophrenia. Issues Ment Health Nurs. 1998;19(5):419–31.

81. Jönsson PD, Nunstedt H, Berglund IJ, Ahlström BH, Hedelin B, Skärsäter I, et al. Problematization of perspectives on health promotion and empowerment in mental health nursing—within the research network "MeHNuRse" and the Horatio conference, 2012. Int J Qual Stud Health Well Being. 2014;9(22945):6. https://doi.org/10.3402/qhw.v9.22945.

82. Svedberg P, Hansson L, Svensson B. The attitudes of patients and staff towards aspects of health promotion interventions in mental health services in Sweden. Health Promot Int. 2009;24(3):269–76. https://doi.org/10.1093/heapro/dap019.

83. Langeland E, Gjengedal E, Vinje HF. Building salutogenic capacity: a year of experience from a salutogenic talk-therapy group. Int J Ment Health Promot. 2016;18(5):247–62. https://doi.org/10.1080/14623730.2016.1230070.

84. Skjelstad DV, Norheim I, Reiersen GK, Mjøsund NH. Psykoedukasjon i gruppe for personer med bipolar lidelse. En presentasjon av kursmodellen, deltagernes tilfredshet, og implementeringserfaringer. (Group psychoeducation for people with bipolar disorders). Tidsskrift for Norsk psykologforening (J Norwegian Psychol Assoc). 2015;52(12):1041–50. http://www.psykologtidsskriftet.no/pdf/2015/1041-1050.pdf.

85. Norheim I, Mjøsund NH. Psykoedukative flerfamiliegrupper for unge med psykose: familien som ressurs i bedringsprosessen. Ergoterapeuten. 2010;(Årg. 53, nr. 6):22–7.

86. WHO. Mental health action plan 2013–2020. Geneva: World Health Organization; 2013.

87. Camacho-Gomez M, Castellvi P. Effectiveness of family intervention for preventing relapse in first-episode psychosis until 24 months of follow-up: a systematic review with meta-analysis of randomized controlled trials. Schizophr Bull. 2019;46:98. https://doi.org/10.1093/schbul/sbz038.

88. Shiner B, Whitley R, Van Citters AD, Pratt SI, Bartels SJ. Learning what matters for patients: qualitative evaluation of a health promotion program for those with serious mental illness. Health Promot Int. 2008;23(3):275–82. https://doi.org/10.1093/heapro/dan018.

89. Terry J, Coffey M. Too busy to talk: examining service user involvement in nursing work. Issues Ment Health Nurs. 2019;40:1–9. https://doi.org/10.1080/01612840.2019.1635667.

90. McCormack B, McCance T. Person-centred practice in nursing and health care: theory and practice. 2nd ed. Chichester: Wiley; 2017.

91. Wallcraft J, Schrank B, Amering M. Handbook of service user involvement in mental health research. 1st ed. Chichester: Wiley-Blackwell; 2009.

92. National Institute for Health Research. Good practice guidance for involving people with experience of mental health problems in research. London: Mental Health Research Network; 2013. Accessed 14 Aug 2013.

93. Koushede V, Nielsen L, Meilstrup C, Donovan RJ. From rhetoric to action: adapting the act-belong-commit mental health promotion Programme to a Danish context. Int J Ment Health Promot. 2015;17(1):22–33. https://doi.org/10.1080/14623730.2014.995449.

94. Donovan RJ, Jalleh G, Robinson K, Lin C. Impact of a population-wide mental health promotion

campaign on people with a diagnosed mental illness or recent mental health problem. Aust N Z J Public Health. 2016;40(3):274–5. https://doi.org/10.1111/1753-6405.12514.

95. Santini ZI, Koyanagi A, Tyrovolas S, Haro JM, Donovan RJ, Nielsen L, et al. The protective properties of act-belong-commit indicators against incident depression, anxiety, and cognitive impairment among older Irish adults: findings from a prospective community-based study. Exp Gerontol. 2017;91:79–87. https://doi.org/10.1016/j.exger.2017.02.074.

96. Act-Belong-Commit Campaign. The act-belong-commit. Guide to keeping mentally healthy. Curtin University Perth, Australia. 2013. Accessed 30 Sept 2019.

97. Donovan RJ, James R, Jalleh G, Sidebottom C. Implementing mental health promotion: the act–belong–commit mentally healthy WA campaign in Western Australia. Int J Ment Health Promot. 2006;8(1):33–42. https://doi.org/10.1080/14623730.2006.9721899.

Health Promotion Among Individuals Facing Chronic Illness: The Unique Contribution of the Bodyknowledging Program

16

Kristin Heggdal

Abstract

This chapter offers an oversight of the concept of chronic illness and the meaning of health promotion in this context. Bodyknowledging is a theory describing patients' process of health promotion in chronic illness that has been used as a theoretical frame for a new health intervention; the Bodyknowledging Program (BKP). This program is outlined as the aim of BKP is to activate and strengthen patients' resources for health in chronic illness. Outcomes for patients and implications for practice are discussed.

Keywords

Chronic illness · Health intervention · Patient participation · Health · Well-being

16.1 Introduction

The concept of health promotion has traditionally been associated with preventive measures for healthy people, while health promotion in relation to people already diagnosed is a relatively new idea which is scarcely described in the literature.

K. Heggdal (✉)
Lovisenberg Diaconal University College, Oslo, Norway
e-mail: Kristin.Heggdal@ldh.no

The goal of health promotion is to increase the involved persons' control over their health and to improve it. This includes people diagnosed with chronic illness and involves mobilizing strengths for the promotion of health and well-being [1].

16.1.1 The Concept of Chronic Illness

Although there is no universal consensus about the definition, it is common to apply the term chronic illness when there is a disease with a prolonged trajectory for which there is no curative treatment, and when the condition impacts the persons' life and functioning and requires monitoring and specific management measures [2]. Chronic illness falls under the heading of noncommunicable diseases (NCD), which encompasses a large group of illnesses, such as diabetes, hypertension, stroke, heart disease, pulmonary conditions, cancer, and mental health conditions. The term may also include selected communicable diseases such as HIV [3]. Chronic illness occurs across the lifespan. Due to the advent of new options for treatment, improved disease management, and improved living conditions, children diagnosed with chronic illness are increasingly surviving into adulthood. Similarly, people who would previously have significantly shortened lifespan due to chronic illness are now experiencing increased longevity [4].

G. Haugan, M. Eriksson (eds.), *Health Promotion in Health Care – Vital Theories and Research*,
https://doi.org/10.1007/978-3-030-63135-2_16

Chronic illness is one of the leading health-related challenges across the world and currently the main cause of both death and disability worldwide [4, 5]. The majority of conditions contributing to mortality and morbidity combined in high-income countries like Europe, USA, and Australia include ischemic heart disease, stroke, lung cancer, depression, diabetes, and back and neck pain. In low-income countries like countries in Africa and middle-income countries like China, the major conditions contributing to mortality and morbidity include stroke, diabetes, and depression, and also communicable diseases such as diarrhea, HIV, and malaria, and road traffic injuries [6].The risk of coronary disease, ischemic stroke, diabetes, and cancer increases steadily with increasing body mass index (BMI) and obesity, which has become a major health concern, especially in high- and middle-income countries. In addition, the Institute for Health Metrics Evaluation reports that the number of people suffering from mental illness is relatively large but stable, as one in four people in the world will be affected by mental of neurological disorders at some point in their lives. The prevalence increases with age, but high rates of comorbidity has also been reported in working-age populations [7]. Many patients attending health care today have two or more chronic conditions. In Europe, it has been estimated that multimorbidity (or comorbidity) affects up to 95% of the primary care population aged 65 years and older. Approximately 25.5% of the United States population report to have more than one chronic condition, and the prevalence increases to 50% of adults 45–65 years, and up to 81% of adults older than 65 years. For adults over 50 years, rates of multiple chronic disease will vary from 45% in China to 71% in Russia [6].

About half of the individuals with comorbid chronic conditions report functional limitations and are more likely to have poor self-reported health; therefore, effective interventions are necessary to optimize health outcomes in the presence of chronic illness [8]. While medical treatment can contribute to the reduction of symptoms and to prevention of complications, sometimes no treatment is available. Addressing comorbidity, including mental health problems, emphasizes the importance of developing interventions that attend to the person's health as a whole [5]. Such interventions call for an understanding of patients as resourceful partners for health together with professionals and peers.

16.2 Health Promotion in Chronic Illness

According to Larsen [2], health promotion in chronic illness involves "efforts to create healthy lifestyles and a healthy environment to prevent secondary conditions, including teaching individuals to address their health care needs, increasing opportunities to participate in usual life activities and striving for optimal health. These secondary conditions may include the medical, social, emotional, mental, family, or community problems that an individual with a chronic or disabling condition is likely to experience (p. 367)." While professionals' treatment and care are significant, patients have an important role in learning as much as possible about their conditions and becoming involved in the management of their disease, in prevention of future relapses and in health promotion efforts. This includes taking part in communication with health professionals on health-related matters as well as efforts to avoid risk factors such as poor nutrition, lack of physical activity, smoking, alcohol abuse, and social isolation, because the same risk factors that cause a chronic condition can also make it worse.

It is important to increase patients' ability to manage their conditions and to maintain or improve their levels of functioning [2, 4, 9]. Manageability, comprehensibility, and meaningfulness constitute dimensions of the persons' Sense of Coherence (SOC) and represent central assets for health as they reflect the ability to understand one's existence as organized and the belief that one has the ability to handle one's life and to reestablish meaning while facing chronic conditions [10, 11]. Studies involving patients with chronic illness confirm that patients who have a strong SOC have a greater capacity to manage their chronic illness [12, 13]. For people who live with chronic illness and their support-ers, health promotion is a process of enabling and developing potentials for healing and health. By this means it affords new strategies and actions to strengthen hope among sufferers, to reduce their anxieties, and to facilitate a meaningful life (Chaps. 7 and 8). Its goal is to increase the capacity of people to deal with the consequences of chronic illness and to ensure that this experi-ence does not dictate their lifestyle. The poten-tial for activities for the strengthening of overall health remains largely untapped in many individ-uals with chronic illness and finding new ways of accomplishing health promotion often remains an unfilled goal for health care professionals and their chronically ill patients. Determining chronically ill individuals' perceptions of their condition, their aspirations, and their available resources, and supporting their effort to achieve health promotion is an ongoing process. Efforts must go beyond the individual's chronic illness and limitations to include holistic health that focuses on personal goals, evidence-based treat-ment and care tailored to the person, and a will-ingness to adjust a plan as needed [2]. Self-care combined with health promotion efforts con-ducted together with health care providers (and peers) is necessary to optimize health outcomes [14]. Self-care involves both the ability to care for oneself and the performance of activities nec-essary to achieve, maintain, or promote optimal health [15]. Qualitative studies of the meaning of self-care to patients have identified themes such as "body listening" and monitoring "bodily cues," managing social context and lifestyle, hav-ing control over treatment, taking care of and not harming oneself [15–17]. Self-care is, therefore, an essential part of health promotion in chronic illness [18].

Summaries of research concerning people with various long-term conditions confirm that they have a lot in common as they face the challenges of trying to live as well as possible within the physical, mental, or social discom-fort and limitations [2, 19, 20]. Powerlessness is an essential part of the illness experience and impose challenges for both person and family

[2, 21]. However, research findings also indicate that people who are diagnosed with chronic ill-ness possess resources and strategies for health that are not fully recognized and capacities for health that is not sufficiently utilized in the cur-rent health system [22–24].

Mobilizing patients' intrinsic resources and capabilities for health in chronic illness to be used alongside medical expertise and care will require new interventions to be applied across age, gender, diagnostic categories, clinical set-tings, and health systems. Such interventions will reflect the philosophical perspective of "health within illness," which holds that individuals liv-ing with long-term health problems are capable of experiencing health and well-being despite their conditions [10, 24, 25]. This perspective fits well with the philosophy of empowerment (Chap. 13) and with the key papers from WHO's Health for All 2000 series [26], which emphasizes indi-viduals gaining control over their lives and their health and the importance of active participation. Individuals who are actively involved are likely to experience at least some degree of control, and there is an assumed relationship between degrees of participation, empowerment, and health.

Empowerment programs imply active par-ticipation and can lead to improved health out-comes for individuals like improved self-efficacy, greater sense of control, increased knowledge and awareness, behavior change and greater sense of community, broadened social networks, and social support [27].

Health promotion, with respect to chronic illness then, requires the joint action of those living with illness, their significant others and professionals that exchange their experience and knowledge, including the patients' experience-based knowledge of how best to live with chronic illness [9, 22, 23]. However, health professionals seem to base their practice on the logics of tradi-tional medicine and expert knowledge on com-pliance and not on what the individual (patients) themselves see as a better life [28, 29]. Wagner et al. [30] argue that there is a need for improv-ing practice by means of interventions that allow for person-centered approaches that provide sufficient support for individuals to take charge of their own health. "Person-centeredness" is underpinned by values of respect for persons, individual right to self-determination, mutual respect, and understanding. It is enabled by cultures of empowerment that foster continuous approaches to interprofessional practice development [31]. There is a need for interventions that can operationalize the philosophy of patient-centeredness in such a way that the patients' potentials for health is activated and strengthened. In the next section, a new health promotion intervention in chronic illness is presented. The intervention was developed in close cooperation with patients and health professionals in clinical practice in specialist and community care settings in Norway.

16.2.1 The Bodyknowledging Program (BKP): An Innovative Approach for Health Promotion in Chronic Illness

The Bodyknowledging Program (BKP) is a person-centered health intervention for the strengthening of self-care, health, well-being, and empowerment in chronic illness [32]. This approach challenges current practice in the sense that the focus is not primarily on the problem of chronic illness, lifestyle, or behavioral change nor the methods used by professionals. Instead, the participating patients' experiences, their strengths, and capabilities is taken as the point of departure, while the challenges imposed by illness is a backdrop to search for possibilities for health within illness. In the following sections, the theoretical foundation, structure, content, and means of the intervention are outlined.

16.2.1.1 Theoretical Framework for the Intervention

The grounded theory of Bodyknowledging [23, 33, 34] serves as the main conceptual framework for the intervention (Fig. 16.1). Bodyknowledging theory asserts that people have bodily knowledge that constitute an impor-

tant but little used resource for health in chronic illness. Bodyknowledging was defined as "a fundamental process for the development of personal knowledge about one's body, coping skills, health and wellbeing [23]." Patients' bodily knowledge of health and illness is multidimensional, consisting of personal knowledge of one's limits and tolerances of the type and amount of activity; physical and psychosocial factors in their environment that have a positive or negative impact on the condition; and personal knowledge of symptoms of relapses, and the actions, interactions, and social contexts that contribute to recovery, health, and well-being [34]. It is an inherent and often tacit type of knowledge, often expressed in action i.e. in the affected persons' competence of self-care, self-management, and strategies for wellness.

Bodyknowledging theory elicits that persons' embodied knowledge is developed as a resource for health through a basic psychosocial process in interaction with the environment. The process is constituted by four phases: Uncertainty—escaping the sick body; Losing life space, grieving, and anger; Listening and understanding the body's signs—strengthening hope; and Integrating embodied knowledge—new possibilities for wellness and health [33]. It is a challenging process of learning to live with health problems, understanding the changes and developing strategies for health. Figure 16.1 serves to visualize this process.

Chronically ill patients' process of Bodyknowledging is dynamic and nonlinear as they are moving up and down, in and out of different phases while building "a bridge" between pre-illness life and their life with health-related challenges. This is in line with a salutogenic orientation [10] in the sense that health is perceived as a flexible continuum. Consequently, persons living with health problems may have different degrees of health according to where they are in their process, and the movement up and down, in and out of phases is a normal and necessary part of the persons' health promoting process. Shifting perspectives between having

	Phases	Experiences	Strategies	Consequences	Contexual factors
BODYKNOWLEDGING	■ **INTEGRATING EMBODIED KNOWLEDGE –NEW POSSIBILITIES FOR WELLNESS AND HEALTH**	■ Reconciliation with a changing life situation. Learning the dynamics of the body's limits of tolerance. Uncertainty of future development of health. *"I known what contributes to my wellness."*	■ Not giving in to the illness. Readjusting to a new life. Team-playing with the body. Focusing on possibilities. Taking chances. Conducting personal treatment. Hoping for future improvements of health. *" I have the courage to hope and to handle my life."*	■ Embodied knownledge of health: knowing the symptoms and personal reactions. knowing the body's tolerance for activity, physical, and psychosocial environment. knowing how to prevent relapses. knowledge of self-treatment. Coping, health and wellness. Empowerment	■ Personal biography. The character of the illness. Social context. Time and space
	■ **LISTENING AND UNDERSTANDING THE BODY'S SIGNS –STRENGTHENING HOPE**	■ The bodys as a source of knownledge: Developing knowledge of the body's tolerance for activity, factors in physical and psychosocial environment. Uncertainty related to possible relapses and effects of treatment. *"what is making my illness better or worse?"*	■ Searching for knowlege: Listening to and reflecting on the body's signs. Asking and listening to health care personnel. Reading the literature on health. Talking to fellow patients, family, friends, and others. *"I hope for recovery in the future."*		■ Personal biography. The character of the illness. Social context. Time and space
	■ **LOSING LIFE SPACE –GRIEVING AND ANGER**	■ Limits of life space: Loss of energy. Changed body image. Obstacles in physical environment. Obstacles in society. *"The body rules my life."*	■ Existential questioning. Creating predictability. Setting limits on life space. Staying at home. Fighting at sustain hope. *"Why did this happen, and what will happen, to me?"*	■ Losing and longing for: Activities, working life and social life. Loss of freedom of movement and freedom of space. Loss of time and sense of coherence. Broken hopes and expectations.	■ Personal biography. The character of the illness. Social context. Time and space
	■ **UNCERTAINITY – DENYING AND ESCAPING THE SICK BODY**	■ Losing body control. Loss of security. *"The body stops me."*	■ Hiding symptoms and suffering. Hoping it will pass. *"I don't want to be sick."*		■ Personal biography. The character of the illness. Social context. Time and space

Fig. 16.1 Bodyknowledging theory: patients' process of health promotion in chronic illness

illness or health in the forefront is a part of the process [19]. Therefore, Bodyknowledging is to be understood as an ongoing process and activity in which knowledge of new possibilities for health and well-being is developed and continually renewed. Varied and flexible strategies for the promotion of health are developed through the process, such as not giving in to the illness, readjusting to a new life, team-playing with the body, focusing on possibilities, taking chances, preventing relapses, conducting personal treatment, and hoping for future improvement of health. Strategies are individually expressed and specific to the situation.

Patients' personal process of health promotion goes on even if the illness at times pose obstacles that seem to be hard to handle. The Bodyknowledging process (Fig. 16.1) elicits the danger of the person being trapped in the experiences of uncertainty, losses of life space, grieving, and anger. In such cases, the process is being changed in a pathogenic direction. These groups of patients are exactly those who need an intervention such as the Bodyknowledging Program in order to learn how to move towards the healthy pole again.

Bodyknowledging theory is in line with the phenomenological understanding of the body as introduced by Merleau-Ponty [35, 36] in which the body is understood as an object and subject at the same time and as a primary source of knowledge. The dialectics of the body as subject and object are being used in the person's efforts to promote health when they observe their body and at the same time sense its reactions. In BKP, this dialectic function of the body is being utilized in the physical exercises as well as in the structured dialogue.

The theoretical basis for the intervention also rests on Freire's pedagogical theory of the oppressed [37], which asserts that the person's acknowledgement of their situation and efforts to find solutions is groundbreaking, and that dialogue is a means for the liberation of human resources. More details on the theoretical foundation has been published elsewhere [32]. The next section offers an overview of the intervention components.

16.2.2 Structure, Content and Pedagogical Approaches of the Bodyknowledging Program Intervention (BKP)

The Bodyknowledging Program is a broadly applicable intervention designed for people living with a variety of chronic illnesses. The objective is to facilitate participants' efforts of prevention of deterioration, their capacity for health as well as their possibilities to participate in society [32] by acknowledging and strengthening patients' unique yet undervalued bodily knowledge in chronic illness [23]. The phases described in the layperson-based concepts of Bodyknowledging is used as "process tools" to promote patients' capability for health. This idea is incorporated in the program structure, in the content, and in the pedagogical approaches.

16.2.2.1 Structure

The program is organized in group format consisting of 7 sessions over 12 weeks and conducted in co-ed groups of 8–10 participants diagnosed with a variety of long-term chronic illnesses. This mode of organization aims to facilitate the participant's systematic work on their health over time.

There is one 3-h session (with a 30-min break to eat and socialize) every week during the first 3 weeks. Sessions 4–6 are held every second week, and the final session is held in week 12. Two health care professionals (HCP) representing two different professions (e.g., one nurse paired with one physiotherapist or occupational therapist) receive 40 contact hours +40 self-study hours of specialized training before they engage as course leaders in the program. BKP is accomplished in groups mixed with men and women having different kinds of diagnoses as this was found to be broadly applicable across diagnosis, ages, sexes, and clinical sites through clinical trials in Norway [38]. Active patient participation was fundamental in the development of the intervention and is a prerequisite for program completion in practice.

16.2.2.2 Content

The content is organized according to the phases of Bodyknowledging [33] described by former patients [23, 33, 34] and used as a tool to support the participants whereby professionals invite participants to work on the uncertainty, losses of life space, grieving and anger, listening and understanding the body's signs and the integration of knowledge on new possibilities for well-being and health [23] (s. 16.1). The Bodyknowledging program constitutes a "room for recovery" in which patients can share their narratives about their health condition and strategies for health and wellness with HCP and peers. In this way, the participating patients contribute to constitute an essential part of the content followed by HCP's questions to facilitate reflection on the person's health promotion efforts. This is in line with empowerment models of health promotion [39] as it aims to facilitate action by raising critical consciousness of one's own health while highlighting factors that are subject to change based on actions relevant to the person. Patient's relationship to, and interaction with, significant others is an important part of the program content as these relations may represent both assets and challenges to patients' health promotion efforts.

16.2.2.3 Pedagogical Approaches

The pedagogical approaches in BKP aim at activating and facilitating patients' inherent resources for health. Dialogue and posing open questions are essential pedagogical approaches in this regard. Bodyknowledging theory is a tool in this regard as it offers a structure for the dialogue in the groups. Participants are invited to engage in dialogue and reflection on their health by means of open-ended questions. HCP invite participants to reflect on questions about how they experience their life-situation and their own perception of how their health can be enhanced, working inductively from the point of view of the singular person at the same time as one focuses on the shared experiences in the group.

The involved persons are encouraged to be active participants in researching their health with the following questions in mind: What is it that contributes to your capability to handle the symptoms and the consequences of illness, and what contributes to your wellness in your life situation? When patients are working on such

questions, their answers and the information they are collecting are equally important to the information gathered by HCP. It has to do with developing a partner-relationship with the person and to elicit their tacit knowledge of health as well as to find relevant solutions together on what it is that contributes to the person's movement to the healthy pole of the health ease/dis–ease continuum [10, 37]. Patients' process of health promotion is facilitated by HCP active listening, and by supporting, comforting, and challenging the participants understanding of their situation. In addition, questions inspired by solution-focused therapy are used in order to facilitate the person's perspectives towards health within illness [19].

The written pedagogical tools in BKP that complement the intervention group work include a poster and a booklet/diary. The poster offers an overview of the phases of Bodyknowledging. The 40-page booklet describes the Bodyknowledging process illustrated by citations from former patients who were engaged in the research on the development of the Bodyknowledging framework. Intervention patients are encouraged to review specific parts of the booklet between the sessions and to reflect on study questions. There are blank pages available to write down reflections. The pedagogical tools imply that patients are engaged in dialogue on their self-care and health in a variety of ways, such as the dialogue with the text on the poster and booklet/diary, the dialogue between patients in the group and with HCP.

HCP leading BKP groups, introduce physical exercises at the beginning of each session to support the participants in the recognition of their bodily knowledge as a resource for health. Exercises are inspired by the physiotherapeutic method of basic body awareness therapy, which concentrates on breathing, balance, and movement [40, 41]. Then, the HCP provides a short introduction to the BKP framework and patients are invited to reflect upon, and discuss questions posed in the booklet connected to each phase; drawing on principles of open dialogue and solution-focused therapy [37, 42, 43]. Facilitation of individual resources for health, physical activity, and social participation is emphasized as participants are supported by interdisciplinary HCP to work systematically on their health by attending to the phases described in the theoretical framework [23, 33, 34]. Herein lies the possibility to activate more of the persons' resources for health promotion and to explore challenges they may have with conducting self-care and self-management.

Bodyknowledging theory describe the grieving and anger as a part of an overall health promoting process in people with chronic illness and when used in the BKP intervention, one explicitly turns the attention of both patients and HCP to the importance of working through the uncertainty, losses, grieving, and anger in order to move towards better health. BKP offers the participating patients time and space to share their story and their experience of handling their life with illness, and HCP leading the groups have the responsibility to ensure a balance between the focus on deficits and the focus on health in the sessions.

Participants are also asked to choose a physical activity to do at home twice a week, and questions concerning these activities are posed in subsequent sessions to support them to conduct physical activity as a part of their health promotion efforts [44]. The purpose of the exercises was also to find the balance of stress, activity, and rest to prevent the outburst of relapses.

16.2.3 Methods for the Development and Trials of BKP

Initially, three clinical units were chosen for developing the new intervention: a rehabilitation unit, an outpatient clinic and a center for patient education. An interdisciplinary team of nine health care personnel representing the sites (nurses, occupational therapists, physiotherapist) and patients diagnosed with a variety of long-term chronic health conditions engaged with the principal investigator in the formative research [45, 46]. Criteria for reporting the development and early piloting of complex interventions [47] in health care was applied as a guide to outline each component of the intervention.

A comprehensive description of the foundation for BKP and the formative research has been published elsewhere [32]. The BKP has been piloted and implemented in specialist and community health care settings in several projects in Norway. Qualitative interviews and focus-group interviews with participating patients and HCP were used to collect data to explore their experiences of being engaged in the intervention, for evaluating the intervention structure, content, and means and to identify possible health-related outcomes. Qualitative process evaluation [46], content analysis [48, 49], and Interpretive Phenomenological Analysis (IPA) [50] were applied in different trials of BKP. Quantitative data were collected by means of Antonovsky's Sense of Coherence [51] questionnaire and the Outcome Rating Scale [52]. In addition, a brief evaluation form was filled in by patients. More details on methods and outcomes are provided in the next section.

16.3 Patient-Reported Outcomes of Improvement in Empowerment and Health

16.3.1 Clinical Trials in Specialist Health Care

The Bodyknowledging Program was first implemented in specialist care in Norway; in a specialist Rehabilitation unit, in an Outpatient Clinic for the follow-up of patients with Inflammatory Bowel Disease (IBD), and in a Center for Patient Education in chronic illness (CPE). A study sample of 31 men and 21 women ($n = 52$) ranging in age from 22 to 88 years volunteered to participate in the pilot-implementation. The diagnoses represented in the sample were Chronic Obstructive Pulmonary Disease, Heart Disease, Chronic Inflammatory Bowel Disease, Stroke, Multiple Sclerosis and other neurological or functional limitations without a specific diagnostic label. Patients varied in functional capacity and in time since diagnosis, but all had been ill for 1 year or more and had illness-related problems that were difficult to manage. The BKP was applied in group and in individual formats as a generic program to facilitate self-care, health, and recovery.

The intervention was implemented successfully across gender, ages, diagnostic categories, and clinical sites. The process evaluation included in-depth interviews with 34 patients after completing the BKP; of these, 25 patients engaged in 4 group interviews and 9 patients were interviewed individually. The research questions were: How do participants experience the program? What health-related changes, if any, can be attributed to the program? What are the interventions active ingredients, contributing to change?

Participants described that the BKP allowed them to work systematically on their health as a process and reported that because the Bodyknowledging framework is based on patient narratives, it is easy to understand. They evaluated the structure of the program as appropriate across clinical sites and saw the mix of men and woman and of people with different long-term conditions as positive because it created rich possibilities for sharing experiences and ideas about how to handle challenges and how to promote health while living with chronic illness. Participants emphasized that beginning with weekly sessions helped establish a good process. While the group format made it possible to relate one's own experiences to those of others, the individual format allowed more direct, in-depth work on each person's process.

Five themes captured participants' experiences of change in coping and health promotion abilities: (1) changed perspectives on health and illness, (2) new ways of thinking and acting towards the illness, (3) understanding situations, choices, and actions that make the health condition better or worse, (4) widening one's life space-being more active, and (5) communicating differently about health-related matters [38].

Changes in patient perspectives was connected to having a shared world of experience with others who were struggling with symptoms of illness. Because the BKP and its pedagogical tools contain a description of the life worlds of those with long-term health problems, the program offered comfort and support in the midst of pain. It also relieved a feeling of alienation created by the illness. A man attending individually in the outpatient clinic explained how his perspective of health and illness had changed through BKP:

> I have seen a way through all the pain and anguish. When you read about the other patients' experiences, your own experience is being confirmed and in this way you do not feel so lonely. You understand that there are other persons who have managed and that there is a way through it all.

A woman attending the program individually at the rehabilitation unit described her *new ways of thinking and acting* after program completion:

> The program has helped me to think in another way and to come out and to participate in life again. If I am completely honest with myself, the things I want to do are not impossible. It just takes more time, and that was absolutely not how I was thinking before I entered this program.

By attending to the Bodyknowledging process, participants could compare their own experience and choices to concepts and phases offered in the BKP's "insider" perspective. The theoretical framework helped them assess "where they were at the moment" and use that assessment to move on in their own process of health promotion. While still being well aware of the limitations imposed by illness, they were more aware of the risk of imposing unnecessary limitations upon themselves—how that could worsen their health—and they were able to think differently and more positively about their own capabilities. A man attending the program in a rehab group (stroke survivor) described how his engagement in BKP changed his *understanding of the situations, choices, and actions that make the health condition better or worse.*

> I know my body better now. I listen to my body. I have learned how I feel when I am tired. Then I take a break before I begin again. It's much easier when you have a program to follow, such as this program—it works. I have gotten much more patient with myself. I try to be positive because then, it is easier to manage and to conduct what I want to do. I have learned that there are many possibilities even if I have a handicap. Even if everything goes more slowly than before, I am able to do the same as before.

A woman attending individually in the outpatient clinic described how she had changed her way of handling her life situation with chronic illness:

> It has become clear to me that I have been escaping from the illness, but this summer I have taken a grip of the situation. I have told about the illness in my workplace, and now I am in a process of defining how much I should work and how. I am trying to reduce the demands I put on myself in order to prevent new relapses, because I know that when I work too much, I get exhausted and then the illness is worsened.

Discovering one's "own standards" was an important part of the participants' improved knowledge. Making this discovery was connected to taking one's levels of tolerance—for certain types and magnitudes of social and physical activity—seriously. Participants identified the ability to say no to oneself and to other people as an important strategy for promoting wellness. As the program encouraged participants to reflect critically on their ways of being, they engaged in a sort of "research process" concerning their own health. With the support of the program, their peers, and the health care personnel, they discovered their own strategies for self-care and what they could do to stay healthy. *Widening one's life space-being more active* was an important result in this regard. A woman attending a group at the CPE described how she learned to handle the dynamic balance between accepting one's limits and finding new possibilities for activities:

> I am more conscious that I, in spite of my limitations, I can manage to have a nice time. I cannot climb the mountains anymore, but this summer, I was riding a horse on a camp in the mountains, so it is all about compensation. Now, in the winter holidays, I was on the mountain with my friends. They went skiing and I was walking, and we had a good time together.

Participants said that being in the program was like "coming out of a vacuum." They used the concepts and phases of the Bodyknowledging model to sort out their chaos, find meaning in their experience, and move on to new phases. The search for meaningful substitutes for pre-illness activities was a central strategy for achieving health within illness. *Communicating differently about health related matters* was described as an important outcome. At the onset of BKP, participants were concerned with how to tell people about their health condition and how to handle reactions from coworkers, employers, friends, and family. A man whose functional limitations were "invisible" to others described his experience of this:

> Before, I got angry, and was not able to put my reactions in words. The program has helped me to say something about my experience with the illness and has helped me to have better relations with my family.

Participants appreciated the opportunity to open up and work on the difficult parts of their lives in a safe setting. Getting feedback from HCP (and peers if in a group) challenged their own understanding and constituted a time for learning. As a result, participants described being stronger in social encounters, in the sense that they were learning to tell to others how they felt and what they had to consider in order to stay well.

Patients' active engagement in the Bodyknowledging Program, the HCP's attitudes and approaches, the group work and the conceptual framework of Bodyknowledging were identified as the interventions' active ingredients [38].

16.3.2 Trials of the BKP Intervention in Community Care

Similar findings to those reported in specialist health care, was identified in a study of the feasibility and outcome of the BKP in community care in Norway [53]. In one of the studies, a sample of 3 men and 8 women ($n = 11$) between the ages of 30 and 60 volunteered to participated in 2 BKP groups. Data were collected in individual and group interviews and analyzed according to Interpretative Phenomenological Analysis (IPA). Participants described their engagement in the BKP as an enlightening experience that contributed to positive change, personal growth, and better health. Themes like changes in self-awareness, changes in attitudes, awareness of one's body, accepting one's limited capacity, making priorities and setting boundaries, letting go of shame, and regaining control were themes that came up in the analysis. The patterns of themes indicate that participating in BKP contributed to a change in the participants' perceived locus of control, taking it from external to internal [53]. This is an essential finding, as perceived internal control is necessary in order for patients to be in charge of their own health.

In another study of the efficiency of BKP in community care, the Outcome Rating Scale (ORS) was used to measure patients' self-reported recovery repeatedly at baseline, after four sessions of BKP and after program completion [54]. Four dimensions were assessed: (1) individual (personal or symptomatic distress and well-being), (2) interpersonal (relational distress or well-being), (3) social (patient satisfaction with work, school, and relationships), and (4) overall (general sense of well-being). The sample comprised of 13 men and 14 women who had been diagnosed with a range of long-term conditions. The mean age was 54 years. Participants reported significant changes in recovery and health throughout the program period. The total change in average ORS for the whole sample ($n = 27$) was 4.6 (SD = 7.6; $p < 0.001$). There was an observed improvement from t_0 to t_1 with a mean change of 3.5 (SD = 4.8; $p = 0.005$). The change did not reverse from t_1 to t_2 with a mean improvement from session 4 to session 7 of 1.3 (SD = 5.7; $p = 0.003$). The greatest change was in the personal and general well-being dimension of ORS. These findings demonstrate that the BKP intervention contributed to an improvement of dysfunctional patients from below to above the ORS cut-point of 25.

16.3.3 Comparison of Outcomes in Specialist and Community Health Care

A study evaluated the impact of BKP on SOC in two samples; (1) patients in the specialist health care and (2) patients in community care context. Both samples completed BKP [55]. The baseline sample included 108 Norwegian adults (aged 21–89). A variety of diagnostic categories were represented in the sample such as neurological diseases (i.e. epilepsy, multiple sclerosis, Parkinson's), musculoskeletal pain, stroke, psy-

chological problems like anxiety and depression, diabetes, heart failure, COPD, and IBD diagnosed with somatic and/or psychological health problems. Both community and specialist care participants were equally represented in the sample with a fairly equal distribution of men (51%) and women (57%). Community and specialist care participants were included and equal proportions of men and women were represented (51% v. 57%). SOC mean score in the total sample increased from a baseline of 135.3–137.6 (mean change 2.3) at program completion (after 12 weeks) which confirms the possibility for patients with chronic illness to strengthen their self-care, self-management and health as they engage in BKP sessions. The manageability and comprehensibility dimensions also improved, whereas the meaningfulness dimensions remained relatively stable. Participants' SOC increased in both settings, with a larger mean change found in community care. The paired sample t-test demonstrate strong evidence for a difference in women's manageability subscales from baseline to follow-up ($n = 61$; mean change = 4.7; $p < 0.05$). Significant changes in SOC and manageability subscales were also found for participants with children ($n = 72$). Similar patterns of positive manageability changes were identified for participants living with a partner and public transfer payment (i.e., pension) recipients [55]. These findings indicate that BKP is an intervention that function to strengthen individual resources and strategies for health in chronic illness.

16.4   Discussion

We are facing an epidemic of chronic illness and comorbidity [56, 57] and the situation calls for new perspectives and approaches in health promotion work. However, the field of health promotion *in chronic illness* is still at the start of its development. The challenge is to move our perspective from focusing heavily on the problem of disease, disability, medical treatment, and care towards the person's and their family's strengths and capability for promoting health within illness [24]. This implies a further development of the holistic paradigm suggested by

Engel [58] decades ago, outlined by WHO as the biopsychosocial model [57] and to use more person-centered approaches as this is widely acknowledged as helping people living well with a chronic condition [59]. In this paradigm, the health care system and the HCP function as supervisors and facilitators for health, while the person and their family are in charge of the health promotion endeavor. Now, the person at risk for or diagnosed with chronic illness is placed at the center and in an active position as the most important health promotion agent in their life and as an equal partner in the health promotion team. Significant others are invited to participate in supporting *the person in their health promotion process*. The aim is to facilitate the person's resources for health at the same time as the treatment of the health condition is taken care of. New models and interventions are needed in order to operationalize the values of person-centeredness and empowerment in practice.

The Bodyknowledging program is an example of such new approaches entailing a person-centered approach focusing on activating and utilizing patients' inherent resources for health [23, 60, 61] (i.e. their embodied knowledge of limits of tolerances for activity and factors of the physical and psychosocial environment with an impact on the condition). The research grounding BKP demonstrates that patient's experience-based knowledge constitutes a critical but underutilized resource for the prevention of deterioration and for the promotion of health in chronic illness [22, 29, 34]. The following example illustrates how the BKP functions in this regard:

> Today, my body "told me" that I am not capable of driving a car because my head is not quite fit today. In the past, I was pushing myself to drive and then, something bad could happened. Still, it is important to push oneself forward, but in the right mode, because there are many ways to push oneself. It is like stretching a rubber band. You can stretch it, but if you stretch too hard, it breaks. That has happened to me. I have learned a lot about myself and my reactions. I got the possibility to tell the health care personnel in the program about it and I got a picture of it (the process) and I have learned that I must allow myself to be sad sometimes. It has been so important to me to learn that I don't have to be clever all the time (Woman with disability).

The example above elicits the person's knowledge of dynamic limits of tolerances and the usefulness of the Bodyknowledging model as a tool to assess one's health capacity and position on the health ease/dis–ease continuum in a given moment or period of time [10]. Bodyknowledging theory [23] elicits how movement in the direction of health depends on a balance between deficits and resources and on the person's active engagement in reflection and action towards better health. The dialogue with health professionals is important as the professionals posit medical and scientific knowledge and clinical experience on many of the issues people with chronic illness are facing. When patients and HCP share their knowledge and experience, they discover which factors in the environment (food, drink, social relations, activity, and so on) that one must become less exposed to or avoid, and what factors that contribute to individual health. Equal respect for the patient's and professional's different types of knowledge is a necessary condition for the dialogue to function as a health promoting window of opportunity [62–64].

People living with chronic illness have a lot in common as they try to live their lives as best they can and stay healthy while living with an illness. However, patient education and wellness-interventions in the context of chronic illness are often specific to particular diagnostic groups and not designed to be applied across diagnostic categories [65, 66]. The BKP program fills a gap in this regard as it is designed to be used across different diagnoses, clinical settings, and health disciplines [32].

16.4.1 The Unique Contribution of the Bodyknowledging Program

16.4.1.1 Reflects Patient's Perspective of Living with Chronic Illness and Their Process of Health Promotion

BKP is new and different from other approaches because the theoretical framework reflects the patient's perspective of living with chronic illness and their process of health promotion [23, 33]. It is different because *Health care personnel who are leading BKP groups are working within a patient-based framework which "reflects" the patients' "world," replacing the professionals stand to be facilitators for health within the patient-defined framework.* When Bodyknowledging is used as a backdrop, this functions as a key to open a new door to "a room of recovery" meaning that BKP participants can come forward with their experiences with the illness, health strategies, and hopes for the future as well as their worries and challenges [24, 54]. This provides a foundation for addressing individual challenges of living with chronic illness and to discover individual possibilities for the promotion of health within illness.

16.4.1.2 Focus Is on Activating Individual Resources for Health: Not on Illness

The BKP interventions' main focus is how individual resources for health can be activated and facilitated by attending to the sick body as a resource for health [23, 35, 60, 64]. This adds to the development of the field of health promotion in the sense that the body is thematized as an expressive, meaningful source of knowledge [35, 36]. When participants are working systematically on the phases of Bodyknowledging, they are assisted in recognizing their altered body as a resource for health as well as in finding words to describe their life situation and to find ways of handling the challenges that confront them. The main message is that the ill persons' process of Bodyknowledging strengthens their resources for handling their life with illness.

16.4.1.3 Patients' Bodily Knowledge Is Seen as Part of Their Generalized Resistant Resources

The BKP program adds and incorporates patients' bodily knowledge to the description of Generalized Resistant Resources by Antonovsky [10]. The phenomenological understanding of the body is important in this regard, that is; the body as a foundation for existence and understanding, and the body as a subject that carries the meaning and expression of the person's life [35, 64, 67]. In this holistic paradigm, the person's ongoing process of listening and understanding the body's signs is equally important to biomedical tests and "outside" observations of the physical body [67–69]. The core of the BKP is the acknowledgement, facilitation and utilization of the patients' bodily knowledge of health and illness [32, 60, 61].

16.4.1.4 Sharing of Lay Bodily Knowledge as Part of Self-Management in Chronic Illness

However, this knowledge is not "inserted" or "taught" them by HCP or peers, as the knowledge is created by means of Bodyknowledging which is a natural process that goes on within them [23, 33]. This unique but undervalued knowledge is recognized and strengthened through the person's engagement in the intervention and through a dialogue characterized by knowledge, understanding and hope [33]. Lorig's research [70] has confirmed the importance of the sharing of lay knowledge as a part of self-management in chronic illness. However, patients' bodily knowledge in chronic illness was not described as a resource for health in the Chronic Disease Self-Management Program (CDSM) or the like.

16.4.1.5 Special Attention to the Psychosocial Dimensions of Health and Relational Support

The BKP adds by demonstrating the effects of using a framework that elicits patients' bodily knowledge of health as a resource for self-management [54, 55] and as a tool to promote shifts from having "illness in the foreground" to having "health in the foreground" [19]. Participants described that "to be healthy within illness" implied coming out of a vacuum and to participate in life again. This applied to different areas of life, including family life, working life, and social life. These findings indicate that the BKP attends especially to the psychosocial dimensions of health in individuals with chronic illness and relational support [38, 53, 54]. According to Dwarswaard et al. [71] relational support is at the center of the support needs and fuels all other types of support. This was confirmed in a systematic review concluding that for COPD self-management to be effective, patients' psychosocial needs must be prioritized alongside medication and exacerbation management [72].

16.4.1.6 Provides Tools for Participants to Assess Their Responses to Long-Term Illness

The Bodyknowledging Program contains *tools for participants* to assess their responses to long-term illness and *to discover* how they can impact their health positively by using their own and their environment's resources. The BKP presents inherent patient expertise (the phases of Bodyknowledging) to be interpreted and applied by patients participating in BKP. This approach is in keeping with Paulo Freire's [37] "pedagogy of the oppressed" in which the person defines their situation and in which dialogue serves as the main method for helping people understand their situations and to act in new ways. This seems to have a liberating effect as the solutions are the person's and not based on predefined skills by professionals. By attending to the different phases described in the Bodyknowledging framework, patients are empowered and healthy transitions are facilitated, that is; a person's feeling of being connected and socially supported, as well as their perceived confidence, coping, and subjective well-being are actively restored [73, 74]. These findings align with a review of what difference empowerment makes to the health and well-being of individuals [27].

16.4.1.7 Emphasis Is Laid on Health as a Dynamic Continuum

Patients' engagement in BKP, the health care personnel's attitudes and approaches, the group work, and the conceptual framework of Bodyknowledging were identified as this interventions' active ingredients [38]. Emphasis is put on the participants' process of health as

a dynamic continuum [10] while living with chronic illness. When personal knowledge of health and illness is acknowledged, this affects the assessment of their situation as well as their way of handling the challenges. The experience of symptoms is not so threatening when they know more about the meaning of their ailments (comprehensibility), how to relieve them and how to prevent relapses (manageability). The uncertainty is lessened and their experience of having bodily control and safety gets stronger, which has a positive effect on the person's ability to handle their life situation with chronic illness. This adds to the theory of salutogenesis [10] by eliciting that the person's embodied knowledge of health and illness represents a great but unheeded resource for coping, recovery, and health in chronic illness [23, 33].

16.4.1.8 Evidence of BKP Health Promoting Outcomes

Findings indicate that the Bodyknowledging Program serves as an intervention to strengthen health and empowerment across diagnostic categories, age, and gender and is suitable both in specialist and community health care [55]. Health-related outcomes of BKP like changed perspectives on health and illness, new ways of thinking and acting towards the illness, understanding situations, choices, and actions that make the health condition better or worse, widening one's life space-being more active, and communicating differently about health-related matters [38] indicate that participating in BKP contributed to a change in the participants' locus of control, taking it from external to internal [53]. Based on these findings one can argue that the BKP contributed to perceived control of illness-related strain and circumstances. The findings are in line with the goal of health promotion which is exactly to increase the involved persons' control over their health and to improve it [1]. Patients in the municipality health care expressed that the BKP represented a new and different encounter with the health care system and suggested that the program should be extended with more sessions and a follow-up period lasting for 6 months [53].

16.5   Implications for Practice

The Bodyknowledging theory and program can be used in the education of HCP to elevate their understanding of the lay-perspective and to gain insight into the patients' process of health promotion in chronic illness. The BKP offers shared concepts for interdisciplinary work and patient participation. The model can be applied by HCP and patients diagnosed with chronic illness as a tool to assess the patients' position in their health promotion process and as a tool for patient activation and dialogue in health care encounters. The Bodyknowledging Program is recommended to be used as a broadly applicable intervention in health promotion work in community health care settings as well as in hospitals, in outpatient clinics, or in rehabilitation units as part of the follow-up of patients at risk or diagnosed with chronic illness.

16.6   Conclusion

This chapter emphasizes the need for developing the field of health promotion in chronic illness by developing interventions that operationalize the values of person-centered and holistic health in practice. A change of focus is needed from focusing heavily on disease and behavioral change to mobilizing patients' intrinsic resources and capabilities for health in chronic illness. Patients' bodily knowledge of health and illness are elicited as an unutilized resource in this regard. The Bodyknowledging program (BKP) is introduced as an example and a broadly applicable intervention to support patients to take charge of their own health. Some studies and positive outcome of trials of BKP in Norway are described. There is a need to evaluate the feasibility and acceptability of BKP internationally in patient samples with a range of chronic illnesses. Such studies are well-positioned to contribute key research findings relating to the mobilization of under-utilized patient capacities for health and well-being. These findings will be important for improving the quality of person-centered care within clinical practice and will set the stage for further work

that will be poised to improve longer-term public health outcomes for chronic illness.

Take Home Messages

- The field of health promotion in chronic illness is in need of further development to ensure a strong focus on how to promote health within illness. The Bodyknowledging Program (BKP) is an example of interventions that aim to activate and utilize patients' inherent resources for health while living with chronic illness.

- Bodyknowledging theory serve as the framework for BKP. The theory elicits how experiences of illness and vulnerability can be turned into assets for health, and how the patient becomes empowered by utilization of their inherent resources for health.

- Patients engaged in the BKP report that their ability to handle distress, conduct self-care, and promote health was improved. This had a positive impact on their relationships to significant others and their participation in society.

References

1. Leddy S. Integrative health promotion: conceptual bases for nursing practice. Massachusetts: Jones & Bartlett Learning; 2006.
2. Larsen PD. Lubkin's chronic illness. Impact and intervention. 10th ed. Massachusetts: Jones & Bartlett Learning; 2019.
3. World Health Organization. Global status report on noncommunicable diseases 2010. Geneva: WHO; 2011.
4. Kralik D, Paterson B, Coates V. Translating chronic illness research into practice. Hoboken: Wiley; 2010.
5. World Health Organization. The world health report—primary health care. Geneva: WHO; 2008.
6. Hajat C, Stein E. The global burden of multiple chronic conditions: a narrative review. Prev Med Rep. 2018;12:284–93.
7. Navickas R, Petric VK, Feigl AB, Sychell M. Multimodbidity: what do we know? What should we do? J Comorbid. 2016;6(1):4–11.
8. Benner P. Interpretive phenomenology. Embodiment, caring and ethics in health and illness. Thousand Oaks: Sage; 1994.
9. Kaplun A, editor. Health promotion and chronic illness. Discovering a new quality of health. Cologne: WHO Regional Publications; 1992.

10. Antonovsky A. Unraveling the mystery of health: how people manage stress and stay well. San Fransisco: Jossey-Bass; 1987.

11. Mittelmark MB, Sagy S, Eriksson M, Bauer GF, Pelikan JM, Lindström B, et al. The handbook of salutogenesis. London: Springer Nature; 2017.

12. Lillefjell M, Jakobsen K, Ernsten L. The impact of a sense of coherence in employees with chronic pain. Work. 2015;50:313–22.

13. Nilsen V, Bakke P, Rohde G, Gallefoss F. Is sense of coherence a predictor of lifestyle changes in subjects at risk of type 2 diabetes? Public Health. 2015;129:155–61.

14. Ko D, Bratzke L-C, Roberts T. Self-management assessment in multiple chronic illness: a narrative review of literature. Int J Nurs Stud. 2018;83:83–90.

15. Richards AA, Shea K. Delineation of self-care and associated concepts. J Nurs Scholarsh. 2011;43(3): 255–64.

16. Leenerts MH, Magilvy JK. Investing in self-care: a midrange theory of self-care grounded in the lived experience of low-income HIV-positive white women. Adv Nurs Sci. 2000;22(3):58–75.

17. Thorne S, Paterson B, Russel C. The structure of everyday self-care descision making in chronic illness. Qual Health Res. 2003;13(10):1337–52.

18. Richards AA, Kimberley S. Delineation of self-care and associated concepts. J Nurs Scholarsh. 2011;43(3):255–64.

19. Paterson BL. The shifting perspectives model of chronic illness. J Nurs Scholarsh. 2001;33(1):21–6.

20. Brooks HL, Rogers A, Sanders C, Pilgrim D. Perceptions of recovery and prognosis from long-term conditions: the relevance of hope and imagined futures. Chronic Illn. 2015;11(1):3–20.

21. Miller J. Coping with chronic illness: overcoming powerlessness. 2nd ed. Philadelphia: F.A. Davis; 1992.

22. Wilde MH. Embodied knowledge in chronic illness and injury. Nurs Inq. 2003;10(3):170–6.

23. Heggdal K. Utilizing bodily knowledge in patients with chronic illness in the promotion of their health: a grounded theory study. Calif J Health Promot. 2013;11(3):62–73.

24. Gottlieb LN. Strengths-based nursing care: health and healing for person and family. New York: Springer Publishing Company; 2013.

25. World Health Organization. Health promotion and chronic illness. Discovering a new quality of health. England: WHO Regional Office for Europe; 1992.

26. WHO. Global strategy for health for all by 2000. 1989. Report no.: 3.

27. Woodall J, Raine G, South J, Warwich-Booth L. Empowerment, health and well-being; 2010.

28. Bossy D, Knutsen IR, Rogers A, Foss C. Moving between ideologies in self-management support—a qualitative study. Health Expect. 2018;22:83–92.

29. Thorne SE, Ternulf Nyhlin K, Paterson BL. Attitudes toward patient expertise in chronic illness. Int J Nurs Stud. 2000;37(4):303–11.

30. Wagner EH, Austin BT, Davis C, Hindmarsh M, Schaefer J, Bonomi A. Improving chronic illness care: translating evidence into action. Health Aff. 2001;20(6):64–78.

31. McCormack B, Borg M, Cardiff S, Dewing J, Jacobs G, Janes N, et al. Person-centredness—the 'state' of the art. Int Pract Dev J. 2015;5(Suppl):1–15.

32. Heggdal K. 'We experienced a lack of tools for strengthening coping and health in encounters with patients with chronic illness': bridging theory and practice through formative research. Int Pract Dev J. 2015;5(2):4.

33. Heggdal K. Kroppskunnskaping—En grunnleggende prosess for mestring ved kronisk sykdom [Bodyknowledging—a basic process of coping with chronic illness]. PhD thesis. Bergen: University of Bergen; 2003.

34. Heggdal K. Kroppskunnskaping: pasienten som ekspert i helsefremmende prosesser. [Bodyknowledging—patients as experts in health promotion processes]. Oslo: Gyldendal Academic Publisher; 2008.

35. Merleau-Ponty M. The phenomenology of the body. Oslo: Pax; 1994.

36. Merleau-Ponty M, Smith C. Phenomenology of perception. New Delhi: Motilal Banarsidass Publisher; 1996.

37. Freire P. Pedagogy of the oppressed. 30th anniversary ed. New York: The Continuum; 2006.

38. Heggdal K. Patient's experience of the outcomes of engaging in a broadly applicable health promotion intervention for individuals facing chronic illness. Health. 2015;7:765–75.

39. Naidoo J, Wills J. Health promotion: foundations for practice. 2nd ed. Edinburgh: Elsevier Health Sciences; 2000.

40. Dropsy J. Den Harmoniska Kroppen. Stockholm: Natur och Kultur; 1988.

41. Gard G. Body awareness therapy for patients with fibromyalgia and chronic pain. Disabil Rehabil. 2005;27(12):725–8.

42. Anderson H, Goolishian H. The client is the expert: a not-knowing approach to therapy. In: McNamee S, Gergen K, editors. Therapy as social construction. London: Sage; 1992. p. 25–39.

43. O'Connel B. Solution-focused therapy. 3rd ed. London: Sage; 2012.

44. Healthy People. Healthy people 2020. 2015. https://www.healthypeople.gov/.

45. Möhler R, Bartoszek G, Köpke S, Meyer G. Proposed criteria for reporting the development and evaluation of complex interventions in healthcare (CReDECI): guideline development. Int J Nurs Stud. 2012;49(1):40–6.

46. Patton MQ. Qualitative evaluation and research methods. 3rd ed. Thousand Oaks: Sage Publications; 2002.

47. Campbell M, Fitzpatrick R, Haines A, Kinmonth AL. Framework for design and evaluation of complex interventions to improve health. Br Med J. 2000;321(7262):694–6.

48. Graneheim UH, Lundman B. Qualitative content analysis in nursing research: concepts, procedures and measures to achieve trustworthiness. Nurse Educ Today. 2004;24(2):105–12.

49. Graneheim UH, Lindgren BM, Lundman B. Methodological challengs in qualitative content analysis: a discussion paper. Nurse Educ Today. 2017;56:29–32.

50. Smith JA, Osborne M. Interpretive phenomenology analysis. London: Sage Publications; 2008.

51. Eriksson M, Linstrøm B. Validity of Antonovsky's sense of coherence scale: a systematic review. J Epidemiol Commun Health. 2005;59:460–6.

52. Miller SD, Duncan BL, Brown J, Sparks JA, Claud DA. The Outcome Rating Scale: a preliminary study of the reliability, validity, and feasibility of a brief visual analog measure. J Brief Ther. 2003;2: 91–100.

53. Engevold MH, Heggdal K. Patients'experiences with changes in perceived control in chronic illness: a pilot study of the outcomes of a new health promotion program in community health care. Scand Psychol. 2016;3:e5.

54. Heggdal K, Oftedal B, Hofoss D. The effect of a person-centred and strength-based health intervention on recovery among people with chronic illness. Eur J Person Centered Healthc. 2018;6(2):279–85.

55. Heggdal K, Lovaas B. Health promotion in specialist and community care: how a broadly applicable health promotion intervention influences patient's sense of coherence. Scand J Caring Sci. 2019;32(2):690–7.

56. National Health Council. About chronic diseases. 2014. www.nationalhealthcouncil.org/sites/default/files/AboutChronicDisease.pdf.

57. Martz E. Promoting self-management of chronic health conditions. Theories and practice. Oxford: Oxford University Press; 2018.

58. Engel GL. The need for a new medical model: a challenge for biomedicine. Science. 1977;196(4286): 129–36.

59. Zoffmann V, Hörnsten Å, Storbækken S, Graue M, Rasmussen B, Wahl A, et al. Translating person-centered care into practice: a comparative analysis of motivational interviewing, illness-integration support and guided self-determination. Patient Educ Couns. 2016;99:400–7.

60. Benner P, Wrubel J. The primacy of caring. Stress and coping in health and illness. Menlo Park: Addison-Wesley; 1989.

61. Toombs SK. The meaning of illness: a phenomenological account of the different perspectives of physician and patient. Dordrecht: Kluwer Academic Publishers; 2013.

62. Thorne S. Patient—provider communication in chronic illness: a health promotion window of opportunity. Fam Commun Health. 2006;29(1):4–11.

63. Kirkengen AL. Inscribed bodies. Health impact of childhood sexual abuse. Dordrecht: Kluwer Academic; 2001.

64. Carel H. Phenomenology as a resource for patients. J Med Philos. 2012;37(2):96–113.

65. Lorig KR, Holman HR. Self-management education: history, definition, outcomes, and mechanisms. Ann Behav Med. 2003;26(1):1–7.

66. Stuifbergen AK, Morris M, Jung JH, Pierini D, Morgan S. Benefits of wellness interventions for persons with chronic and disabling conditions: a review of the evidence. Disabil Health J. 2010;3(3):133–45.

67. Carel H, Kidd IJ, Pettigrew R. Illness as a transformative experience. Lancet. 2016;388(10050):1152–3.

68. Frank AW. The wounded storyteller: body, illness, and ethics. Chicago: University of Chicago Press; 2013.

69. Svenaeus F. The hermeneutics of medicine and the phenomenology of health: steps towards a philosophy of medical practice. Linköping: Department of Health and Society, Linköping University; 1999.

70. Lorig KR, Ritter P, Stewart AL, Sobel D, Brown BW, Bandura A, et al. Chronic disease self-management program: 2-year health status and health care utilization outcomes. Med Care. 2001;39(11):1217–23.

71. Dwarswaard J, Bakker EJM, Staa AL, Boeije HR. Self-management support from the perspective of patients with a chronic condition: a thematic synthesis of qualitative studies. Health Expect. 2015;19:194–208.

72. Russel S, Oladapo J, Ogunbayo J, Newham JJ, Marshall-Heslop K, Netts P, et al. Qualitative systematic review of barriers and facilitators to self-management of chronic obstructive pulmonary disease: views of patients and healthcare professionals. Prim Care Respir Med. 2018;28(1):2.

73. Meleis AI, Sawyer LM, Im EO, Hilfinger Messias DK, Schumacher K. Experiencing transitions: an emerging middle-range theory. Adv Nurs Sci. 2000;23(1):12–28.

74. Halding A-G, Heggdal K. Patients' experiences of health transitions in pulmonary rehabilitation. Nurs Inq. 2012;19(4):345–56.

Health Promotion Among Cancer Patients: Innovative Interventions

17

Violeta Lopez and Piyanee Klainin-Yobas

Abstract

There are growing interests in promoting health of patients with cancer targeting on prevention and control as there are several modifiable risk factors that can be controlled to prevent cancer such as smoking, sedentary lifestyle, and unhealthy behaviors. Once diagnosis of cancer has been determined, health promotion interventions can be targeted on helping patients overcome the physiological and psychological effects of the diagnosis. Health promotion interventions should continue during treatment, survivorship, and for those receiving palliative care. More specifically is the promotion of psychological health of patients with cancer. Introduction of the incidence of cancer, cancer risk protection interventions and innovative health promotion interventions along these different periods in the life of patients with cancer are presented. Some theoretical frameworks used in health promotion research with examples of studies are discussed.

Keywords

Acutherapy · Art therapy · Cancer · Exercise · Herbal therapy · Mindfulness · Psychotherapy Salutogenesis · Sense of coherence

17.1 Introduction

Cancer is a group of diseases characterized by uncontrolled growth and spread of abnormal cells. There are many causes of cancer and many risk factors; some are nonmodifiable while some are modifiable, such as smoking. Cancer causes one in six deaths worldwide; the second leading cause of death after cardiovascular diseases [1]. The incidences of cancer globally are 23.4% in Europe, 13.3% in America, 7.3% in Africa, and 57.3% in Asia [2]. It is also estimated that one-in-five men and one-in-six women will develop cancer and one-in-eight men and one-in-eleven women will die from cancer [3]. It has been reported that cancer is the first or second cause of premature deaths in 100 countries worldwide [2]. The five most common cancers in males are lung, prostate, colorectal, stomach, and liver; and in females they are breast, colorectum, lung, cervix, and thyroid.

V. Lopez (✉)
School of Nursing, Hubei University of Medicine, Shiyan, China

School of Nursing, University of Tasmania, Hobart, Australia
e-mail: violeta.lopez@findnetwork.org

P. Klainin-Yobas
Alice Lee Centre for Nursing Studies, Yong Loo Lin School of Medicine, National University of Singapore, Singapore, Singapore
e-mail: nurpk@nus.edu.sg

G. Haugan, M. Eriksson (eds.), *Health Promotion in Health Care – Vital Theories and Research*,
https://doi.org/10.1007/978-3-030-63135-2_17

The global cancer burden is estimated at 18.1 million new cases and 9.6 million deaths in 2018 (ICRC 2018). In 2040, the global burden is expected to increase to 27.5 million new cases and 16.3 million deaths [4]. The increasing cancer burden is due to population growth and aging, economic and social development, unhealthy diet, physical inactivity, and changing lifestyles. It has been reported that cancer risk increases with age especially among age 65 years. According to the Human Development Index (HDI), there are 60% new cancer cases in high HDI compared to those in medium- and low-HDI countries [1, 5, 6].

17.2   Theoretical Frameworks Used in Cancer Health Promotion Research

Theoretical frameworks provide knowledge base for guiding intervention research. It is important that researchers understand the underpinnings of the various theories to enable appropriate selection for the study to be conducted. There are many theoretical frameworks sued in cancer research but only few examples are provided in this chapter. One example is the Salutogenic Model as a theory to guide health promotion which aims at moving people in the direction of the health end of the continuum [7]. As a Salutogenic orientation, the Sense of Coherence (SOC) construct emerges as a generalized orientation in facilitating the movement towards health [8, 9]. SOC is conceptualized as a global orientation to life experiences, including the degree to which life is viewed as comprehensible, manageable, and meaningful [9]. A meta-analysis by Winger and colleagues [10] found that SOC demonstrated significant negative associations with distress in cancer patients. Their analysis supported Antonovsky's model of health that a high SOC suggests that cancer patients who view life as comprehensible, manageable, and meaningful experience less distress. In a systematic review Eriksson and Lindström [11] found that SOC is a health resource influencing quality of life.

The Transtheoretical Model of health (TTM) was developed by Proschaska and Verizer [12] who posited that health behavior change involves progress through six stages of change: precontemplation, contemplation, preparation, action, maintenance, and termination. It was postulated that behavior change is cyclic with some individuals regressing to earlier stages of readiness before behavior change is sustained. TTM-based interventions attempt to tailor the recommendations to a participant's motivational readiness to change. Pinto [13] conducted the Moving Forward Trial, providing a home-based moderate-intensity physical activity program to determine its effects on physical activity fitness, mood, and physical symptoms in patients with breast cancer guided by TTM.

The Theory of Planned Behavior (TPB) is a social-psychological theory developed by Ajzen [14] to explain the link between attitudes and behaviors. It postulates that behavior is predicted by intention. According to this theory, human behavior is guided by behavioral, normative, and control beliefs. Interventions designed to change behavior can be directed to patients' attitudes, subjective norms, and perceptions of behavioral control [15]. Jones and colleagues [16] applied the theoretical tenets of the TPB to understand the effects of two oncologist-based interventions on self-reported exercise in breast cancer survivors. The effects of the oncologists' recommendations to exercise in patients with breast cancer was mediated by their attitude and positive intention thus supporting the tenets of TPB.

Social Cognitive Theories (SCT), behavior change is influenced by several interacting psychosocial, environmental, and behavioral factors on how a person makes choices. SCT was advanced by Bandura [17] from Social Learning Theory. SCT explains how people learn not only through their own experiences, but also by observing the actions of others and the results of those actions. Self-efficacy theory (SET) is a subset of Bandura's social cognitive theory. Bandura defines self-efficacy as the individual's perception of his or her ability to feel, think, motivate, and act to perform behaviors through four processes: (1) cognitive, (2) motivational, (3) affective, and (4) selection. SCT framework was used in a meta-analysis conducted by Graves [18] to evaluate the quality of life among patients with breast cancer. The results of this meta-analysis showed that using SCT-based interventions maximized improvement in overall quality of life (QOL) outcomes for adult cancer. Grimmett [19] examined the patterns of self-efficacy for managing illness-related problems among colorectal cancer patients in the 24 months following diagnosis. They found that there was an increase in self-efficacy mean score overtime. This study provided support of the positive association between self-efficacy and adaptation to cancer diagnosis and reduction of distress in patients with cancer.

17.3 Risk Protection Interventions to Reduce or Eliminate Exposure to Cancer-Producing Agents

Risk protection interventions can be targeted to mainly reduce or eliminate some types of cancer such as skin, breast, cervical, and colorectal cancers. Skin cancer is one of the most prevalent cancers worldwide among those with more sunlight exposure and can be prevented by protecting skin from excessive sun exposure. Detrimental effects of ultraviolet rays can be prevented by wearing thick clothing when exposed to sunlight, applying an appropriate sunscreen and avoiding artificial sources of ultraviolet rays for tanning.

Tobacco smoking causes many types of cancer and is a known risk factor for lung cancer. Several smoking cessation interventions have been implemented worldwide to curb this unhealthy behavior not only to prevent the risk of lung cancer but also to support patients who already have been diagnosed with lung cancer and undergoing treatment to cease smoking. An intervention involving a brief consultation with a nicotine dependence counsellor was used to help the patient develop an individualized treatment plan. The study showed that the 7-day point prevalence abstinence from tobacco at 6-month follow-up was 22% after adjusting for age, sex, and

baseline cigarettes smoked per day [20]. The results in a study by Charlot [21] using an 8-week mindfulness-based smoking cessation intervention by a certified mindfulness trainer and tobacco treatment nurse specialist showed that there was a significant decrease in weekly cigarette intake from 75.1 cigarettes at baseline to 44.3 at 3 months. This 8-week intervention consisted of lessons on the effects of smoking, instructions for smoking cessation and guided instruction. Each participant received audio compact discs and manual on mind-body practices including meditation, body scan, and chair yoga (each 20 min in length) to facilitate home practice. Another study by Li [22] provided face-to-face individualized brief (15–30 min) risk communication to encourage patients with lung cancer to stop smoking. They hypothesized that participants in the intervention group would have a higher smoking cessation rates and have a reduced daily cigarette consumption by at least 50%. The intervention was followed by exhaled carbon monoxide level assessment. The risk communication component focused on the relationships between smoking and lung cancer diagnosis, treatment, and prognosis as a trigger to think about quitting. After 1 week, the experimental group received a booster intervention via telephone to assess the progress of and to identify difficulties faced by patients towards quitting and how to handle withdrawal symptoms. The results showed that the 268 patients with lung cancer had higher biochemically validated quit rate at the 6-month follow-up compared to the control group. The results found that at 6 weeks after treatment, the 7-day point prevalence smoking abstinence rate was 40% [22].

Mobile phone instant messaging apps (e.g., WhatsApp, Facebook Messenger, and WeChat) are popular and inexpensive alternatives to SMS for interactive messaging [23]. Advances in mobile technologies are also now being used for mobile phone-based interventions for smoking cessation. Wang [24] provided a 12-page self-help booklet on smoking cessation as well as chat-based smoking cessation support using WhatsApp mobile messaging twice a week for the first month, and once per week for the next 2 months by smoking cessation ambassadors. At 6 months follow-up the results showed that 77% of the 591 participants had significantly higher abstinence from smoking.

Breast cancer can be prevented through self-breast screening and improvements have been made to increase women's awareness and attitudes towards the importance of screening for early detection of breast cancer. Promoting the attitude of the women toward breast cancer is largely influenced by their screening behaviors. Culture and ethnicity are also critical factors influencing women's attitudes, beliefs, and access to health screening services [25]. Mirzaii [26] investigated the effects of breast cancer screening training based on the Systematic comprehensive Health Education and Promotion (SHEP) model on the attitudes and breast self-examination skills in 120 women in Iran. The three 2-h SHEP-based educational workshops using posters and images provided general explanation of breast structure, breast lumps and their features, risk factors and symptoms of breast cancer, and self-breast screening methods. Participants were asked to practice accordingly at 1-week interval between the first, second, and third workshops. The results showed the efficacy of the SHEP in promoting awareness, attitudes, and self-breast examination among the Iranian women.

Colorectal cancer is the third most common cancer worldwide and it is the second most common factor for death by cancer [27]. The timely and proper colorectal cancer screening is a leading factor to reduce incidence and consequences of this disease. Boogar [28] examined the moderating role of cancer-related health literacy and cancer-related empowerment in colorectal cancer screening using a comprehensive model in 366 participants. Using the Colorectal Screening Questionnaire and Health Education Impact Questionnaire, the results showed that higher perceived susceptibility and the cancer-related literacy was associated with lower defensive avoidance and had increased the tendency of patients to submit to colorectal screening tests [29]. Super [30] posited that both empowerment and reflection processes, which are interdependent, may be relevant for health promotion activities that aim to strengthen SOC. Low health literacy is associated with lack of knowledge about screening for cancer. Health care professionals should therefore knowledge about the benefits of cancer screening as patients' perceived risk and health-promoting behavior such as regular medical check-ups and self-efficacy have been found to be positively correlated with adherence to colorectal screening [31]. The successful application of resources to deal with low literacy affecting adherence to screening for cancer is not only likely to have a positive influence on health but also creates consistent and meaningful life experiences that can positively reinforce SOC levels.

17.4 Health Promotion Interventions to Reduce the Effects of Cancer Diagnosis

A cancer diagnosis is associated with high levels of distress, a multifactorial unpleasant emotional experience in 35–45% of patients with cancer [32]. It causes fear, uncertainty above recovery, and suffering not only to the patients with cancer but also to their families, as life situation changes suddenly affecting the family unit. Although many studies have been conducted using the Salutogenic theory of SOC and its three components of meaningfulness, manageability, and comprehensibility, Ozanne and Graneheim [33] focused their study on the comprehensibility component of SOC when patients' symptoms appeared and diagnosis was confirmed. They found that whether they comprehend or not, the 27 participants felt uncertain before the diagnosis, they lost their foothold during the diagnosis and lived in fear after the diagnosis. The results highlighted that it takes time to find comprehensibility and health professionals should provide support and information to both patients and spouses to answer their questions. Depression is a comorbidity of cancer and more so if the patients is diagnosed with late stage of cancer with metastasis. SOC has long been recognized as an important factor in the psychological adjustment to cancer and a protective factor for depression. Aderhold [34] examined if SOC and post-traumatic growth (coping, struggling or thriving) were predictors of depression in 252 patients in Germany since being diagnosed with cancer. They found that posttraumatic growth (PTG) is a significant predictor of depressive symptoms 1 year after the cancer diagnosis; the higher PTG levels the lower patients' levels of depressive symptoms. They also found that high levels of SOC predicted low levels of depressive symptoms. Patients' experience of having cancer and survival may enhance a feeling of personal strength and a sense of self-efficacy which could be protective psychological factors. Therefore, interventions should promote SOC in patients with cancer by creating a supportive environment for them to be able to reflect on problems faced since diagnosis, focusing on the positive changes they experience and strengthening their coping resources.

17.5 Health Promotion Interventions to Reduce the Effects of Cancer Treatment

Once diagnosis is confirmed and staged, patients undergo specific treatment according to protocols. The treatment modalities are surgery, chemotherapy, radiotherapy, hormone therapy, immune therapy, and/or targeted therapy. No matter what cancer treatment patients receive, they experience various treatment side effects impacting their overall QoL. Cancer and cancer-related treatments trigger such symptoms like pain, insomnia, nausea, and vomiting, chemotherapy-induced peripheral neuropathy, and sexual dysfunction which may lead to psychological symptoms such as stress, depression and anxiety [35]. Overcoming the psychological effects of cancer treatment require patients with cancer to have a clear concept of coping ability to conceptualize their diagnosis and treatment as meaningful, manageable and comprehensible which are the three components of SOC [8].

Fatigue, a subjective feeling of weariness, tiredness or lack of energy, is the most common unmanaged symptom in patients undergoing chemotherapy or radiotherapy which leads to decreased physical daily activity during treatment. Exercise has been shown to be effective in decreasing fatigue and improving activity tolerance in patients during chemotherapy [36, 37]. A study that showed the effectiveness of exercise was conducted by Mock et al. [38] using the walking exercise intervention in female concurrently with the duration of 4–6 weeks of chemotherapy or 6 weeks of radiotherapy. The exercise was conducted at the clinical site and taught by trained staff using the exercise prescription developed by the exercise physiologist which was individualized for each participant based on age, level of physical fitness, and type of cancer treatment. The walking intervention consisted of an initial 10–15 min sessions and 5–6 sessions per week and increased to 30 min per session, 5–6 weeks per week according to their exercise tolerance and responses to treatment. The women were asked to keep diaries of their daily exercise activity. Velthuis [39] conducted a multicentre randomized controlled trial in 150 breast and 150 colon cancer patients undergoing cancer treatment. The intervention was 18-weeks supervised group exercise program and significant beneficial effects of the exercise were visible during cancer treatment, adherence was moderate to excellent and few adverse events occurred.

Nausea and vomiting are the most common side effects of chemotherapy [40]. Without appropriate antiemetic intervention, chemotherapy-induced nausea and vomiting can lead to dehydration, electrolyte disorder, malnutrition, and can negatively affect patients' adherence to treatment as well as quality of life [41]. Acupoint therapies have been recommended as a complementary intervention to prevent chemotherapy-induced nausea and vomiting by the National Institute of Health [42]. Acupoint therapies including acupuncture, acupressure, acupoints injection, massage, and moxibustion which are safe medical procedures have shown promising intervention for the management of chemotherapy-induced nausea and vomiting [43]. Auricular acupressure, another innovative health promotion intervention in preventing and treating nausea and vomiting in patients with cancer, was also used before chemotherapy which has been recognized by the Federal Nursing Council in its 197/97 resolution as being an acceptable professional role of nurses [44]. Eghbali [45] placed the ear seed on the pinna on each ear for 5 day and asked the patients to press the ear seeds for 3 min three times a day in the morning, noon and night during the chemotherapy cycle. Their study found that auricular therapy led to a decrease in the number and intensity of nausea and vomiting in both the acute and delayed phases in the experimental group and suggested that nurses can use this pressure technique as a complementary nonpharmacological, inexpensive, and noninvasive relief of chemotherapy-induced nausea and vomiting.

Chemotherapy-induced peripheral neuropathy (CIPN) is another symptom experienced by patients with cancer who are undergoing chemotherapy [46]. It is a progressive, prolonged, and often irreversible side effect of many chemotherapeutic agents and affects 30–40% of patients undergoing treatment [47]. CIPN affects the peripheral sensory and/or motor systems and causes numbness, pain, burning, tingling, heat and hyperalgesia, and mechanical allodynia, as well as reduced motor function [47]. It has been reported that CIPN may continue to worsen after chemotherapy as 68% of patients with cancer still experience the problems in the first month and 30% in the sixth month after chemotherapy [48, 49]. There is no effective treatment in preventing or managing CIPN, but complementary therapies have been reported to improve the symptoms of CIPN such as acupuncture, foot bath, massage, reflexology, sensorimotor training as well as Chinese, Korean, and Japanese herbal medicines [50]. However, further research is needed to examine the effects of herbal medicine on its efficacy, safety, and cost-effectiveness.

Sexual dysfunction during treatment of early-stage cervical and endometrial cancer has been reported as the most distressing side effect of cancer treatment. The negative effects of chemotherapy result in threats to the women's sexual identity, self-esteem, intimacy, and the end of reproductive capacity. Psychoeducational intervention has been found to significantly improve frequency of coital activity, reduce fear about intercourse, and improve sexual knowledge. For example, Brotto [51] recruited 22 women with gynaecological cancer with sexual dysfunction and asked them to self-report their response to the 3-min neutral and 4-min erotic audiovisual film using the Film Scale. The Film Scale [52] was administered during the sexual arousal assessments that assessed perception of genital sexual arousal, subjective sexual arousal, autonomic arousal, anxiety, positive affect, and negative affect. Items were rated on a 7-point Likert scale from 1 (not at all) to 7 (intensely). Psychoeducational intervention consisting of three 60-min sessions targeting sexual arousal complaints and how to troubleshoot these difficulties was conducted. A combination of information about progressive relaxation, mindfulness, becoming organismic, and making marriage work in a manual was also given to the patients. The results showed significant improvement in women's sexual response, mood, and quality of life [51].

Another innovative health promotion intervention to improve the psychological well-being and quality of life of patients with cancer by lessening of side effects from chemotherapy is the use of art therapy. A study by Bozcuk [53] involving 48 patients attending the outpatient chemotherapy unit in Turkey participated in the painting art therapy using watercolors for 6 weeks. Group discussions were conducted on the symbolic nature of their paintings, and expression of feelings and thoughts. The results showed that art therapy in the form of water-color painting improved their global quality of life and reduced depression through sharing and discussing problems, feelings and thoughts thus enabled coping with their negative feelings about their cancer diagnosis and treatment. Huss and Samson [54] conducted a study to explore the connection between art therapy and SOC in patients their families dealing with cancer. As a health promoting strategy, the participants drew images causing their stress. In a group discussion, participants explained the image to the group and the group then discussed the meaning, manageability, and comprehensiveness components that could help cope with stress. The study provided evidence that methods in creating meaning through art therapy enhanced the patients' SOC by integrating the three components to overcome their stress about cancer diagnosis and treatment.

17.6   Health Promotion Interventions to Support Survivorship and Palliation

Although cancer has been considered as a global public health issue, with continuing improvement in cancer treatment, more individuals diagnosed with cancer are surviving with the disease [55]. Patients who are alive 5 years after the cancer diagnosis and treatment are referred to as survivors. However, although intensive treatments can improve long-term survival, the emotional and physical demands of the diagnosis and treatment experience of cancer survivors are substantial. Several health promotion interventions have been developed, implemented and evaluated to overcome the physiological and psychological problems experienced by cancer survivors. For example, reports found that exercise improves breast cancer survivors' physical and psychological functioning, reduce the risk of cancer recurrence, second primary cancers, as well as prolong survival [56]. Simple, effective, and inexpensive physical activity interventions for cancer survivors can also improve quality of life and reduce the risk of early mortality. An example of intervention to empower survivors was a 12-week home-based walking intervention to breast cancer survivors [57]. The intervention also consisted of telephone counselling of breast cancer survivors to set their goals to walk three times per week for 20–30 min for the first 4 weeks, walking four times a week for 30–40 min for the next 3 weeks followed by walking five times per week for 30–40 min for 5 weeks. Minutes-by-minutes activity was measured by providing them with

pedometer (portable device that counts the number of steps) as well as actigraphy (monitors movement and sleep-wake cycle) and self-report of the walking log. The results showed that the survivors had increased their activity levels as well as improved their quality of life [57].

Nutritional deficiencies are also common problems associated with cancer diagnosis and should be corrected during the survivorship period. Pierce [58]examined the effectiveness of telephone counseling to promote dietary change in the intervention from baseline to 12 months in 2970 breast cancer survivors in the Women's Healthy Eating and Living (WHEL) Study. Individualized telephone counselling with monthly cooking classes and monthly newsletters were provided by qualified counsellors and nutritionists. Each cooking class featured a nutrition theme to promote adherence and understanding of the intervention dietary pattern and gave women an opportunity to taste new foods and learn to prepare recipes. The newsletters featured research updates, nutrition information and recipes to help motivate women to adopt and maintain the intervention dietary pattern. At 12 months, the intervention group reported a significantly increased daily vegetables, fruits, and fiber intake.

Qigong is a Chinese mind-body integrative exercise used to prevent and cure ailments, to improve health and energy levels through regular practice [59]. Two clinical trials suggested its effectiveness in prolonging the life of cancer patients: (1) a study by Hong [60] involving 24 patients with advanced gastric cancer showed that Qigong was an effective nursing intervention to reduce fatigue, difficulty of daily activities and some chemotherapy side effect such as nausea, vomiting, and stomatitis, and (2) an RCT study by Wang [61] including 62 patients with late stage cancer also showed that Qigong plus chemotherapy had extended the tumor-free and better quality of their survival. However, the health promotion effectiveness of Qigong needs to be further evaluated in more rigorous clinical trials.

Another health promoting intervention to support survivorship was the use of mindfulness-based psychoeducation for cancer survivors (MindCAN) which is a psychoeducation program to help cancer survivors learn essential cancer-related knowledge; and to recognize and manage stress, thoughts, and emotions more effectively [62]. Contents of the MindCAN program was adapted from Mindfulness-Based Stress Reduction (MBSR) involving 8 weekly group-based program encompassed two components: Education and Mindfulness Practice. Each session lasted 90 min. Weekly education topics included: introducing mindfulness, recognizing and managing cancer-related stress, dealing with cancer-related symptoms and treatments, promoting mindful calmness and composure, powerful mind, mindful communication, mindful living, building your mindful lifestyle, and consolidating mindfulness practice. Mindfulness practices included: mindful breathing, body scan, mindful eating, standing and walking meditations, mindful emotions, let go of thoughts, loving-kindness medication and STOP breathing space [63]. Furthermore, participants shared their experiences with group members on their journey toward survivorship. A qualitative study involving 15 cancer patients was conducted to examine the patients' perception towards MindCAN. A thematic analysis suggested five major themes including: (1) heightened awareness of self, (2) enriching body experiences through mindfulness practice, (3) cultivating powerful minds and positive emotions, (4) integrating mindfulness to daily life, and (5) embracing interpersonal mindfulness. Furthermore, most participants perceived that MindCAN helped them feel more relaxed, and that they better managed stress, unhealthy thoughts, and emotions [62, 64].

Many children are also diagnosed with cancer and undergo similar treatments as adults. Advances in cancer treatment and cancer treatment efficacy have also improved the prognosis of childhood cancer and long survivorship period [65]. However, childhood cancer survivorship has shown declining levels of physical activity mainly due to fatigue and reduced physical strength and endurance as well parental view that children must take more rest [65]. In the past two decades, there has been an increase in the promotion of regular physical activity among childhood cancer survivors as it enhances their physical and psychological well-being [66]. There has been an increase in the use of adventure-based training to promote the psychological well-being of primary school children which can be used also in childhood cancer survivors [67]. For example, a 4-day integrated adventure-based training and health education program in the day-camp centre was conducted by 2 professional adventure-based trainers in 71 Hong Kong childhood cancer survivors. The results showed that the intervention promoted increased levels of physical activity, self-efficacy, and QoL in childhood cancer survivors [68].

Cancer also have long-term and lasting adverse effects on the psychological well-being and neurocognitive functioning of childhood cancer survivors. Dietz [65] provided a weekly 45-min lesson on musical training for 52 weeks among 60 children aged 5–8 years. These children were survivors with brain tumor; the program aimed to transform their lives and instill positive values through music. Training was conducted by a group of professional musicians of the nongovernment Music Children Foundation in Hong Kong. One-to-one musical training was conducted by qualified orchestral performers at the participants' homes. The participants were assigned a specific musical instrument to learn based on their interests as well as their fine motor skills and expiratory function which were assessed by the training musician. Training began at the lowest level up to the highest level where children were able to play an entire music. The results showed that children brain tumor survivors reported statistically significant fewer depressive symptoms, higher levels of self-esteem and better quality of life.

Many patients with advanced-stage cancer will only require palliative care and thus will continue to live with the cancer and cancer treatment-related symptoms such as fatigue, paraesthesia and dysesthesias, chronic pain, anorexia, insomnia, limbs oedema, and constipation [69]. For patients with advanced-stage cancer, one option is to provide effective care through pain relief and palliative care. Sometimes, surgery, chemotherapy and radiotherapy are also effective measures for effective palliative care especially for pain relief. Living with persistent pain is always associated with poor life satisfaction and is one of the factors that cause comorbidity and mortality [70]. When cancer patients experience persistent pain, this has negative influence on their well-being. In cancer survivors, pain treatment needs to meet the expectation. Opioids is still the major drug used. In view of the risks of overuse of opioids and the balance between the positive benefit to the survivors, this creates a real challenge to the health care system and the health care providers. The psychological effect of pain is an inner emotional experience of suffering in patients with cancer. As a result of being sick, palliative care patients begin to question the meaning of life and death. As such the salutogenic framework is useful in helping palliative care patients to find meaning and enable them who are living in this difficult situation to have better health and well-being [71]. Roditi and Robinson [72] suggested that promoting SOC in cancer survivors can help empower them to deal with, and acquire new meaning of persistent pain. Other nonpharmacological interventions such as massage, acupuncture, mind and body techniques are evidence-based interventions that can be used to relieve cancer pain, as these techniques are inexpensive, safe, and have no side effects [73]. Promoting palliative care aside from helping patients to feel comfortable by providing pain relief also need psychological and spiritual support. Health promoting interventions are also important. A longitudinal study by Park [74] on survivors of various cancers found that meaning-making efforts were related to less distress through meanings made to their negative emotions which corresponds to Antonovsky's SOC three tenets. Persons with palliative phase of cancer and their families experience low hope, anxiety, and symptoms of depression. In an observational, cross-sectional multiple study Mollenberg [75] found that both the patients and

their families with stronger SOC were associated with higher hope, lower anxiety, and symptoms of depression. Health professional should strive to assess patients and families who have low SOC and offer support to promote their comprehensibility, manageability, and meaningfulness during the palliative phase of cancer.

17.7 Mindfulness Interventions for Psychological Health of Patients with Cancer

Promoting overall psychological health of patients with cancer has been a focus of much research and one of the promising and innovative health promoting intervention is the use of mindfulness-based training among people with cancer [32, 76]. The concept of mindfulness was derived from the term "Sati," which has its original root from Theravada Buddhism. Mindfulness refers to awareness, which can be achieved through focusing and sustaining attention on the current moment on purpose with a nonjudgmental attitude [77, 78]. Mindfulness practice, including formal and informal meditations, are main approaches to cultivate the mindfulness levels among individuals. The formal mindfulness practice requires a person to perform regular meditations for a certain time period (such as body scan), whereas informal practice signifies how persons integrate awareness or "cautious attention" in their daily life activities (such as mindful eating and mindful walking). During the mindfulness practice, the individuals would be able to: (a) recognize the full range of their internal and external experiences, (b) regulate their attention and energy levels, and (c) connect to people around them [78]. People with high levels of mindfulness pay their attention on the current tasks and activities, disengage from unhealthy beliefs, thoughts and/or emotions, and maintain emotional balance and psychological well-being [77]. Mindfulness practice encompasses seven attitudinal foundations, including acceptance, beginner's mind, letting go, nonjudging, nonstriving, patience, and trust [78]. Mindfulness interventions were developed for people with physical and psychological conditions. Subsequently, those interventions have been applied to patients with cancer. Examples of the program are MBSR, MBCT, and MBCR, all of which are explained in the following.

17.7.1 Mindfulness-Based Stress Reduction (MBSR)

The first mindfulness program was developed at the University of Massachusetts Medical Centre's stress reduction clinic for people who experienced pain and stress [78]. The group-based MBSR contains 8 weekly sessions, each one lasts two and a half hours. A 1-day retreat is also included, and participants are asked to perform daily mindfulness practice for 30–45 min. Topics for each week include: (1) simple awareness, (2) attention and the brain, (3) dealing with thoughts, (4) stress: responding versus reacting, (5) dealing with difficult emotions or physical pain, (6) mindfulness and communication, (7) mindfulness and compassion, and (8) conclusion: developing a practice of your own [79]. Participants also learn different mindfulness practices such as meditation, body scan, loving kindness, and yoga [79]. In the field of oncology, specific breast cancer MBSR has been implemented. Studies showed that the mindfulness improved physical symptoms (fatigue and interference) [80], emotional problems (depression, anxiety, fear of occurrence), and QoL in patients with breast cancer [81, 82].

17.7.2 Mindfulness-Based Cognitive Therapy (MBCT)

MBCT is a group-based program originally created as a relapse-prevention treatment for patients with depression [83]. Participants would learn to be more aware of their physical sensations, thoughts and emotions from moment to moment and then respond to unpleasant sensations, thoughts and emotions in more skillful approaches [84]. It is perceived that people with full aware-

ness would have more freedom and choices whilst those in an autopilot mode often engage in unhealthy habits, which may trigger negative moods [84]. MBCT, with much influence from MBSR, contains 8 weekly sessions. For each week, the topics are: (1) Awareness and automatic pilot, (2) Living in our heads, (3) Gathering the scattered thoughts, (4) Recognizing aversion, (5) Allowing/Letting be, (6) Thoughts are not fact & Relapse signature, (7) How can I best take care of myself, and (8) Maintaining and extending new learning [84]. Similar to MBSR, various mindfulness practices are introduced encompassing raisin exercise, body scan practice, mindfulness of the breath, sitting meditation, and mindful walking. Home practices are required whereby participants do daily practice of mindfulness guided by provided CDs. Two RCTs involving participants diagnosed with cancer revealed that MBCT improved mindfulness, depression, anxiety, distress, and QoL in comparisons to control participants [85, 86]. Among women with breast cancer, participants in the MBCT group reported significantly lower pain intensity, nonprescription pain medication use, and function disability, and greater quality of life, posttraumatic growth, and self-management compared to the control group [87, 88].

17.7.3 Mindfulness-Based Cancer Recovery (MBCR)

MBCR is offered to people with cancer as a healing practice, which enables them to enrich their daily life, cope with cancer-related symptoms and treatments, improve an immune system, reduce harmful effects of stress hormones and thus enhance QoL [89]. Mindfulness is represented in two categories: Big-M and Little-m [90]. The former signifies living in the world mindfully whereas the latter represents allocating certain time slots to practice mindfulness [89]. Adapted from MBSR, MBCR comprises 90-min, 8-week intervention sessions, a weekend retreat and home practice. Weekly themes entails: (1) mindfulness attitudes, (2) stress responding versus reacting, (3) mindful movement, (4) balancing breath, (5) stories we tell ourselves (trouble mind), (6) meditation with imagery, (7) a Day of Silence, and (8) deepening and expanding [89]. Certain contents are incorporated into MBCR, including coping with cancer-related symptoms (such as pain, insomnia and fear of reoccurrence) and cognitive coping strategies. Participants are instructed to practice mindful breathing, body scan, sitting meditation, yoga, mindful walking, and mountain and loving kindness meditation. Empirical evidence showed that, in comparison with control groups, MBCR reduced stressed symptoms and mood disturbance [91] and enhanced QoL and post-traumatic growth among distressed breast survivors [92].

17.7.4 Innovation: Technology-Based Mindfulness Interventions

Traditional face-to-face mindfulness programs are beneficial in terms of preventing and reducing physical and psychological symptoms among people with cancer [93]. However, there are some challenges concerning the traditional method of learning. Specifically, some patients may have limited mobility due to cancer-related fatigue and pain, geographical distance and program schedule and setting. As such, technology-based platforms (such as internet and mobile phone) may be the alternatives as they help overcome challenges encountered by traditional face-to-face programs.

A *mobile phone* mindfulness-based stress reduction intervention for breast cancer was examined among 15 breast cancer survivors in USA [94]. A single-group, quasi-experimental design was implemented. The MBSR was created to deliver 6 weekly, 2-h intervention sessions through iPad. Weekly modules covered formal meditative techniques (sitting and walking meditation, body scan and Hatha yoga) and informal meditation (integrating mindfulness into daily life). Participants practiced formal and informal mindfulness for 15–45 min and recorded the practice on the iPad. Results indicated

improvement in psychological symptoms (stress, anxiety and depression), health status (fatigue), QoL, and cognitive abilities (mindfulness and cognitive functioning) [94].

A 10-week, *internet-based* group intervention was developed with elements from MBSR and cognitive-behavioral stress management for ovarian cancer survivors in USA [95]. Participants logged in to a web platform to access weekly a videoconference, relaxation and meditation practice (such as deep breathings mindfulness meditation, and guided relaxation and visualization) and journal to record daily reflection. Session topics encompassed awareness of stressors and strengths, automatic thoughts, rational thoughts, acceptance, social support, effective communication, anger, meaning of life, and wrap up. The study revealed that the internet-based program was highly usable and acceptable with moderate feasibility for ovarian cancer survivors [95].

In the Netherlands, a pilot single-group study tested the effects of a 9-week, internet-based, therapist-guided, individual MBCT (iMBCT) on fatigue among cancer survivors [96]. Each week, patients would log in to the website, read information specific for mindfulness, write down their experiences in the log boxes and practice mindfulness using audio files. On an agreeable day of the week, the therapist would reply to the patients' log and guide them through the program. An online forum allowed participants to share their experiences on mindfulness practice. Patients who attended the iMBCT reported significant reduction in fatigue severity and distress [96].

In Denmark, researchers created an internet-delivered MBCT program (iMBCT) for breast and prostate cancer survivors [97]. In this RCT, cancer survivors included those who completed primary treatments at least 3 months until 5 years. Potential participants were randomized into either an intervention (receiving iMBCT) or control group (receiving care-as-usual). The iMBCT program comprised 8 weekly modules with written materials, audio-guided exercise, examples of cancer-specific patients and videos. Participants were required to submit a weekly training diary to their therapist, who would provide comments each week. Nine therapists, who received MBCT training, involved in such tasks. Findings suggested that patients in both MBCT and iMBCT groups had long-term reduction in psychological and distress; and long-term increase in positive mental health and mental health-related QoL [98].

In Canada, researchers conducted an RCT to test the "synchronous" or "real time" online MBCR on distressed cancer survivors [99]. The online MBCR encompasses eight 2-h weekly sessions with a didactic approach, live group interaction, online 6-h retreat and home practice (hatha yoga, qigong movement and sitting, walking, and loving-kindness meditations). During the mindfulness sessions, all participants interacted in real time with the therapist and other group members. The home practice was achieved through guided recordings and videos. The program demonstrated feasibility and effectiveness in reducing stress, mood disturbances, enhancing mindfulness and spirituality [76]. Similarly, another study in Canada revealed the effectiveness of the real time online MBCR on cancer survivors. Age and gender differences were documented whereby younger participants reported greater improvement in stress, spirituality, and nonreactivity (one component of mindfulness); and men reported greater posttraumatic growth [99]. Results indicated that participants in the iMBCT group had significant improvement in anxiety.

Another pilot study in USA was carried out to test a *Headspace application* (a self-paced commercial program) via website or smart phone [100]. The 8-week program comprised a 30-days foundation course (basic mindfulness meditation) followed by condition-specific sessions (stress, anxiety, sleep and acceptance). Each session took 10–20 min encompassing a short lecture video and progressive audio instruction. The Headspace helped reduce distress, depression, anxiety, and improved mental health and quality of sleep among cancer patients with active cancer treatments and their caregivers [100].

17.8   Chapter Summary

Cancer is a global concern as the incidence rates of cancer continue to increase despite new treatment modalities. The number of cancer survivors are also on the rise prolonging their life beyond the 5-year period. From being aware of the risk for cancer to results of screening, definitive diagnosis, undergoing treatment and survivorship, patients experience physiological as well as psychological ill health and reduced well-being. There are growing health promotion strategies to support patients with cancer. Most of these interventions focused on increasing patients' knowledge, attitudes, and behaviors in changing their lifestyle as well as managing the problematic and debilitating treatment-related symptoms they continue to experience as cancer survivors. The Salutogenic model of health and specifically the SOC has been widely and effectively used in health promotion interventions. It is suggested that health care professionals use these evidence-based interventions appropriately within their sociocultural context. Table 17.1 provides a summary of health promoting interventions presented in this chapter.

Table 17.1 Summary of health promotion interventions for cancer patients

Cancer health issues	Health promotion interventions
Smoking cessation [22]	An 8-week mindfulness-based smoking cessation intervention consisting of lessons on the effects of smoking, instructions for smoking cessation, guided instruction, and an audio compact discs and manual on mind-body practices including meditation, body scan, and chair yoga (each 20 min in length)
Smoking cessation [23]	Face-to-face individualized brief (15–30 min) risk communication followed by a booster intervention via telephone to assess the progress of, and to identify difficulties faced by patients towards quitting and how to handle withdrawal symptoms.
Smoking cessation [25]	Chat-based cessation support delivered through an instant messaging app (WhatsApp) for 1, 2, and 3 months. Smoking cessation counsellor interacted with a participant in real time and provided personalized, theory-based cessation support.
Colorectal cancer patients [29]	An 8-week audio-based mindfulness meditation program using MP3 player preloaded with eight mindfulness meditation tracks, study booklet containing a practice diary. An email was sent each week containing practice instructions, a motivational quote linked to a discussion Of the weekly theme. Participants were instructed to practice 15 ± 20 min per day, 5 days per week, during the 8-week study. They received a text message to their personal cell phone daily at 4 pm with messages containing motivational quotes or practice suggestions.
Fatigue [38]	Walking intervention consisting of an initial 10–15 min sessions and 5–6 sessions per week and increased to 30 min per session, 5–6 weeks per week according to their exercise tolerance and responses to treatment. The women were asked to keep diaries of their daily exercise activity.
Nausea and vomiting [45]	Acupressure by placing ear seed on the pinna on each ear for 5 day and asked the patients to press the ear seeds for 3 min three times a day in the morning, noon and night during the chemotherapy cycle.
Chemotherapy-induced peripheral neuropathy [50]	Eight treatments of foot bath and massage for 30 min every other day for 2 weeks.
Nutritional deficiencies [58]	Twelve months individualized telephone counselling with monthly cooking classes and monthly newsletters provided by qualified counsellors and nutritionists. Each cooking class featured a nutrition theme to promote adherence and understanding of the intervention dietary pattern and gave women an opportunity to taste new foods and learn to prepare recipes. The newsletters featured research updates, nutrition information and recipes to help motivate women to adopt and maintain the intervention dietary pattern.
Stress-related treatment [78]	A group-based, mindfulness-based stress reduction (MBSR) contains 8 weekly sessions, each one lasts two and a half hours. A 1-day retreat is also included, and participants are asked to perform daily mindfulness practice for 30–45 min. Topics for each week include: (1) simple awareness, (2) attention and the brain, (3) dealing with thoughts, (4) stress: Responding versus reacting, (5) dealing with difficult emotions or physical pain, (6) mindfulness and communication, (7) mindfulness and compassion, and (8) conclusion: Developing a practice of your own.
Sexual dysfunction [51]	Self-report response to the 3-min neutral and 4-min erotic audiovisual film, psychoeducational intervention consisting of three 60-min sessions targeting sexual arousal complaints and how to troubleshoot these difficulties and manual of information about progressive relaxation, mindfulness, becoming organismic, and making marriage work followed by group discussion.
Stress of being diagnosed with cancer [54]	Using art therapy, participants drew images causing their stress followed by group discussion, where participants explained the image to the group and the group then discussed the meaning, manageability, and comprehensiveness components that could help cope with stress. The study provided evidence that methods in creating meaning through art therapy enhanced the patients' sense of coherence by integrating the three components to overcome their stress about cancer diagnosis and treatment.
Supporting childhood cancer survivors [67]	Children attended a 4-day integrated adventure-based training and health education program in the day Camp Centre conducted by two professional adventure-based trainers from the sports and recreation management and oncology.

(continued)

Table 17.1 (continued)

Cancer health issues	Health promotion interventions
Neurocognitive functioning in children with cancer [66]	A weekly 45-min lesson on musical training for 52 weeks in 60 5–8 years old children survivors with brain tumor to transform their lives and instill positive values through music. Training was conducted by a group of professional musicians of the nongovernment music children Foundation in Hong Kong. One-to-one musical training was conducted by qualified orchestral performers at the participants' homes. The participants were assigned a particular musical instrument to learn based on their interests as well as their fine motor skills and expiratory function which was assessed by the training musician. Training began at the lowest level up to the highest level where children were able to play an entire music.
Survivorship [62]	The 8-weekly group-based programs encompassed two components: Education and mindfulness practice. Each session lasted 90 min. Weekly education topics included: Introduction of mindfulness, recognizing and managing cancer-related stress, dealing with cancer-related symptoms and treatments, mindful emotions: Calmness and composure, mindfulness: The powerful mind, mindful communication, mindful living: Building your mindful life style, and consolidation of mindfulness practice. Mindfulness practices included: Mindful breathing, body scan, mindful eating, standing and walking meditations, mindful emotions, let go of thoughts, loving-kindness medication and STOP breathing space.
Psychological well-being [76]	Six weekly 2-h mindfulness intervention sessions using mobile application iPad. Weekly modules covered formal meditative techniques (sitting and walking meditation, body scan, and hatha yoga) and informal meditation (integrating mindfulness into daily life). Participants practiced formal and informal mindfulness for 15–45 min and recorded the practice on the iPad.

Take Home Messages

- Cancer patients have reduced psychological well-being and increased stress, anxiety, and depressive symptoms.
- The Salutogenic health theory that focuses on the origins of health and psychological well-being can be used to guide health promotion interventions in patients with cancer.
- A high SOC reflects a coping capacity of cancer patients to deal with everyday life stressors and consists of three elements: comprehensibility, manageability, and meaningfulness.
- Innovative health promotion interventions such as art therapy, auricular therapy, mindfulness, web-based instant messaging, physical exercise, psychoeducational manuals, and other nonpharmacological therapies are needed to strengthen SOC in patients with cancer.

References

1. American Cancer Society. Global cancer facts and figures. 4th ed. Atlanta: American Cancer Society; 2018.
2. Bray F, Ferlay J, Soerjomataram P, Siegel RL, Torre LA, Jemal A. Global cancer statistics 2018: GLOBACAN estimates of incidence and mortality worldwide for 36 cancers in 185 countries. CA Cancer J Clin. 2018;68(6):394–424. https://doi.org/10.3322/cacc.21492.
3. International Agency for Research in Cancer. Latest global cancer data. Press release, no. 263. 2018. https://www.iarc.fr/wp-content/uploads/2018/09/pr263_E.pdf.
4. Ferlay J, Soerjomataram I, Dikshit R, et al. Cancer incidence and mortality worldwide: sources, methods and major patterns in GLOBOCAN 2012. Int J Cancer. 2015;136:E359–86.
5. United Nations Development Program. Human Development Index (HDI). Human Development report. 2019. http://hdr.undp.org/en/content/human-development-index-hdi.
6. American Cancer Society. Global cancer facts & figures. 4th ed. Surveillance research. 2018. https://www.cancer.org/content/dam/cancer-org/research/cancer-facts-and-statistics/global-cancer-facts-and-figures/global-cancer-facts-and-figures-4th-edition.pdf.
7. Antonovsky A. The salutogenic model as a theory to guide health promotion. Health Promot Int. 1996;11:11–8.
8. Antonovsky A. Health, stress, and coping: new perspectives on mental and physical well-being. San Francisco: Jossey-Bass Therapy; 1979.
9. Antonovsky A. Unraveling the mystery of health. How people manage stress and stay well. San Francisco: Jossey-Bass Publishers; 1987.
10. Winger JG, Adams N, Mosher CE. Relations of meaning in life and sense of coherence to distress

in cancer patients: a meta-analysis. Psychooncology. 2016;25:2–10.

11. Eriksson M, Lindström B. Antonovsky's sense of coherence scale and its relation with quality of life: a systematic review. J Epidemiol Community Health. 2007;61:938–44.

12. Proschaska JO, Verizer WF. The transtheoretical model of change. Am J Health Promot. 1997;12(1):38–48.

13. Pinto BM, Friersin GM, Rabin C, Trunzo JJ, Marcus BH. Home-based physical activity intervention for breast cancer patients. J Clin Oncol. 2005;23:3577–86.

14. Ajzen I. The theory of planned behavior. Organiz Behav Human Dec Proc. 1991;50:179–211.

15. Ajzen I. Attitudinal versus normative messages: AN investigation of the differential effects of persuasive communication on behaviour. Sociometry. 1971;34:263–80.

16. Jones LW, Courneya KS, Fairey AS, et al. Does the theory of planned behavior mediate the effects of an oncologist's recommendation to exercise in newly diagnosed breast cancer survivors? Results from a randomized controlled trial. Health Psychol. 2005;24:189–97.

17. Bandura A. Social foundations of thought and action. A social cognitive theory. Prentice Hall: Englewood Cliffs; 1986.

18. Graves KD. Social cognitive theory and cancer patients' quality of life: a meta-analysis of psychosocial intervention components. Health Psychol. 2003;22(2):210–9. https://doi.org/10.1037/0278-6133.22.2.210.

19. Grimmett C, Haviland J, Winter J, Calman L, Din A, Richardson A, Smith PWF, Foster C. Colorectal cancer patient's self-efficacy for managing illness-related problems in the first 2 years after diagnosis, results from the ColoREctal Well-being (CREW) study. J Cancer Surviv. 2007;11(5):634–42. https://doi.org/10.1007/s11764-017-0636-x.

20. Cox LS, Patten CA, Ebbert JO, Drews AA, Croghan GA, Clark MM, Wolter TD, Decker PA, Hurt RD. Tobacco use outcomes among patients with lung cancer treated for nicotine dependence. J Clin Oncol. 2002;20:3461–9.

21. Charlot M, D'Amico S, Luo M, Gemei A, Kathuria H, Gardiner P. Feasibility and acceptability of mindfulness-based group visits for smoking cessation in low-socioeconomic status and minority smokers with cancer. BMC Complement Med Ther. 2019;25(7):762–9.

22. Li HC, Wang MP, Ho KW, Lam KW, Chueng YT, Yannes YT, Chueng TH, Lam TH, Chan SC. Helping cancer patients quit smoking using brief advice based on risk communication: a randomized controlled trial. Sci Rep. 2018;8:2712. https://doi.org/10.1038/s41598-018-21207-1.

23. Zhang X, Zheng X, Chai S, Lei M, Feng Z, Liu J, Lopez V. Effects of using WeChat-assisted perioperative care instructions for parents of pediatric

patients undergoing day surgery or herniorrhaphy. Patient Educ Couns. 2018;101:1433–8.

24. Wang MP, Luk TT, Wu Y, Li WHC, Cheung YTD, Kwong ACK, Lai VWY, Chan SSC, Lam TH. Chat-based instant messaging support integrated with brief interventions for smoking cessation: a community-based, pragmatic, cluster-randomised controlled trial. Lancet Digital Health. 2019;1(4):e183–92. https://doi.org/10.1016/S2589-7500(19)30082-2.

25. von Wagner C, Knight K, Steptoe A, Wardle J. Functional health literacy and health-promoting behaviour in a national sample of British adults. J Epidemiol Community Health. 2017;61:1086–90.

26. Mirzaii K, Ashkezari SN, Khadivzadeh T, Shakeri MT. Evaluation of the effects of breast cancer screening training based on the systematic comprehensive health education and promotion model on the attitudes and breast self-examination skills of women. Evidence Based Care Journal. 2016;6(3):7–18.

27. Jemal A, Siegel R, Ward E, Hao Y, Xu J, Thun MJ. Cancer statistics. CA Cancer J Clin. 2009;59(4):225–49. https://doi.org/10.3322/caac.20006.

28. Boogar IR, Talepasand S, Norouzi H, Mozafari S, Hosseini SJ. The Prediction of colorectal cancer screening based on the extended parallel process model: moderating the role of health literacy and cancer-related empowerment. Int J Cancer Manag. 2018;11:3625–39.

29. Adams SA, Rohweder CL, Leeman J, Friedman DB, Gizlice Z, Vanderpool RC, Askelsom N, Best A, Flocke SA, Glanz K, Ko LK, Legler M. Use of evidence-based interventions and implementation strategies to increase colorectal screening in federally qualifies health centres. J Community Health. 2018;43:1044–52.

30. Super S, Wagemakers MAE, Picavet SHJ, Verkooijen KT, Koelen MA. Strengthening sense of coherence: opportunities for theory building in health promotion. Health Promot Int. 2016;31:869–78. https://doi.org/10.1093/heapro/dav071.

31. Peterson NB, Dwyer KA, Mulvaney SA, Dietrich MS, Rothman RL. The influence of health literacy on colorectal cancer screening knowledge, beliefs and behaviour. J Natl Med Assoc. 2008;99:1105–12.

32. Carlson LE, Angen M, Cullum J, Goodey E, Koopmans J, Lamont L, et al. High levels of untreated distress and fatigue in cancer patients. Br J Cancer. 2004;90(12):2297–304. https://doi.org/10.1038/sj.bjc.6601887.

33. Ozanne A, Graneheim UH. Understanding the incomprehensible—patients' and spouses' experiences of comprehensibility before, at and after diagnosis of amyotrophic lateral sclerosis. Scand J Caring Sci. 2018;32:663–71. https://doi.org/10.1111/scs.12492.

34. Aderhold C, Morawa E, Paslakis G, Erim Y. Protective factors of depressive symptoms in adult cancer patients: the role of sense of coherence and posttraumatic growth in different time spans since

diagnosis. J Psychosoc Oncol. 2019;37:616–35. https://doi.org/10.1080/07347332.2019.1631931.

35. Carlson LE. Mindfulness-based interventions for coping with cancer. Ann N Y Acad Sci. 2017;1373(1):5–12. https://doi.org/10.1111/nyas.13029.

36. Kessels E, Husson O, van der Feltz-Cornelis CM. The effects of exercise on cancer-related fatigue in cancer survivors: a systematic review and meta-analysis. Neuropsychiatr Dis Treat. 2018;14:479–94.

37. Van Vulpen JK, Velthuis MJ, Bisschop CNS, Travier N, Van Den Buijs BJW, Backx FJG, et al. Effects of an exercise program in colon cancer patients undergoing chemotherapy. Med Sci Sports Exerc. 2016;48(5):767–75.

38. Mock V, Pickett M, Kopka ME, et al. Fatigue and quality of life outcomes of exercise during cancer treatment. Cancer Pract. 2001;9(3):119–27.

39. Velthuis MJ, May AM, Koppejan-Rensenbrink RAG, Gijsen BCM, van Breda E, de Wit GA, Schröder CD, Monninkhof EM, Lindeman E, van der Wall E, PHM P. Physical activity during cancer treatment (PACT) study: design of a randomised clinical trial. BMC Cancer. 2010;10:272.

40. Miller M, Kearney N. Chemotherapy-related nausea and vomiting: past reflections, present practice and future management. Eur J Cancer Care (Engl). 2004;13:71–81.

41. Jordan K, Gralla R, Jahn F, et al. International antiemetic guidelines on chemotherapy induced nausea and vomiting (CINV): content and implementation in daily routine practice. Eur J Pharmacol. 2014;722:197–202.

42. Morey SS. NIH issues consensus statement on acupuncture. Am Fam Physician. 1998;57:2545–6.

43. Tipton JM, McDaniel RW, Barbour L, et al. Putting evidence into practice: evidence-based interventions to prevent, manage, and treat chemotherapy-induced nausea and vomiting. Clin J Oncol Nurs. 2007;11:69–78.

44. Kurebayashi LFS, Gnatta JR, Borges TP, Silva MJPD. Applicability of auriculotherapy in reducing stress and as a coping strategy in nursing professionals. Rev Latino-Am Enferm. 2012;20(5):980e987.

45. Eghbali M, Yekaninejad MS, Varaei S, Jalalinia SF, Samimi MA, Sa'atchi K. The effect of auricular acupressure on nausea and vomiting caused by chemotherapy among breast cancer patients. Complement Ther Clin Pract. 2016;24:189–94.

46. Molassiotis A, Cheng HL, Leung KT, Lopez V. Risk factors for chemotherapy-induced peripheral neuropathy in patients receiving taxane- and platinum-chemotherapy. Brain Behav. 2019;9(6):e01312. https://doi.org/10.1002/brb3.1312.

47. Wolf S, Barton D, Kottschade L, et al. Chemotherapy-induced peripheral neuropathy: prevention and treatment strategies. Eur J Cancer. 2008;44(11):1507–15.

48. Boyette-Davis JA, Walters ET, Dougherty PM. Mechanisms involved in the development of chemotherapy-induced neuropathy. Pain Manag. 2015;5(4):285–96.

49. Hile ES, Fitzgerald GK, Studenski SA. Persistent mobility disability after neurotoxic chemotherapy. Phys Ther. 2010;90(11):1649–57.

50. Wu B-Y, Liu C-T, Su Y-L, Chen S-Y, Chen Y-H, Tsai M-Y. A review of complementary therapies with medicinal plants for chemotherapy-induced peripheral neuropathy. Complement Ther Med. 2019;4:226–32.

51. Brotto LA, Heiman JR, Goff B, Greer B, Lentz GM, Swisher E, Tamimi H, Van Blaricom A. A psychoeducational intervention for sexual dysfunction in women with gynecologic cancer. Arch Sex Behav. 2008;37:317–29.

52. Heiman JR, Rowland DL. Affective and physiological sexual response patterns: the effects of instructions on sexually functional and dysfunctional men. J Psychosom Res. 1983;27:105–16.

53. Bozcuk H, Ozcan K, Erdogan C, et al. A comparative study of art therapy in cancer patients receiving chemotherapy and improvement in quality of life by watercolor painting. Complement Ther Med. 2017;30:67–72.

54. Huss E, Samsom T. Drawing on the arts to enhance salutogenic coping with health-related stress and loss. Front Psychol. 2018;9:1612–25. https://doi.org/10.3389/fpsyg.2018.01612.

55. Chan RJ, Yates P, Quiping L, Komatsu H, Lopez V, Thandar M, Chako ST, So W, Pongthavornkamol K, Yi M, Pittayapan P, Butcon J, Wyld D, Molassiotis A. Oncology practitioners' perspectives and practice patterns of post-treatment cancer survivorship care in the Asia-Pacific region, results from the STEP study. BMC Cancer. 2017;17(1):715.

56. Courneya KS, Friedenreich CM, Sela RA, Quinney HA, Rhodes RE. Correlates of adherence and contamination in a randomized controlled trial of exercise in cancer survivors: an application of the theory of planned behavior and the five factor model of personality. Ann Behav Med. 2002;24(4):257–68.

57. Matthews CE, Wilcox S, Hanby CL, Ananian CD, Heiney SP, Gebretsadik T, Shintaniarmacol A. Evaluation of a 12-week home-based walking intervention for breast cancer survivors. Support Care Cancer. 2007;15:203–11. https://doi.org/10.1007/s00520-006-0122-x.

58. Pierce JP, Newman VA, Flatt SW, Faerber S, Rock CL, Natarajan L, et al. Telephone counseling intervention increases intakes of micronutrient- and phytochemical-rich vegetables, fruit and fiber in breast cancer survivors. J Nutr. 2004;134:452–8.

59. Lee MS, Chen KW, Sancier KM, Earst E. Qigong for cancer treatment: a systematic review of controlled clinical trials. Acta Oncol. 2007;46:717–22.

60. Hong EY. The effect of Yudongkong exercise in fatigue, difficulty of daily activities and symptoms of side effect in advanced gastric cancer patients receiving chemotherapy. PhD dissertation. Seoul, Korea: Yonsei University; 2003.

61. Wang CH, Wang BR, Shao MY, Li ZQ. Clinical study if the routine treatment of cancer coordinated by qigong. In: 2nd world conference for academic exchange of medical qigong, Beijing, China; 1993.

62. Klainin-Yobas P, Goei LP, Chng WJ, Ang NKE, Lopez V, Cheng M, Lau Y. Efficacy of the mindfulness-based psychoeducation programme among adult cancer survivors: the preliminary findings. Oral presentation at the NCIS annual research meeting (NCAM) on 2–3 August at National University Health System, Singapore; 2019.

63. Klainin-Yobas P. The development of mindfulness-based psychoeducation for cancer survivors: an evidence-based practice. Oral presentation at the 2nd international meeting on nursing research & evidence-based practice, 19–20 March, Singapore; 2018.

64. Goei L-P. Preventing psychological symptoms and enhancing psychological well-being among adult cancer survivors through the mindfulness-based psychoeducation programme: a feasibility study. Unpublished Honours thesis. Alice Lee Centre for Nursing Studies, Young Loo Lin School of Medicine, National University of Singapore, Singapore; 2019.

65. Dietz AC, Mulrooney DA. Life beyond the disease: relationships, parenting, and quality of life among survivors of childhood cancer. Haematologica. 2011;96(5):643–5.

66. Stolley MR, Restrepo J, Sharp LK. Diet and physical activity in childhood cancer survivors: a review of the literature. Ann Behav Med. 2010;39:232–49.

67. Li HCW, Chung OKJ, Ho KYE. Effectiveness of an adventure-based training programme in promoting the psychological well-being of primary school children. J Health Psychol. 2013;18(11):1478–92. https://doi.org/10.1177/1359105312465102.

68. Li HCW, Chung OKJ, Ho KYA, Chiu SY, Lopez V. Effectiveness of an integrated adventure-based training and health education program in promoting regular physical activity among childhood cancer survivors. Psychooncology. 2013;2:2601–10.

69. Pachman DR, Barton DL, Swetz KM, et al. Troublesome symptoms in cancer survivors: fatigue, insomnia, neuropathy, and pain. J Clin Oncol. 2012;30:3687–96.

70. Sibille KT, Bartsch F, Reddy D, Fillingim RB, Keil A. Increasing neuroplasticity to bolster chronic pain treatment: a role for intermittent fasting and glucose administration. J Pain. 2016;17:275–81.

71. Oliveira CC. Suiffering and salutogenesis. Health Promot Int. 2014;30:222–7.

72. Roditi D, Robinson ME. The role of psychological interventions in the management of patients with chronic pain. Psychol Res Behav Manag. 2011;4:41–9. https://doi.org/10.2147/PRBM.S15375.

73. Cassileth BR, Keefe FJ. Integrative and behavioral approaches to the treatment of cancer-related neuropathic pain. Oncologist. 2010;15(Suppl 2):19–23. https://doi.org/10.1634/theoncologist.2009-S504.

74. Park CL, Edmondson D, Fenster JR, Blank TO. Meaning making and psychological adjustment following cancer: the mediating roles of growth, life meaning, and restored just-world beliefs. J Consult Clin Psychol. 2008;76:863–75. https://doi.org/10.1037/a0013348.

75. Möllerberg M-L, Årestedt K, Swahnberg K, Benzein E, Sandgren A. Family sense of coherence and its associations with hope, anxiety and symptoms of depression in persons with cancer in palliative phase and their family members: a cross-sectional study. Palliat Med. 2019;33(10):1310–8. https://doi.org/10.1177/0269216319866653.

76. Zernicke KA, Campbell TS, Speca M, McCabe-Ruff K, Flowers S, Carlson LE. A randomized wait-list controlled trial of feasibility and efficacy of an online mindfulness-based cancer recovery program: the eTherapy for cancer applying mindfulness trial. Psychosom Med. 2014;76(4):257–67. https://doi.org/10.1097/PSY.0000000000000053.

77. Kabat-Zinn J. Full catastrophe living: using the wisdom of your body and mind to face stress, pain, and illness. New York: Delta; 2009.

78. Kabat-Zinn J. Mindfulness for beginners: reclaiming the present moment and your life. Sounds True: Boulder; 2012.

79. Palouse mindfulness. Mindfulness-based stress reduction. n.d. https://palousemindfulness.com/index.html.

80. Zernicke KA, Campbell TS, Speca M, McCabe-Ruff K, Flowers S, et al. The eCALM Trial-eTherapy for cancer applying mindfulness: online mindfulness-based cancer recovery program for underserved individuals living with cancer in Alberta: protocol development for a randomized wait-list controlled clinical trial. BMC Complement Altern Med. 2013;13(1):13–34.

81. Lengacher CA, Johnson-Mallard V, Post-White J, Moscoso MS, Jacobsen PB, et al. Randomized controlled trial of mindfulness-based stress reduction (MBSR) for survivors of breast cancer. Psychooncology. 2009;18(12):1261–72.

82. Wurtzen H, Dalton SO, Elsass P, Sumbundu AD, Steding-Jensen M, et al. Mindfulness significantly reduces self-reported levels of anxiety and depression: results of a randomised controlled trial among 336 Danish women treated for stage I-III breast cancer. Eur J Cancer. 2013;49(6):1365–73.

83. Segal Z, Teasdale J, Williams M. Mindfulness-based cognitive therapy for depression. New York: Guilford Press; 2002.

84. Segal Z, Teasdale J, Williams M. Mindfulness-based cognitive therapy for depression. 2nd ed. New York: Guilford Press; 2013.

85. Foley E, Baillie A, Huxter M, Price M, Sinclair E. Mindfulness-based cognitive therapy for individuals whose lives have been affected by cancer: a randomized controlled trial. J Consult Clin Psychol. 2010;78(1):72–9. https://doi.org/10.1037/a0017566.

86. Kingston T, Collier S, Hevey D, McCormick MM, Besani C, Cooney J, O'Dwyer AM. Mindfulness-based cognitive therapy for psycho-oncology patients: an exploratory study. Ir J Psychol Med. 2015;32(3):265–74. https://doi.org/10.1017/ipm.2014.81.

87. Johannsen M, O'Connor M, O'Toole MS, Jensen AB, Hojris I, Zachariae R. Efficacy of mindfulness-based cognitive therapy on late post-treatment pain in women treated for primary breast cancer: a randomized controlled trial. Int J Clin Oncol. 2016;34(28):3390–9. https://doi.org/10.1200/JCO.2015.65.0770.

88. Norouzi H, Rahimian-Boogar I, Talepasand S. Effectiveness of mindfulness-based cognitive therapy on posttraumatic growth, self-management and functional disability among patients with breast cancer. Nurs Pract Today. 2017;4(4):190–202.

89. Carlson LE, Speca M. Mindfulness-based cancer recovery. New Harbinger: Oakland; 2010.

90. Shapiro SL, Carlson LE. The art and science of mindfulness: integrating mindfulness into psychology and the helping professions. Washington, DC: American Psychological Association; 2009. https://doi.org/10.1037/11885-000.

91. Carlson LE, Doll R, Stephen J, Faris P, Tamagawa R, Drysdale E, Speca M. Randomized controlled trial of mindfulness-based cancer recovery versus supportive expressive group therapy for distressed survivors of breast cancer (MINDSET). J Clin Oncol. 2013;31(25):3119–26. https://doi.org/10.1200/jco.2012.47.5210.

92. Carlson LE, Tamagawa R, Stephen J, Drysdale E, Zhong L, Speca M. Randomized-controlled trial of mindfulness-based cancer recovery versus supportive expressive group therapy among distressed breast cancer survivors (MINDSET): long-term follow-up results. Psychooncology. 2016;25(7):750–9. https://doi.org/10.1002/pon.4150.

93. Xunlin NG, Lau Y, Klainin-Yobas P. The effectiveness of mindfulness-based interventions among cancer patients and survivors: a systematic review and meta-analysis. Support Care Cancer. 2020;28(4):1563–78. https://doi.org/10.1007/s00520-019-05219-9.

94. Lengacher CA, Reich RR, Ramesar S, Alinat CB, Moscoso M, et al. Feasibility of the mobile mindfulness-based stress reduction for breast cancer (mMBSR(BC)) program for symptom improvement among breast cancer survivors. Psychooncology. 2018;27(2):524–31. https://doi.org/10.1002/pon.4491.

95. Kinner EM, Armer JS, McGregor BA, Duffecy J, Leighton S, Corden ME, Lutgendorf SK. Internet-based group intervention for ovarian cancer survivors: feasibility and preliminary results. JMIR Cancer. 2018;4(1):e1. https://doi.org/10.2196/cancer.8430.

96. Everts FZB, Van der Lee MI, Meezenbroek EJ. Web-based individual mindfulness-based cognitive therapy for cancer-related fatigue: a pilot study. Internet Interv. 2015;2:200–13.

97. Nissen ER, O'Connor M, Kaldo V, Højris I, Borre M, Zachariae R, et al. Internet-delivered mindfulness-based cognitive therapy for anxiety and depression in cancer survivors: a randomized controlled trial. Psycho-Oncology. 2020 29(1):68–75. OI: https://doi.org/10.1002/pon.5237.

98. Cillessen L, Schellekens MPJ, Van de Ven MOM, Donders ART, Compen FR, Bisseling EM, et al. Consolidation and prediction of long-term treatment effect of group and online mindfulness-based cognitive therapy for distressed cancer patients. Acta Oncol. 2018;57(10):1293–302.

99. Zernicke KA, Campbell TS, Speca M, et al. The eCALM Trial: eTherapy for Cancer Applying Mindfulness. Exploratory analyses of the associations between online mindfulness-based cancer recovery participation and changes in mood, stress symptoms, mindfulness, posttraumatic growth, and spirituality. Mindfulness. 2016;7:1071–81.

100. Kubo A, Altschuler A, Kurtoovich E, Hendlish S, Laurent C, Kolevska T, Li YA. A pilot mobile-based mindfulness intervention for cancer patients and their informal caregivers. Mindfulness. 2018;9:1885–94.

Hege Selnes Haugdahl, Ingeborg Alexandersen, and Gørill Haugan

Abstract

Few patients are as helpless and totally dependent on nursing as long-term intensive care (ICU) patients. How the ICU nurse relates to the patient is crucial, both concerning the patients' mental and physical health and well-being. Even if nurses provide evidence-based care in the form of minimum sedation, early mobilization, and attempts at spontaneous breathing during weaning, the patient may not have the strength, courage, and willpower to comply. Interestingly, several elements of

H. S. Haugdahl (✉)
Nord-Trøndelag Hospital Trust, Levanger, Norway

Faculty of Medicine and Health Science, Department of Public Health and Nursing, NTNU Norwegian University of Science and Technology, Trondheim, Norway
e-mail: hege.selnes.haugdahl@hnt.no

I. Alexandersen
Faculty of Medicine and Health Science, Department of Public Health and Nursing, NTNU Norwegian University of Science and Technology, Trondheim, Norway
e-mail: ingeborg.alexandersen@ntnu.no

G. Haugan
Department of Public Health and Nursing, NTNU Norwegian University of Science and Technology, Trondheim, Norway

Faculty of Nursing and Health Science, Nord University, Levanger, Norway
e-mail: gorill.haugan@ntnu.no, gorill.haugan@nord.no

human connectedness have shown a positive influence on patient outcomes. Thus, a shift from technical nursing toward an increased focus on patient understanding and greater patient and family involvement in ICU treatment and care is suggested. Accordingly, a holistic view including the lived experiences of ICU care from the perspectives of patients, family members, and ICU nurses is required in ICU care as well as research.

Considerable research has been devoted to long-term ICU patients' experiences from their ICU stays. However, less attention has been paid to salutogenic resources which are essential in supporting long-term ICU patients' inner strength and existential will to keep on living. A theory of salutogenic ICU nursing is highly welcome. Therefore, this chapter draws on empirical data from three large qualitative studies in the development of a tentative theory of salutogenic ICU nursing care. From the perspective of former long-term ICU patients, their family members, and ICU nurses, this chapter provides insights into how salutogenic ICU nursing care can support and facilitate ICU patients' existential will to keep on living, and thus promoting their health, survival, and well-being. In a salutogenic perspective on health, the ICU patient pathway along the ease/dis-ease continuum reveals three stages; (1) The breaking point, (2) In between, and (3) Never in my mind to

G. Haugan, M. Eriksson (eds.), *Health Promotion in Health Care – Vital Theories and Research*,
https://doi.org/10.1007/978-3-030-63135-2_18

give up. The tentative theory of salutogenic long-term ICU nursing care includes five main concepts: (1) the long-term ICU patient pathway (along the salutogenic health continuum), (2) the patient's inner strength and willpower, (3) salutogenic ICU nursing care (4), family care, and (5) pull and push. The salutogenic concepts of inner strength, meaning, connectedness, hope, willpower, and coping are of vital importance and form the essence of salutogenic long-term ICU nursing care.

Keywords

Critical care nursing · Family care · Health promotion · ICU care · Long-term ICU patient

18.1 Introduction

The main difference between patients in the intensive care unit (ICU) and other patients is that the former are severely critically ill and need advanced life-sustaining care, including mechanical ventilation. ICU patients need fundamentals of care such as keeping clean, warm, fed, hydrated, dressed, comfortable, mobile, and safe. ICU patients who need mechanical ventilation are unable to talk. They are therefore totally dependent on others, including having others interpret their symptoms and feelings. This means that advanced medical treatment and technology need to be accompanied by advanced nursing care. In this chapter, we argue for the relevance of a health promotion perspective in the care of acutely/critically ill patients. The aim of this chapter is to enhance understanding of the essence of long-term ICU care in a health promotion perspective. We build our analysis on qualitative data on former long-term ICU patients' experiences of their struggle to survive, together with the experiences of ICU nurses and patients' family members. This chapter is written from our home-offices since all universities are locked down due to the COVID-19 infec-

tion worldwide. The present Covid-19 pandemic demonstrates that a health promotion approach in the care of long-term ICU patients is ever more important in the years to come. The pathophysiology of severe viral pneumonia (as in COVID-19) is acute respiratory distress syndrome, which is associated with a prolonged ICU stay [1]. A retrospective study from the Lombardy region in Italy demonstrated that 5 weeks after the first admission to the ICU, most of the COVID-19 patients (58%) were still in the ICU showing a higher need for mechanical ventilation than other ICU patients [2]. ICU care of COVID-19 patients is challenged by isolating regimes with limited human contact. ICU nurses caring for the patients are wearing medical masks, gowns, gloves, and face shields, and visits from family members are banned [1]. From a health promotion perspective, these factors might cause stress for patients, family members, and nurses, and negatively affect the patients in the recovery process.

This chapter starts with an outline of research on long-term ICU patients. Following this, a specific nurse–patient situation with data from observations in an ICU (the story of Peter) is used to give the reader insight into the key aspects of care for the long-term ICU patient. The story runs like a thread throughout the chapter, leading the reader through the phases of ICU nursing with a focus on salutogenesis and health promotion. Our aim is to demonstrate how clinical skills are context-specific, and how these skills are manifested in a specific encounter with an individual patient. This chapter is placed in a health promotion perspective and is based in the salutogenic health theory. The chapter is divided into sections on theoretical perspectives, purpose, methodology, results, and discussion of the findings.

18.2 Background

Recent years have seen an increasing focus on the long-term consequences for ICU patients after hospital discharge. Former ICU patients may suffer from physical and mental health problems with a negative impact on quality of life and daily functioning [3]. The term post-intensive care syndrome (PICS) describes new or worsening problems in physical, cognitive, or mental health status arising after a critical illness and persisting beyond acute care hospitalization [4]. Possible mechanisms of PICS are insufficient supply of oxygen (hypoxia), treatment such as a tube is inserted into the patients' airway (endotracheal intubation), frequent use of benzodiazepines, immobilization, and interruption of the sleep-wake cycle [4]. Health promoting and rehabilitation efforts should therefore already be initiated during the ICU stay [3].

A growing evidence suggest that the ABCDEF bundle (A, assess, prevent, and manage pain; B, both awakening and spontaneous breathing trials; C, choice of analgesic and sedation; D, delirium: assess, prevent, and manage; E, early mobility and exercise; and F, family engagement and empowerment) improves ICU patient-centered outcomes and promotes interprofessional teamwork and collaboration [5, 6]. A multicenter prospective cohort study among 15,226 adults concluded that ABCDEF bundle performance showed significant and clinically meaningful improvements in outcomes including survival, mechanical ventilation use, coma, delirium, restraint-free care, and ICU readmission [7]. It was suggested that the bundle components including several elements of human connectedness (waking patients, holding their hand and patients regaining a feeling of control over actions and their consequences) had a positive influence on patient outcomes. However, these nursing interventions cannot easily be quantified; a recent Scandinavian study suggests a shift from technical nursing toward an increased focus on patient understanding, and greater patient and family involvement in ICU treatment and care [8]. Therefore, future studies could benefit from a more holistic view, including the lived experiences of ICU care from the perspectives of patients, family members, and ICU nurses.

The suggestion that patients and their family members be involved in care was first introduced by the Picker Institute in 1988. Since then, family inclusion has evolved into a model of collaboration between and among patients, families, and health care providers [9]. The guidelines for family-centered care [10] highlight the importance of future research to improve collaboration with patient and family in ICU care [10].

Although considerable research has been devoted to long-term ICU patients' experiences from their ICU stays [11], less attention has been paid to health promoting factors [12, 13] that encourage ICU patients' existential will to keep on living [14]. Knowledge of health promotion in ICU care from the perspectives of ICU patients, their family members, and ICU nurses may improve the quality and efficiency of long-term ICU care. Therefore, we suggest the need to develop a tentative theory of salutogenic ICU nursing care to describe long-term ICU care and the health promotion process of getting through the illness trajectory.

18.3 Theoretical Foundation

The choice of theoretical perspectives, models, interventions, and reflections included in this chapter are based on their usefulness for ICU nursing and health care. Further, this chapter emphasizes ICU patients' and their families' perspectives on ICU health promotion. This chapter is based on our own empirical research [14–18], as well as our extensive clinical experience in ICU nursing and nursing of the chronically ill, including palliative patients. The literature we build on is grounded in both qualitative and quantitative research. In a health promoting perspective, we draw on the salutogenic theory of Antonovsky [19–21] and the philosophy of nursing care formulated by the Norwegian nurse and philosopher Kari Martinsen [22, 23]. Additionally, this presentation was substantiated with a literature search using the terms "intensive care patients," "critical care patients," "family," "family member," "next of kin," "health promotion," "salutogenesis," and "long-term ICU care." Since we live in Norway, and have studied and worked there, our examples from clinical practice are drawn from the Norwegian context.

18.3.1 Health Promotion in the Health Care

In 1986 the World Health Organization (WHO) arranged the first international conference on Health Promotion, resulting in the Ottawa Charter. This charter defined health promotion as *"the process of enabling people to increase control over, and to improve their health,"* and identified basic strategies for health promotion. An international network of health promotion hospitals (HPH) was later established, with an aim of reorienting the hospitals in a health promoting direction. However, in order to succeed in doing so, knowledge and evidence on health promoting nursing centering on patients' health and resources were needed. Several theories of health promotion have been developed, among which the salutogenic health theory by Antonovsky [19, 24] is central. Available evidence guiding long-term ICU nursing care into a more health promoting direction is scarce. Hence, this chapter aims at developing a tentative theory of salutogenic ICU nursing care.

18.3.2 The Salutogenic Understanding of Health

Aron Antonovsky (1923–1994) challenged the conventional paradigm of pathogenesis and its dichotomous classification of persons as being either healthy or diseased [19]. He coined the concept of salutogenesis, which means the origin of health. Basically, salutogenesis—the salutogenic understanding of health and the gradually evolving salutogenic concepts—signifies knowledge about the origin of health, i.e. about what provides, facilitates, and supports health. The concept of salutogenesis has matured since 1986 and has become a core theory of health promotion [21]. From a salutogenic perspective, health is a positive concept involving social and personal resources, as well as physical capacities. Hence, the salutogenic theory of health offers a resource-oriented and strength-based perspective, i.e. a broad focus on the genesis or sources of health, as well as circumstances promoting or undermining health.

Figure 1.1 in Chap. 1 in this book illustrates how Antonovsky saw health as a movement along a continuum on a horizontal axis between health-ease (H+) and dis-ease (H−) [25]. Health promotion and salutogenic ICU nursing care intend to move the patient along this continuum toward the positive end, termed H+. According to Antonovsky, sense of coherence (SOC) is a vital health resource moving the individual toward good health. While facing stressors in life, such as, e.g., serious illness, tension appears. To avoid breakdown, and instead move along the continuum in the positive direction, the patient must cope with the tensions. A strong SOC as well as generalized resistance resources (GRRs) will help the seriously ill person to cope, to stand out with the suffering, to survive and recover. Looking at Fig. 18.1, GRRs are important to hinder breakdown and move the ICU patient along the ease/dis-ease continuum toward best possible health. The salutogenic approach to long-term ICU patients is resource-oriented and focuses on the patient's ability to manage the stressors in this specific life situation to recover and stay healthy.

The SOC and the GRR represent key concepts of the salutogenic health theory. SOC is defined as *"a global orientation that expresses the extent to which one has a pervasive, enduring through dynamic feeling of confidence that: (1) the stimuli from one's internal and external environments in the course of living are structured, predictable and explicable; (2) the resources are available to one to meet the demands posed by these stimuli; and (3) these demands are challenges, worthy of investment and engagement"* ([24], p. 19). SOC includes the three dimensions of comprehensibility, manageability, and meaningfulness (ibid.). Comprehensibility represents the cognitive aspect of SOC, including the capacity to appraise one's reality and to understand what is going on. A seriously ill ICU patient might struggle to grasp what is taking place around him. The second aspect, manageability covers an individual's instrumental and behavioral capacity to manage and cope with the situation. Coping is difficult if you do not understand what is happening with you. Finally, the meaningfulness aspect involves an individual's feelings that life makes sense emotionally, and that the present challenges are worth investing one's effort and energy in; that is, one's commitment and engagement. Meaningfulness is seen as the motivation aspect of SOC. Finding meaningfulness and thus motivation to fight for survival might be hard to the long-term ICU patient who is at "a breaking point" (Figs. 18.2 and 18.3). These three aspects of SOC—comprehensibility, manageability, and meaningfulness—are involved when an individual experiences a long-term ICU stay. As illustrated by the example of Peter down under, long-term ICU patients experience several and huge stressors, and thus much tension. The need for resistance resources is obvious. GRR represents a set of resources promoting meaningfulness, comprehensibility, and thus manageability (SOC). GRRs are present in an individual's personal capacities, but also in the immediate and distant environment [24, 26]. A strong SOC enables one to recognize, pick up, and utilize the available GRRs. Salutogenic ICU nursing care supports the patient's awareness and use of the resources available. The patient's family and the ICU nurses should perform as GRR resources during the long-term ICU stay. Specifically, close family members can help to identify and facilitate personal GRRs for their ICU patient.

Furthermore, Antonovsky understood the relationship between the two orientations of pathogenesis and salutogenesis as complementary [20]. We therefore emphasize that health promotion approaches do not imply a disregard of pathogenesis. Knowledge of pathogenesis, i.e. knowledge of disease, risk, and prevention, is important in all health disciplines, and naturally in health care, particularly in the ICU context. When people become injured or seriously ill, whether it be an accident, heart disease, lung disease, cancer, mental illness or the need for a surgical intervention, knowledge of illnesses, injuries and trauma, and their treatment, is crucial to their lives. However, instead of juxtaposing pathogenesis and salutogenesis, it is pertinent to assimilate these two paradigms into a manifestly holistic way of understanding and working with health. Health is always present, while illness and injury occur from time to time. Thus, health is the basis and the origin, and should therefore be the foundation of health care, also in the ICU. We use Peter throughout this chapter to depict the movement along the health continuum during the long-term ICU patient's pathway.

Background: Peter was in a road accident 2 days ago with complicated fractures of his back, femur and ankle. He also has serious rib fractures and bleeding in his chest cavity, requiring mechanical ventilation. Peter's bed is by the window. Over his head hangs a monitor. Right next to the head of his bed, the ventilator produces a rhythmic sound. On the monitor a graph moves, looking like a row of mountain peaks. Suddenly a lung appears at the top of the screen, and then disappears again. We can also see numbers that keep changing. Peter moves his arms and head, and suddenly a sharp sound is heard and a light flashes on the ventilator. Then it goes quiet again just as quickly. Next to the bed are infusion pumps for medication. Several chains with a hook on the end hang from a rail in the ceiling. On one of them is a photo of a man and a little child. A photo that links Peter to a life outside this room.

Peter's reflections on his stay in the ICU (comprehensibility, meaning, manageability):
I was more like a rocket that was shot up into the sky, there was lots of noise, lots of loud noises and steel, rockets are full of steel, aren't they? Then when it was going up into the sky, bits of it began to fall off and then when it reached a certain level, it stopped, and it began to fall again. It was a terribly long and tiresome trip! And on the way down, the bits of metal came back on again and then it fell to the ground. And I think … I think the connection is that the day after I arrived at the ICU, I was operated on. They put steel in my back, it was stiffened, and I heard that noise and everything that was going on, I think … I'm quite sure about that!

The family member's reflections:
There was no communication the days he was on the ventilator. So, then we just made short visits. I went in and looked at him and stroked his cheek and then I talked a bit to the nurses.

Peter is an entity of body-mind-soul who is at a breaking point: will he survive his huge injuries, or will he pass away? We do not know yet. In this early unstable phase, medical treatment is urgent. The patient needs stabilizing, organ support like mechanical ventilation and dialysis, and symptom treatment like pain relief and sedation. However, a health promotion approach also includes family members' presence and nursing care, as well as awareness toward Peter's sense of comprehensibility, manageability and meaning. How can the nurses help him to understand what is going on? How much information is he able to take? What can make him find meaningfulness, and a sense of manageability in the midst of ailments and fatigue?

While people face various life stressors, such as serious illness leading to a long-term stay in an ICU, research has shown that those who, despite the difficulties, experience meaning-in-life cope better and report more well-being than those who experience meaninglessness. Meaning is an important psychological variable that promotes well-being [27–29], protects individuals from negative outcomes [30, 31], and serves as a mediating variable in psychological health [32–36]. The concept of meaningfulness is also crucial in the salutogenic theory of health [19, 24] that focuses on health promoting resources, among which sense of coherence (SOC) is vital. Individuals with a strong SOC tend to perceive life as being manageable and believe that stressors are explicable; thus, they have confidence in their coping capacities [37]. Several studies link SOC with patient-reported and clinical outcomes such as perceived stress and coping [38], recovery from depression [37], physical and mental well-being [39, 40], and satisfying quality of life and reduced mortality [41, 42]. SOC has thus been recognized as a meaningful concept for patients with a wide variety of medical conditions.

caring situation in nursing is by nature concrete and contextual. Care has a relational, practical and moral dimension ([22], pp. 14–20). A central ontological feature of Martinsen's theoretical work is the assumption that human beings are interconnected and dependent upon each other; humans are born as relational individuals. Thus, without a relationship with a "you," there cannot be an "I." The individual can only become a living person in a relationship with a "you" [23, 43, 44]. This dependence on others must not be seen as negating independence; however, people can never understand and realize themselves alone or independently of others. Care is fundamental and natural, but also difficult because in relationships with others we are vulnerable to the other's gaze, mood, and body language. We may ignore or reject what the other is expressing. This implies that human relationships are ethical. Care is to relate to the other and to be able to recognize and respond to the patient's needs [44]. The specific encounter with the long-term ICU patient thus has a moral dimension. As nurses, we can look, and overlook.

A recent Danish study argued for the development of theory in clinical nursing to meet the needs of patients and relatives [45]. Consequently, in the present study we explore and illuminate central concepts in health promoting family-centered long-term ICU care. The focus is not on giving the actual concepts fixed meanings, but on creating a useful understanding of the shared meaning of concepts within a specific context [46]. A conceptual framework aims at prescribing broad, open-textured (structured) assumptions of how phenomena in a field are to be understood [47]. Within the framework of health promotion, we aim to articulate the values and goals of nursing by making aspects of this practice explicit and analyzing patients' needs [48].

18.3.3 Health Promoting Long-Term ICU Nursing

The theoretical perspective is based on a view of nursing as a practical discipline and on professor Kari Martinsen's philosophy of nursing care. The

18.4 Purpose

The purpose of this study was to gain a deeper understanding of the essence of long-term ICU care in a health promotion perspective. A more specific aim was to identify central salutogenic concepts in long-term ICU patients' lifeworld. From the perspective of former long-term ICU patients, their family members, and ICU nurses, this study provides insights into how salutogenic resources can be used to support and facilitate ICU patients' existential will to keep on living. Finally, we aim to propose a tentative theory of salutogenic long-term ICU nursing care.

18.5 Design and Methods

A hermeneutic phenomenological approach was applied, illuminating the meaning embraced in people's experiences and forms of expression [49, 50].

18.5.1 Settings and Sample

This study was based on three different qualitative datasets about long-term ICU patients' struggle to survive, as experienced by (1) the patients themselves, (2) their family members, and (3) ICU nurses. Data were collected from two university hospitals and two local hospitals in Norway between 2004 and 2017.

18.5.2 Data Collection

The three datasets included (1) six in-depth interviews of experienced ICU nurses before and after observations of nurse–patient interactions in mechanical ventilation, collected in 2004, (2)

interviews of ICU patients 5–14 months after ICU discharge (collected in 2012–2014), and (3) interviews of ICU patients, family members, and ICU nurses involved in long-term ICU care (collected in 2016–2017) (Table 18.1). A total of 28 long-term ICU patients, 13 family members, and 13 ICU nurses participated in the study. Further details are published elsewhere [14, 16–18].

18.5.3 Data Analysis

The datasets were handled as a whole and analyzed by the following steps: First, the authors presented and reflected on the results from the first analysis of all datasets using themes and subthemes. Second, a reflective discussion was guided by the following questions: What are the characteristics of long-term ICU patients? What is the essence of long-term ICU care and the health promotion process of getting through the illness trajectory? Third, the original empirical data were reread to identify real life examples of the health promotion process and were further interpreted as phases. Fourth, the reading of literature in the fields of lifeworld research and health promotion concepts based on salutogenic theory [20, 21] inspired further interpretation of data. Fifth, essential concepts describing the health promotion process of getting through the illness trajectory in long-term ICU care and suggested relationships among these concepts were developed [51]. The concepts were framed within

Table 18.1 Characteristics of datasets from ICU patients, family members, and ICU nurses

	Informant characteristics	Data collection	Data collection characteristics
Dataset 1	ICU nurses ($n = 3$, 2 female) >10 years ICU experience	Observations ($n = 3$) In-depth interviews ($n = 6$)	Nurse–patient interaction (24 h) Before and after observation
Dataset 2	ICU patients ($n = 11$, 4 female) Age (years) median 60 (57–72) MV (days) median 10 (6–27)	In-depth interviews ($n = 11$)	5–14 months after ICU discharge
Dataset 3	ICU patients ($n = 17$, 4 female) Age (years) median 57 (27–76) MV (days) median 10 (7–16)	In-depth interviews ($n = 17$)	6–18 months after ICU discharge
	Family members ($n = 13$, 11 female)	In-depth interviews ($n = 13$)	6–18 months after ICU discharge
	ICU nurses ($n = 13$, 9 female)	Focus group interview ($n = 3$)	

Note: ICU intensive care unit, *MV* mechanical ventilation

the salutogenic theory and the ABCDEF bundle approach [6].

18.5.4 Characteristics of the Researchers

Two authors (IA, HSH) are ICU nurses, with expertise in teaching, clinical practice, and research, while the third author (GH) is a specialist in the nursing care of chronically ill patients and end-of-life care and has published widely in health promotion research among different populations.

18.5.5 Ethical Considerations

Ethical approval was not sought, as the study is based on a secondary analysis of data from published studies.

18.6 Results

The health promotion process of getting through the illness trajectory during the ICU stay was interpreted as three overlapping phases: (1) A body at a breaking point, (2) In between, and (3) Never in my mind to give up (Table 18.2). This

Table 18.2 Essential concepts describing the process of getting through the illness trajectory from a health promotion perspective

Process H–	A body at a breaking point	In between	Never in my mind to give up	Salutogenic concepts H +
Observable signs	Unconscious, no contact	Awakening, increasing awareness	Awake and alert	Coherence
Essential concepts derived from long-term ICU patients	Exhaustion, weakness and discomfort Between life and death The patient's inner strength Living in the worst horror movie Vivid dream experiences that ignite willpower	An amorphous and boundless body existential threat Feeling trapped Tiring delusions I wasn't human Connectedness to life: Feeling alive and present	No doubts about coming back to life Meaning and purpose: Feeling valuable to somebody Practical solutions: Coping skills from previous life experiences Provocative and inspiring experiences (info/talk with doctor. Diet) Transforming gloomy weather into a sunny day	Inner strength Meaning Connectedness Hope Willpower Coping
Essential concepts derived from family members	Sitting by the bed No response—an empty gaze Breaking through Knowing the patient Trying to understand Facilitating hope			Knowing the patient Facilitating hope
Essential concepts derived from nurses	Taking responsibility Tuning in to the other person Looking for reasons (for deterioration) Allowing the body to do what it is meant to do Knowing the patient Having experience in the situation and experience over time Pulling and pushing Bearing the patient's suffering Facilitating well-being Supporting the patient where he is Acknowledging family support Using one's skills Bringing back to normal Creating a positive environment			Facilitating well-being Knowing the patient Pull and push

process is not linear, but depends upon the severity of the disease, the patient's progress and setbacks, courage and despondency, hope and despair. Inner strength [52], perceived meaning-in-life [53, 54] as well as meaningfulness [19], connectedness [55], hope [56, 57], willpower [58], and coping [59] appeared to be vital salutogenic resources for long-term ICU patients, particularly in phases 2 and 3, after the first critical phase ("A body at a breaking point"). *Knowing the patient* was important to both family members and ICU nurses. The concepts of *pull and push* used by the nurses were found to be important in all three phases and seemed to be associated with the other health promotion resources identified.

18.6.1 A Body at a Breaking Point

Observation during morning care:
The nurse speaks directly to Peter: "Please bend your foot when we turn you over." He can't do that. He's completely limp when we raise his arms and wash him. The nurse suctions the endotracheal tube before we turn the patient to prevent him coughing badly when he lies on his side during care and changing the sheets. Following the care, Peter is placed up in bed, supported with four pillows. The curtains are pulled aside to let in the light. They put a blanket over him and air the room. The nurse takes a blood gas. When she returns, he's coughing up white foamy phlegm. His face is red and sweaty, and his respiratory rate is 30 breaths per minute. We move him more over on his side as we can smell stool. Then we close the door, pull down the curtains and change his diaper. When he's put back on his back, his face is still red and sweaty, his breathing is rather superficial, and his blood pressure is rising.

Peter's reflections (comprehensibility, meaning, manageability):

The moment when I crashed, I lost consciousness. Before I woke up, three people who have been very close to me came to see me on a mountain. We were lifted together in four pillars of light into heaven—they explained to me that this life was over, and I had to choose where to live my next life! But suddenly I was in the ICU, looking down at myself for a moment, and suddenly I was inside myself again!—An extraordinary experience!

The nurse's reflections:
Although we had no contact with him yesterday, he was lying there with his eyes open and looking around. And then I use the care situation to assess him more closely. Mainly, I look at the patient, and form a mental picture of how well he is based on how he looks and feels. That's the main thing I do. Then I look at what he's getting from the ventilator, look at the monitor values and then I sometimes also take a blood gas to have some figures to lean on.

In principle, it's important for the patient to have rest periods, and it's especially important at night. There shouldn't be bright light and activity around the patient all the time. You have to find a balance, but it depends on how much there is to do around the patient. How long the care takes, if you have to change e.g. the central venous catheter, arterial catheter and the wounds. How much rest we can achieve depends on the particular situation and the individual patient. And it depends a bit on us too, how much we allow a patient to rest.

The situation reveals a sensory presence in which the nurse uses all her senses (looking, listening, touching, smelling) to assess and understand the patient's condition: *"Yesterday, his eyes were open and he was looking around"* is interpreted as a sign of health which the nurse sees as a resource to build on. The nurse's presence, attention and care are health promoting resources, supporting and facilitating the health-giving processes taking place in the patient as an entity of body-mind-spirit. The body is at a breaking point. Thus, the mind and spirit are also in a state that may be termed a "breaking point." In a health promotion perspective, the ICU nurse is aware of every sign of health (his eyes are open, looking around) on which she can build her presence, attention and care. Hence, if we adapt Fig. 1.1 in Chap. 1 to Peter's situation, it may be portrayed as in Fig. 18.1.

Figure 18.1 shows the health ease/dis-ease continuum: a huge stressor appears, and Peter's body is suddenly at a breaking point in the ICU. Peter's situation is characterized by unconsciousness, sedation, exhaustion, weakness, and discomfort, which are experiences also described in other studies as tiring delusions, feeling trapped, and being on an edge between life and death [60–62]. At this point, both pathogenesis and salutogenesis are vital perspectives and approaches in the ICU. Peter may move along the health continuum: either toward breakdown or in the positive direction. Along with medical treatment, the intensive nursing care involves facilitating the salutogenic resources embedded in Peter's situation and the context. By actively supporting and strengthening the salutogenic resources, the nurses may push Peter along the health continuum in the positive direction toward recovery and health. Based on the three datasets, we identified the following salutogenic resources: (1) connectedness to life, (2) feeling alive and present, (3) meaningfulness and purpose, (4) feeling valuable to someone, (5) practical solutions, (6) previous coping experiences, and (7) provoking and inspiring experiences [14, 16–18]. By means of creative approaches that support and enhance these salutogenic resources, Peter is pulled and pushed along the continuum, reaching the stage termed "In between."

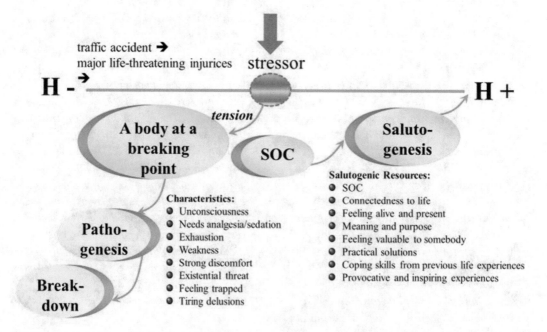

Fig. 18.1 The health ease/dis-ease continuum. (Reproduced and adapted for the ICU context with permission from Folkhälsan Research Center, Helsinki) © Gørill Haugan, 2021

18.6.2 In Between

Peter was transferred to the ICU of a local hospital, where he eventually had secretion stagnation and therefore needed mechanical ventilation again. He has had high fever and severe diarrhea. Now he is recovering and the goal is to disconnect the ventilator, extubate him and let him breathe himself.

Observation:
The doctor on duty indicates that Peter can be allowed to breathe completely on his own. The nurse disconnects him from the ventilator, mucus is suctioned from the breathing tube into a bag and the air is removed from the cuff before the breathing tube in his throat is removed. A sterile compress is applied to the hole in his throat and Peter receives oxygen via a nasal cannula. The nurse sits down by his bed and can see that he's breathing effortlessly. Then he opens his eyes and tries to focus on her. He coughs and the nurse puts her finger over the compress to prevent air leakage to enable him to cough more powerfully. Then he falls asleep again and he seems to be ok. Suddenly he wakes up, opens his eyes and turns his head.

Peter's reflections (comprehensibility, meaning, manageability):
I'm not sure, really, if it was just when I came to or if it was in the coma phase itself ... I think it was when I was coming out of the coma that I felt very nervous ... and scared, but I also felt that things had kind of worked out all right. The fact that it was a bit up and down, that might be a way of reacting when you're woken up again, I don't know, it's hard to say. ... Yes, it was just like it was very hot and it was kind of a lousy feeling to be alive, as it was so hard ... that's a bit weird.

The nurse's reflections:
He seems to have a thousand questions in his head: "My God, who, what, where?" He realizes that I'm here and falls asleep again. He's still so sick that he can't relate to what we're doing. He opens his eyes when we talk to him, but I don't think he would say "I'm cold" of his own accord unless I asked him. He's a man who's been very sick and he'll need a lot of help to get going again. Now he'll be spending most of his energy on breathing and coughing and eventually communicating.

Today when I brushed his teeth, he opened his mouth and stuck out his tongue. Peter follows what I say, or tries to. I asked if he could answer "yes" or "no", but I don't know whether what he said was yes or no. But I don't think he has the look of a person who's completely out of it. He seems to be looking at me as if he's asking: "What are you doing?" But I don't feel that he's afraid. Not now. He might be in a dream, who knows? I try to appeal to him and see if he reacts to anything. See if I can get a smile. I got one yesterday evening. I haven't had one today.

In the "In between" phase, patients were awakened and became gradually more alert. However, at the same time they often experienced their body as amorphous and boundless, and some even felt that they were not human. The patients described this phase as marked by an existential threat and a feeling of being trapped. It was like living the worst horror movie with tiring delusions. Others found that vivid experiences in dreams ignited their willpower.

The ICU nurses were close to the patients during the awakening period (In between) and provided reassurance and well-being:

I remember they were turning me, talking and asking: 'Are you lying comfortably now?' and they had gentle and mild voices. That was all nice, really. My experience was that the nurses were very clever. They were confident in their work. It seemed like they knew what they were doing, no hesitation – that made me feel very safe!

However, the relatives were obviously most important to the patients, and were the first people they remembered when they woke up; they transformed "gloomy weather into a sunny day." Family members were essential for the ICU patient to feel important and have future hopes.

I was happy every time they came. And they brought my five grandchildren from time to time, and that helps to get your spirits up too.

Although visits from family and friends were appreciated, there was a limit where the visit became burdensome. Several talked about the communication problems linked to being intubated. Others wanted someone to tell them how long it would take before they would make enough progress to move out of the ICU. Although this was not easy to predict, it would have reassured the patient if someone had talked about it and explained why they could not give a definite answer. It also seems important to find time to provide care to the patient's relatives in the form of information and advice on how to support the patient.

18.6.3 Never in My Mind to Give Up

The nurse's reflections:
Yesterday Peter was so alert that I went through what had happened with him again. Because if they're capable of thinking in a phase like that, it must be a terrible experience to wake up and not understand anything, because I'm sure he doesn't. So, I prefer to use short phrases like "It's ok" and "You're getting better". Maybe you saw it today too: it's hard to tell if he's trying to say something or if he's trying to swallow. And to make sure he doesn't panic, I emphasized that he has a voice and that he'll get it back and everything will be the way it was before.

Peter's reflections (comprehensibility, meaning, manageability):
The doctor told me to try to scratch my nose and I couldn't do it, only got half-way up with my index finger, I didn't have the strength. Not a single muscle in my body was working then... I probably thought it was a lot easier than it was. Like if I just had a few more days, I could just get on my feet again and get a walker, but in fact it wasn't that easy … There was nothing else in my head except to get up on my feet and be active again, that was all I thought about! ... I had good care and I was looked after properly by competent people, so I felt reassured that I was getting the best treatment you could get.

It was the progress I was making all the time ... and the words of the nurse: "When you finally turn the corner, you'll really notice it and then things will really start to move", and that's what happened. Once I started to make progress, the first thing was stand in front of the bed for 20 seconds, then one step forward and one back and then I could take two steps forward and then I could walk round the room, and then finally I could walk by myself with the walker. So, it was the progress all the time that gave me the courage and motivation to make a bit more effort.

Clearly, disease and illness are more prominent than *well-being* among ICU patients. At the same time, both clinicians and relatives are striving for and looking (consciously or unconsciously) for signs of well-being in the patient. Our data also showed that many patients, despite serious illness, experience inner strength, meaning, comprehensibility, manageability, connectedness, hope, and willpower. The most important aspect of this phase from the patient's point of view was that the salutogenic forces were not distrusted or contradicted (by nurses wishing to present the reality), even though the patient's hopes, meanings and comprehensibility may have seemed completely unrealistic to doctors and nurses.

Most ICU patients felt safe, grateful, and satisfied with nurses and physicians. However, some experienced a lack of respect and understanding of their situation and too little information about things that were obvious to the staff, but not to the patient. Despite exhaustion, weakness and discomfort, most patients expressed no doubts about coming back to life. Their daily life in the ICU was both challenging and monotonous and one way to cope with it all was to dream about one's future life.

18.6.3.1   How Do Family Members Support Patients?

For relatives it was important to be with the patient. Sitting close to a loved one was a burden for many of them, but they still wanted to be there. Family members described a specific sensitivity for the patient's body language and needs, and for what was meaningful in the situation.

I had to keep an eye on things a bit. I don't know anything about the medical stuff, about nursing and so on and what it takes to get him healthy, but I felt I had to be there anyway to ... make sure he didn't miss anything. ... and then I had to do what I could to help him get better, putting skin cream on his legs when they were dry and so on. There wasn't much I could do, but I do know he was pleased I was there!
And because Mom was producing a lot of mucus and she was on the ventilator for so long, they gave her a tracheostomy. And it was very difficult for Mom when she woke up that she had no voice. So, we had to explain that repeatedly.

The presence of family members was important because they could look ahead and encourage the patient by saying that this was something they would cope with together. Relatives knew what motivated the patient, such as family, a pet, a soccer game on television or talking about going hunting again. They could motivate and push the patient by saying: *"If you're going to get out of here, you have to keep going even though it's hard."*

The patient's experience of the presence of relatives was described as follows:

I could recognize her smell, I knew it. And she has a special way of doing things, in a way only she

does, my brain managed to register that. It was very good for me. Small impulses that give me a good feeling ... like stroking my cheek. I didn't hear any voices, just felt that touch!
I remember the visits made me very tired. But when my wife came, it was like I'd had gloomy weather for a long time and then suddenly there was a sunny day! You see? This happened every time she arrived!

18.6.3.2   How Do ICU Nurses Support Patients?

The nurses supported the patients by taking responsibility for both patients and visiting family members. The ability to "tune in" to the patient was important and was expressed through attention and sensitivity to the patient's body language:

I don't know if there's anything we do subconsciously ... if we give the impression that we've given up or not? It's kind of scary to think about ... whether they can feel that we believe they'll pull through or not. We had a patient who said that everyone had kind of given up hope for her ... and she'd understood a lot of what was said. Afterwards, she said to the nurse who had said she would recover: 'You were the one with the kind hands'. And then I thought: Is it possible, really? Do we convey things without realizing it?

In this case, the way the ICU nurse provided reassurance and well-being helped to promote the patient's willpower to fight for recovery. The following case underlines the importance of knowing the patient:

Of course, we can often tell when the patient's at the turning point. When you do familiar things like morning care and talk about everyday life, their children and their family, the dog for example, well then you make contact that may be good for the patient and help prevent delirium. Familiar things and loved ones are important to motivate patients to move forward. I think it's important that it's the same nurses who come back, so you can build on what we achieved yesterday, that has a positive effect. And that you have contact with the patient, that good relationship is very important. My daughter once said: 'Oh, do you need to put on makeup before you go to work?' I answered: 'Well yes, because today I'm almost the only person the patient's going to see.' Not that it makes any difference, but ... we should believe in things for them many times, and we must push them. Some of them often don't want to get up. And precisely that step of getting out of bed and into a chair seems quite out of the question when you've been in bed for weeks and can't even lift your finger. But then we need to believe on their behalf: 'Yes, but this is something we've got to do … I understand you don't want to, but it's for your own good.' Because we see that many times… we have to put in much more effort than they can manage themselves.

Knowing the patient seems important to create meaning. The good relationship and the nurse's efforts in transferring belief and hope to the patient provided support in the rehabilitation process during the illness trajectory.

The above examples may be said to describe model cases. But nurses have also experienced actions that did not go according to plan. One experienced ICU nurse talked about a patient who was a well-known pianist:

Sometimes you think … I'm sure this will be ok! … I remember once when I had a patient called Geir, who had been on the ventilator for a very long time, he was very depressed and heavy-hearted… and eventually he got a tracheostomy. Then I could take him around in a wheelchair, with his oxygen bottle and bag. I thought: he was a very well-known pianist, if I go round past the switchboard … there's a piano there … then I can wheel him there … then he can play! Music was his whole life! But

it was just a big disappointment, because Geir couldn't control his fingers properly. What I thought would be a great motivating factor … it didn't really work out too well.

That was a borderline case where the nurse tried to use the patient's potential health-promoting resources. She regarded him as more than "just a patient," realized his personal qualities and put in an extra effort to help him to "light the spark of life." The patient was probably just as disappointed as she was, despite her good intentions and dedication. Oscillation between success and failure was typical of not only long-term ICU patients but also their nurses and their relatives.

18.6.3.3   Summing Up

Based on the three datasets from long-term ICU patients, their family members, and experienced ICU nurses, three stations along the ease/disease continuum were identified: (1) The breaking point, (2) In between, and (3) Never in my mind to give up. Figure 18.2 portrays the health continuum, illustrating the three different stages along the pathway toward survival and health. Here we see how the ICU nurses make great efforts to relieve Peter's ailments, such as pain, exhaus-

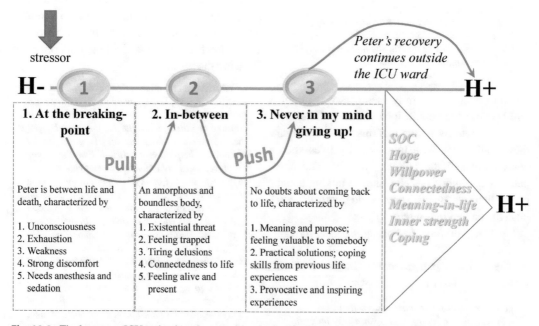

Fig. 18.2 The long-term ICU patient's trajectory along the health disease/ease continuum. © Haugan, 2021

tion, and tiring delusions. Using the identified salutogenic resources, the nurses and Peter's family members are gently pulling and pushing him in the positive direction, toward survival and functioning.

18.7 Discussion

The aim of this study was to enhance understanding of the essence of long-term ICU care in a health promotion perspective. This means that nurses can be both generalized and specific resistance resources against the stress caused by ICU care. Further, they enable patients to find meaningfulness and gain control over their life situation. From the perspectives of former long-term ICU patients, their family members, and ICU nurses, this study provides insights into how salutogenic resources can be used to support and facilitate ICU patients' existential will to keep on living. The salutogenic concepts of inner strength, meaning, connectedness, hope, willpower, and coping are central and form part of the essence of salutogenic long-term ICU care. Below we will discuss the benefit of ICU nurses using a health promotion perspective to support care based on the ABCDEF bundle in relation to a tentative theory of salutogenic long-term ICU nursing care.

18.7.1 The ABCDEF Bundle, Health Promotion, and the Missing Salutogenic "G"

Although intensive care has made great strides in recent years [4], patients and their relatives may experience discomfort and mental and physical health symptoms as a result of examinations, treatment, and the way clinicians relate to them [5, 63]. According to Ely [5], this may partly be due to an ICU culture where physicians and nurses have focused strongly on the technical aspects of patient care at the expense of patients' dignity, self-respect and identity: "The most productive aspect of the philosophy of ICU liberation for us as clinicians is that it

shifts our focus from the monitors, beeps, and buzzers to a human connection" ([5], p. 327). In recent years, international research has therefore called for a shift in ICU culture from heavy sedation and the use of restraint to more open units with patients who are more alert and active [5], and where relatives are given a more active role in patient care [63].

After the patient is stabilized, evidence-based measures in the form of the ABCDEF bundle are recommended. "The ABCDEF bundle is a tool to promote the assessment, prevention, and integrated management of pain, agitation, and delirium, while also facilitating weaning from mechanical ventilation and maximizing early mobility and exercise and family engagement and empowerment" [6]. This bundle is an international framework aiming at flexibility and the incorporation of new evidence-based recommendations. Although an important goal of intensive care is to reduce pain, anxiety and ICU delirium threatening the patient's dignity and self-respect, it appears difficult to achieve this in practice [5]. Ely argues that the ABCDEF bundle is not a cookbook recipe, but requires lasting changes bedside, where the implementation process must include both philosophy and culture ([5], p. 326). Important barriers to ABCDEF bundle compliance are; patient safety, lack of knowledge, workload, turnover (clinicians and managers), poor staff morale, and lack of respect between the professional groups involved in implementing the bundle [6].

In the ICU, points B and E are emphasized as particularly important, meaning that the patient receives pain relief, has minimum or no sedation, and is mobilized despite still being on mechanical ventilation ([5], p. 325). However, our study shows the importance of providing good clinical nursing, the missing salutogenic "G," where ICU nurses know the patient, include the family (F) and know which salutogenic resources are important to long-term ICU patients. This is, however, often underestimated as a health promotion factor in the ABCDEF bundle. The ICU nurse's skills in tuning in to the needs of the patient and relatives and in focusing on salutary factors are regarded as important generalized resistance resources (GRR) that can strengthen patients' SOC and resilience at the physical, psychological, and spiritual levels ([21, 64], p. 289).

18.7.2 A Tentative Theory of Salutogenic ICU Nursing Care

The tentative theory [65] of ICU nursing care has five main concepts: (1) the long-term ICU patient pathway, (2) the patient's inner strength and willpower, (3) salutogenic ICU nursing care, (4) family care, and (5) pull and push. In Fig. 18.3 we suggest a structure of the phenomenon that includes essential concepts describing the health promotion process of long-term ICU care and suggested relationships among the concepts. The concepts of the tentative theory, shown in Fig. 18.3, indicate that the patient goes through three stages (The breaking point, In between, and Never in my mind to give up), and can potentially experience inner strength and willpower in all the stages. Family care and nursing care represent key salutogenic resources for the patient's trajectory. The salutogenic resources are linked

to the concept of pull and push factors. Pull factors help/entice the patient toward an existential "here" (connectedness, meaning, well-being) to enable nurses and relatives to gradually push (encourage) the patient in the continued ICU trajectory.

18.7.3 The Long-Term ICU Patient Pathway: SOC and GRRs

The SOC and GRRs are key concepts that are interrelated in the salutogenic model. But how can we understand the SOC and the salutogenic concept of manageability in ICU patients where fatigue and serious illness requiring life support mean that their bodies are dependent on and connected to ventilators and invasive catheters? What is the relevance of the salutogenic concepts of "meaning" and "comprehensibility" for patients who are totally exhausted and sometimes hallucinating, having experiences of travelling, flying, standing upside down and not knowing where their body begins and ends? For many intensive care patients, these are frightening experiences that are not "comprehensible"

Salutogenic Resources for moving the ICU-patient along the health continuum

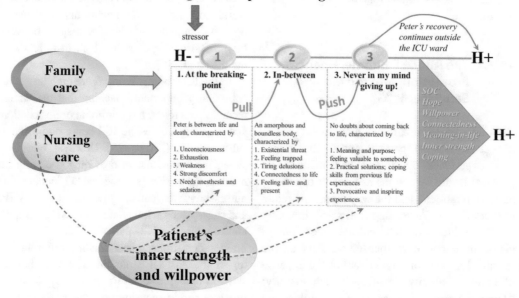

Fig. 18.3 The salutogenic concepts of salutogenic long-term ICU nursing care. © Haugan, 2021

and have no "meaning." Some patients deal with the situation by withdrawing into themselves, while others become very agitated, fight against the ventilator, pull the endotracheal tube and want to get out of bed at the risk of disconnecting vital equipment. In such situations, it is common in many countries to tie patients down [66] and/or use sedatives [67]. Both measures are debated, because they are considered as abuse and because they make patients passive and thus prolong ventilation, leading to an increased risk of complications [68].

Below, we argue that both family members and nurses represent important salutogenic resources to support and facilitate manageability, meaningfulness and comprehensibility to help patients through their stay in the ICU. But firstly, we will show that, despite their disease, delusions, exhaustion, and fatigue, long-term ICU patients have important salutogenic resources (GRRs) themselves.

18.7.4 Patients' Inner Strength and Willpower

Previous studies have shown experiences on the borders of consciousness to be filled with personal meaning as well as healing potential [60–62]. In the present study, long-term ICU patients also told about experiences at the borders of unconsciousness that represented both personal meaning and vitalizing energy. They experienced meeting deceased relatives in their dreams or delusions. Initially, the ICU patients perceived the meeting as if the deceased relatives had come to fetch them, which was felt to be liberating. But without verbal communication, they immediately understood this as a message that seemed to represent a turning point at which the patients were pushed to make a choice about life and death, and an experience of, after all, having inner strength and willpower to go on living. This salutogenic perspective of the ICU patients' dreams and delusions as having healing potential represents a complementary view to the pathogenic perspective that interprets delusional experiences as a symptom of ICU delirium [69].

18.7.5 Salutogenic ICU Nursing Care

Nursing care is to be concrete and present in a relationship where nurses use their senses and bodies. This implies that nurses direct attention away from themselves and toward patients in such a way that patients receive help, feel respected, and enabled to become participants in their own lives.

ICU nurses have close contact with their patients, and in Norway they are responsible for the practical everyday care of patients. Practical nursing, including everyday personal hygiene, provides ample opportunity for clinical observations and for the nurse to assess and respond to changes in the patient's situation. In the close care relationship lies the potential to get to know the patient and build trust. Trust can be built by looking attentively at the patient, being sensitive to the patient's body language and by handling the patient gently and correctly. From the perspective of the phenomenology of the body [70], this involves "pulling" the patient to an existential "here," by the nurse creating a situation where the patient can experience connectedness and meaning in meaninglessness (cf. "gentle hands" and the patient's feeling of hope).

Nurses are recommended to design interventions to enhance the SOC in early phases of hospitalization for patients [64]. Losing the feeling of one's own body is common among ICU patients, as in the story about Peter. "Without" a body, finding meaningfulness in life might prove difficult. The nurse's touch can help the patient to realize the limits of where the body begins and where it ends. Further, in personal hygiene situations it is important that the nurse includes the patient and encourages the use of the body again such as in brushing teeth and assists the patient with body movements (cf. "meaningfulness" and "comprehensibility" in the story about Peter). For the patient who is bedridden and attached to equipment, it provides hope and meaning to feel the floor under one's feet. The nurse can "ground" patients by helping them to sit on the edge of the bed with their feet on the floor, or by offering patients the use of a bed bike so that they can feel resistance in their legs and perform familiar bodily movements, cf. "manageability." It seems important to let the body do what it is meant to do (Table 18.2). Anything familiar seems health promoting, whether it be a familiar sound, smell, voice, touch, movement, or presence. Allowing for patient participation to help patients perceive life as comprehensive, manageable and meaningful is central in salutogenic ICU nursing care [21, 71]. Building a relationship with the patient and thereby gaining insight into the patient's dreams and future plans (impacting meaningfulness, hope, and willpower) can be health-promoting when the nurse encourages patients and helps them to keep those dreams alive through the challenges of gradual rehabilitation, such as mobilization and ventilator weaning.

Since early 1990s, nurses in Norway started writing diaries for ICU patients to offer patients a tool for processing memories of their ICU stay [72]. Diaries are valuable for both patients and their family members [73] and were in a methasynthesis found to decrease anxiety and depression and improve health-related quality of life among ICU survivors [74]. One explanation might be that the diary has the potential to give a better understanding of the ICU period by providing an opportunity for discovery of meaning in experiences and memories. Finding existential meaning seems to be of decisive significance for how far people reach in their lives after having lived through intensive care treatment [80].

18.7.6 Family Care

The present study illuminates how family members are key to the patient's breakthrough because their actions are tailored to the patient's specific personality as well as the patient's lifeworld [17]. The presence of family members helps to awaken and release the patient's inner strength, which has the potential of providing a turning point and breakthrough to life. In the perspective of the body as interpretive and meaningful [70], also at the breaking point between life and death, the

ICU patient might sense the situation to be more comprehensible, manageable and meaningful in the presence of family members.

The presence of a family member means that the patient hears a familiar voice, smells a scent that evokes pleasant memories and feels a familiar hand. Such experiences are resources that can embolden the patient ([44], p. 174) and thus stimulate the patient's inner strength and will to survive. Familiar faces, voices and smells, and a familiar and gentle hand, can help to reassure the patient and make the situation more manageable. The presence of family members provides comprehensibility through their behavior: their forms of communication and their recognition, interpretation, and acknowledgement of the patient's body language.

A meta-analytic review shows that people with stronger social relationships have a 50% greater likelihood of survival than those who have weaker social relationships [75]. In the cross-disciplinary field of psycho-neuro-endocrine-immunology, interaction has been found between biological, genetic, and environmental factors [76]. Studies show that one impact of close relationships on health is through inflammatory response [77]. When people are ill, it is hypothesized that the risk for mortality increases substantially when they lack social support [78]. The importance of social contact is not easy to quantify, but a study of cardiac patients showed that social support reduced the negative effects of stress on their mental and physical well-being [79]. Flexible visiting hours for relatives in ICUs appear to reduce delirium and symptoms of anxiety among patients and increase family member satisfaction [80]. In summary, being socially connected affects psychological and emotional well-being, and has a significant positive effect on physical well-being and survival [78]. ICU nurses thus have an important part to play in including relatives and facilitating their presence in the ICU.

18.7.7 Pull and Push

When the patient is "at breaking point" between life and death, the relationship to family members is important. Knowing the patient was essential to understand what she or he was trying to express [17]. Pull factors involve linking the patient to an existential "here" (connectedness, meaning, well-being), which will enable nurses and relatives to gradually push (encourage) the patient to progress in the ICU trajectory. This study shows that nurse–patient interaction based on the ICU nurse's attunement and sensing can help to provide an understanding of the patient's situation, by acknowledging the patient through eye contact, gentle touch and telling news from home.

18.8 Limitations

How can we determine whether the description of the phenomenon of health promotion in long-term ICU nursing care is valid and relevant? Nurse and professor Karin Dahlberg [49] states that an essence or structure is what constitutes a phenomenon. She uses the horse as an example and asks: What makes a horse a horse, and not a donkey or a mule? Although horses may be large or small and be of many different colors, there is something essential about the horse that makes us immediately realize that a particular animal is a horse. A phenomenon is not mysterious or hidden, but something we immediately see and understand. Essence is not something we add to research; it is not the researcher who makes the phenomenon meaningful. The essence is already there, in the intentional relationship between us and the phenomenon, between nurse and patient, between patient and relatives ([49], p. 249).

In this chapter, therefore, we have focused on presenting descriptions containing various nuances and aspects from the ICU context. The starting point has been the particular and the concrete. Since every phenomenon is related to everything else in the world, it is sometimes difficult to see the specific phenomenon one is looking for. Dahlberg refers to Merleau-Ponty [70] in stating that all phenomena and meanings are interconnected and that it can be difficult to see where one phenomenon ends, and another begins. To return to the horse: although the variety of horses is end-less, there is a kind of model that sets a limit, an essence that says that this is a horse and not a mule. It is a general form, an essential meaning or essence that makes the phenomenon what it is. If the essential meaning changes, it is another phenomenon [49]. Many clinicians already know the essence of long-term ICU nursing care, and how a health promotion approach is already an integral part of the ICU context. For this reason, many ICU nurses can identify factors of particular importance to patients and take appropriate health-promoting measures. For others, such as intensive care students and less experienced ICU nurses, the theoretical analysis and tentative theory in this chapter may lead to reflection on their role and enable them to view their practice in a new light.

A potential weakness of this study is that we as researchers and ICU nurses belong to the same world as the phenomenon we have explored. Consequently, it can be difficult to separate the phenomenon from its context, but also to separate ourselves from the phenomenon. Using phenomenological reduction, which Dahlberg calls "bridling," we have employed critical reflection to discuss "what we take for granted," such as our clinical experience and our theoretical perspective.

A potential strength of this study is that a health promotion approach in ICU nursing is in line with the new paradigm in ICU care where the trend is toward a greater number of awake patients [81–83], with minimal or no sedation [84]. This will further challenge interaction and communication with patients [85]. With the aim of helping patients through the ICU stay, we thus consider it a strength that our empirical data include the voices of the patient, relatives and ICU nurses.

18.9 Conclusion

Few patients are as helpless and totally dependent on nursing as ICU patients. How the ICU nurse relates to the patient is of vital importance to the patient, both mentally and physically. Even if nurses provide evidence-based care in the form of minimum sedation, early mobilization and attempts at spontaneous breathing during weaning, the patient may not have the strength, courage and willpower to comply. From the perspective of former long-term ICU patients, their family members and ICU nurses, this study provides insights into how salutogenic resources can be used to support and facilitate ICU patients' existential will to keep on living. The salutogenic concepts of inner strength, meaning, connectedness, hope, willpower and coping are of vital importance and form part of the essence of salutogenic long-term ICU nursing. The ICU nurse has independent responsibility to include family members in care and thus plays a key role in coordinating and implementing evidence-based measures for patients in a health promotion perspective.

The tentative theory of salutogenic long-term ICU nursing care presented here has five main concepts: (1) the long-term ICU patient pathway, (2) the patient's inner strength and willpower, (3) salutogenic ICU nursing care, (4) family care, and (5) pull and push. These concepts show that the patient goes through three stages (The breaking point, In between, and Never in my mind to give up), in all of which the patient potentially experiences inner strength and willpower. Family care and nursing care represent vital salutogenic resources for the patient, and a key concept related to these resources is that of "pull and push." Pull factors involve facilitating/enticing/linking the patient to an existential "here" (connectedness, meaning, well-being), which will enable nurses and relatives to gradually push (encourage) the patient to progress in the ICU trajectory.

This tentative theory can be used to reflect on one's own clinical practice, and in teaching intensive care students and in research.

Take Home Messages

- ICU patients who need mechanical ventilation are unable to talk and need fundamentals of nursing care. They are therefore totally dependent on others, including having others interpret their symptoms and feelings. This means that advanced medical treatment and technology need to be accompanied by advanced nursing care.

- There is growing evidence to suggest that the ABCDEF bundle (A, assess, prevent, and manage pain; B, both awakening and spontaneous breathing trials; C, choice of analgesic and sedation; D, delirium: assess, prevent, and manage; E, early mobility and exercise; and F, family engagement and empowerment) improves ICU patient-centered outcomes and promotes interprofessional teamwork and collaboration. However, this chapter entails that the bundle misses the salutogenic "G."

- This chapter shows the importance of salutogenic ICU nursing care, termed "the missing G," where ICU nurses know the patient, include the family, and uses salutogenic resources to promote long-term ICU patients' inner strength, health, survival, and well-being.

- The ICU nurse's skills in tuning in to the needs of the patient and relatives and in focusing on salutary factors represent vital generalized resistance resources (GRR) that can strengthen patients' SOC, resilience and well-being physically, psychologically, and spiritually.

- A shift from technical nursing toward an increased focus on patient understanding, and greater patient and family involvement in ICU treatment and care is needed.

- This chapter is based on the three datasets from long-term ICU patients, their family members and experienced ICU nurses, and three stations along the ease/dis-ease continuum were identified: (1) The breaking point, (2) In between, and (3) Never in my mind to give up.

- The tentative theory of salutogenic long-term ICU nursing care includes five main concepts: (1) the long-term ICU patient pathway, (2) the patient's inner strength and willpower, (3) salutogenic ICU nursing care, (4) family care, and (5) pull and push. These concepts demonstrate that the long-term ICU patient goes through the three stages (The breaking point, In between, and Never in my mind to give up), during which the patient potentially experiences inner strength and willpower.

- Family care and nursing care represent vital salutogenic resources for the patient, and a key concept related to these resources is that of "pull and push." Pull factors involve facilitating/enticing/linking the patient to an existential "here" (connectedness, meaning, well-being), which will enable nurses and relatives to gradually push (encourage) the patient to progress in the ICU trajectory.
- The salutogenic concepts of inner strength, meaning, connectedness, hope, willpower, and coping are the central essences of salutogenic long-term ICU care.

References

1. Phua J, Weng L, Ling L, Egi M, Lim CM, Divatia JV, et al. Intensive care management of coronavirus disease 2019 (COVID-19): challenges and recommendations. Lancet Respir Med. 2020;8(5):506–17. https://doi.org/10.1016/S2213-2600(20)30161-2.
2. Grasselli G, Zangrillo A, Zanella A, Antonelli M, Cabrini L, Castelli A, et al. Baseline characteristics and outcomes of 1591 patients infected with SARS-CoV-2 admitted to ICUs of the Lombardy Region, Italy. JAMA. 2020;323(16):1574–81.
3. Mehlhorn J, Freytag A, Schmidt K, Brunkhorst FM, Graf J, Troitzsch U, et al. Rehabilitation interventions for postintensive care syndrome: a systematic review. Crit Care Med. 2014;42(5):1263–71. https://doi.org/10.1097/CCM.0000000000000148.
4. Needham DM, Davidson J, Cohen H, Hopkins RO, Weinert C, Wunsch H, et al. Improving long-term outcomes after discharge from intensive care unit: report from a stakeholders' conference. Crit Care Med. 2012;40(2):502–9. https://doi.org/10.1097/CCM.0b013e318232da75.
5. Ely EW. The ABCDEF bundle: science and philosophy of how ICU liberation serves patients and families. Crit Care Med. 2017;45(2):321–30. https://doi.org/10.1097/CCM.0000000000002175.
6. Stollings JL, Devlin JW, Pun BT, Puntillo KA, Kelly T, Hargett KD, et al. Implementing the ABCDEF bundle: top 8 questions asked during the ICU liberation ABCDEF bundle improvement collaborative. Crit Care Nurse. 2019;39(1):36–45. https://doi.org/10.4037/ccn2019981.
7. Pun BT, Balas MC, Barnes-Daly MA, Thompson JL, Aldrich JM, Barr J, et al. Caring for critically ill patients with the ABCDEF bundle: results of the ICU liberation collaborative in over 15,000 adults. Crit Care Med. 2019;47(1):3–14. https://doi.org/10.1097/CCM.0000000000003482.
8. Egerod I, Kaldan G, Lindahl B, Hansen BS, Jensen JF, Collet MO, et al. Trends and recommendations for critical care nursing research in the Nordic countries: triangulation of review and survey data. Intensive Crit Care Nurs. 2019;56:102765. https://doi.org/10.1016/j.iccn.2019.102765.
9. Ciufo D, Hader R, Holly C. A comprehensive systematic review of visitation models in adult critical care units within the context of patient- and family-centred care. Int J Evid Based Healthc. 2011;9(4):362–87. https://doi.org/10.1111/j.1744-1609.2011.00229.x.
10. Davidson JE, Aslakson RA, Long AC, Puntillo KA, Kross EK, Hart J, et al. Guidelines for family-centered care in the neonatal, pediatric, and adult ICU. Crit Care Med. 2017;45(1):103–28. https://doi.org/10.1097/CCM.0000000000002169.
11. Parker AM, Sricharoenchai T, Raparla S, Schneck KW, Bienvenu OJ, Needham DM. Posttraumatic stress disorder in critical illness survivors: a meta-analysis. Crit Care Med. 2015;43(5):1121–9. https://doi.org/10.1097/CCM.0000000000000882.
12. Al-Mutair AS, Plummer V, O'Brien A, Clerehan R. Family needs and involvement in the intensive care unit: a literature review. J Clin Nurs. 2013;22(13–14):1805–17. https://doi.org/10.1111/jocn.12065.
13. Eriksson M, Lindstrom B. Antonovsky's sense of coherence scale and the relation with health: a systematic review. J EpidemiolCommunity Health. 2006;60(5):376–81.
14. Alexandersen I, Stjern B, Eide R, Haugdahl HS, Engan Paulsby T, Borgen Lund S, Haugan G. "Never in my mind to give up!" A qualitative study of long-term intensive care patients' inner strength and willpower-promoting and challenging aspects. J Clin Nurs. 2019;28(21–22):3991–4003. https://doi.org/10.1111/jocn.14980.
15. Haugdahl HS. Mechanical ventilation and weaning: roles and competencies of intensive care nurses and patients' experiences of breathing. Doctoral thesis. UiT The Arctic University of Norway; 2016.
16. Haugdahl HS, Dahlberg H, Klepstad P, Storli SL. The breath of life. Patients' experiences of breathing during and after mechanical ventilation. Intens Crit Care Nurs. 2017;40:85–93. https://doi.org/10.1016/j.iccn.2017.01.007.
17. Haugdahl HS, Eide R, Alexandersen I, Paulsby TE, Stjern B, Lund SB, Haugan G. From breaking point to breakthrough during the ICU stay: a qualitative study of family members' experiences of long-term intensive care patients' pathways towards survival. J Clin Nurs. 2018;27(19–20):3630–40. https://doi.org/10.1111/jocn.14523.
18. Haugdahl HS, Storli SL. 'In a way, you have to pull the patient out of that state ...': the competency of ventilator weaning. Nurs Inq. 2012;19(3):238–46.
19. Antonovsky A. Health, stress, and coping. San Fransisco: Jossey-Bass; 1979.
20. Antonovsky A. The salutogenic model as a theory to guide health promotion. Health Promot Int. 1996;11(1):11–8.

21. Mittelmark MB, Sagy S, Eriksson M, Bauer GF, Pelikan JM, Lindström B, Espnes GA. The handbook of salutogenesis. Berlin: Springer; 2017.
22. Martinsen K. Omsorg, sykepleie og medisin: historisk-filosofiske essays [Care, nursing and medicine]. Oslo: TANO; 1989.
23. Martinsen K. Care and vulnerability, vol. 1. Oslo: Akribe; 2006.
24. Antonovsky A. Unraveling the mystery of health: how people manage stress and stay well. San Fransisco: Jossey-Bass; 1987.
25. Lindström B, Eriksson M. The Hitchhiker's guide to salutogenesis: salutogenic pathways to health promotion. Helsinki: Folkhälsan Research Centre; 2010.
26. Idan O, Eriksson M, Al-Yagon M. The salutogenic model: the role of generalized resistance resources. In: Mittelmark MB, Sagy S, Eriksson M, Bauer GF, Pelikan JM, Lindström B, et al., editors. The handbook of salutogenesis. Cham: Springer International Publishing AG; 2017. p. 57–70.
27. Bonebright CA, Clay DL, Ankenmann RD. The relationship of workaholism with work–life conflict, life satisfaction, and purpose in life. J Couns Psychol. 2000;47(4):469.
28. Fry P. The unique contribution of key existential factors to the prediction of psychological well-being of older adults following spousal loss. Gerontologist. 2001;41(1):69–81.
29. Melton AM, Schulenberg S. On the measurement of meaning: logotherapy's empirical contributions to humanistic psychology. Humanist Psychol. 2008;36(1):31–44.
30. Haugan G. Meaning-in-life in nursing-home patients: a valuable approach for enhancing psychological and physical well-being? J Clin Nurs. 2014;23(13–14):1830–44. https://doi.org/10.1111/jocn.12402.
31. Pearson PR, Sheffield B. Psychoticism and purpose in life. Pers Individ Diff. 1989;10(12):1321–2.
32. Chan DW. Orientations to happiness and subjective well-being among Chinese prospective and in-service teachers in Hong Kong. Educ Psychol Rev. 2009;29(2):139–51.
33. Halama P, Dedová M. Meaning in life and hope as predictors of positive mental health: do they explain residual variance not predicted by personality traits? Stud Psychol. 2007;49(3):191.
34. Ho MY, Cheung FM, Cheung SF. The role of meaning in life and optimism in promoting Well-being. Pers Individ Diff. 2010;48(5):658–63.
35. Holahan CK, Holahan CJ, Suzuki R. Purposiveness, physical activity, and perceived health in cardiac patients. Disabil Rehabil Literature. 2008;30(23):1772–8.
36. Kleftaras G, Psarra E. Meaning in life, psychological well-being and depressive symptomatology: a comparative study. Psychol Health. 2012;3(4):337.
37. Skärsäter I, Rayens MK, Peden A, Hall L, Zhang M, Ågren H, Prochazka H. Sense of coherence and recovery from major depression: a 4-year follow-up. Arch Psychiatr Nurs. 2009;23(2):119–27.

38. Zirke N, Schmid G, Mazurek B, Klapp BF, Rauchfuss M. Antonovsky's sense of coherence in psychosomatic patients-a contribution to construct validation. Psychosoc Med. 2007;4:Doc03.
39. Li W, Leonhart R, Schaefert R, Zhao X, Zhang L, Wei J, et al. Sense of coherence contributes to physical and mental health in general hospital patients in China. Psychol Health Med. 2015;20(5):614–22. https://doi.org/10.1080/13548506.2014.952644.
40. Nygren B, Alex L, Jonsen E, Gustafson Y, Norberg A, Lundman B. Resilience, sense of coherence, purpose in life and self-transcendence in relation to perceived physical and mental health among the oldest old. Aging Ment Health. 2005;9(4):354–62. https://doi.org/10.1080/1360500114415.
41. Eriksson M, Lindström B. Antonovsky's sense of coherence scale and its relation with quality of life: a systematic review. J Epidemiol Community Health. 2007;61(11):938–44.
42. Surtees P, Wainwright N, Luben R, Khaw K-T, Day N. Sense of coherence and mortality in men and women in the EPIC-Norfolk United Kingdom prospective cohort study. Am J Epidemiol. 2003;158(12):1202–9.
43. Buber M. On intersubjectivity and cultural creativity. Chicago: University of Chicago Press; 1992.
44. Martinsen K. Fra Marx til Løgstrup. Om etikk og sanselighet i sykepleien [From Marx to Løgstrup]: TANO A.S.; 1993.
45. Hoeck B, Delmar C. Theoretical development in the context of nursing-the hidden epistemology of nursing theory. Nurs Philos. 2018;19(1) https://doi.org/10.1111/nup.12196.
46. Duncan C, Cloutier JD, Bailey PH. Concept analysis: the importance of differentiating the ontological focus. J Adv Nurs. 2007;58(3):293–300. https://doi.org/10.1111/j.1365-2648.2007.04277.x.
47. Mikkelsen KB, Delmar C, Sørensen EE. Fundamentals of care in time-limited encounters: exploring strategies that can be used to support establishing a nurse-patient relationship in time-limited encounters. J Nurs Stud Patient Care. 2019;1:8–16.
48. Risjord M. Nursing knowledge. Science, practice, and philosophy. London: Wiley-Blackwell; 2010.
49. Dahlberg K, Dahlberg H, Nyström M. Reflective lifeworld research. Lund: Studentlitteratur; 2008.
50. Van Manen M. Phenomenology of practice : meaning-giving methods in phenomenological research and writing, vol. 13. Walnut Creek: Left Coast Press; 2014.
51. Smith MJ, Liehr PR. Middle range theory for nursing. Berlin: Springer; 2018.
52. Lundman B, Alex L, Jonsen E, Norberg A, Nygren B, Santamaki Fischer R, Strandberg G. Inner strength—a theoretical analysis of salutogenic concepts. Int J Nurs Stud. 2010;47(2):251–60. https://doi.org/10.1016/j.ijnurstu.2009.05.020.
53. Frankl VE. Man's search for meaning. New York: Simon and Schuster; 1985.
54. Haugan G, Dezutter J. Meaning-in-life—a vital salutogenic resource for health (Chapter 8). In: Health

promotion in health care—vital theories and research. Berlin: Springer Nature; 2020.

55. Cooney A, Dowling M, Gannon ME, Dempsey L, Murphy K. Exploration of the meaning of connectedness for older people in long-term care in context of their quality of life: a review and commentary. Int J Older People Nursing. 2014;9(3):192–9. https://doi.org/10.1111/opn.12017.

56. Dufault K, Martocchio BC. Symposium on compassionate care and the dying experience. Hope: its spheres and dimensions. Nurs Clin N Am. 1985;20(2):379–91.

57. Rustøen T. Hope—a health promotion resource. Chapter 7. In: Haugan G, Eriksson M, editors. Vital salutogenic theories and research salutogenic nursing. Berlin: Springer; 2020.

58. Henden E. What is self-control? Philos Psychol. 2008;21(1):69–90. https://doi.org/10.1080/09515080701874092.

59. Lazarus RS, Folkman S. Stress, appraisal, and coping. New York: Springer; 1984.

60. Egerod I, Bergbom I, Lindahl B, Henricson M, Granberg-Axell A, Storli SL. The patient experience of intensive care: a meta-synthesis of Nordic studies. Int J Nurs Stud. 2015;52(8):1354–61. https://doi.org/10.1016/j.ijnurstu.2015.04.017.

61. Storli SL, Lindseth A, Asplund K. "Being somewhere else"-delusion or relevant experience? A phenomenological investigation into meaning of lived experience from being in intensive care. Int J Qual Stud Health Well Being. 2007;2:144–59.

62. Storli SL, Lindseth A, Asplund K. A journey in quest of meaning: a hermeneutic-phenomenological study on living with memories from intensive care. NursCrit Care. 2008;13(2):86–96.

63. Olding M, McMillan SE, Reeves S, Schmitt MH, Puntillo K, Kitto S. Patient and family involvement in adult critical and intensive care settings: a scoping review. Health Expect. 2016;19(6):1183–202. https://doi.org/10.1111/hex.12402.

64. Dietscher C, Winter U, Pelikan JM. The application of salutogenesis in hospitals. In: The handbook of salutogenesis. Cham: Springer; 2017. p. 277–98.

65. Smith MJ, Liehr PR. Understanding middle range theory by moving up and down the ladder of abstraction. In: Middle range theory for nursing. Berlin: Springer; 2018.

66. Perez D, Peters K, Wilkes L, Murphy GJA. Physical restraints in intensive care—an integrative review. Aust Crit Care. 2019;32(2):165–74.

67. Teece A, Baker J, Smith HJJ. Identifying determinants for the application of physical or chemical restraint in the management of psychomotor agitation on the critical care unit. J Clin Nurs. 2020;29(1–2):5–19.

68. Crutchfield P, Gibb TS, Redinger MJ, Ferman D, Livingstone J. The conditions for ethical application of restraints. Chest. 2019;155(3):617–25.

69. Barr J, Fraser GL, Puntillo K, Ely EW, Gelinas C, Dasta JF, et al. Clinical practice guidelines for the management of pain, agitation, and delirium in adult patients in the intensive care unit. Crit Care Med. 2013;41(1):263–306. https://doi.org/10.1097/CCM.0b013e3182783b72.

70. Merleau-Ponty M. Phenomenology of perception. Delhi: Motilal Banarsidass Publisher; 1996.

71. Ringdal M, Warren Stomberg M, Egnell K, Wennberg E, Zatterman R, Rylander C. In-bed cycling in the ICU; patient safety and recollections with motivational effects. Acta Anaesthesiol Scand. 2018;62(5):658–65. https://doi.org/10.1111/aas.13070.

72. Holme AN, Halvorsen K, Eskerud RS, Lind R, Storli SL, Gjengedal E, Moi AL. Nurses' experiences of ICU diaries following implementation of national recommendations for diaries in intensive care units: a quality improvement project. Intensive Crit Care Nurs. 2020;59:102828. https://doi.org/10.1016/j.iccn.2020.102828.

73. Inoue S, Hatakeyama J, Kondo Y, Hifumi T, Sakuramoto H, Kawasaki T, et al. Post-intensive care syndrome: its pathophysiology, prevention, and future directions. Acute Med Surg. 2019;6(3):233–46. https://doi.org/10.1002/ams2.415.

74. McIlroy PA, King RS, Garrouste-Orgeas M, Tabah A, Ramanan M. The effect of ICU diaries on psychological outcomes and quality of life of survivors of critical illness and their relatives: a systematic review and meta-analysis. Crit Care Med. 2019;47(2):273–9. https://doi.org/10.1097/CCM.0000000000003547.

75. Holt-Lunstad J, Smith TB, Layton JB. Social relationships and mortality risk: a meta-analytic review. PLoS Med. 2010;7(7):e1000316. https://doi.org/10.1371/journal.pmed.1000316.

76. Osorio C, Probert T, Jones E, Young AH, Robbins I. Adapting to stress: understanding the neurobiology of resilience. Behav Med. 2017;43(4):307–22. https://doi.org/10.1080/08964289.2016.1170661.

77. Kiecolt-Glaser JK, Gouin JP, Hantsoo L. Close relationships, inflammation, and health. Neurosci Biobehav Rev. 2010;35(1):33–8. https://doi.org/10.1016/j.neubiorev.2009.09.003.

78. Holt-Lunstad J, Smith TB, Baker M, Harris T, Stephenson D. Loneliness and social isolation as risk factors for mortality: a meta-analytic review. Perspect Psychol Sci. 2015;10(2):227–37. https://doi.org/10.1177/1745691614568352.

79. Wiesmaierova S, Petrova D, Arrebola Moreno A, Catena A, Ramirez Hernandez JA, Garcia-Retamero R. Social support buffers the negative effects of stress in cardiac patients: a cross-sectional study with acute coronary syndrome patients. J Behav Med. 2019;42(3):469–79. https://doi.org/10.1007/s10865-018-9998-4.

80. Nassar Junior AP, Besen B, Robinson CC, Falavigna M, Teixeira C, Rosa RG. Flexible versus restrictive visiting policies in ICUs: a systematic review and meta-analysis. Crit Care Med. 2018;46(7):1175–80. https://doi.org/10.1097/CCM.0000000000003155.

81. Karlsson V, Bergbom I. ICU professionals' experiences of caring for conscious patients receiving

MVT. West J Nurs Res. 2015;37(3):360–75. https://doi.org/10.1177/0193945914523143.

82. Laerkner E, Egerod I, Hansen HP. Nurses' experiences of caring for critically ill, non-sedated, mechanically ventilated patients in the Intensive Care Unit: a qualitative study. Intensive Crit Care Nurs. 2015;31(4):196–204. https://doi.org/10.1016/j.iccn.2015.01.005.

83. Vincent JL, Shehabi Y, Walsh TS, Pandharipande PP, Ball JA, Spronk P, et al. Comfort and patient-centred care without excessive sedation: the eCASH concept. Intensive Care Med. 2016;42(6):962–71. https://doi.org/10.1007/s00134-016-4297-4.

84. Strom T. Sedation in the ICU. DanMedJ. 2012;59(5): B4458.

85. Karlsen MW, Olnes MA, Heyn LG. Communication with patients in intensive care units: a scoping review. Nurs Crit Care. 2019;24(3):115–31. https://doi.org/10.1111/nicc.12377.

Health Promotion and Self-Management Among Patients with Chronic Heart Failure

Ying Jiang and Wenru Wang

Abstract

Heart failure is a chronic and complex clinical syndrome. It is one of the common causes of hospitalization and readmission among the older population. Patient self-management is essential to maintaining health and avoiding disruption of life caused by frequent hospitalizations. However, many patients lack self-care skills. This chapter provides a review on evidence for the importance of self-management and strategies to educate patients and promote self-care while living with the limitations on physical function.

Keywords

Health promotion · Self-management Self-efficacy · Heart failure

19.1 Introduction

Heart failure (HF) is not a specific disease, but a chronic and complex clinical syndrome that developed as the end-result of a variety of cardiovascular diseases [1]. Broadly speaking, the car- diac function of patients with HF may be impaired in two ways: (1) when cardiac contraction (ejection) is reduced and the heart is unable to pump the blood well, also known as "systolic dysfunction"; and (2) when relaxation of the ventricles is impaired and the heart is unable to fill the blood well, also known as "diastolic dysfunction." Both conditions lead to a decreased cardiac output which is insufficient to meet the body's metabolic demands [1], therefore, other compensatory mechanisms must be employed to offset the reduction in cardiac performance. These include activation of the neurohormonal and adrenergic pathways, as well as remodeling of the heart and blood vessels. The systemic and persistent over-activation of multiple neurohormonal and adrenergic pathways that aims at normalizing cardiac output may offer short-term benefits, but in a long run, the continued stimulatory effects on the heart will eventually worsen the HF progress [1]. Clinically, the typical symptoms of HF include symptoms caused by excessive fluid retention, such as dyspnea due to pulmonary congestion, abdominal distention from ascites, weight gain and peripheral edema, and symptoms caused by decreased cardiac output, such as activities intolerance, fatigue, hypotension, poor mentation, and weakness [1, 2].

As a chronic condition, HF imposes great burdens on the society. Around 38 million people worldwide are living with HF and the condition is becoming more common in both developing

Y. Jiang (✉) · W. Wang
Alice Lee Centre for Nursing Studies, Yong Loo Lin School of Medicine, National University of Singapore, Singapore, Singapore
e-mail: nurjiy@nus.edu.sg; nurww@nus.edu.sg

© The Author(s) 2021
G. Haugan, M. Eriksson (eds.), *Health Promotion in Health Care – Vital Theories and Research*,
https://doi.org/10.1007/978-3-030-63135-2_19

and developed countries [2–4]. The incidence and prevalence of HF increase with age. With the rising prevalence of cardiovascular risk factors, as well as improved survival rate in heart attacks and other cardiovascular diseases, the number of people with HF is expected to continue to surge [5, 6]. The growing burden of HF is taking its toll on the society, particularly on the health care systems. HF is one of the most common causes of hospitalization and readmission [7–10]. In Singapore, age-adjusted HF hospital admission rate rose by 38% from 1991 to 1998 [9]. More recently, local data from public institutions show that HF readmission rate is 18%, with an average length of stay of 5.2 days per admission [11], which is similar to the average length of hospital stay (5–10 days) across the globe [2]. The lengthy and recurring hospital stays required by the patients not only account for the majority of health care expenditure but also pose additional challenges for hospital administrators to plan and allocate the scarce manpower and medical resources [7].

For the individuals, HF is a long-term condition that involves one or more hospitalizations. Living with HF is fraught with challenges. The distressing symptoms reduce the patients' independence and ability to perform many activities of daily living [12]. Also, recent health care reforms have increasingly shifted the self-management responsibility to patients and families, as hospital stays are becoming shorter and less frequent. Therefore, the critical role of patients in their own care is receiving increasing attention. Self-care refers to specific behaviors that patients perform of their own accord to control their disease and maintain health [13]. As with many other chronic diseases, there is no cure for HF, but through treatment and self-care management, the impact on quality of life and disease progression can be abated.

The Salutogenic model of health considers health to be on a continuum between ease and dis-ease [14], instead of merely the absence of disease. Based on this model, most individuals are somewhere between the imaginary poles of complete wellness and complete illness [15]. An individual may have many physical ailments, but

he or she can be relatively healthy if he or she is asymptomatic and fully functioning. Conversely, an individual who is physically healthy may also have moments of sickness or emotional distress. Health promotion requires the active participation of individuals in their contexts and, ultimately, moving towards the healthy pole [15]. To do this, individuals need to have the ability to understand the whole situation in which they find themselves, and to use the resources available to them to move in a direction that promotes health.

There are three key concepts in the Salutogenic model of health, namely, the generalized resistance resource (GRR), the specific resistance resource (SRR), and the sense of coherence (SOC) [16]. According to Antonovsky, GRR refers to an attribute of a person, a group, or a community that contributes to successfully coping with the inherent tensions of human existence [16, 17]. In contrast, SRR is a specific resource used when a particular stressor is encountered [17]. GRR are resources with broad utility, such as wealth, ego strength, and social network, while SRR are resources with situation-specific utility, such as medical emergency number to access ambulance. Similarly, Sullivan [18] made a distinction between GRR and SRR and indicated that nursing is the GRR, while the nurse providing specific care to a particular health problem of the patient is the SRR. GRR is important for the development of a strong SOC [17]. Antonovsky [14] believed that a person with a strong SOC is more likely to mobilize the SRR and GRR in any given situation to overcome stressors. And through such a mechanism, SOC eventually translates into better health.

The concept SOC is a global life orientation, referring to a way of seeing the world as manageable, predictable and meaningful [15, 19]. It consists of three essential components: "comprehensibility," "manageability," and "meaningfulness" [14]. SOC has a significant impact on health. In health promotion, SOC reflects a person's ability to identify their internal and external resources and use them in a way that promotes health and well-being [15]. Like personality, SOC is thought to be fairly stable and enduring, with only a margin of malleability [14]. The debate over whether SOC can be improved by interventions continues [20], but some have reported that the three components of SOC can be strengthened by interventions [21]. Nurses have a responsibility to promote patients' understanding of the situation after their diagnosis of HF (i.e. to increase patient's comprehensibility), to help patients reduce the adverse impacts of HF on their quality of life and to ensure patients are able to live as healthily as possible with their physical limitations (i.e. to improve manageability). Self-care is an important part of promoting health in patients with HF. Despite its importance, many patients find it challenging, especially when transitioning from hospital care to home and community care [22, 23]. Patients often feel unprepared to manage their condition in the community due to having to acquire a variety of skills in multiple domains of daily living without the supervision from hospital staff [13, 24]. And many of these changes impose heavy demands on patients' ability to understand and act [13]. This chapter provides a review of some important research on HF self-management in the literature. Particular attention is paid to HF self-care and its associated problems, strategies to improve different aspects of HF self-care, as well as the multifaced psychosocial disease-management interventions to improve overall self-care management.

19.2 Management of Heart Failure (HF)

Overall, the aims of HF management are to (1) reduce morbidity, that is to reduce symptoms and hospital admissions while improving functional status and quality of life, and (2) to improve survival through slowing down the disease progression. In clinical practice, HF management generally includes treating the underlying causes of HF (e.g. coronary heart disease or valve disease) and associated conditions (e.g. hypertension or diabetes), follow-up monitoring and preventative care, case management and care coordination, patient education and support for self-management and health promotion, cardiac rehabilitation, palliative care, implantable device therapy, and in some cases heart transplantation [25, 26].

19.2.1 Heart Failure Self-Management Interventions

Self-management interventions refer to disease-management interventions that focused on improving patients' self-care. Self-care is the cornerstone of HF management and health promotion, which defines as specific behaviors performed by a patient on his or her own accord to manage illness and maintain health [13]. Self-care for HF encompasses a range of specific behaviors, from adhering to medication, reducing excessive fluid and salt intake, monitoring daily weight, exercising, monitoring and identifying exacerbating symptoms, and taking appropriate steps to intervene if symptoms worsened [27]. Studies have shown that if patients practice constant self-care, 30% of hospital admissions and more than half of the readmissions can be prevented [28, 29].

19.2.1.1 Medication Management

Medication is important in HF treatment. Most patients with HF are prescribed a combination of at least three types of agents: angiotensin-converting enzyme inhibitors (ACE-I), angiotensin II receptor blockers (ARB), β-blockers, aldosterone receptor antagonists (AA), and/or diuretics. Although evidences on medication efficacy are clear, studies have found that a significant proportion of patients does not take medication as prescribed [30]. In the literature, medication adherence rates vary widely, depending on how adherence is measured [30]. Zhang et al. [31] reported that on average, only half (52%) of the patients had good medication adherence, which was measured by the ratio of total number of medication the patient had actually taken (numerator) over the total number of medication the patient should have taken (denominator). As medication regimens have become increasingly complex, many patients found medication management challenging. In the qualitative studies, patients reported that the demands to adhering the complex treatment regimens are onerous and difficult to meet. Some patients also reported troubles on learning new medications and dealing with the burden of medication side effects [32, 33].

Previous studies on medication adherence have found an inverse relationship between number of daily doses and adherence rate [34, 35]. However, a recent study attempted to evaluate this strategy of simplifying medication regimen to once-daily dosing on its own did not find any evidence in improving medication adherence in patients with HF [36]. Specifically, there was no statistically significant difference in medication adherence between patients taking once-daily carvedilol controlled-release (CR) and patients taking twice daily carvedilol immediate-release (IR) for a 5-month period. However, this trial may be confounded by the "ceiling effect" resulted from high baseline medication adherence among the participants [36]. In addition, in a systematic review on the relationships between dosage regimens and medication adherence, Claxton et al. [37] compared medication adherence between different dose regimens and found that medication adherence was significantly higher with once daily regimens compared to 3-times-daily or 4-times-daily regimens, and between twice-daily dosing and 4-times-daily dosing. However, there was no significant differences in medication adherence between once-daily and twice-daily regimens or between twice-daily and thrice-daily regimens [37]. These findings suggest that simpler medication regimens may improve patient's medication management and medication adherence, but that simply reducing a single dose (e.g., from twice-daily to once-daily) may have too little impact on patients.

Two systematic reviews have reviewed intervention strategies to promote medication adherence in HF patients [38, 39]. Overall, more than half of the included studies (63% and 50%) shown significant better medication adherence in the intervention arms, suggesting that medication adherence in patients with HF can be improved by effective interventions. Because of the importance of comprehensibility in building SOC and promoting health [40], effective interventions should not only increase patient knowledge of medications, but also be delivered in a way that is easy for patients to grasp. In the literature, most of the effective interventions used a combination of educational, behavioral, and affective inter-ventions, with education being the most widely included component [38]. Studies using intensi-fied patient care included interventions with direct patient contacts and interventions with regular telephone follow ups or tele-monitoring. Face-to-face direct patient contacts were found to be the most effective strategy in improving medi-ation adherence. In contrast, only one of the telephone-based or tele-monitoring interventions has led to enhanced mediation adherence [39]. Similar result was observed in a recently pub-lished systematic review and meta-analysis of the effectiveness of mobile phone-based self-management interventions on medication adher-ence in patients with coronary heart disease [41]. In this review, the meta-analysis result from the pooled data did not find a significant impact of the mobile phone-based interventions on improv-ing medication adherence [41].

More recently, mobile health (mhealth) appli-cations (apps) to support medication adherence have also grown in number, some studies have been conducted to examined its efficacy among cardiovascular patients, including patients with HF [42, 43]. Goldstein et al. [42] performed a four-arm randomized feasibility study of 60 par-ticipants with HF, comparing an e-pill box (tele-health) to a smartphone-based mHealth app on medication adherence and patient's acceptance of the devices. Participants were provided one of the two devices with or without active reminders. No significant difference in medication adherence was found among the four arms. However, patients preferred the mHealth approach [42]. Studies conducted on other cardiovascular patients showed modest benefits in improving medication adherence [43].

Taken together, current evidences suggest that multicomponent interventions conducted face to face may still be the most effective strategy to improve medication adherence in patient with HF. Although some evidences suggests that mHealth app may potentially improve medica-tion adherence in patients with cardiovascular diseases, findings from trials on patients with HF are not consistent. High-quality trials are still needed to confirm its role and justify its use in routine care [43].

19.2.1.2   Sodium Restriction

Restricting daily sodium intake to <2 g has been commonly recommended in patients with HF. However, there is no firm evidence to support this practice [44]. Both observational and experimental studies have shown mixed results [45–47]. Therefore, the efficacy and safety of sodium restriction remain unclear, and there is no consensus on the optimal amount of sodium intake for patients with HF [48]. Updated guideline by the Canadian Cardiovascular Society has recommended patients with HF to restrict their daily dietary salt intake to between 2 and 3 g [49], while the recent American College of Cardiology Foundation (ACCF)/AHA guideline for HF management suggests some degree of sodium restriction (e.g. <3 g/day) in patients with congestive symptoms but does not endorse any specific level of sodium intake [50]. Similarly, the 2016 European Society of Cardiology (ESC) guideline for diagnosis and treatment of HF does not provide any explicit recommendation on sodium restriction but suggesting avoiding excessive salt intake (>6 g/day) [51]. Most of these recommendations are based on expert opinions given the conflicting evidences in the literature, which make it difficult to compare or draw definite conclusions [50, 52–54].

In the context of HF self-care, adhering to a low-sodium diet requires patients to understand the relationship between sodium intake and congestive symptoms (e.g. edema), and make sensible adjustments to their diet based on clinical situation [49]. To do this, the patient would need to have the knowledge and skills to measure daily sodium intake, know how to read food nutrition labels, distinguish low-sodium foods from high-sodium foods, and recognize the "hidden" sources of sodium (e.g. canned foods). In addition, patients are also required to perform actions of choosing low-sodium food and avoiding high-sodium food, reducing salt added in cooking, as well as asking for reduced-salt meal when eating out at restaurants [55]. Therefore, dietary adherence is often difficult.

It was reported that HF patients had an average of 2.7–3.9 g daily sodium intake as measured by 24-h urine sodium [56]. Riegel et al. [57] reported that medication adherence was the highest (95.5%), while dietary adherence (45.5%) was the lowest after hospital discharge, and over-time, both adherences decreased rapidly. Within 3 months, the overall adherence rate for low-sodium diet was 42%, compared to 96.4% for adhering to fluid restriction and 84.7% for adhering to medication [57]. Colin-Ramirez et al. [58] evaluated the dietary patterns of sodium consumption in 237 patients with HF. It was reported that 4.2% of patients who reported "always" being adherent with a low salt diet ate canned or package soups daily, while 22.9% of those who reported "sometimes" being adherent ate fast foods one to three times a week. Among all the participants, one third (30%) reported consuming large amounts of processed meat on a weekly basis, and 52% reported using seasoning such as ketchup, BBQ sauce, soy sauce, or salad dressings in their cooking. On further examination, a number of the participants connected the idea of low-salt diet mainly with not adding salt to cooking, but not with reducing high-sodium processed foods. Similarly, in an earlier study, Chung et al. [59] found that there was no significant difference in the 24-h urine sodium levels between those who reported being adherent to low-sodium diet (4560 mg) and those who reported being nonadherent (4333 mg, $p = 0.59$). The inconsistent findings between self-reported adherence and participants' actual dietary pattern on sodium intake reflected significant gaps in patients' knowledge related to low-sodium diet [59], even when dietary teaching on low-sodium diet was provided to all the participants by a registered dietician [58].

A qualitative study exploring factors associated with not adhering to low-sodium diet has found that "lack of knowledge," "interference with socialization," and "lack of food selections" were the major reasons contributing to nonadherence [60]. Many patients perceived that health care providers did not cover what they wanted to know, and they were given too little information on low-sodium foods or strategies to follow dietary recommendations. For patients with additional dietary restriction, following a dietary regimen can be confusing, and confounded by the limited food choices, for example, patients with diabetes worried that eating fresh fruits that contained low sodium may increase their blood glucose levels [60]. Similarly, in a descriptive study, Ong et al. [61] reported that although patients may understand their diet restriction, but they faced practical problems because of limited food choices and lack of tactics to fit the dietary regimen into their everyday lives.

While health care professionals believe the importance of patient education [62, 63], such belief does not seem to be translated into promoting patients' knowledge or self-care. Riegel et al. [57] observed that although nurses routinely teach patients about importance of treatment adherence and behaviors that are important to adopt, adherence to self-care recommendations decreased rapidly after hospitalization. The finding called into question whether patient education during hospitalization is effective in influencing patients' adherence. Similarly, Bentley et al. [60] raised the question of whether patients truly did not receive diet education, or whether the education delivered was untimely, ineffective, and presented in a way that hinders learning. Some studies have suggested that effective teaching should be provided over several sessions to increase knowledge retention [62]. In addition, it is important to involve family member as their understanding of low-sodium diet may enhance patient's adherence and reduce family conflict [64]. Repetitive reinforcement of diet guidelines seems to have little effect on promoting dietary adherence [61], therefore, interventions would also need to address factors other than lack of knowledge [60].

19.2.1.3 Fluid Restriction

The 2013 ACCF/AHA and the 2016 ESC HF guidelines have suggested fluid restriction of 1.5–2 L/day in patients with refractory or symptomatic HF to relieve congestion [50, 51], and it is best implemented in the context of self-management on symptoms and weight monitoring. Routine fluid restriction in all HF patients regardless of symptoms or other considerations does not show any benefits, therefore it is not recommended [50].

In a recent review on fluid restriction in patients with HF, Johansson et al. [65] found that most of the randomized trials included fluid restriction as one of the components in combined intervention, only two studies assessed the effect of fluid restriction alone [66, 67]. But neither of them found any significant differences in clinical parameters, body weight, or renal markers between patients on fluid restriction and those with a liberal fluid intake [66, 67]. Many of the studies did not report patients' actual fluid intake, but studies did report on this showed most of the patients consumed less than 2 L/day, irrespective of whether they were in the intervention group or control group, suggesting that excessive fluid intake may not be a general problem in the HF population [65–67].

On the contrary, stringent fluid restriction in hot and low-humidity climates may predispose patients with HF to heat stroke [50]. It was also reported that fluid restriction of 1.5 L/day was associated with decreased quality of life and increased sensation of thirst [66]. Elderly patients might even be at risk of dehydration as a result of impairment of thirst sensation, decreased kidney function, medications (e.g. diuretics), depression or dependence on a caregiver to provide fluid [68]. Therefore, the discussion of fluid intake should be placed in a larger context of HF management with consideration of dietary habits, diuretic regimen, and symptoms presentation rather than restricting fluid intake in isolation [66]. In HF self-care, fluid management also requires patients to recognize the needs to alter fluid intake, such as to increase fluid intake during period of high heat, nausea, or vomiting, and to restrict fluid when body weight increases and/or presence of congestive symptoms [50, 51].

19.2.1.4 Daily Symptoms Monitoring

Changes in signs and symptoms often precede further changes in clinical status that may require intervention. For example, weight gain is commonly regarded as a marker of HF decompensation. In a nested case-control study among 268 patients with HF, Chaudhry et al. [69] reported that weight gain was associated with a subsequent hospitalization for HF and started at least 1 week before admission. Daily monitoring of signs and symptoms is a pragmatic way for patients to track their health status and identify high-risk period, during which timely interventions could be rendered to avert episodes of decompensation. Major clinical guidelines have recommended symptoms monitoring as part of the routine self-care management, specifically, daily weight monitoring, daily check for edema, and daily check for symptoms severity are the typical self-care strategies to monitor signs and symptoms [55, 70].

Despite the importance of symptoms monitoring, Zeng et al. [63] reported that HF patients lacked the knowledge on HF symptoms recognition. Among 187 Singaporean HF patients, only 55.6% were able to associate increased weight with change in HF condition, and less than half (40.1%) knew that they should weigh themselves every day. More than half of the patients were not able to recognize signs and symptoms of worsening HF [63]. Similarly, Ong et al. [61] investigated the learning needs among hospitalized Singaporean patients with HF and found that education topics on HF signs and symptoms were ranked as the most important learning need by the patients. These findings echoed the result of an earlier qualitative study that local patients wanted to know more about their conditions and symptom management, but physicians preferred to discuss their conditions with their family more than with them. Consequently, patients felt less empowered to manage their conditions [71].

Studies conducted in other countries found similar challenges in symptoms monitoring and detection [13, 72–74]. Moser et al. [75] reported that symptoms monitoring was the least well-performed self-care activities, with only 14% weighing themselves every day and 9% monitoring for symptoms of worsening HF. Adequate self-monitoring and symptoms management impose heavy demands on patients' ability to understand and act on their knowledge. However, poor memory on basic concepts of HF, misattribution of symptoms to other conditions, and low comprehension of links between symptoms and HF are common among patients [72]. Older patients often discount the early-warning signs as

normal aging [76, 77]. Some evidences have reported that HF is associated with changes in cognitive function, therefore diminishing patients' ability on symptoms perception [78, 79]. Furthermore, inadequate explanation by the health care professionals is perceived as another barrier. Even when patients are provided with educational brochures, they do not feel sufficiently informed [24]. Most of the patients are not ready to receive education at the time of initial diagnosis due to the fears and worries stemming from the new diagnosis of HF. On the other hand, education given at the time of hospital discharge is often overwhelming and hard to follow, especially when a big chunk of information needs to be communicated to the patient at one go [80]. Consequently, the windows of opportunity to treat the early symptoms of HF decompensation may be hindered by the difficulties that patients faced in monitoring and recognizing the symptoms [81]. Therefore, strategies to improve the "comprehensibility" and "manageability" in symptom monitoring remain essential. For example, comprehensibility can be supported by teaching patients on how to make sense of their subjective symptoms (e.g. feeling of fatigue) and objective assessment (e.g. weight record and edema assessment), providing easy-to-understand graphic illustrations, and breaking down information into digestible chunks by using simple language and short sentences. Manageability can be improved by providing technical solutions on how to incorporate symptom monitoring into the patient's daily routine.

Similar to medication management, interventions based on remote telemonitoring, mobile phone-based monitoring and mHealth apps have grown significantly in the field of symptoms monitoring over the past two decades [82]. The deployment of these technologies has provided a powerful tool to look for early warning symptoms and to prevent hospitalization [83]. However, evidences from the literature show inconsistent results on the effectiveness of these technologies.

In an earlier Cochrane systematic review and meta-analysis, Inglis and colleages [84] reported that remote telemedical surveillance through telemonitoring significantly reduced all-cause mortality (RR 0.66, 95% CI 0.54–0.81) and HF-related hospitalizations (RR 0.79, 95% CI 0.67–0.94). "Structured telephone support" by using a mobile phone to monitor symptoms and provide self-care management without additional home visit or intensified clinic follow-up significantly reduced HF-related hospitalizations (RR 0.77, 95% CI 0.68–0.87), although effect on reducing all-cause mortality was not statistically significant (RR 0.88, 95% CI 0.76–1.01) [84]. In another study, Seto and colleagues [85] tested the effect of a mobile phone-based telemonitoring system on the outcomes of HF patients after a decompensation episode. The mobile phone-based patient terminals were used for data collection and data transmission. Patients in the intervention group were required to have their weight and blood pressure measured daily, single-lead ECG measured weekly, and to answer symptoms check questions on their mobile phones daily for 6 months. Their results showed that participants in the intervention group had significant improvements in self-care maintenance and HRQoL compared to those in the control group after 6 months. However, differences on the hard outcomes, such as hospitalization, mortality, or emergency department visits between the two groups were not significant [85]. Similarly, in a large-scale RCT (the Tele-HF study) involving 1653 patients with HF, Chaudhry et al. [86] testing out a telephone-based interactive voice response (IVR) system that gathered information on symptoms and weight every day, but failed to show any evidence on improving patients' clinical outcomes. Furthermore, the study found that 14% of the patients in the intervention group never used the system, while only 55% of them were using the system at least three times a week. The authors believed that the adherence rate reflected the "best case" scenario which is difficult to replicate in the real-world clinical practice since considerable resources were directed toward optimizing patients' engagement in this clinical trial [86]. The trial by Scherr et al. [83] also reported low adherence rate that 22% of their study participants were "never beginners" due to the difficulty in entering and

sending the data through a mobile phone internet browser.

Many of the technologies being tested in the previous studies are almost obsolete today due to how rapidly technology is changing. For example, in the Tele-HF study, participants needed to call the IVR system daily [86], while in the other two studies, the study interventions were based on the old mobile phone models (BlackBerry Pearl 8130 and Nokia 3510) for data transmission and symptoms reporting [83, 85]. The less user-friendly patient terminal may decrease the usability of an intervention, especially for those elderly and technically unskilled patients [83]. More recently, with the rapid development of mobile technology and the expansion of mobile network coverage, personal mobile devices (smartphone and/or tablets) and mHealth apps seem to be better positioned for monitoring symptoms [82]. In a single-arm prospective pilot study, Zan and colleagues [87] evaluated the feasibility of a remote web- and telephone-based monitoring system, called the "iGetBetter" system. The "iGetBetter" system enables the patients to self-monitor their body weight by a bluetooth weight scale and blood pressure through an auto-inflating blood pressure cuff. Data were transmitted onto the secured web platform. Patients can view their results by logging into the patient portal using an iPad mini at home, while the physician can access patients' data remotely through the clinician portal. Patients who did not complete the self-monitoring activities as planned would receive a reminder phone call from the IVR telephone system. The IVR telephone system served as an alternative means for patients to log their activities and key in their measurements manually through the phone keypad. Over the 90-day study period, the study team found that 19 patients (95%) agreed that the monitoring system was easy to use, and more than half of the participants had 80% or greater adherence to care plan. Most participants engaged the system through patient portal on the iPad mini, but three participants (15%) only used the IVR telephone system exclusively. At the end of the study, participants had an improvement of HRQoL from baseline, but there were no significant differences in hospital utilization and length of hospital stay [87]. The pilot study demonstrated the feasibility of a remote monitoring system that leveraged on latest mHealth technology and portable digital devices. It offered a potential low-cost solution on timely symptoms monitoring [87]. However, its effect on clinical outcomes were yet to be confirmed. To date, there is still a lack of evidence from high-quality large-scale randomized controlled trial (RCT) on clinical effectiveness of these technologies [55].

19.2.1.5 Other Lifestyle Modifications

Physical inactivity, cigarette smoking and excessive alcohol consumption are the highly avoidable lifestyle risk factors for worsening HF. Therefore, exercise, smoking cessation and limit alcohol intake are the other recommended self-care strategies.

Many studies have demonstrated consistent benefits for a range of outcomes with exercise training in patients with HF, including improved quality of life, improved functional capacity, decreased mortality and reduced hospitalization [88–90]. Exercise training or regular physical activity is the Class I recommendation to improve functional status among patients with HF according to the 2013 ACCF/AHA guideline [50]. Nonetheless, exercise adherence is hard to maintain. Some studies reported that overall exercise adherence rate ranged from 9% to 53% [13]. In a large RCT with 2331 stable HF patients (the HF-ACTION trial), exercise adherence of the participants in the intervention group decreased over time, from a median of 95 min per week during 4–6 months follow-up to 74 min per week during 10–12 months follow up, even though the patients were provided a structured exercise program and were supervised closely [88].

Smoking and excessive alcohol consumption are associated with higher risk of HF mortality in patient with HF [91, 92]. Smoking cessation is as effective as drug treatment in reducing mortality among smokers with HF, with benefits of prevention death and hospitalization emerging quickly in less than 3 years [91, 93]. Therefore smoking cessation is an important part of HF self-care and should be encouraged in all HF patients who are current smokers [55].

Earlier guideline has stated that patients with HF should limit their alcohol intake to two standard drinks or less per day for men and one standard drink or less per day for women, while patients with suspected alcohol-induced cardiomyopathy should abstain from alcohol [94]. More recent guidelines only recommend counseling and/or treatment to reduce alcohol intake in patients who have consumed excessive amounts of alcohol, especially in patients with alcohol-induced cardiomyopathy [50, 51]. It should be noted, however, that the effects of small amounts of alcohol are still controversial [95, 96]. Therefore, for those who were nondrinkers, health care provider should not endorse alcohol to them [97].

In summary, HF self-care consists of a variety of skills across multiple domains on a daily basis [13, 72]. It is a dynamic and complex process, in which some of the required actions may conflict with patients' preferences. Despite its importance, HF self-care remains challenging for many patients. While several studies focus exclusively on improving a single aspect of HF self-care, such as medication management or symptoms monitoring, most studies adopt a multifaceted approach to improve patient's overall self-care management. The following section will provide a review on these interventions.

19.3 Psychosocial Self-Management Interventions

In the literature, there are many disease management programs developed to help patients to manage their HF condition and to improve overall self-care and promote health [88, 98–102]. Most of these programs are instructional with a focus on the value of exercise training, pharmacological care and lifestyle modifications [88, 98, 99, 102, 103]. While evidences acknowledge that patient education is a necessary and important component to promote effective self-care [104–106], it is also noted that education alone is insufficient to support behavioral changes [107]. Efforts to promote successful self-care should consider patients' knowledge, skills and engagement [55].

Over the past decades, there has been increasing attention to the role of psychosocial factors in the etiology and prognosis of cardiac disease, including HF [108, 109]. Psychosocial interventions, as part of the nonpharmacological interventions, have been increasingly used to enhance the health outcomes of patients with HF [110]. Besides disease education, a psychosocial education program is usually an intervention that combines psychological (e.g. cognitive behavioral therapy, relaxation, motivational interviewing, nondirective counseling, or supportive therapy) and social (e.g. social support) components. It is a multicomponent intervention that aims to promote patients' understanding of knowledge and encourage behavioral changes for an effective self-management [111]. It is also a holistic approach to improving health literacy, strengthening a person's psychological and social resources, enabling patient's resistance to illness, and mitigating the negative impacts of HF on their quality of life.

In a recent systematic review and meta-analysis, Samartzis et al. [110] examined the effectiveness of psychosocial interventions on quality of life in patients with HF. The review included 16 RCTs involving 2180 participants. The combined data showed that psychosocial interventions improved patients' quality of life (standardized mean difference [SMD] 0.46, 95% CI 0.19–0.72), among which, face-to-face interventions showed greater quality of life improvement compared to telephone-based interventions ($p < 0.02$). However, in terms of length of the intervention, or whether the intervention adopted a multidisciplinary team approach, or whether used telemedicine technology, or whether involved patients' caregivers in the intervention, there was no evidence favoring any specific type of these psychosocial interventions. In addition, education on disease aspects and/or psychoeducation were presented in most of the interventions, which are often given by a nurse, suggesting that patient education still played a significant role in improving patients' quality of life [110].

Patient engagement plays a pivotal role in designing an effective self-management intervention. Without patient's engagement, knowledge and skills are less effective to enhance HF self-care [55]. Psychological techniques, such as motivational interviewing techniques and cognitive behavioral strategies, may improve patients' engagement and psychological outcomes. However, the effect of psychological intervention on self-care and psychological outcomes among patient with HF are less clear. An earlier Cochrane systemic review and meta-analysis on psychological intervention for depression in patients with HF found no studies that met their inclusion criteria [112]. Although a later systemic review and meta-analysis supported the efficacy of some psychological interventions, such as psychotherapy, progressive muscle relaxation techniques, counselling or mindfulness-based intervention in improving psychological outcomes among patients with coronary heart disease, but none of the included studies was conducted on patients with HF [113]. Our recent systematic and meta-analysis on the efficacy of psychological interventions on self-care, psychological and health outcomes in patients with HF has found that psychological interventions improve health-related quality of life at 3 months of follow-up [114]. However, there was no statistically significant effect detected after 3 months of follow-up. The intervention effects on the participants' anxiety level was not statistically significant. In addition, evidences from appraised literature revealed possible positive but short-term effects on HF self-care. Cognitive behavioral therapy tends to improve depression levels [114].

As one of the psychological factors, SOC refers to one's enduring attitude towards life, which is the basis for successfully coping with life's ups and downs. It is also thought to motivate individuals to stay healthy during the trajectory of a worsening illness [115, 116]. Gallagher [116] reported that a strong SOC is one of the predictors for better self-management in patient with HF living in the community. However, Ferreira and colleagues [117] did not find any significant difference in SOC in relation to performing any self-care behavior or not among hospitalized HF patients. Other studies have suggested that SOC may associate with better HRQoL and life satisfaction in patients living with HF [115, 118]. Nevertheless, after searching the literature, it was found that there is still a lack of studies in the literature to date on the effectiveness of interventions based on the Salutogenic approach or the concept of SOC in improving self-management of HF.

19.3.1 mHealth-Based Multicomponent Self-Management Intervention

Most recently, with rapid evolution of technology over the past few decades, there has been an increasing trend in using mHealth to promote chronic disease self-management in the literature [119–121]. There is evidence suggesting that mHealth offers prospects for providing effective and affordable health care services to a widespread population, reducing geographical inconvenience and socioeconomic disparities [119]. In HF self-management, mHealth provides a new way to improve patient participation in self-care by constantly reminding patients about key aspects of self-care and symptoms tracking [122]. Compared to the older technology, the newer generation of personal mobile devices (smartphone and/or tablets) and mHealth apps also have better usability and integration into patient's everyday lives [82]. Therefore, it has a great potential to be adopted in the multifaceted HF self-management.

Nevertheless, as aforementioned, many of the initial mHealth technologies are deployed to primarily support a single aspect of HF self-care, such as medication management or symptoms monitoring. There are very few studies on mHealth-based interventions aimed at improving overall self-care, even though the number of commercially available mobile apps is growing rapidly [123]. In the most recent study, Athilingam and her team [124] have developed a new smartphone app (the HeartMapp) to improve overall self-care and quality of life in patients with HF. The smartphone-based intervention leveraged on mobile phones and heart rate sensor (chest strap) to provide individualized alerts on symptom checking, symptom management and

medication adherence, as well as real-time vital signs monitoring. The components of the HeartMapp app covered all the essential aspects of HF self-care, including patient education, medication management, symptoms monitoring and management, relaxation technique (deep breathing exercise), and physical activity (walking) [124]. Their results revealed that participants in the HeartMapp group had significant improvement in self-care management, self-care confidence, and HF knowledge. But results on medication adherence, quality of life, and depression were not significant. Over 30-day study period, 43% (4/9) used the app daily and completed daily symptoms assessment and exercise, 56% (5/9) accessed HeartMapp features over 80% of the time (24/30 days). However, the study attrition rate was close to 30% [124], which was higher than previous studies adopting a face-to-face multicomponent psychosocial educational disease management approach [110]. The small sample size and high attrition rate has limited the generalizability of their findings [124]. In addition, the review of existing commercially available apps for HF self-care management has found that very few apps met the prespecified criteria for quality, content, or functionality. Therefore, these findings underscore the need for further clinical validation and mapping evidence-based guidelines to improve the overall quality of self-care-related apps [123].

19.4 Conclusion

In summary, this chapter provides a review of research on HF self-management interventions aimed at improving self-care and promoting health. HF is a disabling and life-limiting condition. Living with HF is challenging, with many patients expressing frustration when they were unable to perform their daily work or social roles due to symptom burden or decreased physical function. Effective self-management may help to stabilize their life while living with the limitations on functional abilities and disease burden.

Today, the medical perspective and approaches are highly developed and emphasized, which is good. However, patients are whole human beings, a person consisting of different dimensions; individuals comprise of a wholeness of body-mind-spirit. Thus, a holistic physical-psychological-social-spiritual model of care is required in order to provide high-quality and effective health care. The health care industry still largely follows a pathogenesis paradigm. Integrating and applying salutogenesis into specific disease management can be challenging. The successful application of salutogenesis in this area cannot accomplished by only introducing it into the clinical practice, but it has to demonstrate its evidence-based properties. Therefore, research in this area is still very much needed if the salutogenic model of health is to gain greater acceptance in the health care field [17].

Take Home Messages
- Heart failure is a chronic, disabling, and life-limiting condition. The Salutogenic model of health focuses on the origins of health and emphasizes efforts towards health promotion.
- Effective self-management and self-care skills help patients to stabilize their life while living with the limitations on functional abilities (i.e. moving towards the healthy pole).
- Heart failure self-care required skills across multiple domains of life. Many patients find it difficult to manage.
- Effective interventions should be multifaced and adopt a holistic approach to improve patients' health literacy and strengthen their psychological and social resources.
- Nurses play a significant role in empowering patients to self-manage their condition and move in the health-promoting direction.

References

1. Krum H, vod Lueder T. Advances in heart failure management. London: Future Medicine Ltd; 2012.
2. Ponikowski P, Anker SD, AlHabib KF, Cowie MR, Force TL, Hu S, et al. Heart failure: preventing disease and death worldwide. ESC Heart Fail. 2014;1(1):4–25.
3. Heidenreich PA, Trogdon JG, Khavjou OA, Butler J, Dracup K, Ezekowitz MD, et al. Forecasting the future of cardiovascular disease in the United States: a policy statement from the American Heart Association. Circulation. 2011;123(8):933–44.
4. Reyes EB, Ha JW, Firdaus I, Ghazi AM, Phrommintikul A, Sim D, et al. Heart failure across Asia: same healthcare burden but differences in organization of care. Int J Cardiol. 2016;223:163–7. https://doi.org/10.1016/j.ijcard.2016.07.256.
5. Rajadurai J, Tse HF, Wang CH, Yang NI, Zhou J, Sim D. Understanding the epidemiology of heart failure to improve management practices: an Asia-Pacific perspective. J Card Fail. 2017;23(4):327–39. https://doi.org/10.1016/j.cardfail.2017.01.004.
6. Richards AM, Lam C, Wong RC, Ping C. Heart failure: a problem of our age. Ann Acad Med Singap. 2011;40(9):392–3.
7. Bundkirchen A, Schwinger RHG. Epidemiology and economic burden of chronic heart failure. Eur Heart J Suppl. 2004;6(Suppl D):D57 LP–D60. http://eur-heartjsupp.oxfordjournals.org/content/6/suppl_D/D57.abstract.
8. Kannel WB. Incidence and epidemiology of heart failure. Heart Fail Rev. 2000;5(2):167–73. https://doi.org/10.1023/A:1009884820941.
9. Ng TP, Niti M. Trends and ethnic differences in hospital admissions and mortality for congestive heart failure in the elderly in Singapore, 1991 to 1998. Heart. 2003;89(8):865–70.
10. Santhanakrishnan R, Ng TP, Cameron VA, Gamble GD, Ling LH, Sim D, et al. The Singapore heart failure outcomes and phenotypes (SHOP) study and prospective evaluation of outcome in patients with heart failure with preserved left ventricular ejection fraction (PEOPLE) study: rationale and design. J Card Fail. 2013;19(3):156–62. https://doi.org/10.1016/j.cardfail.2013.01.007.
11. Chan WX, Lin W, Wong RCC. Transitional care to reduce heart failure readmission rates in South East Asia. Card Fail Rev. 2016;2(2):85–9.
12. Jeon Y-H, Kraus SG, Jowsey T, Glasgow NJ. The experience of living with chronic heart failure: a narrative review of qualitative studies. BMC Health Serv Res. 2010;10(1):77. http://bmchealthservres.biomedcentral.com/articles/10.1186/1472-6963-10-77.
13. Evangelista LS, Shinnick MA. What do we know about adherence and self-care? J Cardiovasc Nurs. 2008;23(3):250.
14. Antonovsky A. The structure and properties of the sense of coherence scale. Soc Sci Med. 1993;36(6):725–33.
15. Eriksson M. The sense of coherence in the salutogenic model of health. The handbook of salutogenesis. Berlin: Springer; 2017. p. 91–5.
16. Antonovsky A. Health, stress, and coping. London: Jossey-Bass; 1979.
17. Mittelmark MB, Sagy S, Eriksson M, Bauer GF, Pelikan JM, Lindström B, et al. The handbook of salutogenesis. Berlin: Springer; 2017.
18. Sullivan GC. Evaluating Antonovsky's salutogenic model for its adaptability to nursing. J Adv Nurs. 1989;14(4):336–42.

19. Nesbitt BJ, Heidrich SM. Sense of coherence and illness appraisal in older women's quality of life. Res Nurs Health. 2000;23(1):25–34.

20. Volanen S, Suominen S, Lahelma E, Koskenvuo M, Silventoinen K. Negative life events and stability of sense of coherence: a five-year follow-up study of Finnish women and men. Scand J Psychol. 2007;48(5):433–41.

21. Eriksson M. Unravelling the mystery of salutogenesis: the evidence base of the salutogenic research as measured by Antonovsky's sense of coherence scale. Turku: Åbo Akademi; 2007.

22. Lainscak M, Keber I. Patient's view of heart failure: from the understanding to the quality of life. Eur J Cardiovasc Nurs. 2003;2(4):275–81.

23. Mahoney JS. An ethnographic approach to understanding the illness experiences of patients with congestive heart failure and their family members. Heart Lung. 2001;30(6):429–36. http://www.ncbi.nlm.nih.gov/pubmed/11723447.

24. Currie K, Strachan PH, Spaling M, Harkness K, Barber D, Clark AM. The importance of interactions between patients and healthcare professionals for heart failure self-care: a systematic review of qualitative research into patient perspectives. Eur J Cardiovasc Nurs. 2015;14(6):525–35. http://journals.sagepub.com/doi/10.1177/1474515114547648.

25. Yancy CW, Jessup M, Bozkurt B, Butler J, Casey DE, Colvin MM, et al. 2017 ACC/AHA/HFSA focused update of the 2013 ACCF/AHA Guideline for the Management of Heart Failure: a report of the American College of Cardiology/American Heart Association Task Force on Clinical Practice Guidelines and the Heart Failure Society of America. Circulation. 2017;136(6):e137–61.

26. Colucci WS, Gottlieb SS, Yeon SB. Use of diuretics in patients with heart failure. UpToDate. 2019. https://www.uptodate.com/contents/use-of-diuretics-in-patients-with-heart-failure?search=diureticin heartfailure&source=search_result&selectedTitle=1~150&usage_type=default&display_rank=1#H1.

27. Lainscak M, Blue L, Clark AL, Dahlstrom U, Dickstein K, Ekman I, et al. Self-care management of heart failure: practical recommendations from the patient care committee of the heart failure association of the European Society of Cardiology. Eur J Heart Fail. 2011;13(2):115–26.

28. Ma H, Lum C, Woo J. Readmission of patients with congestive heart failure: the need for focused care. Asian J Gerontol. 2006;1(1):59–60.

29. Phillips CO, Wright SM, Kern DE, Singa RM, Shepperd S, Rubin HR. Comprehensive discharge planning with postdischarge support for older patients with congestive heart failure: a meta-analysis. JAMA. 2004;291(11):1358–67.

30. van der Wal MHL, Jaarsma T. Adherence in heart failure in the elderly: problem and possible solutions. Int J Cardiol. 2008;125(2):203–8.

31. Zhang Y, Wu S-H, Fendrick AM, Baicker K. Variation in medication adherence in heart failure.

32. JAMA Intern Med. 2013;23173(6):468–70. https://www.ncbi.nlm.nih.gov/pmc/articles/PMC3624763/pdf/nihms412728.pdf.

32. Horowitz CR, Rein SB, Leventhal H. A story of maladies, misconceptions and mishaps: effective management of heart failure. Soc Sci Med. 2004;58(3):631–43.

33. Nordfonn OK, Morken IM, Bru LE, Husebø AML. Patients' experience with heart failure treatment and self-care—a qualitative study exploring the burden of treatment. J Clin Nurs. 2019;28(9–10):1782–93.

34. Greenberg RN. Overview of patient compliance with medication dosing: a literature review. Clin Ther. 1984;6(5):592–9.

35. Pullar T, Birtwell AJ, Wiles PG, Hay A, Feely MP. Use of a pharmacologic indicator to compare compliance with tablets prescribed to be taken once, twice, or three times daily. Clin Pharmacol Ther. 1988;44(5):540–5.

36. Udelson JE, Pressler SJ, Sackner-Bernstein J, Massaro J, Ordronneau P, Lukas MA, et al. Adherence with once daily versus twice daily carvedilol in patients with heart failure: the compliance and quality of life study comparing once-daily controlled-release carvedilol CR and twice-daily immediate-release carvedilol IR in patients with heart failure (CASPER) trial. J Card Fail. 2009;15(5):385–93. https://doi.org/10.1016/j.cardfail.2008.12.010.

37. Claxton AJ, Cramer J, Pierce C. A systematic review of the associations between dose regimens and medication compliance. Clin Ther. 2001;23(8):1296–310.

38. Andrews AM, Russell CL, Cheng AL. Medication adherence interventions for older adults with heart failure: a systematic review. J Gerontol Nurs. 2017;43(10):37–45.

39. Molloy GJ, O'Carroll RE, Witham MD, McMurdo MET. Interventions to enhance adherence to medications in patients with heart failure a systematic review. Circ Hear Fail. 2012;5(1):126–33.

40. Bergman E, Malm D, Ljungquist B, Berterö C, Karlsson J. Meaningfulness is not the most important component for changes in sense of coherence; 2012.

41. Sua YS, Jiang Y, Thompson DR, Wang W. Effectiveness of mobile phone-based self-management interventions for medication adherence and change in blood pressure in patients with coronary heart disease: a systematic review and meta-analysis. Eur J Cardiovasc Nurs. 2020;19(3):192–200.

42. Goldstein CM, Gathright EC, Dolansky MA, Gunstad J, Sterns A, Redle JD, et al. Randomized controlled feasibility trial of two telemedicine medication reminder systems for older adults with heart failure. J Telemed Telecare. 2014;20(6):293–9.

43. Gandapur Y, Kianoush S, Kelli HM, Misra S, Urrea B, Blaha MJ, et al. The role of mHealth for improving medication adherence in patients with cardiovascular

disease: a systematic review. Eur Heart J Qual Care Clin Outcomes. 2016;2(4):237–44.

44. McMurray JJV, Adamopoulos S, Anker SD, Auricchio A, Böhm M, Dickstein K, et al. ESC guidelines for the diagnosis and treatment of acute and chronic heart failure 2012. Eur J Heart Fail. 2012;14(8):803–69. http://doi.wiley.com/10.1093/eurjhf/hfs105.

45. Colin-Ramirez E, Ezekowitz JA. Salt in the diet in patients with heart failure: what to recommend. Curr Opin Cardiol. 2016;31(2):196–203.

46. Arcand J, Ivanov J, Sasson A, Floras V, Al-Hesayen A, Azevedo E, et al. A high-sodium diet is associated with acute decompensated heart failure in ambulatory heart failure patients: a prospective follow-up study. Am J Clin Nutr. 2011;93:332–7.

47. Song EK, Moser DK, Dunbar SB, Pressler SJ, Lennie TA. Dietary sodium restriction below 2 gram per day predicted shorter event-free survival in patients with mild heart failure. Eur J Cardiovasc Nurs. 2014;13(6):541–8.

48. Butler J, Papadimitriou L, Georgiopoulou V, Skopicki H, Dunbar S, Kalogeropoulos A. Comparing sodium intake strategies in heart failure: rationale and design of the PROHIBIT sodium (PRevent adverse Outcomes in Heart failure By LimITing Sodium) study. Circ Heart Fail. 2015;8(3):636–45.

49. Ezekowitz JA, Meara EO, Mcdonald MA, Abrams H, Chan M, Ducharme A, et al. 2017 Comprehensive update of the Canadian Cardiovascular Society Guidelines for the management of heart failure. Can J Cardiol. 2017;33(11):1342–433.

50. Yancy CW, Jessup M, Bozkurt B, Butler J, Casey DE, Drazner MH, et al. 2013 ACCF/AHA guideline for the management of heart failure: a report of the American College of Cardiology Foundation/American Heart Association Task Force on practice guidelines. Circulation. 2013;128(16):240–327.

51. Ponikowski P, Voors AA, Anker SD, Bueno H, Cleland JGF, Coats AJS, et al. 2016 ESC guidelines for the diagnosis and treatment of acute and chronic heart failure. Eur Heart J. 2016;37(27):2129–200.

52. Konerman MC, Hummel SL. Sodium restriction in heart failure: benefit or harm? Curr Treat Options Cardiovasc Med. 2014;16(2):286.

53. Colin-Ramirez E, McAlister FA, Zheng Y, Sharma S, Armstrong PW, Ezekowitz JA. The long-term effects of dietary sodium restriction on clinical outcomes in patients with heart failure. The SODIUM-HF (Study of Dietary Intervention under 100 mmol in Heart Failure): a pilot study. Am Heart J. 2015;169(2):274–281.e1. https://doi.org/10.1016/j.ahj.2014.11.013.

54. Paterna S, Gaspare P, Fasullo S, Sarullo FM, Di Pasquale P. Normal-sodium diet compared with low-sodium diet in compensated congestive heart failure: is sodium an old enemy or a new friend? Clin Sci. 2008;114(3–4):221–30.

55. Horwitz L, Krumholz H, Hunt SA, Yeon SB. Heart failure self-management. UpToDate.

2019. https://www.uptodate.com/contents/heart-failure-self-management.

56. Dunbar SB, Clark PC, Reilly CM, Gary RA, Smith A, McCary F, et al. A trial of family partnership and education interventions in heart failure. J Card Fail. 2012;23(1):1–7.

57. Riegel B, Lee S, Hill J, Daus M, Baah FO, Wald JW, et al. Patterns of adherence to diuretics, dietary sodium and fluid intake recommendations in adults with heart failure. Hear Lung. 2019;48(3):179–85.

58. Colin-Ramirez E, McAlister FA, Woo E, Wong N, Ezekowitz JA. Association between self-reported adherence to a low-sodium diet and dietary habits related to sodium intake in heart failure patients. J Cardiovasc Nurs. 2015;30(1):58–65.

59. Chung ML, Lennie TA, de Jong M, Wu JR, Riegel B, Moser DK. Patients differ in their ability to self-monitor adherence to a low-sodium diet versus medication. J Card Fail. 2008;14(2):114–20.

60. Bentley B, De Jong MJ, Moser DK, Peden AR. Factors related to nonadherence to low sodium diet recommendations in heart failure patients. Eur J Cardiovasc Nurs. 2005;4(4):331–6.

61. Ong SF, Foong PPM, Seah JSH, Elangovan L, Wang W. Learning needs of hospitalized patients with heart failure in Singapore: a descriptive correlational study. J Nurs Res. 2018;26(4):250–9.

62. Kuehneman T, Saulsbury D, Splett P, Chapman DB. Demonstrating the impact of nutrition intervention in a heart failure program. J Am Diet Assoc. 2002;102(12):1790–4.

63. Zeng W, Chia SY, Chan YH, Tan SC, Low EJH, Fong MK. Factors impacting heart failure patients' knowledge of heart disease and self-care management. Proc Singapore Healthc. 2017;26(1):26–34.

64. Wilson DK, Ampey-Thornhill G. The role of gender and family support on dietary compliance in an African American adolescent hypertension prevention study. Ann Behav Med. 2001;23(1):59–67.

65. Johansson P, Van Der Wal MHL, Strömberg A, Waldréus N, Jaarsma T. Fluid restriction in patients with heart failure: how should we think? Eur J Cardiovasc Nurs. 2016;15(5):301–4.

66. Holst M, Strömberg A, Lindholm M, Willenheimer R. Liberal versus restricted fluid prescription in stabilised patients with chronic heart failure: result of a randomised cross-over study of the effects on health-related quality of life, physical capacity, thirst and morbidity. Scand Cardiovasc J. 2008;42(5):316–22.

67. Travers B, O'Loughlin C, Murphy NF, Ryder M, Conlon C, Ledwidge M, et al. Fluid restriction in the management of decompensated heart failure: no impact on time to clinical stability. J Card Fail. 2007;13(2):128–32.

68. Hooper L, Abdelhamid A, Attreed NJ, Campbell WW, Channell AM, Chassagne P, et al. Clinical symptoms, signs and tests for identification of impending and current water-loss dehydration in older people. Cochrane Database Syst Rev 2015;(4).

69. Chaudhry SI, Wang Y, Concato J, Gill TM, Krumholz HM. Patterns of weight change preceding hospitalization for heart failure. Circulation. 2007;116(14):1549–54.

70. Riegel B, Lee CS, Dickson VV, Carlson B. An update on the self-care of heart failure index. J Cardiovasc Nurs. 2009;24(6):485–97.

71. Malhotra C, Cheng Sim Wong G, Tan BC, Ng CSH, Lee NC, Lau CSL, et al. Living with heart failure: perspectives of patients from Singapore. Proc Singapore Healthc. 2016;25(2):92–7.

72. Clark AM, Spaling M, Harkness K, Spiers J, Strachan PH, Thompson DR, et al. Determinants of effective heart failure self-care: a systematic review of patients' and caregivers' perceptions. Heart. 2014;100(9):716–21.

73. Costello JA, Boblin S. What is the experience of men and women with congestive heart failure? Can J Cardiovasc Nurs. 2004;14(3):9–20. https://www.scopus.com/inward/record.uri?eid=2-s2.0-7244224845&partnerID=40&md5=bcd548737deab960031324587433e477.

74. Vaughan Dickson V, Lee CS, Riegel B. How do cognitive function and knowledge affect heart failure self-care? J Mix Methods Res. 2011;5(2):167–89.

75. Moser DK, Doering LV, Chung ML. Vulnerabilities of patients recovering from an exacerbation of chronic heart failure. Am Heart J. 2005;150(5):984.e7–13.

76. Miller CL. Cue sensitivity in women with cardiac disease. Prog Cardiovasc Nurs. 2000;15(3):82–9.

77. Patel H, Shafazand M, Schaufelberger M, Ekman I. Reasons for seeking acute care in chronic heart failure. Eur J Heart Fail. 2007;9(6–7):702–8.

78. Alves TCTF, Rays J, Fráguas R Jr, Wajngarten M, Meneghetti JC, Prando S, et al. Localized cerebral blood flow reductions in patients with heart failure: a study using 99mTc-HMPAO SPECT. J Neuroimaging. 2005;15(2):150–6.

79. Woo MA, Macey PM, Fonarow GC, Hamilton MA, Harper RM. Regional brain gray matter loss in heart failure. J Appl Physiol. 2003;95(2):677–84.

80. Moser DK, Dickson V, Jaarsma T, Lee C, Stromberg A, Riegel B. Role of self-care in the patient with heart failure. Curr Cardiol Rep. 2012;14(3):265–75.

81. Jurgens CY, Hoke L, Byrnes J, Riegel B. Why do elders delay responding to heart failure symptoms? Nurs Res. 2009;58(4):274–82. https://www.scopus.com/inward/record.uri?eid=2-s2.0-68349095171&doi=10.1097%2FNNR.0b013e3181ac1581&partnerID=40&md5=6da4adfddb8b1dc4006b92375b216525.

82. Creber RMM, Hickey KT, Maurer MS. Gerontechnologies for older patients with heart failure: what is the role of samrtphones, tablets, and remote monitoring devices in improving symptom monitoring and self-care management? Curr Cardiovasc Risk Rep. 2016;10(10):1–15.

83. Scherr D, Kastner P, Kollmann A, Hallas A, Auer J, Krappinger H, et al. Effect of home-based tele-monitoring using mobile phone technology on the outcome of heart failure patients after an episode of acute decompensation: randomized controlled trial. J Med Internet Res. 2009;11(3):1–12.

84. Inglis SC, Clark RA, McAlister FA, Ball J, Lewinter C, Cullington D, et al. Structured telephone support or telemonitoring programmes for patients with chronic heart failure. Cochrane Database Syst Rev. 2010;4(8):CD007228.

85. Seto E, Leonard KJ, Cafazzo JA, Barnsley J, Masino C, Ross HJ. Mobile phone-based telemonitoring for heart failure management: a randomized controlled trial. J Med Internet Res. 2012;14(1):1–14.

86. Chaudhry SI, Mattera JA, Curtis JP, Spertus JA, Herrine J, Lin Z, et al. Telemonitoring in patients with heart failure. N Engl J Med. 2011;364(24):2301–9.

87. Zan S, Agboola S, Moore SA, Parks KA, Kvedar JC, Jethwani K. Patient engagement with a mobile web-based telemonitoring system for heart failure self-management: a pilot study. JMIR Mhealth Uhealth. 2015;3(2):e33.

88. O'Connor CM, Whellan DJ, Lee KL, Keteyian SJ, Cooper LS, Ellis SJ, et al. Efficacy and safety of exercise training in patients with chronic heart failure: HF-ACTION randomized controlled trial. JAMA. 2009;301(14):1439–50.

89. Taylor RS, Sagar VA, Davies EJ, Briscoe S, Coats AJS, Dalal H, et al. Exercise-based rehabilitation for heart failure. Cochrane Database Syst Rev. 2014;2014(4):CD003331.

90. Pearson MJ, Smart NA. Exercise therapy and autonomic function in heart failure patients: a systematic review and meta-analysis. Heart Fail Rev. 2018;23(1):91–108.

91. Suskin N, Sheth T, Negassa A, Yusuf S. Relationship of current and past smoking to mortality and morbidity in patients with left ventricular dysfunction. J Am Coll Cardiol. 2001;37(6):1677–82. https://doi.org/10.1016/S0735-1097(01)01195-0.

92. Sidorenkov O, Nilssen O, Nieboer E, Kleshchinov N, Grjibovski AM. Premature cardiovascular mortality and alcohol consumption before death in Arkhangelsk, Russia: an analysis of a consecutive series of forensic autopsies. Int J Epidemiol. 2011;40(6):1519–29.

93. Lightwood J, Fleischmann KE, Glantz SA. Smoking cessation in heart failure: it is never too late. J Am Coll Cardiol. 2001;37(6):1683–4. https://doi.org/10.1016/S0735-1097(01)01188-3.

94. Heart Failure Society of America. Nonpharmacologic management and health care maintenance in patients with chronic heart failure. J Card Fail. 2006;12(1):29–37.

95. Aguilar D, Skali H, Moyé LA, Lewis EF, Gaziano JM, Rutherford JD, et al. Alcohol consumption and prognosis in patients with left ventricular systolic dysfunction after a myocardial infarction. J Am Coll Cardiol. 2004;43(11):2015–21.

96. Salisbury AC, House JA, Conard MW, Krumholz HM, Spertus JA. Low-to-moderate alcohol intake

and health status in heart failure patients. J Card Fail. 2005;11(5):323–8.

97. O'Keefe JH, Bhatti SK, Bajwa A, DiNicolantonio JJ, Lavie CJ. Alcohol and cardiovascular health: the dose makes the poison...or the remedy. Mayo Clin Proc. 2014;89(3):382–93. https://doi.org/10.1016/j.mayocp.2013.11.005.

98. Powell L, Calvin J, Richardson D, Janssen I, de Mendes LC, Flynn K, et al. Self-management counseling in patients with heart failure: the heart failure adherence and retention randomized behavioral trial. JAMA. 2010;304:1331–8. http://onlinelibrary.wiley.com/o/cochrane/clcentral/articles/813/CN-00762813/frame.html.

99. Shao J, Chang A, Edwards H, Shyu Y, Chen S. A randomized controlled trial of self-management programme improves health-related outcomes of older people with heart failure. J Adv Nurs. 2013;69:2458–69. http://onlinelibrary.wiley.com/o/cochrane/clcentral/articles/850/CN-00987850/frame.html.

100. Smeulders E, Haastregt J, Ambergen T, Janssen-Boyne J, Eijk J, Kempen G. The impact of a self-management group programme on health behaviour and healthcare utilization among congestive heart failure patients. Eur J Heart Fail. 2009;11:609–16. http://onlinelibrary.wiley.com/o/cochrane/clcentral/articles/763/CN-00720763/frame.html.

101. Smeulders E, Haastregt J, Ambergen T, Uszko-Lencer N, Janssen-Boyne J, Gorgels A, et al. Nurse-led self-management group programme for patients with congestive heart failure: randomized controlled trial. J Adv Nurs. 2010;66:1487–99. http://onlinelibrary.wiley.com/o/cochrane/clcentral/articles/016/CN-00773016/frame.html.

102. Dracup K, Evangelista LS, Hamilton MA, Erickson V, Hage A, Moriguchi J, et al. Effects of a home-based exercise program on clinical outcomes in heart failure. Am Heart J. 2007;154(5):877–83.

103. Yu DSF, Thompson DR. What makes a disease management programme for heart failure different: results of a meta-regression analysis. Int J Cardiol. 2008;125:S45–6.

104. Boren SA, Wakefield BJ, Gunlock TL, Wakefield DS. Heart failure self-management education: a systematic review of the evidence. Int J Evid Based Healthc. 2009;7(3):159–68.

105. Boyde M, Peters R, New N, Hwang R, Ha T, Korczyk D. Self-care educational intervention to reduce hospitalisations in heart failure: a randomised controlled trial. Eur J Cardiovasc Nurs. 2018;17(2):178–85.

106. Boyde M, Peters R, Hwang R, Korczyk D, Ha T, New N. The self-care educational intervention for patients with heart failure. J Cardiovasc Nurs. 2017;32(2):165–70. http://insights.ovid.com/crossref?an=00005082-201703000-00012.

107. Arlinghaus KR, Johnston CA. Advocating for behavior change with education. Am J Lifestyle Med. 2018;12(2):113–6.

108. Rozanski A, Blumenthal JA, Davidson KW, Saab PG, Kubzansky L. The epidemiology, pathophysiol-ogy, and management of psychosocial risk factors in cardiac practice: the emerging field of behavioral cardiology. J Am Coll Cardiol. 2005;45(5):637–51. https://doi.org/10.1016/j.jacc.2004.12.005.

109. Williams RB. Psychosocial and biobehavioral factors and their interplay in coronary heart disease. Annu Rev Clin Psychol. 2008;4:349–65.

110. Samartzis L, Dimopoulos S, Tziongourou M, Nanas S. Effect of psychosocial interventions on quality of life in patients with chronic heart failure: a meta-analysis of randomized controlled trials. J Card Fail. 2013;19(2):125–34. https://doi.org/10.1016/j.cardfail.2012.12.004.

111. Thompson DR, Ski CF. Psychosocial interventions in cardiovascular disease—what are they? Eur J Prev Cardiol. 2013;20(6):916–7. http://cpr.sagepub.com/lookup/doi/10.1177/2047487313494031.

112. Lane D, Chong A, Lip G. Cochrane review psychological interventions for depression in HF. 2005;(1). file:///C:/Users/acer/Documents/Mendeley Desktop/Cochrane review psychological interventions for depression in HF.pdf.

113. Klainin-Yobas P, Ng SH, Stephen PDM, Lau Y. Efficacy of psychosocial interventions on psychological outcomes among people with cardiovascular diseases: a systematic review and meta-analysis. Patient Educ Couns. 2016;99(4):512–21. https://doi.org/10.1016/j.pec.2015.10.020.

114. Jiang Y, Shorey S, Seah B, Chan W, Tam WWS, Wang W. The effectiveness of psychological interventions on self-care, psychological and health outcomes in patients with chronic heart failure—a systematic review and meta-analysis. Int J Nurs Stud. 2018;78:16–25. https://doi.org/10.1016/j.ijnurstu.2017.08.006.

115. Gustavsson A, Bränholm IB. Experienced health, life satisfaction, sense of coherence, and coping resources in individuals living with heart failure. Scand J Occup Ther. 2003;10(3):138–43.

116. Gallagher R. Self management, symptom monitoring and associated factors in people with heart failure living in the community. Eur J Cardiovasc Nurs. 2010;9(3):153–60. https://doi.org/10.1016/j.ejcnurse.2009.12.006.

117. Ferreira VMP, Silva LN, Furuya RK, Schmidt A, Rossi LA, Dantas RAS. Self-care, sense of coherence and depression in patients hospitalized for decompensated heart failure. Rev da Esc Enferm. 2015;49(3):387–93.

118. Ekman I, Fagerberg B, Lundman B. Health-related quality of life and sense of coherence among elderly patients with severe chronic heart failure in comparison with healthy controls. Heart Lung. 2002;31(2):94–101.

119. Chow CK, Ariyarathna N, Islam SMS, Thiagalingam A, Redfern J. mHealth in cardiovascular health care. Hear Lung Circ. 2016;25(8):802–7. https://doi.org/10.1016/j.hlc.2016.04.009.

120. Dansky KH, Vasey J, Bowles K. Impact of telehealth on clinical outcomes in patients with heart failure.

Clin Nurs Res. 2008;17(3):182–99. http://journals. sagepub.com/doi/10.1177/1054773808320837.

121. Arora S, Peters AL, Burner E, Lam CN, Menchine M. Trial to examine text message-based mhealth in emergency department patients with diabetes (TExT-MED): a randomized controlled trial. Ann Emerg Med. 2014;63(6):745–754.e6. https://doi.org/10.1016/j.annemergmed.2013.10.012.

122. Buck H, Pinter A, Poole E, Boehmer J, Foy A, Black S, et al. Evaluating the older adult experience of a web-based, tablet-delivered heart failure self-care program using gerontechnology principles. Geriatr Nurs (Minneap). 2017;38:537–41. https://doi.org/10.1016/j.gerinurse.2017.04.001.

123. Creber RMM, Maurer MS, Reading M, Hickey KT, Iribarren S. Review and analysis of existing mobile phone apps to support heart failure symptom monitoring and self-care management using the mobile application rating scale (MARS). JMIR mHealth uHealth. 2016;4(2):e74.

124. Athilingam P, Jenkins B, Johansson M, Labrador M. A mobile health intervention to improve self-care in patients with heart failure: pilot randomized control trial. JMIR Cardiol. 2017;1(2):e3.

Older Adults in Hospitals: Health Promotion When Hospitalized

20

Anne-S. Helvik

Abstract

The population of older adults (≥60 years) is currently growing. Thus, in the years to come it is expected that a high proportion of patients hospitalized will be in the older age range. In western countries, the proportion of older inpatients is about 40% in the medical and surgical hospitals units. Older people with illness is vulnerable to both physical and cognitive impairments as well as depression. Therefore, a health-promoting perspective and approach are highly warranted in clinical nursing care of older adults in medical hospitals. This chapter focuses on health promotion related to depressive symptoms, impairment in activities of daily living, and cognitive impairment in older hospitalized adults.

Keywords

Cognition · Coping · Discharge · Elderly · Functioning · Inpatient · Mood · Screening

20.1 Introduction

The increasing proportion of older adults (≥60 years) [1–3] represents a heterogeneous group of people often characterized by a complex health situation [4], with several diseases and limitations compared to younger adults [5, 6]. Furthermore, older adults (≥60 years) may be more vulnerable for negative health outcomes connected to hospitalization than younger adults. In addition, they may have symptoms of disease that are less typical than for younger adults. Older adults being hospitalized have or may get depressive symptoms, reduced functioning in activities of daily living and/or reduced cognitive functioning, all of which affecting the older individual's coping and health-promoting actions negatively.

To provide good quality nursing care, it is important to have several aspects of care in mind at the same time. In a hospital setting, health-promoting nursing care improves the medical condition causing hospitalization, strengthens the individual's health-promoting resources, and support well-being and quality of life. Thus,

A.-S. Helvik (✉)
Department of Public Health and Nursing, NTNU Norwegian University of Science and Technology, Trondheim, Norway

Norwegian National Advisory Unit on Ageing and Health, Vestfold Hospital Trust, Tønsberg, Norway
e-mail: anne-sofie.helvik@ntnu.no

G. Haugan, M. Eriksson (eds.), *Health Promotion in Health Care – Vital Theories and Research*,
https://doi.org/10.1007/978-3-030-63135-2_20

focusing on the medical condition(s), promotion of mental health along with cognitive and physical functioning in activities of daily living are equally important.

Health promotion is built on the salutogenesis model proposed by Antonovsky in 1979 [7]. The salutogenic approach to health includes other aspects than the pathogenic model, leading to a more nuanced understanding of health. Salutogeneses includes a shift from solely focusing on the pathogenesis related to the medical reasons for hospitalization and risk factors, toward capabilities and potential of the person. Despite hospitalization and disease, the individuals posess resources which are fundamental for health and well-being. The salutogenic approach to health includes reflection of the patient's life situation, a review of available resources and active adaptation to life stressors, challenges, and a changing situation or environment [7, 8]. How you cope and adapt to life stressors and challenges are affected of available coping resources. Both general resistant resources (GRR) and sense of coherence (SOC) are of importance [7]. SOC express an individual's ability to comprehend the whole situation, the capacity to use the resources available to move in a health-promoting direction and finding life to be meaningful [7, 9]. Thus, the way people are able to perceive structures, create coherence and manage change in a meaningful manner has a central impact on health [8]. Resources available include both internal and external resources [7], and nurses and other health professionals should be valuable resources for health promotion among hospitalized older persons.

20.2 Methods

This chapter focuses on hospitalized older adults in general and does not focus on any specific medical condition. The research literature used here has been published in review-based journals reporting results from cross-sectional and longitudinal studies about depression, impairment, and functioning in activities of daily living and cognitive functioning and impairment during and after

acutely hospitalization due to medical conditions. The author has published several observational studies focusing on depression, activities of daily living and cognitive functioning during and after acutely hospitalization of older adults [10–17]. Thus, this chapter is based on the authors' former studies, along with previous evidence published up to June 2019. The search terms were: elderly/older adults/older patients, depression/depressive symptoms, physical functioning/personal functioning/basic functioning/activities of daily living, cognitive functioning/cognitive impairment/dementia/Alzheimer disease/mild cognitive impairment, and lastly, in patients/hospitalization/medical ward/geriatric unit and combinations of these terms were also used.

20.3 Health Promotion During Hospitalization

Nursing care should contribute to improve the medical condition causing hospitalization as well as promote the patients' health resources. This chapter focuses on health promotion related to depressive symptoms, impairment in activities of daily living and cognitive impairment in older hospitalized adults. The consequences of depression, cognitive impairment, and reduced physical functioning for potential health outcome and well-being are described. Health-promoting care will map existing and limited health resources as basis for care actions. This chapter will also include simple methods to uncover existing and evolving symptoms of depression, cognitive impairment, and limitations of physical activities of daily living.

20.3.1 Depression

Depression is a frequent cause of emotional suffering in old age causing negative health consequences such as reduced physical functioning and quality of life [18–20], increased risk of nursing home admission [21], and lower life expectancy [22, 23]. Depression in old age is also related to higher health care costs [24].

Depression, also known as major depressive disorder or clinical depression, is a common and serious mood disorder, which is diagnosed based on specific diagnostic criteria e.g., ICD-10 or DSM-V [25, 26]. Symptoms related to depression are feelings of sadness, hopelessness and loss of interest in activities they once enjoyed, involuntary weight change, sleep disturbance, changes in psychomotor activity, fatigue or loss of energy, feelings of worthlessness or excessive or inappropriate guilt, diminished ability to think or concentrate and recurrent thoughts of death. In accordance to diagnostic criteria, symptoms of (1) depressed mood, or (2) loss of interest or pleasure have to be present to define a person's state as a depression disease [25]. In addition, several of the symptoms mentioned above must be present simultaneously in a 2 weeks period. The severity of the symptoms has to significantly reduce the person's ability of functioning in one's daily living [25].

Older adults may have more uncharacteristic symptoms of depression than younger people. For example, the experience of sadness may be missing, but they may have pronounced medical symptoms such as fatigue, pain, sleeping difficulties, and loss of appetite [27, 28]. In older people depression may be mistaken for dementia, or grief due to losses, as well as a reaction of disease or functional impairment. Depression limits your resilience and resources available to cope with stressors and difficulties as well as to maintain and promote health.

A population-based meta-analysis found the diagnostic pooled prevalence of depression in older adults to be 7% [29]. Reviews of epidemiological community studies in Europe and worldwide have estimated the prevalence of significant depressive symptoms to be a bit higher and to vary between 8% and 15% among older adults [30, 31]. Poor physical health is a known risk factor for depression [32]. The prevalence of depression or significant depressive symptoms are reported higher in older adults with medical diseases and reduced ability to perform activities of daily living, compared to more healthy older adults [33]. Furthermore, the prevalence of depression is reported higher in older adults

being hospitalized [34]. In a review of international studies involving elderly medical inpatients, the prevalence of significant depressive symptoms ranged between 10% and 73% [10]. In a Norwegian study of acutely hospitalized older persons coming from rural municipalities, the prevalence of significant depressive symptoms was low (10%). However, 78% of those 10% with significant depressive symptoms had no information in their medical record that they ever had experienced some kind of mental health difficulties, problems or diagnoses of any kind previously in their life [10]. Thus, 78% of those detected with screening would probable not been uncovered or diagnosed with depression if depression was not systematically screened for at that study. Uncovering existing and evolving symptoms of depression is a necessary step for treatment of the condition.

As said previously, the prevalence of depression is higher in those with medical conditions, is increasing with age [33], and is influenced by gender, ethnicity, place of living, income, and social support [33]. However, hospitalized older adults with reduced ability to perform activities of daily living (ADL), in need of in-home nursing care before hospitalization, and using several prescribed drugs, are more likely to experience depressive symptoms than those without such difficulties or use of drugs [10]. Accordingly, those hospitalized with several and/or considerable health limitations and fewer resources are more likely to experience depressive symptoms. Health personal must be aware of the complex relation between gender, ethnicity, place of living, income, social support, and different health aspects. The older person's total situation as well as his or her background and life experiences are relevant. Health professionals' knowledge about the older adult's thoughts, expectations, wishes and hopes for the stay and future has importance when tailoring care to promote her/his mental state. A person-focused approach with an earnest interest in the person's total situation, including psychological health and mental well-being, includes health-promoting care facilitating perceived meaning-in-life, hope, self-transcendence, and sense of coherence. Moreover, in this context health-promoting nursing care includes assessment and awareness of the older person's experience of self-confidence, sense of worthiness/worthlessness, as well as needs and wishes in the present situation. In all phases of the hospitalization, health-promoting nursing is based on respect of the patient's integrity. Health-promoting nurse–patient interaction contributes to a sense of being welcome and safe, and to make the situation comprehensible as well as manageable and thereby easing emotional distress. Health-promoting nursing facilitates hope and resilience in the patient and his family.

For older adults, depression may be experienced as being in a vice, with little power of resistance for depressive thoughts, not being able to make peace in life, with limited resilience and reduced ability to experience hope and difficulties finding meaning-in-life [35]. Thus, the salutogenic health processes are impeded. Even so, emotional support as well as respectful attitudes are ground pillars for regaining resilience and meaning-in-life and to boost well-being and health. However, depressive symptoms constrain the old individual's ability to see a positive outcome of the situation. Consequently, identifying depressive symptoms and supporting the older adult's coping resources are essential. This is essential in order to arrange for salutogenic health processes. Even so, depression in older adults may be unrecognized, untreated, and thus reducing the health outcome [36]. This may obstruct health promotion in terms of developing resilience, experiencing coherence, hope, and finding meaning-in-life. Both milder and more severe depressive symptoms may provoke and increase functional limitations in older adults [12, 37]. Furthermore, the cognitive functioning and quality of life may decrease [16, 38], both in a short and long-term perspective. Therefore, the following section focuses on the importance of uncovering depressive symptoms using valid screening tools.

20.3.1.1 Uncovering Depressive Symptoms by Use of Screening Tools

To ask about depression and to screen for depressive symptoms are relevant in order to promote older adults' health while hospitalized. In addition, use of established screening tools may contribute to a joint understanding among health professionals treating and caring for the individual, and be the first step for further examination and eventually a diagnostic workup. Registered nurses may use simple screening tools to reveal depressive symptoms. Several screening tools are available.

The Geriatric Depression Scale for older adults (GDS) [39] is a well-known screening tool and translated to several languages [40, 41]. This tool is used in older adults with minor or no cognitive impairment, but is not suitable among people with dementia [42]. The GDS has several shorter versions; a short version with 15 items [39] is frequently used. Other short versions include four or five items [43, 44]. All versions of the GDS have two response options for each question. The cutoff values indicating clinically relevant symptoms of depression are based on the number of items of the GDS version in use [39, 43, 44]. The GDS screening tools are freely available and deemed suitable for use in hospitals as well as in primary health care.

Another screening tool often used in hospitals is the "Hospital Anxiety and Depression Scale" (HADS) [45] including 14 items with 4 response options (scoring goes from 0 to 3). This tool assesses both symptoms of depression and anxiety (7 items within each area) and does not include any questions about physical symptoms related to these conditions. The scale was developed for use in medical hospitals among all ages of adults, including older hospitalized adults. Lately, a study in older adults including persons both with and without poor physical health and need of care assistance found that the cutoff suggested for symptoms indicating depression in the general populations of hospitalized adults (≥ 8) was too high for older adults. In this validation of the HADS, the best cutoff score to indicate a clinical relevant depressive symptom load was 4 [43]. In clinical practice, it is important to note that the score indicating depression may be lower in older adults than for younger adults. Thus, it is important to use screening tools validated for the same type of population. Otherwise, clinically relevant depressive symptoms may be under-reported and untreated. The items used to assess symptoms of depression and anxiety are found adequate also in older adults [11, 46, 47]. An advantage with use of HADS is that it also assesses anxiety symptoms. Older adults with clinically relevant load of depressive symptoms may also have symptoms of anxiety [48]. HADS is a self-report questionnaire and has several advantages. However, with reduced physical health in combination with reduced cognitive capacity, it may be challenging to answer a questionnaire with four response options at each question. HADS is translated and validated in several languages and settings and have for years been used without charge eff. However, now there may be restricts related to its use [49].

As demonstrated above, the choice of screening tool may depend not only on the preferred use in a care unit, but also on the characteristics of the hospitalized person. The health professionals could preferably know a couple of screening inventories to make the conditions favorable for health promotion.

20.3.2 Activities of Daily Living (ADL)

The concept of 'Activities of daily living' (ADL) includes necessary activities to maintain self-care. ADL consists of basic activities (B-ADL) and more complex actions (I-ADL) that are necessary to be independent of help from others [50]. Even though there are some variations on the definition of B-ADL, this concept normally includes: (1) personal hygiene including bathing/showering, grooming, nail care, and oral care, (2) dressing including the ability to make appropriate clothing decisions and physically dress/undress oneself, (3) eating including having the ability to feed oneself, though not necessarily the capability to prepare food, (4) handling toilet visits including maintaining continence, having both the mental and physical capacity to use a restroom, including the ability to get on and off the toilet and cleaning oneself, and lastly, (5) transferring/mobility including having the ability for moving oneself from seated to

standing, getting in and out of bed, and the ability to walk independently from one location to another. The B-ADL is necessarily performed every day.

The more complex actions, named instrumental activities of daily living (I-ADL), are not necessarily required every day, but are related to independent living. The I-ADL includes: (1) using communications technology such as a regular phone, mobile phone, email, or the Internet, (2) using transportation either by driving oneself, arranging rides, or taking public transportation, (3) meal preparation with regard to meal planning, cooking, clean up, storage, and safely use kitchen equipment and utensils, (4) doing shopping and making appropriate food and clothing purchase decisions, (5) housework performance such as doing laundry, washing dishes, dusting, vacuuming, and maintaining a hygienic place of residence, (6) managing medications with regard to taking accurate dosages at the appropriate times, as well as managing re-fills, and finally, (7) managing personal finances with regards to operating within a budget, writing checks, paying bills, and avoiding scams [50].

Concerning functionality, loss of I-ADL is maybe not as noticeable in the beginning as loss of B-ADL, either not for the person self, next of kin and/or health personal. I-ADL functioning generally starts to decline prior to B-ADL functioning. Loss of both I-ADL and B-ADL reduces your ability to maintain self-care and may influence your experience of hope, meaning in life and well-being. Thus, it is important to detect any impairment early and by means of for instance empowerment, to promote individuals' coping, finding new solutions and a new or reinforced understanding of life, hope and meaning, despite that physical health is exposed. Loss of B-ADL functioning may enforce a change of life style followed by lower quality of life and increased mortality [51–57]. In addition, loss of B-ADL will increase health care costs due to care assistance [56–58].

Regardless of the cause of hospitalization, an essential part of nursing is to support and facilitate patients' B-ADL functionality, enhancing self-care during and after the hospitalization and thereby to promote health in general. Thus, the nurses focus on assessment, care and treatment and not only on treating the primary cause of hospitalization.

20.3.2.1 Decline of B-ADL in Connection with Hospitalization

Over some years it has been known that functional change in older people is a complex dynamic process where B-ADL may change, both before admission to hospital and during the hospital stay due to their illness and health condition [59] as well as after discharge [12].

The type and degree of B-ADL resources may vary considerably in older adults admitted to a medical hospital [60]. An American study reported that about 30% of older adults at admission to the medical unit had difficulties with dressing, hygiene, and transferring, and that about 40% of all patients had experienced a decline in B-ADL within 2 weeks before hospitalization [60].

A health-promotion approach to hospitalized older adults is essential, since a semi-acute or acute illness or condition increases the risk for B-ADL decline [61, 62]. This is the case for older adults, both with and without reduced functioning prior to the hospitalization. A study of more than 2000 older Americans hospitalized in general medical wards reported that about 20% of the patients had a decline in B-ADL during the hospitalization period [60]; the oldest old revealed the highest loss of B-ADL at discharge [60]. A recent large longitudinal hospital study found three trajectories of B-ADL in older patients admitted to acute medical ward units; (1) functionally decline (17%), (2) functionally recovering (41%), and (3) functionally stable (42%) over the hospital stay, with a mean of 10.5 days. In this American study, functional decline was explained by nursing and hospital care factors such as less daily care, larger hospital size, and lower care qualifications [63]. Accordingly, adequate time to interact with older hospitalized patients and health-promoting care competency are crucial. Even so, this is not enough. Health-promoting interaction is needed. This means that the health care professionals must engage in the relationship with patients. The professional strives to see, recognize and confirm the patient as the person he is and not only the patient with diagnoses, symptoms, needs and physiological conditions (see Theoretical section). This contributes to a personalized care that is accommodated to the patient's wishes promoting B-ADL and health.

Immobility has long been recognized as a hazard of hospitalization causing loss of body strength and B-ADL functions [61]. Maintaining and improving mobility and body strength as much as possible during hospitalization will improve the patient's ability to perform B-ADLs after discharge. In addition, patients who report unsteadiness while walking at hospital admission are more likely to experience functional decline after a stay in hospital [64]. Furthermore, unsteadiness may contribute to reduced mobility or falls during hospitalization. Thus, it is important to assess unsteadiness in order to give a care adapted to existing resources and support available B-ADL functioning rather than handling consequences of potential new difficulties, illness or impairments.

In general, older people need longer time to recover from illness and B-ADL decline. It is reported that among those with a new B-ADL decline during hospitalization, more than one-third needed 3 months or longer after discharge to regain normal B-ADL [52]. Furthermore, a decline in B-ADL is found to relate with mortality; about one fifth of those discharged with a new or additional decline in B-ADL during hospitalization stayed alive only 3 months after hospitalization [52]. Another study reported that the odds to regain normal B-ADL functioning both at 2 and 12 months after hospitalization was reduced by increasing number of B-ADL limitations [65]. A Norwegian observational study of medically hospitalized older adults showed that the mean B-ADL was significantly poorer 1 year after hospitalization compared to the functioning during the hospitalization [12]. In this study, the B-ADL decline 1 year after was explained by poorer baseline B-ADL [12].

A study of more than 500 acutely hospitalized older adults in medical wards reported that those with higher decline in B-ADL during hospital stay were more likely to be readmitted to the hospital within 30 days after discharge [66]. Furthermore, a Norwegian study of hospitalized older adults in medical wards found that those with one or more B-ADL difficulties while hospitalized were five times more likely to become nursing home residents within the first year after hospitalization [13]. Thus, in a health-promotion perspective, it is important to promote B-ADL functions while hospitalized. It may contribute to well-being not only in the moment, but also to improved health, well-being, and quality of life over time. Using a health promotion nursing perspective implies that in addition to a focus on supporting and improving B-ADL resources and functioning, the nursing care should be given in a health-promoting manner. Health-promoting interactions are fundamental in nursing care. By use of health-promoting interactions when supporting the patient with his or her B-ADL functioning, health professional may promote an experience of hope and meaning-in-life in the older adults. It may be a hope for managing the situation or hope that with help he or she has the strength to overcome difficulties and experience coherence in life.

Several factors may contribute to a B-ADL decline before, during, and after hospitalization. B-ADL decline may be explained by generally reduced health, loss of weight, chronical disease or multi-morbidity, pain, a high number of drugs taken, and/or visual impairment [67, 68]. A study revealed that decline in B-ADL after hospitalization, in addition to lower baseline B-ADL, were linked to higher age, reduced cognitive function during and after hospitalization as well as poorer psychological health after hospitalization [12]. The above study demonstrates that B-ADL is one of several areas for health promotion in hospitalized older adults; mental health (depression) and cognitive functioning need nursing attention and health-promoting interventions as well.

Nevertheless, regaining older individuals' B-ADL function requires effective treatment of the underlying conditions. Thus, a further decline of B-ADL during and after hospitalization may be due to ineffective treatment. Furthermore, the

health conditions forcing hospitalization may represent the beginning of a health condition that independently of treatment will contribute to a poorer B-ADL functioning. In such cases, health-promoting interventions by nurses and an interdisciplinary team of health care professionals in the hospital may contribute to reduced speed of the B-ADL decline during, but also after the hospitalization. In a health-promoting approach which is based in a holistic understanding of health, the older individual's situation, available resources and capacity to support self-care and B-ADL must be assessed, and actions taken to sustain B-ADL functioning during hospitalization and thereby contribute to best possible self-care after the discharge. This can for example be support of unsteadiness, reducing consequences of immobility due to bed rest. Furthermore, it is important to prepare and organize care such as personal hygiene, dressing, toileting, transferring, and other such activities in line with available B-ADL- resources. This may over time be health promoting.

Another reason for B-ADL decline after the hospitalization may be that the older adults themselves do not manage or know how to handle their health problems and their B-ADL deficits after discharge. In a health-promoting perspective, it is important to prepare the patient for the discharge from hospital, to strengthen their coping resources, and contribute to adequate arrangements and support afterwards. An optimal B-ADL function based on the individuals' premises during the hospitalization will also promote health and B-ADL functioning after discharge. For example, studies have found that B-ADL during hospitalization is linked to depression and cognitive function after discharge. Those, with little or no B-ADL deficits during hospitalization have reduced risk of depression and cognitively impairment 1 year after discharge [14, 15]. The phenomenon of persistent morbidity and functional disability after hospitalization may be labeled as a "post-hospital syndrome" and is accompanied by impaired quality of life of older people [69].

Some care units are organized, and the staff trained, to take care of acutely hospitalized older adults. Geriatric care units have for long been known to support and maintain patients' functionality during hospitalization compared to regular units [62]. Regardless of the hospital care unit or ward, health-promoting nursing should be based in a person-oriented approach; this way of interacting with the individual supports the patient's independency and self-care resources, increases hope, meaning, and resilience and thereby facilitates B-ADL performance from admission to discharge [70, 71] (see also Theoretical section). This may, in addition to a well-planned discharge, contribute to well-being and resilience over time. The Acute Care for Elders Unit (ACE) model [70] uses person-oriented care, applies a structured process including interdisciplinary teams, and uses systematic screening assessments of B-ADL following clinical guidelines to restore coping resources, resilience, and self-care [70], all of which are important for well-being and quality of life. Three randomized clinical trials using ACE interventions have found reduced B-ADL during hospitalization and reduced risk of nursing home admission among those in ACE units, and furthermore, a somewhat lower cost of hospitalization, due to shorter stay in the group randomized to ACE units [72–74]. The ACE principles could be implemented to improve care of hospitalized older adults, independently of which hospital ward or unit they are admitted to. A step toward including ACE principles is for nurses to be competent in systematic screening of B-ADL.

20.3.2.2 Systematically Screening of B-ADL Functioning

Systematically screening of B-ADL at admission, throughout the hospitalization and at discharge of older hospitalized adults will uncover areas of concern. Previously, the screening tools most often were used in research studies, but clinical experience have shown that systematically use of B-ADL tools improves the quality of nursing care. Nursing assessment is based in a systematic and joint framework to assess change. This framework gives a good basis to minimalize B-ADL decline due to illness, treatment, and hospital stay, and to improve level of

functioning. Based in the screening results, adequate nursing actions can be provided. Furthermore, identifying an individual's available B-ADL-resources, possible support and the individuals' will is crucial. Use of screening tools provides a joint framework of the interdisciplinary hospital team for high quality treatment. Consequently, such screening tools will not go out of fashion [50].

Several screening tools assess B-ADL, both short inventories and longer more complex versions exist [75–78]. Such tools have shown to capture small but important changes in an individual's ability to perform B-ADL [50]. Lawton and Brody's scale to assess ability self-care is often used and is among the relatively shorter tools that screen for B-ADL, such as personal hygiene, dressing, toileting, eating, and transferring [75]. This tool is easy to use; a higher score indicates higher B-ADL difficulties. In choosing a screening tool, whether the tool is fitted and validated for the language and culture of the specific country should be considered [70]. The problem in some countries is not a lack of adequate measures, but that there is no national agreement of which measure of B-ADL should be used in ward units and hospitals. This dearth makes it difficult to follow change in B-ADL for individuals with several steps through their treatment chain. It also makes it hard to compare change of B-ADL between institutions and care wards. A consensus about one appropriate tool to measure B-ADL may contribute to quality assurance of treatment and to improvement of care over time.

20.3.3 Cognitive Functioning

Decline in cognitive performance is commonly linked to aging [79, 80]. The cognitive functioning encompasses our ability to receive and process information, remember, learning new stuff, to organize information when we are thinking, using a language and communicate, to write/calculate/draw, have discernment, calculate distances (spatial awareness), take initiative and perform actions, thinking abstract, and to have attention. The ability to have attention is also affecting the above areas.

In cognitively intact older adults, an acute medical illness needing hospitalization may lead to reduced cognitive functioning in the acute phase of the disease [81, 82]. The cognitive decline may for some patients be caused by delirium which is an organically caused decline developed over a short period of time, typically hours to days [83]. Delirium is a syndrome encompassing disturbances in attention, consciousness, and cognition [26]. Nurses' knowledge and ability to observe cognitive function and signals of change are essential for the diagnostic process and treatment. Treatment of delirium requires treatment of the underlying disease processes [84]. Nursing care is important to comfort the person with delirium and to avoid additional complications of the disease. Those older adults experiencing delirium has an increased risk of mortality within 12 months [85, 86]. In older hospitalized persons with cognitive decline during the hospitalization, but not delirium, the cognitive function may improve after hospitalization and during the first year after discharge [81, 82]. In a health-promoting perspective, it is vital to reduce stress related to hospitalization, illness, and new environments. Health-promoting interactions may contribute to reducing the risk of delirium and reduced cognitive functioning, even if the medical illness and biological cause for the illness also are important contributors to reduced cognition.

An increasing number of studies report that older people hospitalized with stroke, heart failure, lung disease, or surgery procedures, have an increased risk for cognitive decline. A review suggested that the hospital processes may partially be responsible for the cognitive decline during and after a hospital stay, beyond the effects of the acute illness(es) [87]. The health-promoting care philosophy and nurse-patient interaction aim to facilitate coping and health resources and thereby supporting cognitive health and well-being during and after hospitalization.

Also, some older adults have preexisting cognitive impairment prior to the hospitalization [88], including both mild cognitive impairment (MCI) and dementia. MCI is an intermediate clinical state between normal cognitive aging and dementia, and it precedes and leads to dementia in many cases, but not always [89, 90]. Dementia is a clinical syndrome causing long term and often gradually loss of cognitive functioning and impairment in activities of daily living [91]. MCI or dementia may not be diagnosed prior to hospitalization or recognized by the older adult him/her-selves or their next of kin. Despite that preexisting cognitive impairment among older adults may contribute to an overall poorer outcome of the hospitalization, which is also related to an increased risk of delirium [85, 86, 92], preexisting cognitive impairment and limited cognitive resources are often unrecognized by the hospital staff [93]. The use of cognitive screening detecting cognitive limitations and available resources might disclose vulnerability for delirium. Such screening provides information necessary for adequate support and health-promoting actions. Dependent on the context and situation, health-promoting actions could be to promote sleep and diurnal rhythm, to secure nutrition, to reduce the stressors that may exist in the hospital environment and to minimize side-effects of treatment. Such health-promoting actions can reduce an individual's vulnerability concerning delirium and cognitive decline.

A Norwegian 1-year follow-up study assessed cognitive functioning among older adults without cognitive impairment or dementia. They were screened using the Mini-Mental State Examination (MMSE) [94] and all participants had a score found to be within the normal range (MMSE 24–30) when discharged from a medical hospital unit. Those hospitalized had a wide range of medical diagnoses. This study found that older adults without any known or screened cognitive impairment prior to discharge had a significantly declined function 1 year after [15]. A cognitive decline was found among those with low normal cognitive functioning (MMSE 24–26) as well as in those with high functioning (MMSE 27–30) prior to discharge. ADL impairments, independent of basic or instrumental ADL activities, were associated with an increased risk for reduced cognitive functioning 1 year after hospitalization. This finding was independent of age, gender, and severity of the disease among those hospitalized [15]. In line with other studies [87] this study demonstrated that cognitive function is interrelated with ADL functioning. Hence, despite that some cognitive decline results from the actual disease, it is important to counteract decline in the B-ADL functioning, also, among those with normal cognitive functioning. Given that a normal B-ADL among older adults is linked to a better cognitive functioning 1 year after the hospitalization, the importance of maintaining ADL functions seems apparent.

The risk of decline in B-ADL is increased in those with cognitive impairment compared to those without such impairment [12, 95, 96]. Thus, it is essential to counteract limitation of B-ADL functioning due to hospitalization when the patient has cognitive impairment. The nursing care planning needs to consider the disease, as well as both the physical and cognitive functioning resources. Health-promoting nursing utilizes the individual's existing health resources to support well-being and health. In doing so, a care plan is a valuable tool. Also, information collected by screening the patient's cognitive functioning will guide the health-promoting nursing care. Care actions should be based on the patient's resources, both while in hospital and when identifying needs of assistance after discharge from the hospital. Screening of cognitive resources as well as B-ADL functioning, aims to strengthen health resources, compensate for loss of functions, limit decline, and promote well-being. After discharge each patient should be provided the best premises to cope at home, as well as receiving care and support at home, in a rehabilitation unit or in a care facility. Summarized, screening of cognitive functioning represents a fundamental basis for health-promoting care during a hospital stay as well as in supporting the individual to cope at home after hospitalization.

20.3.3.1 Systematic Screening of Cognitive Functioning

A reliable assessment of patients' cognitive functioning cannot be based on a single clinical observation and/or the patient's self-report. Therefore, it is important to routinely screen

older adults' cognitive functioning when hospitalized. Most often, the screened areas are memory (short term and working), attention, concentration, orientation, language skills, interpret sense impressions, ability to follow simple instructions, and processing information [94, 97]. However, the different screening tools differ concerning which cognitive areas they include. Two commonly used screening tools are Montreal Cognitive Assessment tool (MoCA) [97] and Mini-Mental State Examination (MMSE) [94]. MoCA is a suitable measure assessing persons with mild cognitive complaints [97] and a mild degree of dementia. The maximum sum score of MoCA is 30 points, where higher scores indicate a better cognitive functioning. A score between 26 and 30 points indicates normal cognitive functioning [97].

The Mini-Mental Status Examination (MMSE) is frequently used to assess cognitive functioning both for clinical and research purposes. The MMSE is a 30-point scale, where higher scores indicate a better cognitive functioning [10]. While used for screening purposes, a score below 20 indicates cognitive impairment, whereas the interval between 20 and 24 indicates a mild cognitive impairment. Even so, the reported cutoff points for abnormality have varied considerably [98]. However, it is important to be aware that the MMSE is not a diagnostic tool, but a screening tool that indicates whether an individual's cognitive functioning needs a special attention during the hospital stay.

The most frequently noted disadvantage of the MMSE relates to its lack of sensitivity to mild cognitive impairment [99]. Another disadvantage of the MMSE is that the score may be affected by demographic factors; age and education exert the greatest effect [100]. In addition, the MMSE is protected by copyright and authorized use of the test is linked to costs [101–103] which has forced clinicians to use other tests [98]. Nevertheless, independently of which screening tool one chose it is important to gain knowledge and practice before the tool is used in clinical settings or for research purposes. The mentioned screening tools are easy to use and implement; thus, utilizing such screening tools provides a common understanding and reference for cognitive functioning promoting systematic care and treatment.

20.4 Conclusion - Health-Promoting Assets and Actions

Older adults are often vulnerable for complications and loss of coping resources when hospitalized. While facing physical disease, good coping resources such as sense of coherence and trusting one's coping capacity is important for well-being and perceived health [17]. Thus, care supporting both improvement of the medical condition contributing to the hospitalization and coping resources is important.

In this chapter, we have been looking at three factors related to high age that are contributing to vulnerability when hospitalized: depression, B-ADL decline, and cognitive impairment. These conditions limit coping resources, well-being, and health.

Clinically significant depressive symptoms need to be uncovered and treated, if not they may have negative consequences for the treatment, cognitive functioning and B-ADL functioning. Thus, a general assessment should preferably include screening of depressive symptoms.

Older adults in needs of assistance to ensure B-ADL functioning, such as personal hygiene, toileting, walking, eating, etc., should be given assistance supporting present resources and abilities. To do so, the health professionals need to observe the level of functioning and develop a plan for how they can support the patient's health resources and compensate for lacking abilities.

The utilization of tools assessing cognitive functioning, depressive symptoms, and B-ADL functioning will equip health professionals with a common understanding which will contribute to a systematic approach to care in a health-promoting way.

Additionally, there are several other health conditions important for coping and health promotion during and after hospitalization. In older adults, securing or maintaining a healthy pattern of sleep and proper nutrition during the hospital stay are vital. Furthermore, existential and religious needs might be actualized due to hospitalization and declining health. While hospitalized, family and social resources available to support living at home after hospitalization needs to be mapped. Thus, it is imperative to prepare, plan, and organize the transition to home or to a care home in advance of the discharge. However, these areas are not covered in this chapter.

Take Home Messages
- Depression is a frequent cause of emotional suffering in old age causing negative health consequences.
- Unrecognized and untreated depression may obstruct health promotion, thus, uncovering depressive symptoms using valid screening tools is important.
- In older adults, a hospitalization increases the risk for decline of physical functioning and ADL.
- Based in a holistic understanding of health, the older individual's situation, available resources and capacity to support self-care and ADL must be assessed, and actions taken to sustain ADL functioning during hospitalization.
- In older adults, an acute medical illness needing hospitalization may lead to reduced cognitive functioning in the acute phase of the disease.
- Limited cognitive resources are often unrecognized by the hospital staff if not screened for.
- Common understanding of available cognitive, mental and physical resources in older adults may contribute to a systematic approach to care in a health-promoting way.

References

1. Syse A, Pham D, Keilman N. Befolkningsframskrivinger 2016–2100: Dødelighet og levealder. In: Økonomiske analyser 3/2016. Oslo: Statistisk sentralbyrå; 2016.
2. Vincent GK, Velkoff VA. The next four decades: the older population in the United States: 2010–2050.

Washington, DC: United States Census Bureau; 2010. p. 15. https://www.census.gov/content/dam/Census/library/publications/2010/demo/p25-113.

3. US Centers for Disease Control and Prevention. Number, percent distribution, rate, days of care with average length of stay, and standard error of discharges from short-stay hospitals, by sex and age: United States. 2010. https://www.cdc.gov/nchs/data/nhds/2average/2010ave2_ratesexage.pdf Accessed 20 Aug 2019.

4. SAMDATA2013 Spesialisthelsetjenesten. Helsedirektoratet. 2014. https://www.helsedirektoratet.no/search?searchquery=SAMDATA%202013.

5. Rø, O. Gamle i sykehus. Innlagte 75 år og over i medisinsk avdeling 1998. In: Helsetilsynets utredningsserie; 7/99; 1999.

6. Marengoni A, et al. Prevalence of chronic diseases and multimorbidity among the elderly population in Sweden. Am J Public Health. 2008;98(7):1198–200.

7. Antonovsky A. Unraveling the mystery of health. San Francisco: Jossey-Bass; 1987.

8. Eriksson M, Lindström B. A salutogenic interpretation of the Ottawa charter. Health Promot Int. 2008;23(2):190–9.

9. Lindstrom B, Eriksson M. Salutogenesis. J Epidemiol Community Health. 2005;59(6):440–2.

10. Helvik AS, Skancke RH, Selbaek G. Screening for depression in elderly medical inpatients from rural area of Norway: prevalence and associated factors. Int J Geriatr Psychiatry. 2010;25(2):150–9.

11. Helvik AS, et al. A psychometric evaluation of the hospital anxiety and depression scale for the medically hospitalized elderly. Nord J Psychiatry. 2011;65:338–44.

12. Helvik AS, Selbaek G, Engedal K. Functional decline in older adults one year after hospitalization. Arch Gerontol Geriatr. 2013;57(3):305–10.

13. Helvik AS, et al. Nursing home admission during the first year after hospitalization - the contribution of cognitive impairment. PLoS One. 2014;9(1):e86116.

14. Helvik AS, Engedal K, Selbaek G. Depressive symptoms among the medically hospitalized older individuals - a 1-year follow-up study. Int J Geriatr Psychiatry. 2013;28(2):199–207.

15. Helvik AS, Selbaek G, Engedal K. Cognitive decline one year after hospitalization in older adults without dementia. Dement Geriatr Cogn Disord. 2012;34(3–4):198–205.

16. Helvik AS, Engedal K, Selbaek G. The quality of life and factors associated with it in the medically hospitalised elderly. Aging Ment Health. 2010;14(7):861–9.

17. Helvik AS, et al. Factors associated with perceived health in elderly medical inpatients: a particular focus on personal coping recourses. Aging Ment Health. 2012;16(6):795–803.

18. Sivertsen H, et al. Depression and quality of life in older persons: a review. Dement Geriatr Cogn Disord. 2015;40(5–6):311–39.

19. Charlson ME, et al. Outcomes of community-based social service interventions in homebound elders. Int J Geriatr Psychiatry. 2008;23(4):427–32.

20. Reid MC, et al. Depressive symptoms as a risk factor for disabling back pain in community-dwelling older persons. J Am Geriatr Soc. 2003;51(12):1710–7.

21. Lohman MC, Mezuk B, Dumenci L. Depression and frailty: concurrent risks for adverse health outcomes. Aging Ment Health. 2017;21(4):399–408.

22. Moise N, et al. Observational study of the differential impact of time-varying depressive symptoms on all-cause and cause-specific mortality by health status in community-dwelling adults: the REGARDS study. BMJ Open. 2018;8(1):e017385.

23. Aziz R, Steffens DC. What are the causes of late-life depression? Psychiatr Clin North Am. 2013;36(4):497–516.

24. Katon WJ, et al. Increased medical costs of a population-based sample of depressed elderly patients. Arch Gen Psychiatry. 2003;60(9):897–903.

25. WHO. International statistical classification of diseases and related health problems, 10th Revision. Geneva: World Health Organisation; 2016. https://icd.who.int/browse10/2016/en

26. Arlington V. Diagnostic and statistical manual of mental disorders : DSM-5 (Fifth ed.). Washington, DC: American Psychiatric Association; 2013.

27. Gallo JJ, Rabins PV. Depression without sadness: alternative presentations of depression in late life. Am Fam Physician. 1999;60(3):820–6.

28. Carpenter L, Winnett A. Depression in hospitalized elderly people. Br J Hosp Med (Lond). 2014;75(8):C126–8.

29. Luppa M, et al. Age- and gender-specific prevalence of depression in latest-life--systematic review and meta-analysis. J Affect Disord. 2012;136(3):212–21.

30. Copeland JR, et al. Depression in Europe. Geographical distribution among older people. Br J Psychiatry. 1999;174:312–21.

31. Rosenvinge BH, Rosenvinge JH. Forekomst av depresjon - systematisk oversikt over 55 prevalens studier fra 1990-2001. [Occurrence of depression in the elderly--a systematic review of 55 prevalence studies from 1990-2001. In Norwegian]. Tidsskr Nor Laegeforen. 2003;123(7):928–9.

32. Blazer DG. Depression in late life: review and commentary. J Gerontol A Biol Sci Med Sci. 2003;58(3):249–65.

33. Stordal E. Aspects of the epidemiology of depression based on self-rating in a large general health study (The HUNT-2 study). Trondheim: Department of Neuroscience, Faculty of Medicine, University of Science and Technology; 2005.

34. Alexopoulos GS, et al. Assessment of late life depression. Biol Psychiatry. 2002;52(3):164–74.

35. Bjørkløf GH, et al. Being stuck in a vice: the process of coping with severe depression in late life. Int J Qual Stud Health Well-being. 2015;10:27187.

36. Frasure-Smith N, et al. Social support, depression, and mortality during the first year after myocardial infarction. Circulation. 2000;101(16):1919–24.

37. Covinsky KE, et al. Relation between symptoms of depression and health status outcomes in acutely ill hospitalized older persons. Ann Intern Med. 1997;126(6):417–25.

38. Kørner EA. Forekomst av depression hos ældre over 65 år i Karlebo kommune. [Prevalence of depression in elderly over 65 years in Karlebo Municipality. In Danish]. København: Foreningen af Danske Lægestuderendes Forlag; 1998.

39. Sheikh J, Yesavage J. Geriatric depression scale (GDS): recent evidence and development of a shorter version. In: Clinical gerontology: a guide to assessment and intervention. Philadelphia: The Haworth Press; 1986. p. 165–73.

40. Berentsen VD, Schirmer H. Depresjon hos geriatriske pasienter. In: Sosial og Helsedepartementet og Statens Helsetilsyns utviklingsprogram om alderspykiatri, Rapport 2; 1995.

41. Baker FM, Espino DV. A Spanish version of the geriatric depression scale in Mexican-American elders. Int J Geriatr Psychiatry. 1997;12(1):21–5.

42. Burke WJ, et al. Use of the geriatric depression scale in dementia of the Alzheimer type. J Am Geriatr Soc. 1989;37(9):856–60.

43. Eriksen S, et al. The validity of the hospital anxiety and depression scale and the geriatric depression scale-5 in home-dwelling old adults in Norway. J Affect Disord. 2019;256:380–5.

44. Weeks SK, et al. Comparing various short-form geriatric depression scales leads to the GDS-5/15. J Nurs Scholarsh. 2003;35(2):133–7.

45. Montgomery S, Asberg M. A new depression scale designed to be sensitive to change. Br J Psychiatry. 1979;134:382–9.

46. Haugan G, Drageset J. The hospital anxiety and depression scale-dimensionality, reliability and construct validity among cognitively intact nursing home patients. J Affect Disord. 2014;165:8–15.

47. Djukanovic I, Carlsson J, Arestedt K. Is the hospital anxiety and depression scale (HADS) a valid measure in a general population 65-80 years old? A psychometric evaluation study. Health Qual Life Outcomes. 2017;15(1):193.

48. Beattie E, Pachana NA, Franklin SJ. Double jeopardy: comorbid anxiety and depression in late life. Res Gerontol Nurs. 2010;3(3):209–20.

49. Hospital anxiety and depression scale (HADS); 2019.

50. Bennett JA. Activities of daily living. Old-fashioned or still useful? J Gerontol Nurs. 1999;25(5):22–9.

51. Inouye SK, et al. Importance of functional measures in predicting mortality among older hospitalized patients. JAMA. 1998;279(15):1187–93.

52. Boyd CM, et al. Recovery of activities of daily living in older adults after hospitalization for acute medical illness. J Am Geriatr Soc. 2008;56(12):2171–9.

53. Buurman BM, et al. Geriatric conditions in acutely hospitalized older patients: prevalence and one-year survival and functional decline. PLoS One. 2011;6(11):e26951.

54. Fortinsky RH, et al. Effects of functional status changes before and during hospitalization on nursing home admission of older adults. J Gerontol A Biol Sci Med Sci. 1999;54(10):M521–6.

55. WHO. International classification of functioning, disability and health. Geneva: World Health Organization; 2001. p. 251.

56. Campbell SE, Seymour DG, Primrose WR. A systematic literature review of factors affecting outcome in older medical patients admitted to hospital. Age Ageing. 2004;33(2):110–5.

57. Millan-Calenti JC, et al. Prevalence of functional disability in activities of daily living (ADL), instrumental activities of daily living (IADL) and associated factors, as predictors of morbidity and mortality. Arch Gerontol Geriatr. 2010;50(3):306–10.

58. Chuang KH, et al. Diagnosis-related group-adjusted hospital costs are higher in older medical patients with lower functional status. J Am Geriatr Soc. 2003;51(12):1729–34.

59. Hirsch CH, et al. The natural history of functional morbidity in hospitalized older patients. J Am Geriatr Soc. 1990;38(12):1296–303.

60. Covinsky KE, et al. Loss of independence in activities of daily living in older adults hospitalized with medical illnesses: increased vulnerability with age. J Am Geriatr Soc. 2003;51(4):451–8.

61. Creditor MC. Hazards of hospitalization of the elderly. Ann Intern Med. 1993;118(3):219–23.

62. Zelada MA, Salinas R, Baztan JJ. Reduction of functional deterioration during hospitalization in an acute geriatric unit. Arch Gerontol Geriatr. 2009;48(1):35–9.

63. Palese A, et al. Hospital-acquired functional decline in older patients cared for in acute medical wards and predictors: findings from a multicentre longitudinal study. Geriatr Nurs. 2016;37(3):192–9.

64. Lindenberger EC, et al. Unsteadiness reported by older hospitalized patients predicts functional decline. J Am Geriatr Soc. 2003;51(5):621–6.

65. Wu AW, et al. Predicting functional status outcomes in hospitalized patients aged 80 years and older. J Am Geriatr Soc. 2000;48(5 Suppl): S6–15.

66. Tonkikh O, et al. Functional status before and during acute hospitalization and readmission risk identification. J Hosp Med. 2016;11(9):636–41.

67. Stuck AE, et al. Risk factors for functional status decline in community-living elderly people: a systematic literature review. Soc Sci Med. 1999;48(4):445–69.

68. Vermeulen J, et al. Predicting ADL disability in community-dwelling elderly people using physical frailty indicators: a systematic review. BMC Geriatr. 2011;11:33.

69. Krumholz HM. Post-hospital syndrome--an acquired, transient condition of generalized risk. N Engl J Med. 2013;368(2):100–2.

70. Palmer RM. The acute care for elders unit model of care. Geriatrics (Basel). 2018;3(3):59.

71. Flood KL, et al. Acute Care for Elders (ACE) Team Model of Care: a clinical overview. Geriatrics (Basel). 2018;3(3):50.

72. Barnes DE, et al. Acute care for elders units produced shorter hospital stays at lower cost while maintaining patients' functional status. Health Aff (Millwood). 2012;31(6):1227–36.

73. Landefeld CS, et al. A randomized trial of care in a hospital medical unit especially designed to improve the functional outcomes of acutely ill older patients. N Engl J Med. 1995;332(20):1338–44.

74. Counsell SR, et al. Effects of a multicomponent intervention on functional outcomes and process of care in hospitalized older patients: a randomized controlled trial of acute care for elders (ACE) in a community hospital. J Am Geriatr Soc. 2000;48(12):1572–81.

75. Lawton MP, Brody EM. Assessment of older people: self-maintaining and instrumental activities of daily living. Gerontologist. 1969;9(3):179–86.

76. Mahoney F, Barthel D. FUNCTIONAL EVALUATION: THE BARTHEL INDEX. Md State Med J. 1965;14:61–5.

77. Katz S, et al. Progress in development of the index of ADL. Gerontologist. 1970;10(1):20–30.

78. Buurman BM, et al. Variability in measuring (instrumental) activities of daily living functioning and functional decline in hospitalized older medical patients: a systematic review. J Clin Epidemiol. 2011;64(6):619–27.

79. Zuccala G, et al. The effects of cognitive impairment on mortality among hospitalized patients with heart failure. Am J Med. 2003;115(2):97–103.

80. Chodosh J, et al. Cognitive decline in high-functioning older persons is associated with an increased risk of hospitalization. J Am Geriatr Soc. 2004;52(9):1456–62.

81. Inouye SK, et al. Recoverable cognitive dysfunction at hospital admission in older persons during acute illness. J Gen Intern Med. 2006;21(12):1276–81.

82. Lindquist LA, et al. Improvements in cognition following hospital discharge of community dwelling seniors. J Gen Intern Med. 2011;26(7):765–70.

83. Ahmed S, Leurent B, Sampson EL. Risk factors for incident delirium among older people in acute hospital medical units: a systematic review and meta-analysis. Age Ageing. 2014;43(3):326–33.

84. Wong CL, et al. Does this patient have delirium?: value of bedside instruments. JAMA. 2010;304(7):779–86.

85. Israni J, et al. Delirium as a predictor of mortality in US Medicare beneficiaries discharged from the emergency department: a national claims-level analysis up to 12 months. BMJ Open. 2018;8(5):e021258.

86. McCusker J, et al. Delirium predicts 12-month mortality. Arch Intern Med. 2002;162(4):457–63.

87. Dasgupta M. Cognitive impairment in hospitalized seniors. Geriatrics (Basel). 2016;1(1):4.

88. Pisani MA, McNicoll L, Inouye SK. Cognitive impairment in the intensive care unit. Clin Chest Med. 2003;24(4):727–37.

89. Thompson SA, Hodges JR. Mild cognitive impairment: a clinically useful but currently ill-defined concept? Neurocase. 2002;8(6):405–10.

90. Petersen RC. Clinical practice. Mild cognitive impairment. N Engl J Med. 2011;364(23):2227–34.

91. Burns A, Iliffe S. Dementia. BMJ. 2009;338:b75.

92. Kukreja D, Gunther U, Popp J. Delirium in the elderly: current problems with increasing geriatric age. Indian J Med Res. 2015;142(6):655–62.

93. Pisani MA, et al. Underrecognition of preexisting cognitive impairment by physicians in older ICU patients. Chest. 2003;124(6):2267–74.

94. Folstein MF, Folstein SE, McHugh PR. "Mini-mental state". A practical method for grading the cognitive state of patients for the clinician. J Psychiatr Res. 1975;12(3):189–98.

95. Helvik AS, et al. A 52 month follow-up of functional decline in nursing home residents - degree of dementia contributes. BMC Geriatr. 2014;14(1):45.

96. Helvik A-S, et al. A 36-month follow-up of decline in activities of daily living in individuals receiving domiciliary care. BMC Geriatr. 2015;15:47. https://doi.org/10.1186/s12877-015-0047-7.

97. Nasreddine ZS, et al. The Montreal Cognitive Assessment, MoCA: a brief screening tool for mild cognitive impairment. J Am Geriatr Soc. 2005;53(4):695–9.

98. Holsinger T, et al. Does this patient have dementia? JAMA. 2007;297(21):2391–404.

99. Arevalo-Rodriguez I, et al. Mini-Mental State Examination (MMSE) for the detection of Alzheimer's disease and other dementias in people with mild cognitive impairment (MCI). Cochrane Database Syst Rev, 2015;(3):CD010783.

100. Crum RM, et al. Population-based norms for the Mini-Mental State Examination by age and educational level. JAMA. 1993;269(18):2386–91.

101. Powsner S, Powsner D. Cognition, copyright, and the classroom. Am J Psychiatry. 2005;162(3):627–8.

102. Folstein M, Folstein S, McHugh P. Mini-Mental State Examination. Psychological assessment resources, Inc. https://web.archive.org/web/20070929001727/http://www.minimental.com/.

103. de Silva V, Hanwella R. Why are we copyrighting science? BMJ. 2010;341:c4738.

Sociocultural Aspects of Health Promotion in Palliative Care in Uganda

21

James Mugisha

Abstract

Despite its vital importance, health promotion has not occupied its due place in public health in Uganda. The country is engulfed into a rising wave of both communicable and non-communicable conditions. This rising burden of both communicable and non-communicable conditions turns health promotion and palliative care essential health care packages; though there is little to show that these two important programs are getting vital support at policy and service delivery levels. A new theoretical framework that is anchored into sociocultural issues is essential in guiding the design and delivery of both health promotion and palliative care in Uganda. The salutogenic theory puts socio-cultural issues at the centre of developing health promotion and palliative care and, seems to solve this dilemma. In this chapter, illustrations from indigenous communities in Uganda are employed to demonstrate the challenges to the health promotion and palliative care agenda in the country and how they can be addressed. Uganda Ministry of Health should develop robust structures within public health for development of health promotion and palliative care in the country.

Research should be conducted on the effectiveness of the current strategies on health promotion and palliative care and their cultural sensitivity and appropriateness. Given the limited resources available for development of health care in Uganda, as an overall strategy, health promotion and palliative care should be anchored in public health and its (public health) resources.

Keywords

Social aspects · Salutogenesis · Health promotion · Palliative care · Uganda

21.1 Background

There is a dramatic shift in low-income countries from communicable to non-communicable diseases [1–3]. As noted, by 2030, the burden of non-communicable diseases, including neuropsychiatric disorders, will constitute seven of the ten leading causes of disease burden globally and its impact will be more felt in low-income countries where health systems are more fragile as compared to the ones in high-income countries [1, 4, 5]. It is estimated that within a generation, the share of disease burden attributed to non-communicable diseases in some poor countries of the world will exceed 80%, rivalling that of rich countries

J. Mugisha (✉)
Faculty Arts and Social Sciences, Department of Sociology and Social Administration, Kyambogo University, Kampala, Uganda

© The Author(s) 2021
G. Haugan, M. Eriksson (eds.), *Health Promotion in Health Care – Vital Theories and Research*,
https://doi.org/10.1007/978-3-030-63135-2_21

[3]. And, this burden is likely to affect more the younger generation in poorer resource contexts than in the high-income countries [3].

The most prevalent globally of these non-communicable conditions are: cardiovascular diseases, cancers, chronic respiratory disease and diabetes [6]. And, a similar trend seems to be unravelling in Africa [6]. Globally, it is estimated that these conditions, contribute to large mortality, accounting for 36 million deaths in 2008 (63% of total fatalities) [7]. Majority (four-fifths) of these deaths occur in LMICs [7]. It is also estimated that, if these trends go unchecked (as it is the case in most LMCs), by 2030, deaths due to NCDs will be the most common causes of mortality in low-income countries. More specifically, diabetes cases in sub-Saharan Africa are projected to increase from 4.8% prevalence (19.8 million) in 2013, to 5.3% (41.5 million) in 2035 (IDF, 207). In the same vein, cancer cases are also projected to nearly double (1.28m new cases and 970,000 deaths) by 2030 (in 2012 there were 645,000 new cases and 456,000 cancer-related deaths in Africa) [8]. The most obvious risk factors are a combination of increasing and ageing populations, the adoption of risk-factor lifestyles (largely due to sedative life style), and deficient diagnostic, preventative and curative treatment services [9].

Unfortunately, in many of the low-income countries that have started to witness this shift, the health system is not prepared enough to deal with this challenge [2, 3]. Many of the non-communicable conditions are chronic in nature necessitating the need for a fundamental reprograming of the public health sector and palliative care.

21.2 The Public Health and Palliative Care Context in Africa

The need for palliative care in low-income countries in general and Africa in particular is already overwhelming [10, 11]. Evidence is available that there is a large gap between the number of people in need of palliative care services and those who are able to actually receive it [12]. At present, only a few countries have any form of palliative care program and this gap may be larger in Africa [7]. There are no obvious strategies to meeting this need due to already over-stretched health systems in low-income countries and the ever-increasing political dilemmas (such as political turmoil and mismanagement) that affect service delivery.

Suggestions have been made that public heath can effectively work in tandem with palliative care [13]. It is possible for public health to enter deeply into palliative care narratives and establish strong relationships to improve the current service delivery mechanisms of both programs (public health and palliative care) [13]. The essence here is using a public health approach in palliative care. This presupposes fundamentally building community capacity to own and work on its health issues. Such approaches have large benefits of being cost effective, empowering; improve coverage of services to the general population and are sustainable [13]. All that is needed is conceptual clarity [13]. The revised WHO definition of palliative care is anchored into public health and seems to take care of these concerns [13]. Palliative care is defined as:

> Palliative care is an approach that improves the quality of life of patients and their families facing the problems associated with life-threatening illness, through the prevention and relief of suffering by means of early identification and impeccable assessment and treatment of pain and other problems, physical, psychosocial, and spiritual (Whitelaw and Clerk [13], p. 4).

The notion of prevention and early detection of suffering is highlighted in this definition and is key to the public health agenda. This understanding did not get the due emphasis in the previous public health efforts [13]. Current public health efforts should have a new outlook that focuses on a comprehensive person with psychical, psychosocial and spiritual needs.

Taking as comprehensive approach to health service delivery demands for a lot of resources. In many low-income settings however, public health has relatively compelling volume of resource as compared to other sectors and these resources could be used in shaping the future direction of the palliative care policy [2, 13]. Deep reflections are needed here to create a secondary deployment (where palliative care is "infused" into public health) to create better synergies [13]. Moreover, within this new thinking, the need for palliative care should be understood as a public health issue [13]. This evidence (of infusing palliative care into public health care) is already available in some countries; though still in a few of them [13].

21.3 Health Promotion and Salutogenesis: Concepts and Theory

The concept health promotion has had more extensive use in the developed world as compared to the low-income countries. Health promotion in Africa in general and Uganda in particular is not well articulated in the public health agenda. In this chapter we shall adopt the World Health Organisation (WHO) definition of health promotion: *"Health promotion is the process of enabling people to increase control over, and to improve, their health"* [14]. The biggest challenge for health promotion in Africa and Uganda in particular has been: (a) lack of frameworks and models for classifying activities and determine the scope of health promotion [15] and, (b) most people in Africa have poor health status and therefore it is difficult to sustain development and economic viability of most health programs [2]. Due to the above-mentioned challenges, to a larger extent, most countries in Africa have had their focus on curative care, they have minimal resources to satisfy this sector (curative sector) and because of this reason, health promotion has been forgotten.

21.4 Salutogenesis in Health Promotion and Palliative Care in Uganda: Theoretical and Status Issues

Within the field of health promotion, perspectives have emerged. Some of these include positive psychology and salutogenesis. The interest in this

chapter will be salutogenesis though positive psychology, which is also of much relevance here. The originator of salutogenesis (Aaron Antonovsky) described health systems in the Western world as "pathogenic" [16]. His description seems to be of much relevancy to the health systems in the developing world such as Uganda. Simply put, Antonovsky [17] referred to this malaise in the health system as "disease care system" ([17], p. 12). His perspective is a sharp opposition to the pathogenic orientation, which is dominant in Western medical thinking [18]. "Antonovsky rejected a dichotomous categorisation of the health status (e.g., well vs. diseased, healthy vs. ill as inappropriate) to represent the complexity of health status" [18]. His view was that health is more reasonably understood as a continuum; every person is at a given point in time somewhere between health and disease poles in the continuum [18]. In this regard, he coined the "construct of generalised resources against stress" (which is defined as a property of the person, a collective or situation which, as evidence or logic has indicated, facilitated successful coping with inherent stressors of human existence" ([17], p. 15; [18], p. 326). Related to this the construct of "sense of coherence", which is a generalised orientation towards the world, which perceives it, on ease/health continuum, as comprehensible, manageable and meaningful ([17], p. 15). "When confronted with a stressor, people with a strong sense of coherence are likely to be motivated to cope (meaningfulness), to believe that coping resources are accessible" (manageability) [18]; also see Antonovsky [17]. This thinking is useful for those at the dyeing stage of their life.

Since hospitals are traditionally characterised by an orientation to diagnosing, curing and caring for severely ill people [19] they have a limited contribution to the public health agenda. This understanding calls for new frameworks for health promotion and palliative care in Uganda. The curative approach fails to recognise that death, dying, loss and care giving exist to some extent beyond the domains of individualistic therapeutic intervention and a public health care approach brings better results [13]. It requires the reorientation of health services in Uganda into more public health and health promotion domains; as demanded by the Ottawa Charter [14]. This has not happened to a remarkable degree yet in many countries.

21.5 The Cultural Context and Issues Related to Death and Dying in Uganda

21.5.1 Meaning of Death

During the dyeing process, many people within indigenous communities are preoccupied with the meaning of *Good Death*. Drawing from sociality, good death culturally means dying while surrounded by people, especially, your children, wives(s) and close relatives. Though having less pain is part of good death this is not the most important consideration of good death as emphasised by modern health workers. In our study in Mpigi [20], we saw our informants having a negative attitude against long periods of hospitalisation that are normally synonymous with chronic diseases (also see [20, 21]). Long stay in hospital is seen as affecting sociality since the patient is normally away from his/her children, spouse and close family members. What was evident from the narratives expressed by people in our project in Mpigi is that the cultural conception of death was different from the "scientific view" of good death and this has implications on the way health promotion and palliative care should be delivered. Searching for meaning in life is part of the salutogenic approach and this makes it important for any health service to focus on the subjective experience of the people targeted. Within salutogenesis, it is postulated that there is a connection between spirituality (religion and meaning making) and health. Within salutogenic and the health promotional framework, dimensions of health are referred to in terms of the physical, mental, social and spiritual; a notion of huge relevance to health and palliative care programs in Uganda [22, 23]. This calls for comprehensive and integrated programs that can address physical, mental, social, and spiritual aspects of human functioning and, these are inextricably intertwined.

Though Uganda is getting more urbanised (over 76% of the Ugandans live in rural area), the influence of culture (and tradition) is still so strong among indigenous communities in Uganda. Health promoters have to manage diversity; the patient, family and the community where they live [24]. The cultural values of the patient and family within the locations/contexts must be given attention [24]. Uganda is quite cosmopolitan in terms of tribes (over 50 tribal groupings), age, gender and other socioeconomic variables. In many of the societies, health promotion and palliative care should pay attention to these multiple components including race, ethnicity, gender, age, differing abilities, sexual orientation, religion, spirituality, and socioeconomic status [24]. The beliefs, norms and practices should be the target of the health promotion activities as they are likely to guide behavioural responses, decision-making and action and other key variables related to acceptability of health promotion and palliative care.

21.6 Aetiology and Cultural Frameworks

Within the salutogenic theory, existential issues are given due attention. One goes into meaning making, contact inner feels in order to mobilise generalised resources. The subjective experience of diseases such as cancer and HIV/AIDS is cultural based [25]. They are cognitively and linguistically expressed within cultural frameworks and therefore the medical model (pathogenesis) becomes less meaningful to those afflicted by disease. Among indigenous communities, causality of disease is largely attributed to external factors or different aspects in the natural environment, both living and/or non-living [25]. Studies undertaken in the field of mental health indicate that over 80% of the people in Uganda seek help from spiritual/traditional healers [20, 26, 27]. Because of the differences in perspectives between modern and traditional healers, there develops polarised relationships between the two (modern and traditional healers). This polarisation normally delays appropriate treatment seeking:

Cancer is about a neighbour who might not be happy with your achievements. The medical stories don't make sense to our people and that is why they keep home till death (Personal Communication, Anthropologist Makerere University Medical School).

There is always a failure by the health system to undertake a meaningful co-construction between the patient, the family, the traditional healers and the modern health systems. The palliative care and health promotion field fail to deal with medical domination of the traditional system. Many of the people they are targeting within indigenous communities have existential needs for which they have little trust in the modern health system. With the salutogenic field, it is postulated that the way people view themselves and the world has implications for their health and more importantly, their quality of life. Hence, the need to shift attention to the subjective experience of the people and to change their existing perspectives to health care. We cannot afford to ignore the backyard issues that seat at deepest part of people's values and belief systems. Our study in northern Uganda; the Wayo-Nero Strategy (https://www.mhinnovation.net/innovations/wayo-nero-strategy) aimed at reducing the treatment gap for mental disorders by utilising indigenous institutions in post-conflict areas. Many people targeted in the three districts in northern Uganda were able to access services using this strategy. The Wayo (aunti)-Nero (uncle) are traditional counsellors and their services were harnessed to deliver modern health care but also spiritual care. This made the interventions more acceptable to the people since we were using a cultural resource.

21.6.1 Communication About Death

The subjective experience of diseases such as cancer and HIV/AIDS is culturally based [25]. They are cognitively and linguistically expressed within cultural frameworks. Again in our research work in Mpigi, we see a challenge where indigenous communities have great fear and respect for death and never refer to *death*

directly. Instead, they circumvent around its (death) meaning using their oral skills. In our study in Mpigi among indigenous communities in Uganda (see [19, 20]), our research topic was on the meaning of completed suicide. We as researchers were not born in this culture and never knew that "Baganda" do not refer to death directly. Once we did that cultural tension emerged. Death as a subject cannot easily be avoided in palliative care. However, discussing it among indigenous communities must be done with a lot of cultural sensibility [20]. In our project, we adapted the concepts that could mean death but less offence to culture and tradition (see [19, 20]). This experience is of high relevance to the current health promotion and palliative care workers in Uganda.

21.6.2 Masculinity and Help Seeking

Society always sets different expectations for men and women [20]. The cultural meaning of a "real man" sets expectations that men even under great pain should undertake controlled emotional expression (should suppress pain inwards) (see [19, 20]). But this may again come with other risks as the pain may become more severe; patients may become depressed or traumatised by diseases among other risks [20]. Culturally, accepting uncontrolled emotional expression is turning into a "woman". The most obvious challenge with masculinity in this context is that it limits sharing of information between the client and the palliative health care worker because of the high possibly of normalising pain; one has to be a man. The man is expected to be tough and this has to be demonstrated even in situations of great pain. Interestingly, strict adherence to masculine norms in indigenous communalities is rewarded by society with respect before and after death. "The man is praised for being a man and not a woman and that means keeping quite over most of the pain" (Personal Communication with Senior Lecturer Anthropology Makerere University). Too much emotional outpour is culturally disrespected and only expected of women. "For a woman it is ok to cry before the public but for the man you are expected to do otherwise" (Senior Lecturer Anthropology Makerere University).

Masculinity also comes with a belief in self-reliance, the need to do things by yourself and these trends can be seen in urban areas where communalism has lost grip on society and there is more individualism. In our study in Mpigi [20], we established individualistic traits in urban areas where people are more inclined to self-efficacy. Researches in mental health indicated that, those inclined to masculine ideology and, have strong individualistic construes rarely seek formal health care. Palliative care to them has a connotation of communalism-sharing your problems with others. "Yah, there are those who want to die with their private life and the way our palliative care is structured with several nurses and village health workers, it cannot work for such people" (Lecturer Social Work Kyambogo University).

21.6.3 Community Gate-Keeping and Health Promotion

Most studies largely undertaken in the developed world have looked at the notion of gatekeeping in terms of research-the structures, which the researcher(s) has to deal with to access potential respondents for the study [20]. In this study I take a different view. I look at gate-keeping agencies as community structures, which the program has to deal with to access clients [20]. In indigenous communities, cultural institutions/structures are the custodians of culture and play a major role in its survival [20]. They also play a major role in the survival of community members including infirmities that might befall individuals, families or the larger community and they are always called upon when negative life events befall a community [28]. Many of the cultural leaders are at the same time the political leaders of the community as they play multiple roles [29, 30]. Several studies conducted in Uganda indicated that they increase acceptability and coverage of community programs [29, 30]. They have been instrumental in popularising HIV/AIDS [31] and

malaria campaigns at community level. Though palliative care has exploited some of the community leaders attached to the HIV/AIDS programs, this has been undertaken to a limited extent and many of them have not been trained in palliative care as a methodology. In many communities in Uganda, there are no community-based palliative care workers despite the program having a national coverage. "The coverage of community workers is still marginal and needs to be addressed. And many of them lack the core palliative care skills and health promotion. HIV/AIDS is not necessarily palliative care" (Personal Communication, Lecturer Palliative Care Kyambogo University, Uganda).

In our Wayo-Nero Mental Health Care Project, we managed to bridge the treatment gap for common mental disorders using the Wayo (aunt)-Nero (uncle) as traditional institutions (https://www.mhinnovation.net/innovations/wayo-nero-strategy). The Wayos and Neros used their influence as cultural leaders to deliver the program including health messages. There are lessons to learn from the Wayo-Nero project by the health promoters in palliative care in Uganda in increasing addressing sociocultural issues in health.

21.7 Looking at the Future

The salutogenic field provides an important theoretical framework for health promotion in Uganda. "Africans are notoriously religious, and each people has its own religious system with a set of beliefs and practices" [32]. Mbiti further observed that "religion permeates into all the departments of life so fully that it is not easy or possible always to isolate it" [32]. And most of the time African people are entangled in both modern and traditional religious systems [20, 32]. Quite more modern religious writers such as Gyekye [33] observed that African heritage is intensely religious. "The African lives in a religious universe: all actions and thoughts have a religious meaning and aspired or influenced by a religious point of view ([33], p. 3). The views expressed above by the two African writes Mbiti [32] and Gyekye [33] though have been in print for a while still largely represent the religious systems of African people. They indicate the religious standpoint of African people and any effective program should address their spatial needs [20]. There is a possibility to use the current cultural resources (both modern and traditional) to improve public health and the delivery of health promotion and palliative care. HIV/AIDS, malaria and other communicable diseases have attracted quite a lot of resources from the donor community. Some of these resources can be used to develop a national framework for delivery of health promotion and palliative care in the country. Indigenous (e.g. spiritual healers and herbalists) and modern cultural (e.g. churches and church leaders) resources could be tapped into to deliver both health promotion and palliative care more effectively and with a high level of cultural acceptability. Drawing again from our salutogenesis framework, these historical roots that are embedded on religion and religious associations have implications in strengthening the members of these societies in their sense of coherence [34]. Cultures seem to define the resources that are appropriate to deal with a stressful situation [34]. The cultural context is likely to shape the type of the stressor experienced by the individual and also the choice of appraisal and coping strategy employed [34]. The spiritual/religious social networks can be important sense of community coherence.

The Ottawa conference in 1986 called for reorientation of health services. It was further observed that there has been slow progress in making health promotion a core business for health services and there was a need to reframe, reposition and renew efforts in this field [35]. Part of these efforts includes being more active in health systems development [35, 36]. This slow development is more felt in Africa and Uganda in particular. The Uganda Ministry of Health needs to make pragmatic steps in making health promotion a priority sector within the ministry. This is more critical today with the aging of the population in Uganda and the rising impact of chronic diseases in the country [35]. New policies and budget frameworks that are sufficient and efficient should be developed and operationalised.

Unfortunately, many Ministries of Health in Africa and this is also the case with Uganda lack a health promotion structure [15]. As noted these Ministries always have an IEC Unit, perform traditional health education functions and not tied to the overall global framework of health promotion [15]. Health promotion should not be seen as an added cost but as a cost saving strategy (especially when one focuses on disease prevention, patient empowerment and community management and participation).

Research should be undertaken to establish the cost and effectiveness of health promotion activities that are part of the health promotion and palliative care agenda currently and in future [35]. Government agencies such as universities and especially schools of Public Health should take leadership in this. The World Health Organisation's Ottawa Charter for Health Promotion from 1986 is still the gold standard for health promotion worldwide [36]. Academic institutions (though none exists in Uganda) can set up centres of excellence on health promotion to foster critical thinking about health promotion in the country. They can also ensure that the gold standard envisaged in the Ottawa charter is engendered though this has to be done with caution [15]. The Alma Ata Declaration is deemed more impactful on the continent due to its strong focus on primary health care [15] while the Ottawa conference is quite lacking in this since its focus was more on industrialised countries. It has argued that that there is a possiblity for the two instruments (Alma Ata Declaration and Ottawa Charter) to cross-fertilise each other. The Alma Ata Declaration can be used for comprehensive primary health care while the Ottawa Charter can be more useful in tacking the double burden of emerging non-communicable and communicable diseases [15]. This also requires changing the political will and ideology in many countries [36].

While local government are rich in local context which can improve the cultural sensitivity of their programs, they at the same time lack the required resources especially funds to deliver public health interventions [15]. However, a public-private partnership can boost the amount of resources available at the local government level (Alma Ata Declaration).

Overall, efforts should be made to ensure that health promotion is embedded into all aspects of life, including home, work leisure and within health care [36]. A special focus on the social aspects of health promotion and palliative care makes this agenda feasible. Watson [37] suggested that those involved in health promotion should ensure: (a) creation of a healthy working environment (c) integrating health promotion into daily activities and (c) reaching out into the community. The crosscutting theme in all these three aspects is culture and social aspects of health promotion, becomes an important theme. Given the limited resources in Uganda, it might be difficult to work with all units in the health sector at the same time. However, we could go piecemeal until all vital units in the heath sector are covered. Even in the developed countries, these variations exist despite having a relatively larger volume of resources. Hospitals still take a lion's share of the Uganda health sector budget and primary health care where much of the health promotion takes place is still neglected. This should be reversed. The words of John Catford are also very informative here, "We look in eager anticipation to see how Africa moves ahead in closing the implementation gap in health promotion…Although Africa may light the way, the rest of the world will also need to shoulder the task" ([35], p. 3). These words have been interpreted to imply that the international community should play a major role in helping Africa to close the gap in health promotion [15]. While understanding is important, the Western world should not *transpose* health promotion packages from their countries as it normally happens with many of the development assistance programs in the health sector [15]. As noted, high-income countries differ a lot from low-income countries in key aspects especially in their individualist/communitarian orientations [15]. A home grown package that takes into account the social aspects in health promotion and palliative care should be developed and propagated. As seen in our findings, communalism is still the mainstay in social organisation of our study communities. The health promotion

agenda should be based on communalism rather than an individualist Eurocentric health promotion discourse and practice [15]. This thinking does not serve to connote that there should be only an African public or health promotion agenda. However, it is an attempt to look at public health and health promotion in Africa with contextual eyes, cultural sensitivity and lastly in its own right.

21.8 Conclusion

Uganda's quest for palliative care national wide is based on false premises and constitutes a categorical fallacy. The current model spearheaded by hospitals to deliver health promotion and palliative care misses the critical components that are vital in this field. Individuals and families are not empowered to take charge of their health needs and resources to support care. The salutogenic theory takes care of these dilemmas and takes health promotion and palliative care into communities. The existing resources for public health in Uganda should be synergistically tapped into to develop health promotion and palliative care through a community based model.

Take Home Messages
- The need for palliative care in Uganda and other low-income countries is real and growing.
- The existing medical model(s) that have historically informed the development and delivery of health service in Uganda are faced with insurmountable challenges and therefore there is need for a paradigm shift.
- Culture stands in the road to providing effective palliative care and this challenge should be addressed through designing programs that are culturally sensitive and acceptable to individuals and communities.
- Uganda Ministry of Health needs to move away from tokenistic approaches to health promotion and palliative care to comprehensive programs. Health promotion and palliative care should be accorded their due right-not to remain small units in the health education

sector at the Uganda Ministry of health but become fully-fledged departments.

• Education institutions in the country should build capacity for research in this field and also train specialists in health promotion and palliative care.

References

1. Marais DL, Petersen I. Health system governance to support integrated mental health care in South Africa: challenges and opportunities. Int J Ment Health Syst. 2015;9:14. https://doi.org/10.1186/s13033-015-0004-z.

2. Mugisha J, Ssebunnya J, Kigozi FN. Towards understanding governance issues in integration of mental health into primary health care in Uganda. Int J Ment Health Syst. 2016;10(1):25.

3. Bollyky TJ, Templin T, Cohen M, Dieleman JL. Lower-income countries that face the most rapid shift in noncommunicable disease burden are also the least prepared. Health Aff (Millwood). 2017;36(11):1866–75. https://doi.org/10.1377/hlthaff.2017.0708.

4. Mugisha J, Abdulmalik J, Hanlon C, Petersen I, Lund C, Upadhaya N, Ahuja S, Shidhaye R, Mntambo N, Alem A, Gureje O, Kigozi F. Health systems context(s) for integrating mental health into primary health care in six Emerald countries: a situation analysis. Int J Ment Health Syst. 2017;11:7. https://doi.org/10.1186/s13033-016-0114-2.

5. World Health Organization. The global burden of disease: 2004 update. Geneva: WHO; 2004.

6. WHO. Mental health action plan 2013–2020, Geneva; 2013.

7. Alwan A, et al. Monitoring and surveillance of chronic noncommunicable diseases: progress and capacity in high-burden countries. Lancet. 2010;376:1861–8.

8. International Agency for Cancer Research. Latest world cancer statistics – GLOBOCAN 2012: estimated cancer incidence, mortality and prevalence worldwide in 2012, Geneva; 2012.

9. Peters R, Ee N, Peters J, Beckett N, Booth A, Rockwood K, Anstey KJ. Common risk factors for major noncommunicable disease, a systematic overview of reviews and commentary: the implied potential for targeted risk reduction. Ther Adv Chronic Dis. 2019;10:2019. https://doi.org/10.1177/2040622319880392.

10. World Health Organisation. Global status report on non-communicable diseases 2014. Geneva: World Health Organisation; 2014.

11. Currow DC, Allingham S, Bird S, Yates P, Lewis J, Dawber J, Eager K. Referral patterns and proximity to palliative care inpatient services by level of socio-economic disadvantage. A national study using spatial analysis. BMC Health Serv Res. 2012;12:42.

12. Hawley P. Barriers to access to palliative care. Palliat Care Res Treat. 2017;10:1178224216688887. https://doi.org/10.1177/1178224216688887.

13. Whitelaw S, Clerk D. Palliative care and public health: an asymmetrical relationship? Palliat Care Res Treat. 2019;12:1178224218819745. https://doi.org/10.1177/1178224218819745.

14. WHO. Ottawa charter for health promotion. In: First international conference on health promotion, Ottawa 21 November, 1986. WHO/HPR/HEP/95.1. 1986. [Last accessed on 2014 May 10]. http://www.who.int/healthpromotion/conferences/previous/ottawa/en/index4.html.

15. Dixey R. After Nairobi: can the international community help to develop health promotion in Africa? Health Promot Int. 2014;29(1):185–94. https://doi.org/10.1093/heapro/dat052.

16. Joseph S, Sagy S. Positive psychology in the context of salutogenesis. In: The handbook of salutogenesis. Cham: Springer; 2017. Chapter 10.

17. Antonovsky A. The salutogenic model as a theory to guide health promotion. Health Promot Int. 1996;11:11–8.

18. Quehenberger V, Krajic K. Applications of salutogenesis to aged and highly-aged persons: residential care and community settings. In: The handbook of salutogenesis. Cham: Springer; 2017. Chapter 31.

19. Mugisha J. Positioning for safety. Attitudes and cultural responses towards suicide among the Baganda, Uganda. PhD Thesis. Norwegian University of Science and Technology (NTNU), Trondheim, Norway; 2012.

20. Kikule E. A good death in Uganda: survey of needs for palliative care for terminally ill people in urban areas. Br Med J. 2003;327(7408):192–4. https://doi.org/10.1136/bmj.327.7408.192.

21. Eriksson M, Lindström B. Antonovsky's sense of coherence scale and the relation with health: a systematic review. J Epidemiol Community Health. 2006;60(5):376–81.

22. Eriksson M, Lindström B. Bringing it all together: the salutogenic response to some of the most pertinent public health dilemmas. In: Morgan A, Ziglio E, Davies M, editors. Health assets in a global context: theory, methods, action. New York: Springer; 2010. p. 339–51.

23. Kumar S, Preetha GS. Health promotion: an effective tool for global health. Indian J Community Med. 2012;37(1):5–12. https://doi.org/10.4103/0970-0218.94009.

24. Haider S, Ahmad J, Ahmed M. Identifying barriers to implementation of health promoting schools in Pakistan: the use of qualitative content analysis and fuzzy analytic hierarchy process. Int J Adv Appl Sci. 2018;5(4):56.

25. Okello ES. Cultural explanatory models of depression in Uganda. Doctoral dissertation, Karolinska University and Makerere University. 2006. http://mak.academia.edu/ElialiliaSOkello/Papers/634784/

Cultural_explanatory_models_of_depression_in_Uganda.

26. Ovuga O. Depression and suicidal behavior in Uganda: validating the response inventory for stressful life events (RISLE). Doctoral thesis, Karolinska Institutet; 2005.

27. Stockholm, Sweden, and Makerere University, Faculty of Medicine, Kampala, Uganda. http://publications.ki.se/jspui/bitstream/10616/39769/1/thesis.pdf.

28. Menkiti I. Person and community in African traditional thought. In: Wright RA, editor. African philosophy: an introduction. New York: University Press of America; 1984.

29. Katabarwa NM, Richards FO, Ndyomugyenyi R. In rural Ugandan communities the traditional kinship/clan system is vital to the success and sustainment of the African Programme for Onchocerciasis Control. Ann Trop Med Parasitol. 2000;94(5):485–95. https://doi.org/10.1080/00034983.2000.11813567.

30. Katabarwa M, Habomugisha P, Eyamba E, Agunyo S, Mentou C. Monitoring ivermectin distributors involved in integrated health care services through community-directed interventions – a comparison of Cameroon and Uganda experiences over a period of three years (2004–2006). Trop Med Int Health. 2010;15(2):216–23. https://doi.org/10.1111/j.1365-3156.2009.02442.x.

31. Muyinda H, Kengeya J, Pool R, Whitworth J. Traditional sex counselling and STI/HIV prevention among young women in rural Uganda. Cult Health Sex. 2001;3(3):353–61.

32. Mbiti JS. Introduction to African religion. Rev. ed. Botswana: Heineman Educational Publishers; 1991.

33. Gyekye K. African cultural values. An introduction. Ghana: Sankofa Publishing Co; 1996.

34. Braun-Lewensohn O, Sagy S. Salutogenesis and culture: personal and community sense of coherence among adolescents belonging to three different cultural groups. Int Rev Psychiatry. 2011;23(6):533–41.

35. Catford J. Editorial. Turn, turn, turn: time to reorient health services. Health Promot Int. 2014;29(1):1–4.

36. Ziglio E, Simpson S, Tsouros A. Health promotion and health systems: some unfinished business. Health Promot Int. 2011;26(2):216–25.

37. Watson M. InnovAiT. Education and inspiration for general practice principles of palliative care. 2008;1:4. https://doi.org/10.1093/innovait/inn037

Health Promotion Among Home-Dwelling Elderly Individuals in Turkey

22

Öznur Körükcü and Kamile Kabukcuoğlu

Abstract

Although the social structure of Turkish society has changed from a broad family order to a nuclear family, family relations still hold an important place, where traditional elements dominate. Still, elderly people are cared for by their family in their home environment. Thus, the role of family members is crucial in taking care of elderly individuals. In Turkey, the responsibility of care is largely on women; the elderly's wife, daughter, or daughter-in-law most often provides the care. Family members who provide care need support so that they can maintain their physical, psychological and mental health. At this point, Antonovsky's salutogenic health model represents a positive and holistic approach to support individual's health and coping. The salutogenic understanding of health emphasizes both physical, psychological, social, spiritual and cultural resources which can be utilized not only to avoid illness, but to promote health.

With the rapidly increasing ageing population globally, health expenditures and the need for care are increasing accordingly. This increase reveals the importance of health-promoting practices in elderly care, which are important for the well-being and quality of life of older individuals and their families, as well as cost effectiveness. In Turkey, the emphasis on health-promoting practices is mostly focused in home-care services including examination, treatment, nursing care, medical care, medical equipment and device services, psychological support, physiotherapy, follow-up, rehabilitation services, housework (laundry, shopping, cleaning, food), personal care (dressing, bathroom, and personal hygiene help), 24-h emergency service, transportation, financial advice and training services within the scope of the social state policy for the elderly 65 years and older, whereas medical management of diseases serves elderly over the age of 85. In the Turkish health care system, salutogenesis can be used in principle for two aims: to guide health-promotion interventions in health care practice, and to (re)orient health care practice and research. The salutogenic orientation encompasses all elderly people independently of their position on the ease-/dis-ease continuum. This chapter presents health-promotion practices in the care of elderly home-dwelling people living in Turkey.

Ö. Körükcü (✉) · K. Kabukcuoğlu
Faculty of Nursing, Department of Obstetrics
and Gynecological Nursing, Akdeniz University,
Antalya, Turkey
e-mail: oznurkorukcu@akdeniz.edu.tr;
kkamile@akdeniz.edu.tr

Keywords

Elderly in Turkey · Elderly care · Health promotion · Home-dwelling individuals

22.1 Introduction

Exercising, quitting smoking, limiting alcohol consumption, participating in learning and physical activities, and being included in the community as well as preventing losses of functional capacity improve the quality of life and prolong people's longevity [1–3]. Longer life is a valuable resource that provides the opportunity to reconsider not only what older age might be, but how our whole lives might unfold [4, 5]. Therefore, the decade of 2020–2030 has been declared as the "healthy ageing decade" by the World Health Organization (WHO) involving the importance of a healthy lifestyle at every stage of life [6–9]. After WHO emphasized the importance of health-promoting practices for all ages, people have increasingly begun to understand that a healthy lifestyle is important also among older people [5, 6, 9–11]. In many high-income countries, elderly people are spending their "extra years" in innovative and healthy ways, such as a new career, continuing education, life-long learning programs or pursuing a neglected passion, while the understanding of health promotion still is in its infancy in developing countries [5]. Turkey, as a developing country, slowly moves toward the transformation from a pathogenic or disease-oriented paradigm to a paradigm integrating pathogenesis and salutogenesis highlighting how to promote people's health. That is, a health resource-oriented paradigm.

Antonovsky [4] developed the concept of sense of coherence (SOC) representing a person's confidence in having the resources needed to cope with challenges. SOC is linked with personal strength and a person's ability to cope in difficult situations [4, 8]. The first implication of adopting a salutogenic health orientation is the rejection of the dichotomy posited by a pathogenic paradigm: stating that people are either sick or healthy [4].

Despite the changes in the social structure of the Turkish society, family relations still hold an important place, where the traditional family structure prevails [1]. Thus, many older people still live at home and only a small number of elderly adults are staying in Turkish nursing homes [2]. Being able to continue living at home

in old age provides a familiar environment within which to contend with the challenges and changes to lifestyle that occur due to the ageing process [8]. Social support, i.e., from the family, is one of the generalized resistance resources (GRRs) against stress that in turn contributes to the development of a strong SOC [7]. In the Turkish society, this means that elderly living together with their families have access to social support when facing life challenges. This represents a health-promoting resource for the elderly, as well as for their family.

On the other side, although it is a priority for the elderly to live in a society without being isolated from their own living environment, caring for elderly at home can also be experienced as a burden. A large part of the Turkish population considers elderly care as a duty [1]. The burden of care is largely on women; the wife, daughter, or daughter-in-law most often provide the care needed [2, 12]. This can be a demanding life situation to the caregivers. Knowledge of a person's SOC might be one possible way to identify those who may be more vulnerable to stressful situations. Further, a strong SOC is related to quality of life, indicating that perceiving one's life situation as comprehensible, manageable, and meaningful influences on family members' coping strategies in care of older people [11]. SOC is a global orientation that expresses the extent to which one has a pervasive, enduring though dynamic feeling of confidence that (1) the stimuli deriving from one's internal and external environments in the course of living are structured, predictable and explicable; (2) the resources are available to meet the demands posed by these stimuli, and (3) these demands are challenges, worthy of investment and engagement ([7], p. 19). In this chapter, importance of the health-promoting practices for elderly people staying at home in Turkey are presented and discussed.

22.1.1 Aging in Turkey

In the twenty-first century, we now face a significant demographic shift towards an aging population in Turkey and worldwide [9]. Aging, which has been more prominent in developed countries, is now gaining importance also in developing countries; in Turkey, the older population is gradually increasing. While the percentage of population over the age of 65 in Turkey was 8% in 2014, it is estimated to be 10.2% in 2023, 16.3% in 2040, 22.6% in 2060 and 25.6% in 2080 [10]. Life expectancy at birth in 2020 was 73 years for men and 78 years for women in Turkey. According to the Turkish Statistical Institute (TÜİK), the population aged ≥65 was 5.7 million in 2012; this number will rise to 8.6 million in 2023, 19.5 million in 2050 and 24.7 million in 2075 [9, 10]. Due to the increasing rate of elderly people, from 2009 Turkey has established a pro-natalist population policy to increase the rate of young people in society; the social importance of having three children or more is emphasized [7, 9].

Social and cultural factors represent the basis for the perception of elderly care at home as the "basic duty of family members" [11]. Therefore, those who care for family members need to be supported and directed to maintain their physical and mental health [12, 13]. Salutogenic strategies represent health promoting approaches of supporting families and reducing the care-giving burden. Health is a human right. Thus, health promotion and health protection depend upon the promotion and protection of human rights and dignity [13]. Healthy aging seems to be achievable to a certain extent if the older individual can maintain or promote a strong SOC [4].

Prior to the 1950s, the dominant family type was large families due to the patriarchal social structure in Turkey [14]. However, during the recent years the socioeconomic and technological developments have accelerated a shift toward nuclear families. Resulting from changes in the social structure of the Turkish society, rural-urban migration has increased since the 1950s; young people move to urban areas, whereas the elderly remain in rural areas. Hence, the issue of elderly care has begun to emerge also in rural areas [7, 15]. This migration has affected the family structure and accelerated a change from the traditional large family toward the core family [2]. This change includes that the elderly (65 years and older), whom in the traditional large families were valued as a "wise" person in

the family, increasingly are perceived as a "burden" to the family, causing the elderly to feel insignificant and lonely [4, 7].

In some ways, elderly people living in rural areas in Turkey have a greater need for health-promoting support compared to those living in urban areas [16]. Especially in villages, old people who are physically frail might be unable to conduct the needed work at the farm for different reasons; consequently, they are not able to earn money. Due to the migration of young people to the cities elderly people are left alone in villages. As a result, agricultural areas remain idle. Since the elderly people are unable to produce as they did before, they tend to buy ready-made products [7]. Due to population shortage, existing establishments (grocery, mill, coffee, etc.) and health institutions (health centers) are closing, public transport and flights are limited in the rural areas. Initially, the elderly who remain in the village become dependent on their children, relatives, and neighbors, i.e., their environment, for their many socioeconomic needs [7, 8].

With age, the prevalence of chronic diseases is increasing [17]. In recent years, researches and public health practices have shown that chronic diseases can be prevented in elderly individuals and their need of social and medical service can be reduced [14, 17, 18]. However, health promotion is still a relatively unfamiliar concept for health professionals. The most important way to fight chronic diseases in old age is successful aging and health-promoting activities and/or programs [14]. Successful aging is understood not only in terms of good physical health, but also psychologically and socially well-being [13]. Life length, biological and mental health, cognitive and social competence, productivity, personal control and enjoyment of life are common indicators of aging successfully [9, 14, 18]. In this context, successful aging means keeping the social environment and relationships alive while preparing oneself for old age, taking preventive measures to minimize health problems, making efforts to improve memory and physical functions and keeping a positive orientation toward life [6, 19].

Several conditions impact on older people's health [19, 20]. The best-known types of health-related behaviors are smoking, alcohol use, physical exercise, eating, and lifestyle habits [2, 6]. In Turkey, health-promotion practices in the elderly can be financed and organized by donations from individuals or nongovernmental organizations or taxed by national governments [2]. In short, health-promotion activities and initiatives are heterogeneous as the providers of services and support differ by the contribution of the individual, the family, the immediate environment, society, and the local and central government [7]. Biological age is represented by the bodily and cellular changes seen with chronological age [6, 21]. In addition to the increased frequency of chronic diseases, some older people experience losses of functions followed by various degrees of disability [21]. When all these factors occur simultaneously, there is a significant increase in the need for health and social care; in the years to come the care needs of the elderly will continue to increase. Generally, development applications and health-promotion practices for older people in Turkey have three main objectives: (1) continuation and expansion of functional capacity, (2) protection or improvement of health, and (3) social network development and physical activity based in a social group [2].

In the Action Plan of the Turkish Ministry of Health including activities of Health-Promotion and Development in 2009–2013, "reducing threats to the health of people and improving health" in health services were determined as the strategic objectives. For this purpose, the "Health Promotion Department" and "Non-Communicable Diseases and Chronic Conditions Department" were established and started their activities within the General Directorate of Basic Health Services of the Ministry of Health in 2008 [22]. Health professionals can advise and support health behavior of elderly people, improving their well-being and quality of life [9].

22.2 Health-Promoting Approaches in Older People Home Care in Turkey

In order to strengthen the health care system to meet with the increase of older people, the government aims to realize the targets and strategies in accordance with the WHO, European Healthy Aging Strategy and Action Plan (2012–2020) and Health 2020 targets [2]. With the aging population, health care spending and the need for care will increase rapidly, representing a serious responsibility to the future even in countries with a strong social security system [21]. In parallel with the increase of older people, the burden of chronic diseases as part of the total health expenditures is increasing gradually [14].

Maintaining independence and preventing disability among the older population are closely related to rehabilitation and ensuring quality of life [2]. In Turkey, quality of life in the elderly is related to maintaining life without social isolation, appropriate living conditions, timely and easy access to quality health services, maintaining relationships with friends and neighbors, and devoting time to meaningful activities of value to other people and the society [23]. Older adults are still capable of self-reflection, anticipation, and problem solving [24]. Health-promotion practices are an effective way to focus on people's resources and capacities to create and maintain health [23, 24]. A health care approach focused on the individuals' abilities for self-care that promote and maintain health is less costly than the management of diseases [25]. Meaningful relationships, social support, physical activity, healthy eating, vaccination, cessation of harmful habits such as smoking and alcohol, fight against obesity or malnutrition, preventive practices in falls, neurological and mental health protective activities represent areas for health-promotion initiatives [2, 26–28]. In the following, some central areas for health promotion directed to elderly in Turkey are presented.

Health-promotion initiative aims at involving and empowering individuals in the activities and decisions involving their health [6]. At any time during its lifetime, a living system must deal with and withstand negative forces that are on the verge of pushing it to maximum irregularity or entropy [19]. The salutogenic paradigm and practices contribute to health-promotion and public health in terms of quality of life, mental health, psychological resilience, coping with stress, maintaining and improving general health, well-being and healthy aging [6]. Healthy aging is stated as a process—it is the journey, not the end [14]. Fundamental to feeling good is to have a positive outlook on life [15]. Nutrition, lifestyle/habits, genetics, exercises, education, knowledge, skills, mental abilities, family, religion, self-esteem and ideology are social factors affecting healthy aging [8, 14]. The gero-salutogenic approach is shaped by SOC, which is an important factor in successfully coping with the stressful factors of daily life and improving the well-being and health of the elderly [19]. This approach considers the individual as a highly complex bio-psycho-social-spiritual living system, which is self-creating, self-organizing, and self-preserving [4, 19]. Older individuals have good prospects for positive development, if they manage to maintain or even improve their SOC [19]. Antonovsky [4] offered two explanations for the positive association between SOC and well-being, explicitly maintaining that it is not a causal one: (1) a strong SOC is shaped by life experiences that are characterized by the availability of general resistance resources; (2) there are certain resistance resources that contribute to both a strong SOC and well-being. SOC represents the gero-salutogenic core variable, which is fundamental to successful coping with the abundant stressors of everyday life and a key factor for determining an older individual's well-being and health [19]. In this context, we aimed to examine three main aspects of positive aging and SOC among Turkish elderly people: subjective physical health, well-being, and psychological health.

22.2.1 Nutrition Problems and Health-Enhancing Practices

Adequate and balanced nutrition plays an active role in maintaining physical, mental development and functional status as well as preventing, treating and improving diseases in old age [20]. Nutrition problems can be one of the most important reasons underlying chronic diseases [28]. Elderly people living alone in Turkey are particu-

larly at risk for malnutrition [28, 29]. Malnutrition occurs most often in the elderly as a result of insufficient intake or absorption of nutrients [29]. Other factors affecting nutritional status are physiological changes with age, acute and chronic diseases, dental problems, polypharmacy, economic issues, doing shopping alone, preparing meals, and inability to eat [26, 28].

There may be excessive (or unstable) intake of wrong food during old ages [25]. Another common unbalanced eating problem is obesity [30]. Assessment of abdominal obesity, glucose intolerance, hypertension, and dyslipidemia should be performed simultaneously [28]. Inadequate and unbalanced nutrition among elderly individuals is associated with obesity, cardiovascular diseases, cancer, diabetes, osteoporosis, all of which are correlated with high morbidity and mortality [31]. It is recommended that obese elderlies change their lifestyle by developing individual nutrition and physical activity programs [26]. Especially for the elderly with a chronic disease, a specific nutrition program should be developed to support well-being [25].

22.2.2 Cigarette Consumption/ Respiratory System Problems and Health-Enhancing Applications

With high age, a decrease in lung elasticity, increased chest wall stiffness, and decreased lung function due to the weakening of respiratory muscles are seen [26]. These changes result in significant progressive reductions in vital capacity, diffusion capacity, gas exchange, ventilation and respiratory sensitivity [32]. Smoking accelerates these changes considerably, and the prevalence of chronic obstructive pulmonary disease is known to vary between 2% and 9% [26, 32]. Respiratory infections, especially pneumonia, are an important cause of death in both developed and developing countries in people aged 65 years and older [33]. Sitting times in front of the television should be determined and the drawbacks of sitting still for a long time in terms of respiratory and circulatory system should be explained to older people [25]. The effect of smoking on respiratory infections should be explained and elderly people should be supported to quit smoking without creating stress [32]. Since drug use is widespread in the elderly and there may be pharmacokinetic and pharmacodynamic changes due to physiological changes, counseling approaches are recommended instead of pharmacological smoking cessation methods [34]. The health effects of exercising for 30 min every day should be explained [35]. Two hours of decongestant cough and deep breathing exercises should be done especially in bed-dependent individuals [26]. In bed-dependent and confused elderly people, frequent change of position is suggested as it will prevent stagnation in the lungs and the development of pneumonias [32].

22.2.3 Drug Management and Health-Enhancing Practices

The perspective of healthy aging in the medical model is focused on the absence of chronic illness, the ability to overcome chronic illness, or the elimination of risk factors that lead to chronic illness [14]. Unfortunately, globally as well in Turkey, the elderly constitute the majority of the population using drugs to cope with diseases [36, 37]. Polypharmacy drug side effects, drug-drug-disease interactions, treatment noncompliance, increase in cost, weight loss, falls, cognitive dysfunction: medication can lead to many health problems causing an increase in hospitalization and death [38]. Therefore, careful drug use is advised [36]. Older patients and caregivers should be informed about the medicines, vitamins, nutritional support products, and herbal medicines provided [39]. Written and oral information should be given about the preparations given, their frequency of use, their dosage as well as both their generic and market names [36]. Patients and caregivers should be educated about the common side effects of the drugs and informed about where to contact their physician [26]. Drug treatment should be simplified, especially to improve the adaptation to treatment

among elderly people living alone [30]. The focus of the medical model on the absence of chronic illness and physical disabilities does not account for older individuals who, despite chronic illness, consider themselves as healthy and vital human beings [4, 8, 14]. It is well known that to achieve healthy aging, drug management is not enough; the individual must also maintain good exercise patterns, a healthy diet, and good lifestyle habits supporting people's health [14]. Keys for successful and healthy aging are mental stability, social support, and social interaction rather than drugs [14, 30].

22.2.4 Physical Activity and Health-Promoting Practices

The "National Plan of Action on Aging and the Situation of Elderly People" was formed in Turkey in 2007. This national plan contains important recommendations and activities, such as emergency health care, day-care centers, cleaning services, social activities, food services to houses, repair and renovation services for the Turkish population showing increased longevity [40]. Physical activity and movement are seen as one of the most important health-promoting practices in maintaining health in elderly individuals, and the lack of it may set the stage for triggering the most dangerous chronic diseases such as cardiovascular diseases and cancer [34, 41]. Physical activity is found essential to older people's quality of life, and is a therapeutic component in rehabilitation programs, as well as in the treatment and prevention of chronic diseases [20]. It is well known that in elderly individuals the mineral content of the skeletal system is decreasing, causing a decrease in muscle strength and muscle mass and therefore also a decreased ability to move [42]. Moreover, studies have shown a decrease in physical activity with advancing age [35, 43]. There is a direct relationship between increased inactivation with old age and cardiovascular diseases, osteoporosis, and colon cancer [38, 42].

WHO [5] asserts that mobility is the best guarantee of not losing independence and being able to overcome independency. Walking is the most accepted and recommended physical activity by physicians for older people [42, 44]. Walking takes place in social settings (e.g., parks, shopping centers, roads, neighborhood streets), often outdoors, both for leisure and exercise, as well as transportation [45]. In addition, walking or cycling for transportation purposes, dancing, playing, gardening, making housework and similar activities, sports, and physical exercises or activity are recommended [44, 46]. Health care professionals in Turkey recommend active sports, such as walking, slow running, dancing, swimming and cycling, or team games with their own age groups, for active aging [44].

In addition, gardening is recommended as a health-promoting activity for older people staying at home [47]. Gardening provides an opportunity for the elderly to stay outdoors and is described by many as a pleasurable physical activity [47, 48]. In this process, opportunities can be provided for the elderly to care for plants and trees, to weed out leaves or to water plants and trees, to grow their own plants [49]. Seeing the growing of the plants and caring for them both provide physical activity and help to develop a sense of success, meaning, and self-confidence [44, 47]. If there is no garden possibility, plants or flowers grown in the house may also be an alternative [48]. It has been found that elderly individuals who engage in regular physical activity increase their independence and self-confidence, improve sleep quality due to reduced stress, modify depression, and decrease the incidence of chronic diseases [50]. Maintaining autonomy and physical activity are the most important factors of successful aging [14].

22.2.5 Home Accidents/Falls and Health-Promoting Practices

Falling is one of the most common and serious problems causing significant morbidity and mortality [42]. Age-related impairments in walking and cardiovascular function occur in the vestibular system (that is located in the labyrinth in the inner ear together with the cochlea, which is part of the hearing system) and in the ear vestibulum and provides motor coordination and sense of balance [35]. Falls are among the most common causes of injury/death in old age [51]. If looking at the fall rates of individuals over the age of 65 in Turkey, 60% of the falls occur in the home environment, 44% of home accident are on a dry ground and 4% on wet ground [52]. In community-based prospective studies, it is reported that the annual rate of falls in the elderly is between 30 and 60%, about half of the falls are repeated falls and two-third of them are preventable falls [35, 51, 53].

Knowing the risk factors causing falling is important for taking the necessary precautions [53]. Health-promoting activities preventing falls at home include regulating the physical environment of the elderly, teaching measures to prevent falls for the family and the elderly, providing assistance during activities that require skill and eliminating factors that may cause accidents [42, 43].

In Turkey, medical interventions, environmental regulations, training and exercise programs and auxiliary instruments are used to prevent and reduce the frequency of falls [35, 38]. The aim of these initiatives is to reduce the number of recurrent falls and reduce the rates of resulting diseases and deaths [42]. Decreasing the number of drugs in elderly people, especially reducing the number to be less than four, significantly reduces the risk [51]. In old ages, postural hypotension represents a risk of falling; thus, etiology is investigated, drugs are reviewed, diet of those with excessive salt restriction is reorganized and patients are asked to have adequate fluid intake [42]. Balancing arrangements include raising the head of the bed, getting up slowly from the bed, dorsiflexion exercises and pressure-enforcing socks [35, 42].

Environmental regulations are another important issue in preventing falling [35]. In this context, families and elderly individuals are informed about the use of non-slip tiles in the bathrooms, the use of non-slip floor covers and adhesive strips for the floor near the bathtub, washbasin and toilet, the use of slip resistant floor polish for the in-home safety in bathrooms [51]. Less furry carpets are recommended [42]. Lighting needs to be increased in stairs, bathrooms and bedrooms [51]. Dark painted material can be used on the windows for preventing excessive daytime brightness [54]. As there may be a problem of visibility in the dark, electric buttons should be placed on the top and bottom of the stairs, illuminated with night lights; colored adhesive strips should be placed on the step edges and step height should be no more than 15 cm [42, 51, 54]. On both sides of the steps, cylindrical, inward-facing end parts, easy to be grasped and some continuing handrails at the end of the step should be placed [53]. It is recommended to place holding bars on the wall next to the toilet [51], placing pads with non-slip adhesive rubber bands on the bathtub floor, holding bars in the bathtub and shower, as well as using a shower chair and a hand-held flexible shower head for those with reduced balance [54]. Information should be given to measure the distance from the kneecap to the floor for the bed height, not to use low chairs, and to keep the frequently used kitchen and toilet seats within reach [42, 51].

In addition to the regulations of elderly individuals' home environment, there has been increased awareness on the importance of environmental arrangement in the external environment [35]. Research has shown that barriers on sidewalks are primarily responsible for falls happening in the external environment [35, 51, 54]. These barriers are easily damaged during winter months and high narrow-sidewalks, lack of crosswalks, slippery surfaces, stairs without handrails, poor lighting, and traffic seem to be the most important reasons for elderly individuals falling outside their home [45, 51, 53]. In recent years, awareness about the destructive effects of falls on elderly health has increased and interventions that can be made have been planned [51]. In this respect, elimination of architectural deficiencies and careful urban planning represent approaches that will prevent falling among older people [51, 54].

22.2.6 Vitamin D Deficiency and Health-Promoting Practices

Osteoporosis is one of the most threatening conditions in the older population with the progression of age; the most important factor that causes osteoporosis is vitamin D deficiency [55, 56]. Vitamin D is essential for calcium metabolism and bone quality [38, 57, 58]. Although the main source of vitamin D is exposure to sunlight, various factors such as latitude of the area experienced, season, hours of sunlight, and use of sunscreen influence the absorption of vitamin D [55, 57]. Especially elderly people who spend most of their time at home are at risk for vitamin D deficiency due to insufficient sunlight exposure and kidney synthesis of vitamin D and decreased absorption of vitamin D [59, 60]. In this case, calcium absorption decreases, parathyroid hormone works more to compensate this absorption, bone remodeling occurs, bone density decreases, and osteoporosis occurs [55, 60]. Although there is plenty of sunlight in Turkey, insufficient exposure to sunlight and wearing plenty of clothing due to sociocultural/religious beliefs are factors leading to vitamin D deficiency in the elderly [57]. Routine health-promoting practices in this group in Turkey are focused in education and counseling [56]. Recommendations are made to encourage the consumption of seafood, milk and dairy products, to supplement vitamin D and Calcium, and to increase the exposure to sunlight during the day [56, 60]. In particular, health professionals should enhance elderly people's knowledge about the importance of vitamin D, the risks of vitamin D deficiency and the ways to prevent it as well as treatment options [55, 56, 60].

22.2.7 Well-Being, Mental Health and Health-Promoting Practices

Healthy aging is the process of slowing down, physically and cognitively, while resiliently adapting and compensating in order to optimally function and participate in all areas of one's life (physical, cognitive, social, and spiritual) [14]. Individual lifestyle factors, social and community networks, living and working conditions, and general socioeconomic, cultural and environmental factors are some determinants of well-being [3, 4]. The salutogenic approach leads to a more profound understanding through reflection on life situations and a review of available resources and active adaptation to stress-rich environment, which promotes movement toward the "ease" part of Antonovsky's health continuum [19, 61]. Over the life span, negative life events might reduce SOC which includes three interrelated components: comprehensibility of one's world (cognitive aspect), manageability of one's outcomes (behavioral aspect), and meaningfulness of one's life (motivational aspect) [8, 15].

Antonovsky [4] stated that developing SOC requires internal and external generalized resistance resources, including ego identity, social network and social support. The social environment of the elderly individual's such as spouse, family and friends are important support systems for feeling valuable, increased well-being, mental health satisfaction from life and coping with stress [61]. In Turkey, depression is the most important mental health problem that negatively effects SOC: perceived social support is significantly related with depression in old age [62].

The Turkish culture emphasizes the family as a core institution in the Turkish society; accordingly, older individuals live with their families and children [61, 63]. However, the number of elderly people living alone at home or in nursing homes has increased gradually as the nuclear family structure has become widespread in recent years [63]. If the older individual perceives aging as an isolated existence, he or she will tend to isolate him-/herself and begin to fail. However, if the older individual perceives aging as an integral part of the social structure in which he or she lives, thriving will be supported [14]. The quality of social support is considered a crucial resource for SOC and coping [4, 8]. Social support is significant for health and well-being for older people [8]; correspondingly, the physical, mental and emotional health of the elderly living with relatives are significantly better than among elderly

living alone in Turkey [62–64]. Turkish Statistical Institute (TÜİK) [10] reported that family support in old age was closely associated with depression and suicide rates. Bozo et al. [62] found that perceived social support had no effect on life quality and depression: however, depressive symptoms decreased among older individuals with high daily life activity and adequate social support.

In Turkey, which predominantly is a Muslim country, worship and religion play an important role in dealing with loneliness, depression and psychosocial problems [65, 66]. In one study, elders stated that worship raised their morale and gave them peace [67]. Praying, reading the Qur'an, going to a mosque and worshipping with the community are among the most preferred coping methods among Turkish elderlies to fight against depression [66, 67]. According to the salutogenic health model, personal resources may include the following factors: (1) material resources (e.g., money), (2) knowledge and intelligence (e.g., knowing the real world and acquiring skills), (3) ego identity (e.g., integrated but flexible self), (4) coping strategies; (5) social support, (6) commitment and cohesion with one's cultural roots, (7) cultural stability, (8) ritualistic activities, (9) individuals' state of mind, (10) preventive health orientation, (11) genetic and constitutional GRRS, and (12) religion and philosophy (e.g., stable set of answers to life's perplexities) [7, 67]. Just as recommended for many religions, it is an important responsibility for believers in Islam to take care of ones health, avoidance of substance use, healthy eating, and healthy living [66]. Religion might be a gatekeeper that can promote mental health and spirituality among older believers [65].

22.2.8 Sleep/Rest and Health-Promoting Practices

Sleep quality is a big challenge to many old people [68]. Elderly adults may experience daytime sleepiness, waking up earlier in the morning, difficulty falling asleep and maintaining sleep, and a decrease in night sleep time [69]. Sleep problems can cause troubles such as lack of attention, inability to perform daily tasks, falling and it seriously affects individuals' quality of life [70].

A study examining sleep quality among 250 elderly people living at home in Turkey, found that 20.8% of individuals fall asleep within 30 min or longer after going to bed, that women complain more about sleep disorder than men, and that married older individuals pay more attention to sleep quality [68]. In another study, sleep quality was associated with fatigue and quality of life [71].

Elderly people need regular sleep in order to maintain their quality of life and body functions in the best way [72]. Solutions to sleep problems can be found with the correct use of pharmacological and non-pharmacological methods. Music has been widely used as a method for treating diseases in Turkish societies and in many civilizations [73]. Music relaxes the body by lowering heart rate as well as by regulating body temperature, blood pressure and respiratory rate [72, 74]; passive music therapy treatment has been widely used [74]. During passive music therapy people are resting, comfortably sitting or lying down, listening to a relaxing rhythm and the sound of water in accordance with the melody [72, 74]. Sleep and rest are physiologically needed in all individuals, and especially in elderly individuals. Therefore, creating a good sleep environment alongside music might improve older people's sleep quality [75]. Noise should be reduced, and a quiet and safe environment should be provided. The atmosphere must be ventilated, the light should be reduced, the room temperature should be warm and the bed should be comfortable [68].

22.2.9 Quality of Life (QoL) and Health-Promoting Practices

Age, which is an inevitable biological and psychological development process, affects quality of life through changes in the human body such as vision, hearing, skeletal system, brain and prostate, menopause, and andropause periods [72]. In addition, an individual's past experiences, health behaviors, habits, and genetic factors influence quality of life in late ages [76].

Elderly people should be supported to use resources optimally in order to maintain their health and quality of life [72]. The most common problems that affect quality of life associated with aging are changes in the cardiovascular system, respiratory system and the neurological system [64, 76]. In a salutogenic perspective, health, well-being and quality of life should be promoted throughout the life course [2]. The main purpose of preventive health services offered to the elderly in Turkey is to improve the individuals' quality of life by supporting them to live independently and preventing obstacles [72, 76]. The main objective of the preventive health services offered to the elderly people is to improve their quality of life, allowing independent living and preventing disabilities [76].

One of the most important indicators of life quality is social relationships [77]. Developing SOC requires internal and external general resistance resources, including ego identity, social network, and social support [4]. Most elderly people ≥65 retire. As the children leave home, the family lessens, and thus shortening the elderly individuals' social environment. Moreover, the elderly adults may experience physiological changes followed by loss of functionality and mobility. Hence, both social and functional restraints occur [78]. The loss of a spouse may be one of the most devastating factors in elderly individuals [79]. With retirement, the decrease in income causes a decline in social status among most of the elderly followed by a loss of many social activities [80]. WHO defines successful aging as a process of "age-in-place," optimizing opportunities for health, continue to be involved in the community, maintain autonomy, independence and attain physical, social and mental well-being and quality of life [72, 75, 81]. Watching television, listening to the radio, chatting with people, and lounging represent common social activities among elderly people staying at home in Turkey [79]. Research demonstrates that although the elderly generally appreciate their current situation, some older individuals yearn for the activities they were doing while they were younger or healthier [82]. The salutogenic approach leads to a more profound understanding through reflection on life situations and a review of available resources and active adaptation to an irritating and stress-rich environment, which promotes movement toward the "ease" part of the health ease–dis-ease continuum [4, 72]. Aközer and colleagues [77] found that seniors in their free time gave priority to watching television, shopping and visiting family members and relatives. An elderly adult who lives a life isolated from the outside environment may tend to be closed, longing for the past, resistant to innovation and change [3, 83]. Therefore, the ability to maintain social interaction, relationship, autonomy and independence are important determinants of healthy ageing and quality of life [81].

22.3   Home Care Services

Physical, social, and spiritual changes occur with the progression of aging; the functional capacity of elderly individuals decreases and for some this situation causes older people to need help as well as care [78]. Health, welfare, housing, transport, and infrastructure are responsible sectors for healthy aging and quality of life of elderly people [81]. Although increasing needs are met by the families, relatives or communities of the elderly, long-term and regular assistance and services can be provided by health care services [12, 78]. The environment should support the individual's SOC by means of available resources for health, enabling older people to live well despite their limitations [81]. The aims of the health care services are: (1) to support individuals with disabilities, the elderly, people with permanent illnesses during or after the disease recovery period in their environment, (2) to keep up with social life, (3) to ensure their integration with society by maintaining their lives happily and peacefully, and (4) to support the family members who care for the elderly person and especially women in the family [79, 84, 85].

The adaptation of the salutogenic approach as complementing the pathogenic approach is important to health-promotion among home-dwelling elderly individuals: the salutogenic approach highlights to utilize the individual's resources for health in his or her social and physical environment [81] as well as helps to better understand the transitions in old ages and successful aging [4]. The salutogenic approach focuses on movement toward health, whereas the pathologic approach focuses on disease and identifies the person with the disease [4]. Both paradigms are equally important and should be integrated in a holistic salutogenic understanding of health. A central priority by the state should be to meet the needs of the older population including health-promotion and continuity of the social and health care facilities/policies for every individual without any discrimination [2]. A policy based on salutogenic approaches and comprehensive perspectives such as the "Active aging" concept could better improve the well-being of the older population. WHO states that "active aging allows people to realize their potential for physical, social, and mental well-being throughout the life course and to participate in society, while providing them with adequate protection, security and care when they need" [86]. With a strong SOC, people would be more confident about having control over their own choices and their situation by using their resources for health [81]. The European Region of WHO, in which Turkey is a member, has given priority to the facts like enjoying supportive, adapted social environments, having access to high-quality, tailor-made, well-coordinated health and social services, giving support to maintain the maximum health and functional capacity throughout life, and empowering individual while living and providing dignity through the entire life [2, 86].

The professional home-care in Turkey is still in it's infancy; the first studies in this field started in the private sector [87]. Today, home-care services are supported by municipalities, private hospitals, private home-care centers and home-care units of public hospitals [79]. The "elderly-friendly cities" have gained increasing attention by policy makers over the last decade, since the WHO started to promote the concept [88]. In 2010, the Ministry of Health of the Turkish Republic started free home-care services including examination, treatment, nursing care, medical care, medical equipment and device services, psychological support, physiotherapy, follow-up, rehabilitation services, housework (laundry, shopping, cleaning, food), personal care (dressing, bathroom and personal hygiene), 24-h emergency service, transportation, financial advice and training services within the scope of the social state policy [12, 83, 86, 87, 89]. In Turkey, municipalities, social workers, public health workers, policymakers, and researchers work on many activities, facilities or services for older people to promote active ageing; nonetheless, access the to these services is sometimes low [87].

22.4 Conclusion

Ageing is a natural developmental dynamic process of human life and an individual's triumph of accumulated life experiences [88]. As the proportion of older people in Turkey is increasing, the importance of health-promotion among the elderly is increasingly acknowledged. The WHO twenty-first century's theme entitled "Health for all" was directly related to elderly's health [75]. In this context, and in a health-promoting perspective, WHO focuses on strengthening the physical and mental capacities of seniors, as well as creating the environment to allow them to achieve their valued goals [88]. It is necessary to develop elderly friendly communities including aspects related to transportation, housing, public spaces, community and health services [90]. Healthy ageing is influenced by determinants such as social norms, living and working conditions, socioeconomic, cultural, and environmental factors [91]. Health-promotion initiatives in the older population should aim to increase or maintain elders' functionality both socially, cognitively, emotionally, spiritually and physically, improving longevity and well-being. Enhancing functionality, maintaining strength as much as possible, living independently and facilitating well-being are main priorities of health-promotion [84, 92, 93]. Ensuring that older people remain healthy and active is a necessity, not a luxury. It is necessary to regulate the living space of elderly individuals aiming to support their quality of life and health, as well as to improve social relationships.

Take Home Messages

- Healthy ageing is influenced by a variety of interacting determinants, such as belief, living conditions, socioeconomic, cultural and environmental factors.
- There are health gains both for the elderly, their families and health care professionals by integrating a salutogenic orientation as part of the health policy, health care practices and research.
- The salutogenic model of health including the concept of sense of coherence should be implemented in health care practice, research, and health policy.
- Even if health-promotion practices still for most health care settings are limited in Turkey, existing evidence recommends an increased integration of salutogenesis into health care practices as well as a more systematic use of this approach in research on health care settings.
- In Turkey, elderly care is mostly provided by families in the home environment. Thus, there is a need to strengthen the care of the caregivers developed and organized as part of the home-care services.
- WHO has declared the period 2020–2030 as the "healthy ageing decade." The importance of a healthy lifestyle and health-promoting practices during the entire life span is now increasingly understood among older people in Turkey.
- To fulfill the aim of making 2020–2030 "the healthy aging decade," the development of nutritional and health care suitable for elderly people, programs supporting cigarette consumption, physical activity as well as adapting the physical environments to hinder accidents/falls, coping with vitamin D deficiency, supporting self-management of mental health, sleep/relaxation, quality of life and well-being are essential.
- The home-care services should be trained in health-promotion as well as in development and the implementation of health-promoting activities among elderly people in Turkey.

References

1. Yilmaz F, Çağlayan Ç. Effects of healthy life-style on quality of life in the elderly. J Fam Med. 2016;20(4):129–40.
2. Kutsal YG, Kabaroglu C, Aslan D, Sengelen IDM, Eyigor S, Cangoz B. Gerontology in Turkey. Adv Gerontol. 2015;28(1):80–92.
3. Lindström B, Eriksson M. From health education to healthy learning: implementing salutogenesis in educational science. Scand J Public Health. 2011;39(6_Suppl):85–92.
4. Antonovsky A. The salutogenic approach to aging. A lecture held in Berkeley, 21 January 1993. 1993. http://www.angelfire.com/ok/soc/a-berkeley.html. Accessed 24 Feb 2015.
5. Beard JR, Officer A, Araujo de Carvalho I, Sadana R, Pot AM, Michel JP, Lloyd-Sherlock P, Epping-Jordan JE, Peeters GMEE, Mahanani WR, Thiygarajan JA, Chatterji S. The world report on ageing and health: a policy framework for healthy ageing. Lancet. 2016;387(10033):2145–54.
6. World Health Organization Geneva. 1998. http://apps.who.int/iris/bitstream/10665/65230/1/WHO_HPR_AHE_98.1.pdf. Accessed 2 Feb 2020.
7. Antonovsky A. Unraveling the mystery of health. How people manage stress and stay well. San Francisco: Jossey-Bass; 1987.
8. Hatcher D, Chang E, Schmied V, Garrido S. Exploring the perspectives of older people on the concept of home. J Aging Res. 2019;1:1–10.
9. Kıssal A, Tezel A. Aging and health promotion. Turk Klinikleri Publ Health Nurs Spec Top. 2019;5(1):44–9.
10. Turkish Statistical Institute (TÜİK). Seniors with statistics. TÜİK News Bulletin; 2018.
11. Andren S, Elmståhl S. The relationship between caregiver burden, caregivers' perceived health and their sense of coherence in caring for elders with dementia. J Clin Nurs. 2008;17(6):790–9.
12. Adak N. The unofficial caregivers of the elderly are women. J Fam Soc. 2003;2(6):81–91.
13. Mann J. Health and human rights: if not now, when? Am J Public Health. 2006;2(11):113–43.
14. Hanson-Kyle L. A concept analyses of healthy aging. Nurs Forum. 2005;40(2):45–57.
15. Koelen M, Eriksson M, Cattan M. Older people, sense of coherence and community. In: The handbook of salutogenesis. Cham: Springer; 2017. p. 137–49.
16. Please provide complete bibliographic details for Ref. [16]
17. Bilir N, Paksoy-Subaşı N. Old age problems and control of non-communicable diseases. In: Public health basic information. Ankara: Hacettepe University Publications; 2006.
18. Yilmaz F, Çağlayan Ç. Yaşlılarda sağlıklı yaşam tarzının yaşam kalitesi üzerine etkileri. Turk J Fam Pract. 2016;20(4):129–40.
19. Wiesmann U, Hannich HJ. A salutogenic inquiry into positive aging—a longitudinal analysis. Aging Ment Health. 2019;23(11):1562–8.
20. Křížová E, Brzyski P, Strumpel C, Billings J, Lang G. Health promotion for older people in the Czech Republic in a European perspective. Cent Eur J Public Health. 2010;18(2):63–9.
21. Canlı S, Karataş N. A public health nursing approach for the elderly: "physical activity counseling". Ankara Healthc J. 2014;17(2):36–45.
22. Republic of Turkey Ministery of Turkey. Turkey health aging action plan and implementation program 2015–2020. Ankara: Anıl Publication; 2015. http://staging.nationalplanningcycles.org/sites/default/files/planning_cycle_repository/turkey/turkey_health_aging_action_plan_and_implementation_program_2015-2020.pdf.
23. Taskiran N, Demirel F. Quality of life of older people in Turkey: a systematic investigation. İzmir Katip Çelebi Sağlık Bilimleri Üniversitesi Dergisi. 2017;2(1):21–8.
24. Wiesmann U, Hannich H-J. A salutogenic analysis of healthy aging in active elderly persons. Res Aging. 2010;32(3):349–71.
25. Yabancı N, Akdevelioğlu Y, Rakıcıoğlu N. Evaluation of health and nutritional status of elderly individuals. J Nutr Diet. 2012;40(2):128–35.
26. Yıldırım B, Özkahraman Ş, Ersoy S. Physiological changes in old age and nursing care. Duzce Univ J Inst Med Sci. 2012;2(2):19–23.
27. Kalender N, Özdemir L. The use of tele-medicine in the provision of health services to the elderly. J Nurs Health Sci. 2014;17(1):50–8.
28. Ongan D, Rakıcıoğlu N. Nutritional status and dietary intake of institutionalized elderly in Turkey: a cross-sectional, multi-center, country representative study. Arch Gerontol Geriatr. 2015;61(2):271–6.
29. Sanlier N, Yabanci N. Mini nutritional assessment in the elderly: living alone, with family and nursing home in Turkey. Nutr Food Sci. 2006;36:50–8.
30. Aslan D, Ertem M. Elder health: problems and solutions. Ankara: Palme Publishing; 2012.
31. Aslan D. The role of physicians in healthy eating. J Clin Psychol. 2008;39(4):175–80.
32. Özbek Z, Öner P. Geriatric physiological and biochemical changes. J Clin Biochem. 2008;6(2):73–80.
33. Aydin Z. Healthy aging for society and the individual: the role of lifestyle. J Clin Psychol SDU. 2006;13(4):43–8.
34. Çalık İ, Algun C. The relationship between physical activity and sleep quality in the elderly. Physiother Rehabil. 2013;6(2):24–31.
35. Kibar E, Aslan D, Karakoç Y, Kutsal YG. The frequency of falls among the elderly living in an institution in Ankara, risk factors and approaches related to protection. TAF Prev Med Bull. 2015;14(1):23–7.
36. Demirbağ BC, Timur M. Information, attitudes and behaviors of a group of elderly people about drug use. Ankara J Health Serv. 2012;11(1):1–8.
37. Boran ÖF, Bilal B, Bilal N, Öksüz H, Boran M, Yazar FM. Comparison of the efficacy of surgical tracheostomy and percutaneous dilatational tracheostomy with flexible lightwand and ultrasonography in

geriatric intensive care patients. Geriatr Gerontol Int. 2020;20(3):201–5.

38. Karan MA. Assessment of the importance and risk factors of falls in the elderly. Ege J Med Sci. 2018;4(1):4–9.

39. Golinowska S, Groot W, Baji P, Pavlova M. Health promotion targeting older people. BMC Health Serv Res. 2016;16(Suppl 5):345.

40. State Planning Organization. The situation of the elderly in Turkey and National Action Plan on Aging. 2007. http://www.monitoringris.org/documents/tools_nat/trk.pdf.

41. Etgen T, Sander D, Huntgeburth U, Poppert H, Förstl H, Bickel H. Physical activity and incident cognitive impairment in elderly persons: the INVADE study. Arch Intern Med. 2010;170(2):186–93.

42. Naharcı Mİ, Doruk H. Approach to decline in the elder population. TAF Prev Med Bull. 2009;8(5):437–44.

43. Donmez L, Gokkoca Z. Accident profile of older people in Antalya City Center, Turkey. Arch Gerontol Geriatr. 2003;37(2):99–108.

44. Demirtaş Ş, Güngör C, Demirtaş RN. Healthy aging and physical activity: the contribution of individual, psychosocial and environmental features to this. Osmangazi Med Ed. 2017;39(1):100–8.

45. Uslu A, Shakouri N. The concept of independent movement and universal design for disabled/elderly individual in urban landscape. Kastamonu Univ Faculty For. 2014;14(1):7–14.

46. Soyuer F, Soyuer A. Old age and physical activity. J Clin Psychol. 2008;15(3):219–24.

47. Kılınç H, İrez GB, Saygın Ö. Effects of Swissball and theraband exercises on quality of life and some physical characteristics of individuals over 65. Int J Hum Sci. 2014;11(2):678–90.

48. Koçak F, Özkan F. Physical activity level and quality of life in the elderly. Turk Clin J Sports Sci. 2010;2:46–54.

49. Stubbs B, Eggermont L, Soundy A, Probst M, Vandenbulcke M, Vancampfort D. What are the factors associated with physical activity (PA) participation in community dwelling adults with dementia? A systematic review of PA correlates. Arch Gerontol Geriatr. 2014;59(2):195–203.

50. Karadakovan A. Elderly health and care. İstanbul: Academic Medical Bookstore; 2014.

51. Harutoğlu F, Öztürk B. Biomechanics of falling in the elderly and preventive physiotherapy approaches. Turk Clin Physiother Rehabil Spec Top. 2015;1(3):7–14.

52. Atay E, Akeniz M. Falls in elderly, fear of falling and physical activity. GeroFam. 2011;2(1):11–28.

53. Bozdemir N, Özeren A, Koç F, Özcan S, Güzel R, Göçmen C. Çukurova University Faculty of Medicine multidisciplinary approach to elderly individual module: preparation phase. Turk J Fam Med Primary Care. 2011;5(1):45–9.

54. Gümüş E, Arslan İ, Tekin O, Fidancı İ, Eren ŞÜ, Dilber S. Comparison of balance and walking scores

and the risk of falling in elderly people living in their own home and nursing home. Ankara Med J. 2017;2:102–10.

55. Yıldız Hİ, Yalçın A, Aras S, Varlı M, Atlı T, Turgay M. Relationship between serum vitamin D levels and bone mineral density in the geriatric population: a cross-sectional study. Bozok Med J. 2016;6(3):1–7.

56. Şenyiğit A, Orhanoğlu T, Ince B, Yaprak B. Vitamın D levels in routine medical examination. İstanbul Tıp Fakültesi Dergisi. 2018;81(4):115–8.

57. Atli T, Gullu S, Uysal A, Erdogan G. The prevalence of vitamin D deficiency and effects of ultraviolet light on vitamin D levels in elderly Turkish population. Arch Gerontol Geriatr. 2005;40(1):53–60.

58. Kung AW, Lee K-K. Knowledge of vitamin D and perceptions and attitudes toward sunlight among Chinese middle-aged and elderly women: a population survey in Hong Kong. BMC Public Health. 2006;6(1):226.

59. Gürbüz P, Yetiş G. Vitamin D deficiency in the elderly. Inönü Univ Vocational School Health Serv J. 2017;5(2):13–30.

60. Börekçi NÖ. Current information on vitamin D deficiency. J Turk Fam Phys. 2019;10(1):35–42.

61. Tan KK, Vehviläinen-Julkunen K, Chan SWC. Integrative review: salutogenesis and health in older people over 65 years old. J Adv Nurs. 2014;70(3):497–510.

62. Bozo Ö, Toksabay NE, Kürüm O. Activities of daily living, depression, and social support among elderly Turkish people. J Psychol. 2009;143(2):193–206.

63. Ağırman E, Gençer MZ. Comparison of levels of depression, feeling of loneliness in elderly individuals living in nursing homes, at home with family and alone. J Contemp Med. 2017;7(3):234–40.

64. Altun F, Yazici H. The relationships between life satisfaction, gender, social security, and depressive symptoms among elderly in Turkey. Educ Gerontol. 2015;41(4):305–14.

65. Ayten A, Yıldız R. What is the role of religious coping in the relationship of piety, life satisfaction? A study of retirees. J Relig Stud. 2016;16(1):24–9.

66. Turan Y. Coping with loneliness: loneliness, religious coping, religiosity, life satisfaction and social media usage. Rep J Theol. 2018;22(1):395–434.

67. Idan O, Eriksson M, Al-Yagon M. The salutogenic model: the role of generalized resistance resources. In: Mittelmark M, Sagy S, Eriksson M, Bauer GF, Pelikan JM, Lindström B, Espnes GA, editors. The handbook of salutogenesis. New York: Springer; 2017. p. 57–69.

68. Arpacı F, Cantekin ÖF, Demirtola H. Examination of sleep study of elderly people living at home. J Mediterr. 2019;12(68):1032–7.

69. Keleşoğlu A. Normal sleep in old age. Principles of sleep medicine. Ankara: Atlas Kitabevi; 2012.

70. Akkuş AGY, Kapucu S. Sleeping problems in elder individuals. J Intern Med. 2008;15(3):131–5.

71. Pekçetin S, İnal Ö. The relationship of sleep quality with fatigue and quality of life in older individuals. ACU Med J. 2019;10(4):604–8.

72. Khoon-Kiat T, Vehvilainen-Julkunen K, Wai-Chi-Chan S. Integrative review: salutogenesis and health in older people over 65 years old. J Adv Nurs. 2013;70(3):497–510.

73. Somakcı P. Treatment with music in Turks. J Inst Soc Sci. 2003;15:131–40.

74. Altan Sarikaya N, Oğuz S. Effect of passive music therapy on sleep quality in elderly nursing home residents. J Psychiatr Nurs. 2016;7(2):18–24.

75. WHO. About the global network for age-friendly cities and communities [internet]. n.d. https://extranet. who.int/agefriendlyworld/who-network/ Accessed 3 Mar 2020.

76. Arslantas D, Ünsal A, Metintas S, Koc F, Arslantas A. Life quality and daily life activities of elderly people in rural areas, Eskişehir (Turkey). Arch Gerontol Geriatr. 2009;48(2):127–31.

77. Aközer M, Nuhrat C, Say Ş. Research on the expectations of old age in Turkey. J Fam Soc. 2011;27(7):103–29.

78. Akdemir N. Home care service requirements for bed-dependent patient' health problems at home. Dicle Med J. 2011;38(1):57–65.

79. Hisar K, Erdoğdu H. Quality of life in home health care areas and determining the factors affecting. J Gen Med. 2014;24:138–42.

80. Bahar G, Bahar A, Savaş HA. Old age and social services offered to the elderly. Euphrates J Health Serv. 2009;4:86–98.

81. Donmez L, Gokkoca Z, Dedeoglu N. Disability and its effects on quality of life among older people living in Antalya city center, Turkey. Arch Gerontol Geriatr. 2005;40(2):213–23.

82. Altay B, Çavuşoğlu F, Çal A. Health perception of the elderly, quality of life and factors affecting health-related quality of life. TAF Prev Med Bull. 2016;15(3):181–9.

83. Enginyurt O, Öngel K. Sociodemographic characteristics and medical conditions of patients in home care service. İzmir Med J. 2012;2(2):45–8.

84. Sarıipek DB. Demographic shift and elderly care in Turkey. J Soc Security. 2012;6(2):93–112.

85. Bodur S, Filiz E. A survey on patient safety culture in primary healthcare services in Turkey. Int J Qual Health Care. 2009;21(5):348–55.

86. WHO. What is healthy aging? [Internet]. n.d. https://www.who.int/ageing/healthy-ageing/en/. Accessed 11 May 2020.

87. Özer Ö, Şantaş F. Home care services and financing offered by the public. Acibadem J Health Sci. 2012;3(2):96–103.

88. Seah B, Espnes GA, Ang ENK, Kowitlawakul Y, Wang W. Achieving healthy ageing through the perspective of sense of coherence among senior-only households: a qualitative study. Aging Ment Health. 2020:1–10. https://doi.org/10.1080/13607863.2020.1 725805.

89. Dilekçi E, Dilekçi EA, Demirkol ME, Öğün MN. Vitamin D levels in home health patients. J Faculty Med Kırıkkale Univ. 2018;20(2):101–5.

90. Menec V, Brown C. Facilitators and barriers to becoming age-friendly: a review. J Aging Soc Policy. 2018:1–23. https://doi.org/10.1080/08959420.201815 28116.

91. Lezwijn J, Vaandrager L, Naaldenberg J, Wagemakers A, Koelen MA, van Woerkum CMJ. Healthy ageing in a salutogenic way: building the HP 2.0 framework. Health Soc Care Community. 2011;19(1):43–51.

92. Kulakçı H, Kuzlu Ayyıldız T, Emiroğlu ON, Köroğlu E. Evaluation of self-efficacy perceptions and healthy lifestyle behaviors of the elderly living in the nursing home. Dokuz Eylul Univ Hemsirelik Yuksekokulu Electron J. 2012;5(2):53–64.

93. Subaşı N, Öztek Z. A requirement that cannot be met in Turkey: home care service. TSK Prev Med Bull. 2006;5(1):19–31.

SHAPE: A Healthy Aging Community Project Designed Based on the Salutogenic Theory

Betsy Seah and Wenru Wang

Abstract

Salutogenesis introduces a paradigm that requires a perceptual change towards what creates health and how health can be facilitated. Removing the lens of pathogenesis, aging is an achievement to be embraced and older people are valued as assets for their wealth of experiences, resources, skills and knowledge. From the perspectives of older adults, the concept of healthy aging is multidimensional, comprising bio-psycho-social-spiritual health. Evidence shows that sense of coherence via resistance resources promotes health outcomes among older adults. However, very few works have attempted to operationalise the salutogenic theory to promote healthy aging among older community dwellers. This chapter provides a detailed description of the Salutogenic Healthy Aging Program Embracement (SHAPE) intervention for senior-only household dwellers. SHAPE represents an application of the salutogenic concepts: sense of coherence and resistance resources. SHAPE is an integrative person-centric multi-dimensional health resource program that employs an asset-based insight-oriented approach. Illustration of examples in which how the salutogenic concepts were operationalised in developing the SHAPE intervention approach, its content, activities and the conduction of the intervention are presented.

Keywords

Salutogenic health theory · Sense of coherence Resistance resources · Healthy aging · Older adults · Community-based care · Asset-based approach · Health promotion

23.1 Introduction

Normal aging is a precursor of pathology and influence the degree of disease presentation, response to treatment and probability of developing complications [1]. It sets the challenge of approaching aging from the salutogenic perspective in identifying factors that create health among older adults. With aging as a disease and frailty risk factor [2–4], efforts to promote health in older people commonly focus on disease prevention, reducing frailty and disability. In a scoping review performed on past systematic reviews of interventions targeting health maintenance or improvement of older adults, majority of them focused on disease-specific interventions [5].

B. Seah (✉) · W. Wang
Alice Lee Centre for Nursing Studies, Yong Loo Lin School of Medicine, National University of Singapore, Singapore, Singapore
e-mail: nurseah@nus.edu.sg; nurww@nus.edu.sg

© The Author(s) 2021
G. Haugan, M. Eriksson (eds.), *Health Promotion in Health Care – Vital Theories and Research*,
https://doi.org/10.1007/978-3-030-63135-2_23

Removing the lens of pathogenesis, aging is an achievement to be embraced; where older people are valued as assets for their wealth of experiences, resources, skills and knowledge. Advocated in the 2002 Madrid International Plan of Action on Aging, older adults should be continued to be developed, supported by the environment and to live with health [6]. However, there are very few works that attempted to operationalise the salutogenic theory in cultivating such environments by developing interventions for older adults to age healthily. This book chapter documents the development of a health resource program, titled Salutogenic Healthy Aging Program Embracement (SHAPE), for older community dwellers residing in senior-only households using the salutogenic theory.

23.2 Healthy Aging as a Multidimensional Concept

Having an understanding towards older community dwellers' perceptions towards contributing factors of healthy aging allows health professionals to strategize and align health promotion interventions effectively to facilitate this pursuit. A literature search was performed to identify qualitative studies which explored views of healthy aging among independent older community dwellers. Unlike quantitative studies, qualitative evidence synthesis provides an in-depth and nuanced understanding towards the concept of healthy aging across different contexts. The included studies were conducted in Canada [7, 8], Germany [9], Hong Kong [10], Hungary [9], Latvia [9], Malaysia [11], Netherlands [12], New Zealand [13], Sweden [9], Thailand [14, 15], the United Kingdom [9] and the United States [16–19]. The following in Sect. 23.2 presents the synthesized findings of these 13 qualitative studies.

23.2.1 Having Physical and Mental Health

Some older adults referred physical well-being as absence of chronic diseases [10, 15] while oth-

ers acknowledged illness as part of late life [13, 17]. Having physical health meant not suffering from complications or debilitating conditions which impair daily activities [14, 17]. Abilities deriving from physical health allow one to fulfil one's spiritual desires [11], everyday activities [12] and meaningful activities [16]. Having a balanced state of mind was important too as older adults recognized that mental health was connected to physical health [17]. Having good cognitive function was also recognized in five studies and some older adults reported the importance of engaging in cognitive stimulating activities to avoid or delay decline [7, 9, 11, 14, 17].

23.2.2 Positive and Optimistic Outlook

Older adults in five studies reported that having positive and optimistic outlook was an essential element to healthy aging. Maintaining positivity and optimism towards changes in own health and aging experiences influenced how one coped and adapted to these challenges [12], such as through acceptance of situation [7, 17], hope [17], reframing of situation [17], and instilling a sense of self, self-confidence and self-efficacy in knowing what to do with the situation [16]. Having a positive and optimistic outlook gave the older adults a sense of control and willpower over health and own lives [7, 12, 15, 16]. In Thailand, having positive psycho-emotional outlook contributes to one's internal state of mind and it is related to Buddhism [15]. Healthy older adults were perceived to be friendly, humorous and enjoyable too [15].

23.2.3 Being Socially Connected and Supported

Another aspect of healthy aging is social health. A supportive social environment consisted of family members, partner/spouse, friends, neighbours, acquaintances and the presence of social activities [12]. Often, valued relationships involved reciprocity, contact, engagement, caring and companionship [7, 13, 15, 16]. Participation in social activities was reported important as this mitigated feeling of isolation, loneliness abandonment, fostered relationships and promoted sense of fulfilment [17]. Social activities could be related to their social roles [16] and social contributions [13, 15]. Older Malay adults contributed to their families as responsibility towards children and grandchildren was perceived as a lifelong commitment [11]. However, immobility due to pain and disability [7, 16], financial constraints, lack of transport [13], cultural and linguistic background among minorities [17] were reported to limit social opportunities.

23.2.4 Being Spiritual and Religious

Seven studies mentioned that being spiritual and religious contributed to healthy aging. The doctrine of faith offered older adults positive outlook and acceptance towards difficult aging-related encounters [16, 17] and a peace of mind to balance feelings and material desires [11, 14, 15]. Having spiritual and/or religious beliefs freed older adults from worries and anxiety over uncontrolled future, placing their health and late life in the hands of the higher being [14, 17, 18] and preparing them for the end of life and acceptance to death [11, 14]. Being spiritual included having a peaceful life [11, 14], doing good, being a role model and being useful [11, 14, 15]. Having to receive positive feedback from people gave them happiness, pride, meaning in life and higher self-esteem [14]. Moreover, being spiritual and religious was perceived to be associated with healthy lifestyle among African Americans [18]. Spiritual-religious activities involved praying, offering services, donating and going to churches, mosques and temples [11, 15, 19].

23.2.5 Being Active and Committed to Healthy Behaviours

Another key component of healthy aging was to stay active physically, mentally and socially in their daily lives [7, 9, 17, 19]. To engage in activi-

ties which were pleasurable [13], fun [15], meaningful and worthwhile to do was important [7, 13, 16]. These activities varied from physical exercises, volunteering, gardening, puzzles, reading, watching television, lottery and other leisure pursuits [13, 16]. With increased awareness towards ailing health, some reported having difficulties in staying active and had to negotiate competing priorities to continue their pursuit of valued activities [9, 13]. Older adults also identified the importance of committing to healthy behaviours by having self-discipline and making conscious choices to take charge of own health [9, 17]. These behaviours included having balanced and healthy diet, exercising, having enough sleep, not smoking, not drinking, taking medicine as prescribed, attending regular medical check-ups and adhering to doctor's advice [15, 17]. Although taking self-initiative was important [7], some older adults reported the lack of motivation to maintain healthy lifestyle behaviours [19].

23.2.6 Being Independent

Having to maintain and preserve independence was a key contributor to healthy aging in almost all studies. Being independent was a sense of pride and an existential identity in one's home [9, 16]. It meant that the older adults can make their own decisions [7, 13, 14], take care of themselves [13–16, 18], get around on their own [7, 13, 16], and be self-sufficient [7, 9, 17]. Few studies reported their fear of losing independence [7, 16, 17] as it would erode their self-worth and dignity [17]. The studies showed that independence was also a cultural value. Older adults from cultures with strong familism such as Hong Kong, Thailand and Ethiopia, reported having interdependence with family [10, 14, 19] and health care professionals [14] were part of healthy aging.

23.2.7 Being Safe and Secure

Feeling safe and secure, in terms of finances and living environment, played a role in healthy aging as reported in nine studies. This became apparent among older adults who struggled with financial independence to make ends meet and had no substantial savings for late life, bringing them stress, insecurity and uncertainties [13, 17]. Older adults in Latvia and Hungary expressed their fear of becoming homeless while those from Sweden, Germany and United Kingdom reported barriers in accessing or unawareness of financial help for home improvement works [9]. Financial constraints also have consequential effects on health behaviour practices such as limited food choice while on budget [13]. For older adults from Hong Kong and Malaysia, being in a financial state which support a reasonable lifestyle and material needs mattered and would suffice [10, 11].

Being in a living environment that gave older adults daily sense of security and safety was crucial too. It included the house lived in, the people they live with in the neighbourhood and the amenities around [11]. Having physical comfort of a home, which is a basic need, gave older adults warmth [13]. Particularly, older adults whom were formerly homeless reflected that having a home protected them from bad weather, contagious diseases and unsafe physical environment, and brought about access to nutritious food, social support, income support, better hygiene and self-care [8]. With increasing frailty, some older adults felt less safe at home [13]. Others expressed concerns of burglars and unknown neighbours [13]. One study reported that healthy behaviours such as walking as an exercise was limited as African Americans older adults felt unsafe in their neighbourhoods [18]. Moreover, proximity and familiarity towards social support and environmental amenities provided older adults with access and increased their sense of control towards utility of nearby resources [12].

Based on the above literature, older adults' perspectives towards healthy aging spread across multiple aspects of later life, including bio-psycho-social-spiritual health. The above review also suggested that healthy aging interventions need to be cultural-sensitive and explore contextual factors unique to the targeted older population's characteristics.

23.3 The Salutogenic Theory

23.3.1 The Salutogenic Orientation

In the salutogenic health theory, Antonovsky compared salutogenesis and pathogenesis. According to the traditional biomedical approach, homeostasis is the regulation of human life and any occurrence of disease or risk factor disrupts the homeostatic human living environment. The homostasis model focuses on pathogenesis, searching for factors that cause diseases and reduce risk factors [20]. This contrasted with the salutogenesis. It took on the assumption of heterostasis where we live in an environment full of turbulence, stress and instability.

Antonovsky proposed that each of us is on different positions of the health ease/dis-ease continuum, with total health (ease) and total ill health (disease) at the two poles of the continuum. However, this position on the continuum is not static. In the presence of a stressor which creates tension in an individual, one's ability to cope successfully results in salutogenesis, and a movement towards the total health of continuum. Contrarily, failure to cope results in pathogenesis, the movement towards total ill health [20]. Thus, in the salutogenic perspective, health is a process and its scope is non-limiting, multi-faceted and subjective [21].

Antonovsky argued that the focus on diagnoses in the traditional biomedical approach discounted the 'story of the person' (p. 5) or the perspective and context of an individual [20]. This limits the optimisation of one's health potential. While outcomes of pathogenesis are confined to eliminating diseases and minimising deficits, the end-goal of salutogenesis is active adaptation to problems encountered in a stressor-rich environment. The latter provides the possibility of being healthy despite hardship, misfortune and illness. Nonetheless, health care professionals should not boycott the traditional biomedical approach, as managing diseases and risk factors are important. Both salutogenic and pathogenic approaches are complementary and should be embraced and practiced with equal importance [20, 22].

Central to the salutogenic theory are the following concepts of sense of coherence (SOC), and generalised and specific resistance resources.

23.3.1.1 Sense of Coherence

SOC is both a life orientation and a resource. This global perceptual influence affects how one copes cognitively, behaviourally and emotionally with tension caused by stressors [21]. It comprises the following three components: comprehensibility, manageability and meaningfulness.

Comprehensibility refers to how well one perceives the character and phenomenon of the stressor as consistent, expected and clear; Manageability refers to one's capacity to mobilise existing resources at one's disposal to cope with the stressor; and Meaningfulness refers to one's appraisal of the value and experience brought about by the stressor [20]. Thus, an individual with a strong SOC perceives life as comprehensible, manageable and meaningful. He or she will have trust in self to identify resources needed to develop strategies in resolving issues, thereby facilitating active adaptation processes.

Among the three domains, meaningfulness plays a pivotal role in providing the motivation for an individual to engage in the search for understanding and resources within one's contexts. Thus, it can strengthen other components on comprehensibility and manageability. Having to see meaning in what one understands he or she can do matters. Thus, the second important component is comprehensibility, followed by manageability—perceiving which resources could be mobilised. Accordingly, Antonovsky suggested an unequal weight placed on the three SOC components [20].

23.3.1.2 Generalised and Specific Resistance Resources

Generalised resistance resources refer to any characteristic of a person, group or situation which facilitates effective coping of tension caused by stressors. This characteristic can take in any form of 'physical, bio-chemical, artefactual-material, cognitive, emotional, valuative-attitudinal, inter-personal-relational and macro-sociocultural' traits ([20], p. 103). Examples include immunity, money, knowledge, happiness, optimism, social support and cultural stability. In other words,

coping with stressors involves interaction with one's living context, and is related to ecological thinking [21]. Particularly, the scope of GRRs reflected that health is inextricably linked to the community and ecosystem people are situated in, recognising the social or environmental determinants of health which are not within the direct control of the individual [23]. Depending on the context, types of resources needed to meet the demands of stressors can vary. A person with strong SOC has the ability to use available resources to cope with stressors.

According to the salutogenic health theory, interactions with GRRs offer life experiences of consistency, underload overload balance and participation in valued decision-making, all of which contributing to SOC development [20]. Processes of building up an individual's capacity to mobilise resources are more significant than examining the existence of resources [24]. Thus, GRRs are essential ingredients in developing SOC to move one towards the health pole [21].

Compared with GRRs which have a broader range of utility, specific resistance resources (SRRs) are mobilised only in specific situations [20]. SRRs are context bound and they help people to cope with specific stressors in specific circumstances. For example, getting immediate medical attention via ambulance hotline in times of medical emergencies. Not only do GRRs influence the strength of SOC, they enable the mobilisation of SRRs [25]. Despite the distinction of SRRs from GRRs, both types of resources are essential in creating supportive environment for health promotion [25]. The term 'resistance resources', is used in this chapter to refer to both the variants.

Adopting the salutogenic orientation requires a change in how one perceives issues related to health and well-being. Instead of developing solutions to reduce health-related risks, it focuses on how individuals can be encouraged to use resource-based processes to cope with stressors of daily life, thereby generating health. It requires an appreciation and understanding of these stressors and resistance resources, for their interaction brings about repeated life experiences which generate SOC [26].

23.3.2 Sense of Coherence and Resistance Resources Among Older Adults

To strengthen SOC among older adults, it is imperative to identify and mobilise resistance resources which facilitate health-promoting processes.

In an integrative review by Tan et al. [27], factors which correlated with SOC positively were reported as resistance resources among older community dwellers. These resources included one's immune function, appraisal of situations, coping strategies, self-care abilities, social support and income. Similarly, social resources such as having time with children and grandchildren, and relocation within past 5 years were associated with SOC among older adults [28].

Several studies examined how SOC mediated effects of various resources on health-related outcomes and well-being among older adults. These studies found that resistance resources such as education [29], marriage among men [30], self-efficacy [29, 31], self-esteem [29, 31, 32], lesser chronic conditions [32], cognitive function [30], lesser depressive symptoms [31], social support and family relations [31, 33], engagement in physical exercises and daily activities [30, 31], competence in motor activities such as speed walking and swimming, and having sense of autonomy and identity [31] contributed to enhancing SOC among older adults. Additionally, how older adults perceived leisure and their self-efficacy to perform leisure were reported as significant resources influencing SOC, which mediates effects on attitudes towards retirement [34]. These causality studies supported the salutogenic concept of resistance resources facilitating one's SOC which in turn promoted health [20].

Alternatively, resistance resources could provide life experiences which reinforce SOC over time and this could be illustrated using a longitudinal cross-lag study design. Monma, Takeda, and Okura found engaging in frequent leisure-time physical activities, such as walking outside home and participating in sports of various intensities, had longitudinal cross-lagged and synchronous effects on SOC among Japanese seniors [35].

A qualitative study reported that positive and forward-looking attitudes, social contacts with family and others, being physically and mentally active, conscious of maintaining positive lifestyle and being satisfied with own life were health-promoting characteristics exhibited by other adults with strong SOC [36]. These findings corresponded with the characteristics displayed by older adults with high QoL and stronger SOC [37].

Regardless of the method used to identify resources related to SOC, findings from this brief literature synthesis corroborated with the health assets reported in a recent systematic review [38]. These assets included self-appraised health and life satisfaction, psychological well-being, social networks, engagement in leisure and social activities, education and financial resources. While our literature synthesis focused on resources related to SOC, the systematic review examined factors which positively influenced multidimensional health at old age [38]. This confirmed a strong relationship between SOC and health, suggesting that resources for SOC could be pooled together with health assets for older adults.

Evident from the literature, most SOC research conducted among older community dwellers employed quantitative methods to examine relationships between resources, SOC and health-related outcomes. Through these quantitative studies on SOC, resources were identified. However, it is more valuable to understand how resources could be mobilised for utilisation compared to prior resource identification in enhancing SOC [20]. Moreover, SOC is activated when one encounters stressful situations or events in life, and this cannot be observed from the outside [39]. Qualitative studies can capture this process and understand precisely what SOC is according to its components, comprehensibility, manageability and meaningfulness, and how SOC intervenes in different situations and experiences [39]. However, there were few SOC or salutogenic theory related qualitative studies conducted in older community dwellers [12, 16, 36]. Amongst them, two studies used the salutogenic perspective to explore perceptions of healthy aging [12, 16] while the other purposively sampled older adults with high SOC to explore their self-care experiences in health management [36]. Although the third study was not directly related to healthy aging, perspectives of older adults with strong SOC were of key interest to the authors.

All three studies concurred that older adults who were satisfied with their health had positive attitudes and adopted an asset-based perspective. Healthy aging was described in the context of everyday life and interaction with environment, making references to one's physical and mental functions, relationships with people, places and institutions [12, 16, 36]. These findings suggested that salutary factors contributing to healthy aging are embedded in daily life activities of older adults; and these salutary factors involves the mobilisation of one's attitudinal, physical, social and infrastructural resources.

Upon analysis of how the SOC concept was construed, only one of the three qualitative studies reported findings that correspond with the meaningfulness component [16]. This study described health as the ability to engage in meaningful activities but made no reference to comprehensibility and manageability. None of these three studies shed light on the function and application of SOC and its components, which was crucial in understanding SOC-enhancing processes among older adults to advance healthy aging. In relation to resource mobilisation, Naaldenberg et al. [12] revealed challenges encountered by older adults, such as misinterpreted information about resources and negative self-perceived ability to use resources. Such findings on how older adults cope with existing resources are important in identifying problems faced, so that strategies could be undertaken to increase the ease of resource utilisation. The other two qualitative studies merely described health-promoting actions, along with the mention of resources [16, 36].

As such, the authors conducted a qualitative study employing the salutogenic perspective to explore the application of SOC concept [40] and mobilisation of resistance resources [41] among older community dwellers to obtain insights on how healthy aging could be promoted. The key findings from this study were thus applied in the development of the SHAPE intervention as described later in this chapter.

23.3.3 Interventions Enhancing SOC

Despite empirical evidence calling out to strengthen SOC, there are no clear directives in formulating SOC-enhancing interventions. Based on theoretical explanations, Super et al. [42] proposed that SOC can be strengthened by two processes, namely empowerment and reflection. Empowerment, which acts on the behavioural mechanism, can be facilitated by enabling individuals to identify appropriate resources to manage or avoid stressful situations. Reflection involves the perceptual mechanism to enhance individuals' perceived understanding towards situation, perceived knowledge on resources for mobilisation and perceived feeling that addressing the situation is a meaningful process.

Nonetheless, a good way to uncover SOC strengthening strategies is to learn from existing interventions that used SOC as a dependent variable, regardless whether SOC was enhanced, maintained or weakened [39]. Since the targeted population is older adults, interventions conducted in older populations would first be examined, followed by other pertinent interventions which demonstrated effectiveness in SOC enhancement in other populations.

A total of nine interventional studies which evaluated SOC as an outcome variable among older adults were reviewed in this section to understand the potential SOC-enhancing strategies among older populations. These nine studies were identified based on a comprehensive search on PubMed and CINAHL databases using the keywords 'elderly', 'experimental studies' and 'sense of coherence.' While five studies evaluated on health education interventions related to self-management [43–47], three studies focused on exercise training interventions [48–50] and one study evaluated an intergenerational program involving older adults to read picture books to children [51]. Among the five health education interventions, four of them yielded promising findings in enhancing SOC of older adults

[43–45, 47]. The three exercise training interventions differed in the duration of intervention, ranging from 12 [50], 24 [48] and 36 weeks [49]. Significant positive SOC change was reported for the 36-week resistance training intervention only [49]. As for the intervention on intergenerational program, only the meaningfulness component increased significantly for older adults whom read picture books to children [51].

Drawing attention to the health education interventions, the authors identified two common characteristics of the four interventions which yielded significant post-test SOC improvements [43–45, 47]. These two characteristics might shed some light on SOC-enhancing strategies. Firstly, these four health education interventions involved active engagement of older adults to be aware of own abilities, resources and health situations. Such intervention engagement was delivered in the form of interactive group activities [47], individual face-to-face interviews using assessment forms [44, 45] or senior meeting discussions and a home visit [43]. Secondly, these four interventions equipped and empowered older adults with knowledge on coping strategies of various aspects, ranging from managing daily living needs, aging-related issues, home safety and healthy lifestyle behaviours. Three out of four of these health education interventions even provided educational booklets related to these specific topics [43–45]. On side note, the only health education interventional study which reported decreased SOC scores in both intervention and control groups might have minimal face-to-face active engagement to allow for the deep learning of resources and sharing of knowledge on coping strategies [46]. After all, this health education intervention comprised five motivational interviewing self-care telephone talks with health care professionals.

Among the nine reviewed intervention studies, it is noteworthy that Tan et al. [47] used the salutogenic theory as underpinning theoretical framework for a self-care health education program, titled Resource Enhancement and Activation Program (REAP). This self-care program consisted of 24 group activities conducted twice a week, over 12 weeks. The activities focused on topics related to physical well-being, psychosocial well-being, physical activity and motivation; that is, to motivate older adults in using their internal and external resources. REAP addressed resistance resources in their daily activities in hope to enhance comprehensibility, manageability and meaningfulness of SOC, as reported in their study protocol [52]. Participants whom received the REAP program reported enhanced SOC, particularly in the comprehensibility and manageability domains [47].

Apart from examining SOC-enhancing interventions among older adults, other pertinent SOC-enhancing intervention studies conducted in other populations were considered. Notably, the first intervention designed to strengthen SOC was conducted for patients with mental health illnesses [53]. This 19-week talk therapy intervention consisted of 1.5-h weekly group meetings involving 5–9 participants and 1 mental health professional. During which, participants discussed about challenges important to them in relevance to their everyday life, followed by reflective conversations on specific topics which they had prepared as homework. The intervention program was guided by five salutogenic therapy principles and its detailed theoretical application was reported [54]. The five salutogenic principles which were adopted are as follows: (a) the health continuum model, (b) the story of the person, (c) health-promoting (salutary) factors, (d) the understanding of tension and strain as potentially health promoting and (e) active adaptation. Significant improvements in total SOC, comprehensibility and manageability were observed with the talk therapy intervention [53].

Based on the review of the nine interventional studies which evaluated SOC as an outcome variable among older adults as well as the salutogenic talk therapy intervention study conducted on mental health patients, the following are possible SOC strengthening approaches, complementing underlying processes on empowerment and reflection [42]. Firstly, these SOC-enhancing interventions included face-to-face social interaction with peers and/or health care professionals to facilitate discussion and mutual learning. Through them, active participation of 'being present with others' allowed interactive information exchange and reflective awareness of own situation. Secondly, topics discussed were related to managing everyday life affairs and challenges, regardless of the intervention agenda [43–45, 47, 54]. They developed mastery in perceptual understanding towards demands of everyday life and learning the know-how on how to go about with valued coping activities. After all, SOC is about one's global orientation towards life. Thirdly, the interventions are resource programs that provided participants with information beyond health knowledge and resources, they included concrete skills. They focused on devising solutions through problem-solving or learning to be resourceful in managing challenges encountered. Through them, participants are empowered with resources through knowledge acquisition, clarification, experimentation and reflective awareness of own situation and values.

23.3.4   The SHAPE Intervention: A Health Resource Program for Senior-Only Household Dwellers Living in a Resource-Rich Environment

Globally, two in five older adults live independently, either living alone or with spouse only [55]. Owning to changes in marital preferences [56], personal living arrangement preferences [57–59], forced familial circumstances [59] or greater affluence and financial independence among older adults [58], Singapore observed a rise in the number of senior-only households in the recent decade [60]. Where aged care is concerned, familism play an important role in supporting and caring for older adults in Singapore. With lesser familial contact time and exchanges, senior-only household dwellers might receive lesser familial resources that are instrumental to healthy aging in their everyday lives.

Based on the qualitative study the authors conducted on older adults residing in senior-only households in Singapore [41], family members are nevertheless amongst the wealth of health assets they utilised to promote and maintain their health. Apart from residing in a resource-rich external environment where the local government recently channelled considerable capital and support to create an age-friendly living city [61], older adults accrued an internal rich source of personal strengths, life disposition, experiences, self-care skills and knowledge, as well as social resources comprising family, friends, neighbours and social activities [41]. However, these older adults residing in senior-only households displayed variable levels of resourcefulness in gaining access, maintaining and utilising their health resources; some were less proficient in understanding and mobilising them [41]. Furthermore, most of the older adults aged 65 years and above in Singapore received minimal years of education [62] and might not be information savvy. Construction and integration of useful applicable self-care health information and meaningful utility of the older adults' internal and external health assets via a health resource program is thus needed. As such, SHAPE was initiated and designed for senior-only household dwellers to strengthen SOC, better navigate health resources and facilitate them in applying health resources to their own context of health and daily living.

The SHAPE intervention is an integrative multidimensional health resource program with the aim of increasing SOC of senior-only household dwellers. SHAPE focuses on identifying, equipping and strengthening the seniors' existing internal and external resistance resources to adopt health-promoting strategies and cope with aging-related challenges, thereby living a healthy and meaningful life.

The SHAPE-program consisted of 12 weekly group sessions, at least two home visits and a supplementary health resource book. Its curriculum was designed to address the stressors of healthy aging faced by senior-only household dwellers using their health assets/resistance resources [41]. Its content was drawn from the aging experiences of older adults residing in senior-only households to align health-promoting strategies, thereby meeting the demands and needs of their everyday lives. Stressors of healthy aging include physiological decline, shrinking social connections, requiring situational tangible assistance, encountering unpredictable life events and pathogenic health orientation [40].

Instead of being teachers who impart health knowledge and coping strategies, health care professionals leading both the group sessions and home visits are resource facilitators. These health care professionals play a critical role in engaging participants in exploration, knowledge acquisition and reflection. Additionally, the principles of salutogenesis have to be integral to the values and beliefs of these resource facilitators to influence and elicit participants' perceptual awareness towards their worldviews, late life and resources at their disposal.

An intervention manual was developed to provide resource facilitators with clear directives on the implementation of the SHAPE intervention. This manual described the principles of SHAPE intervention, and the detailed conduct of each session; all of which were developed to be consistent with the intervention aim and the salutogenic theory. Outline of each session consisted of specific learning objectives and evaluative outcomes, experiential activities arranged in developmental order and process questions in the form of weekly homework for participants to reflect and connect the content of each session to their lives [63]. The supplementary resource book was designed as a consolidative easy-to-read health information book that complements the content of the group sessions and home visits. Both the intervention manual and the resource book were content validated by a panel of experts and potential users of the program to ensure the appropriateness, comprehensibility and applicability of the SHAPE intervention. The panel comprised two academic experts in salutogenesis, an academic expert in gerontological social work, one senior physician with geriatrics specialty, one senior nurse trained in geriatrics and gerontology and two senior community social workers. They provided ratings using scoring rubrics and gave comments related to the relevancy, comprehensibility, adequacy and organisation of intervention. Revisions were made by the authors in accordance to the feedback received.

23.3.5 Application of the Salutogenic Theory in SHAPE Intervention

The following sections describe and illustrate examples on how the SHAPE intervention approach, content and activities addressed SOC, resistance resources and the salutogenic orientation sequentially. While the authors attempted to delineate the application of the salutogenic theory, the following section contains some overlapping operation of principles and concepts across the aspects on SOC, resistance resources and the salutogenic orientation.

23.3.5.1 Sense of Coherence (SOC)

SOC is a global orientation of how one views the world and individual's stress-rich environment as comprehensible, perceives one's capacity to activate resource utilisation generating health-promoting strategies as manageable, and view the confrontation with stressors as meaningful, with purpose and worth. Having a better understanding of older adults' stressors, health assets and health-promoting strategies provided the contextual knowledge on SOC strengthening processes [40, 41]. Comprehensibility can be strengthened by reducing the unpredictability and incomprehension of aging-related processes and daily living challenges. Manageability can be enhanced by supporting and empowering older adults in using their health assets/resistance resources to adopt health-promoting strategies to deal with or avoid the stressor(s). Lastly, meaningfulness can be fortified by activating older adults to reflect and make sense of old age experiences. Having to contemplate about what life at old age meant gives one a better sense of identity and affirmation of own values and life direction [64].

The curriculum of SHAPE intervention is guided by the three SOC components and strengthening processes to equip older adults with resource information to cope with healthy aging stressors. Figure 23.1 illustrates the categorisation of intervention curriculum according to the three SOC components. They are (1) the cognitive aspect of understanding health and aging-related topics, (2) the behavioural aspect of managing health by adopting health-promoting

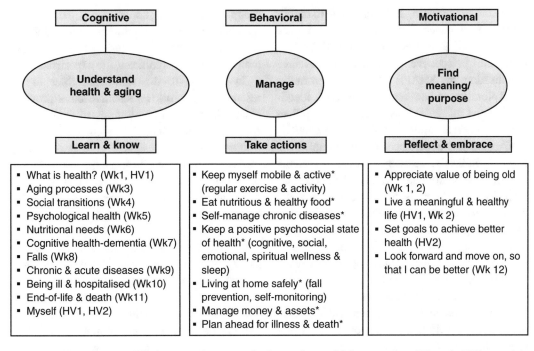

Fig. 23.1 Curriculum of SHAPE intervention categorised according to SOC components. *Wk* week, *HV* home visit, *chapters in resource book

actions and (3) the motivational aspects of finding meaning and self-worth at old age.

The understanding of health and aging acts on cognition to increase comprehension and predictability towards health changes and life events encountered, making life in old age structured and consistent. The 12 weekly group sessions encompass a broad range of health and aging topics, which allow participants to be aware of, and gain understanding towards their physical, psychological, social and spiritual experiences during old age.

Provision and facilitation of awareness towards resource information and experiential mobilisation of resources seek to improve perceived ability to manage stressors through behavioural change. During the group sessions, participants and resource facilitators share with each other coping strategies and practice some of these strategies together to tackle aging-related stressors and daily living challenges. Additional resource information is also provided in the SHAPE resource book, which recommends various health-promoting actions

and includes information on available resources supporting these actions.

Through personal reflection of experiences in life, one can find meaning, value and purpose, providing the motivation to embrace life in old age. The group sessions in week 1, 2 and 12, as well as the home visits allow participants to look back at their past life experiences, connect to their present and project into the future on how they can live a meaningful healthy late life. These reflective sessions help to seek meaning of one's existence from the past to derive meaning for the present and basis for meaning in future [65, 66]. The sessions also create a sense of awareness, identity and a destination or purpose in life for the participant [67]. These reflections bring coherence of story to one's life, contributing to the cognitive, emotional and motivational aspect of SOC [68].

23.3.5.2 Resistance Resources

Both SOC and resistance resources have a dynamic and reciprocal interactional relationship. While resistance resources contribute to SOC-enhancing experiences, SOC contribute to mobilisation of resistance resources to cope with life stressors [69]. To address the three SOC aspects from the perspective of resistance resource mobilisation, the SHAPE intervention promotes the exploration and awareness (cognitive), identification and utilisation (behavioural), and reflection and internalisation of resources to generate SOC-enhancing experiences (motivational) [41]. More specifically, resistance resources create experiences of consistency, load balance, participation in valued decision-making, thereby contributing to comprehensibility, manageability, meaningfulness, respectively [69]. The eco-map of aging assets emerged from the qualitative study provided a visual framework to guide resistance resource mobilisation [41].

Firstly, to create experiences of consistency via SOC comprehensibility, older adults need to process cognitively that there is order and structure in their life. The resource facilitator engages older adults to be aware, apprehend and distinguish the types of appropriate resources to cope with the specific demands of aging-related processes and vulnerabilities during late life.

Secondly, to create experiences of load balance via SOC manageability, older adults need to take on behavioural actions in identifying and utilising the resources available to them. Such experimentation and experiential learning in developing the ability to activate the appropriate resource from their environment allow them to develop the know-how knowledge in initiating and maintaining the utility of the resource. This brings about the adoption of health-promoting actions in their everyday lives. The resource facilitator influences older adults by encouraging, reinforcing and complimenting them for their acts of resource utility.

Lastly, to create experiences of participation in valued decision-making via SOC meaningfulness, older adults' motivation of utilising the specific resources to perform the health-promoting behaviour needs to be intrinsic and based on personal decision-making to shape their health outcomes. Each older adult has to engage him/herself emotionally in making sense of the intended purpose of using the specific resource. During the group sessions and home visits, the resource facilitator probes and prompts older adults to reflect and internalise the insights and meanings drawn from their significant life experiences.

In addition to the significant roles of the resource facilitator, the resource book provides older adults with opportunities to create SOC-enhancing experiences independently. The resource book is designed to make one-stop 'resistance resource' information available and accessible to older adults who are less literate or savvy in information technology. Although the titles of the resource book chapters were targeted at SOC manageability (Fig. 23.1), the contents in the chapters addressed both SOC comprehensibility and manageability. To facilitate adoption of health-promoting strategies more easily via the mobilisation of 'resistance resources', the resource book provides contextual information on the local services, communal activities, and government schemes, as well as practical information on where and how these 'resistance resources' can be accessed. At the end of chapter, additional information sources such as hyperlinks and QR codes are provided to allow interested older adults to explore further. The intent of providing such access information was to impel older adults to search for information when needed, as part of a health-promoting strategy in face of stressors.

23.3.5.3 The Salutogenic Orientation: Five Salutogenic Principles

To reinforce the salutogenic orientation and support the operationalisation of SOC and resistance resources, the aforementioned five salutogenic principles (Sect. 23.3.3) which guided the salutogenic therapy talk intervention [54] were also employed in the development of SHAPE intervention. The following describes the five salutogenic principles and illustrates how these principles were integrated in the approach, contents and activities of the SHAPE intervention.

Health as a Continuum
This salutogenic principle focuses on facilitating older adults to move forward along the health continuum, by addressing health-promoting fac-

tors instead of managing risk factors to avoid diseases. This requires a perceptual change among older adults if they adopt a disease-oriented definition towards health. The adoption of strength-based perspective which focuses on what works well can address this. It shifts frame of reference to redefine issues according to experiences of an individual instead of problems or health deficits [70]. Such perspective views older adults 'by their values, strengths, hopes, aspirations, and capacities, regardless of the stressful or burdensome nature of the situation around them' (p. 642–43). With an assumption that people are capable of growth and change, older adults can be assisted to develop insight to their strengths and resources [71].

To embrace the strengths-based perspective, approaches used in various strength-based models, such as appreciative inquiry, building capacities and solution-focused therapy [70], were incorporated in SHAPE intervention.

Appreciative inquiry uses a way of asking questions to appreciate ideas that have worked and use these ideas to envision and shape the future [72]. The resource facilitator can engage older adults in 'strengths chats' by asking the right questions [70]. Asking about past positive experiences can uncover and draw on individual's strengths while inquiring about the form of support needed to build upon existing strengths, and information about past and present issues influencing or preventing the use of strengths could help in formulating health-promoting strategies [70, 73]. Using the same question in the qualitative interview [40], older adults can be asked to share their healthiest or most energised moments during their late life to elucidate characteristics which create health in them. They could be guided to perceive that these moments of accomplishment on desired pursuits or activities are examples of moving forward along the health continuum. In this way, reframing and redefinition of health from pathogenic to salutogenic perspective is facilitated among the older adults [40]. This also expands their meaning of being healthy.

Scale questions, a solution-focused therapy technique which use scale from 0 to 10, can be used as a tool to simulate and facilitate movement on the health continuum [74]. In the SHAPE intervention, the following question is used: 'On a scale of 0 to 10, where 0 refers to worst imaginable life and 10 as best imaginable life, how would you rate yourself as living meaningfully and healthily now?'. If the older adult rates four, the resource facilitator can ask why the rating is not a two or six to find out possibilities of what the former hopes to achieve and what had been achieved. It allows exploration of possible progress of the older adult's health position in the immediate future [75].

The Story of a Person

Having to learn about the story of an older adult recognises him or her as a person with rich diverse experiences, mould by a set of attitudes, beliefs, values, social cultural norms, daily life activities and interaction with their physical, social and structural environment. It is contextualised and sees a person behind the illness and disease [20], akin to person-centred thinking in contrast to disease-centeredness or the focus on impairment in care delivery [76].

Underpinned by values of respect for person, individual's right to self-determination, mutual understanding and respect [77], person-centred approach traced back to humanistic psychology and person-centred therapy [78]. Elements of person-centred approach involves perceiving a person holistically and as an unique individual, being empathetic towards his/her experiences, needs, values and preferences, having mutual trust and relationship with each other and participative decision-making through information exchange and communication [79–82], with the goal of achieving a meaningful life [79]. It requires openness to experiences, being curious, understanding, having respect and the establishment of trusting, collaborative and egalitarian relationship between older adults and the resource facilitator.

In SHAPE intervention, part of understanding the story of person for the resource facilitator is to use narrative accounts as a tool to understand participants' values in life [80]. Narrative accounts also emanate participants' awareness towards own living situation, facilitating conscious recognition of own internal and external resources to cope with it. This tool uses language expression to organise one's thoughts and feelings, creating and describing a 'pre-understanding' of situations [83]. It is insight-oriented because it sheds light on the participant's coping capacity and strategies to adopt [54].

Health-Promoting Factors

Contrary to deficit orientation, salutogenic thinking focuses on health-promoting factors through resource mobilisation, building and enhancing capacities through process of empowerment [21]. It has been suggested that salutogenesis could provide the underpinning theoretical basis for health assets [84, 85].

The SHAPE intervention adopts an asset-based approach to facilitate aging assets mobilisation. Apart from providing information needed for resource mobilisation, SHAPE encourages older adults to gain insight that they can contribute to their own health by identifying and learning how to access and use resources [86]. The resource facilitator engages older adults to recognise their personal, social, economic and environmental factors as health assets which they could use to pursue desired activities or health goals [38].

In the intervention, simple activities are planned to raise older adults' awareness towards their resources. This includes reflection on identifying their unique strengths/attributes and plotting daily activity routine on a 24-h activity clock to identify activity participation preferences and involvement. Also, having older adults to draw their own social eco-map allows them to have an overview of their existing social capital and reflect on how some of these relationships could be strengthen or improved. Unlike in social work profession, social eco-map is used as an assessment tool to understand client's sources of psychosocial stress and transactional relationships, aiding in development of care interventions such as discharge planning [87]. During the intervention, participants are encouraged to build their social network by establishing and maintaining new social relationships, such as making friends. To further equip older adults with self-care knowledge and relevant external resources

such as community services and government support schemes, exchange of information through printed materials and discussions are facilitated. This involves the resource facilitator to share relevant health knowledge and resource information with older adults too.

Stress and Strain as Potentially Health Promoting

According to Antonovsky, stressors and tension create life experiences of inconsistency, overload and lack of engagement in decision-making, which provide situations for developing coping capacity and generating SOC [20]. Being challenged by tension-causing stressors to adapt is salutary and health promoting.

Confrontation as a form of coping strategy to stressors has been found to have mediating effects on both SOC and self-care behaviours [88]. Having to confront and discuss openly about stressors could reduce older adults' incomprehension, enhance manageability and promote acceptance towards it. This can result older adults in resource activation and adopting positive health behaviours.

In SHAPE intervention, stressors such as unpredictable illness and death are confronted by anticipating experiences of and preparing for illness and death. Examples of activities include hands-on usage of assistive ambulatory aids, exposure to common medical requisites encountered during hospitalisation and introducing advance care plans [52]. Although this approach presents an adverse portrayal to older adults, it can be introduced in a safe learning environment for them to inquire and clarify doubts.

As stressors are omnipresent [20], it is important to universalise feelings of tension by acknowledging normalcy of stressful experiences [54]. This requires the older adults to acknowledge and accept stressors such as physiological and social changes of aging, and times of vulnerability requiring tangible assistance. Having to discuss and hear stories of others who underwent similar experiences help in normalising these feelings of tension. Also, such perception towards stress and tension should be consistently demonstrated in the resource facilitator's attitude and interaction with older adults during the SHAPE intervention [54].

Active Adaptation

Aforementioned, salutogenic processes which involve developing personal capacity for resourcefulness are more important than providing resources as pre-requisites for SOC enhancement [20, 24]. Creating such experiences during SHAPE intervention would allow resources to be internalised by older adults through personal usage, giving them a sense of ownership and control of their own health and aging journey [24]. Activities such as hands-on preparation of nutritious meal, acts of physical exercises and accomplishment of personal health goals using 'resistance resources' could provide experiential and adaptation opportunities for the older adults.

In addition, as one ages and confronts with life experiences, personal meaning to life and health changes [64]. The use of self-reflection is an essential tool to construct participants' personal meaning of health and meaning in life at old age. It creates self-awareness of knowing own self, contributing to meaning-focused health-promoting strategies as part of adaptation. This, however, is a developmental process which requires creation and self-discovery [68]. The use of narrative life stories can contribute to older adults' sense of self, uncover their meaning in life, allow them to accept life, and live with purpose and enthusiasm [64]. A quick life review activity using a life ruler can allow older adults to reminisce and appreciate past experiences of personal development, achievements, loss and hardship in their life journey. It facilitates participants to examine how their stories contribute to their meaning in life, and come to terms with aging [65]. Integrating experiences of past difficult transitions and vulnerabilities help them to accept loss and hardship, preserve their self-worth and adapt to present life stressors [89].

23.4 Conclusion

Salutogenesis introduces a paradigm on the origins of health; what is health and how health can be created. In the context of healthy aging, the salutogenic perspective recognises aging as a positive developmental process of a person and values the life experiences of the person. This perspective involves a conscious reflection of how an individual views life as a whole to cope with the salutary vulnerabilities and stressors in old age. Healthy aging is a multidimensional concept embraced in the SHAPE intervention. Based on the salutogenic principles, SOC and resistance resources, SHAPE is a health resource program that employs an asset-based, person-centric and insight-oriented approach. Apart from the intervention approach, content and activities, the SHAPE intervention places emphasis on the significant role of health professionals conducting the intervention to communicate and elicit the salutogenic perspective to its target audience—senior-only household dwellers. To advance this salutogenic initiative, the SHAPE intervention needs to be piloted to test for its feasibility.

Take Home Messages

- The salutogenic perspective on healthy aging views aging as an achievement; where older people are valued as assets for their wealth of experiences, resources, skills and knowledge.
- The SHAPE intervention embraces the multidimensional concept of healthy aging; It covers a range of comprehensive health and aging topics encompassing physical, psychological, psychological, social and spiritual aspects of aging.
- The concepts on sense of coherence, resistance resources and the salutogenic orientation are operationalised and illustrated in the intervention approach, curriculum and the conduct of SHAPE.
- As a health resource program, the SHAPE intervention aims to strengthen 'resistance resources' of older adults, so as to promote the adoption of health-promoting strategies and coping of stressors at old age; it employs an asset-based, person-centric and insight-oriented approach.
- Health professionals conducting salutogenic theory based interventions such as SHAPE play an important role of communicating and eliciting the salutogenic perspective to the participants.

Acknowledgements This research project was funded by Singapore Ministry of Education Social Science Research Thematic Grant. Any opinions, findings, and conclusions or recommendations expressed in this material are those of the author(s) and do not reflect the views of the Singapore Ministry of Education or the Singapore Government.'

References

1. Rowe JW, Kahn RL. Human aging: usual and successful. Science. 1987;237(4811):143–9. https://doi.org/10.1126/science.3299702.
2. Niccoli T, Partridge L. Ageing as a risk factor for disease. Curr Biol. 2012;22(17):R741–52. https://doi.org/10.1016/j.cub.2012.07.024.
3. Ng TP, Feng L, Nyunt MS, Larbi A, Yap KB. Frailty in older persons: multisystem risk factors and the frailty risk index (FRI). J Am Med Dir Assoc. 2014;15(9):635–42. https://doi.org/10.1016/j.jamda.2014.03.008.
4. Niederstrasser NG, Rogers NT, Bandelow S. Determinants of frailty development and progression using a multidimensional frailty index: evidence from the English Longitudinal Study of Ageing. PLoS One. 2019;14(10):e0223799. https://doi.org/10.1371/journal.pone.0223799.
5. Duplaga M, Grysztar M, Rodzinka M, Kopec A. Scoping review of health promotion and disease prevention interventions addressed to elderly people. BMC Health Serv Res. 2016;16(Suppl 5):278. https://doi.org/10.1186/s12913-016-1521-4.
6. United Nations. Political declarations and Madrid International Plan of Action on Ageing. New York: United Nation; 2002.
7. Bacsu J, Jeffery B, Abonyi S, Johnson S, Novik N, Martz D, et al. Healthy aging in place: perceptions of rural older adults. Educ Gerontol. 2013;40(5):327–37. https://doi.org/10.1080/03601277.2013.802191.
8. Waldbrook N. Exploring opportunities for healthy aging among older persons with a history of homelessness in Toronto. Can Soc Sci Med. 2015;128:126–33. https://doi.org/10.1016/j.socscimed.2015.01.015.
9. Sixsmith J, Sixsmith A, Fange AM, Naumann D, Kucsera C, Tomsone S, et al. Healthy ageing and home: the perspectives of very old people in five European countries. Soc Sci Med. 2014;106:1–9. https://doi.org/10.1016/j.socscimed.2014.01.006.
10. Lee LY, Fan RY. An exploratory study on the perceptions of healthy ageing among Chinese adults in Hong Kong. J Clin Nurs. 2008;17(10):1392–4. https://doi.org/10.1111/j.1365-2702.2007.02273.x.
11. Tohit N, Browning CJ, Radermacher H. 'We want a peaceful life here and hereafter': healthy ageing perspectives of older Malays in Malaysia. Ageing Soc. 2011;32(3):405–24. https://doi.org/10.1017/s0144686x11000316.
12. Naaldenberg J, Vaandrager L, Koelen M, Leeuwis C. Aging populations' everyday life perspectives on healthy aging: new insights for policy and strategies at the local level. J Appl Gerontol. 2011;31(6):711–33. https://doi.org/10.1177/0733464810397703.
13. Stephens C, Breheny M, Mansvelt J. Healthy ageing from the perspective of older people: a capability approach to resilience. Psychol Health. 2015;30(6):715–31. https://doi.org/10.1080/08870446.2014.904862.
14. Manasatchakun P, Chotiga P, Roxberg A, Asp M. Healthy ageing in Isan-Thai culture--a phenomenographic study based on older persons' lived experiences. Int J Qual Stud Health Well Being. 2016;11:29463. https://doi.org/10.3402/qhw.v11.29463.
15. Thanakwang K, Soonthorndhada K, Mongkolprasoet J. Perspectives on healthy aging among Thai elderly: a qualitative study. Nurs Health Sci. 2012;14(4):472–9. https://doi.org/10.1111/j.1442-2018.2012.00718.x.
16. Bryant LL, Corbett KK, Kutner JS. In their own words: a model of healthy aging. Soc Sci Med. 2001;53(7):927–41. https://doi.org/10.1016/S0277-9536(00)00392-0.
17. Nguyen H, Lee JA, Sorkin DH, Gibbs L. "Living happily despite having an illness": perceptions of healthy aging among Korean American, Vietnamese American, and Latino older adults. Appl Nurs Res. 2019;48:30–6. https://doi.org/10.1016/j.apnr.2019.04.002.
18. Waites C. Examining the perceptions, preferences, and practices that influence healthy aging for African American older adults: an ecological perspective. J Appl Gerontol. 2013;32(7):855–75. https://doi.org/10.1177/0733464812446020.
19. Waites CE, Onolemhemhen DN. Perceptions of healthy aging among African-American and Ethiopian elders. Ageing Int. 2014;39(4):369–84.
20. Antonovsky A. Unraveling the mystery of health: how people manage stress and stay well. 1st ed. San Francisco: Jossey-Bass; 1987.
21. Lindstrom B, Eriksson M. The Hitchhiker's guide to salutogenesis. Salutogenic pathways to health promotion. Folhalsan Research Centre: Helsinki; 2010.
22. Mittelmark MB, Bull T. The salutogenic model of health in health promotion research. Glob Health Promot. 2013;20(2):30–8. https://doi.org/10.1177/1757975913486684.
23. Harris N, Grootjans J. The application of ecological thinking to better understand the needs of communities of older people. Australas J Ageing. 2012;31(1):17–21. https://doi.org/10.1111/j.1741-6612.2010.00501.x.
24. Cowley S, Billings JR. Resources revisited: salutogenesis from a lay perspective. J Adv Nurs. 1999;29(4):994–1004. https://doi.org/10.1046/j.1365-2648.1999.00968.x.
25. Mittelmark MB, Bull T, Daniel M, Urke H. Specific resistance resources in the salutogenic model of health. In: Mittelmark MB, Sagy S, Eriksson M, Bauer GF, Pelikan JM, Lindstrom B, et al., editors.

The handbook of salutogenesis. Cham: Springer; 2017. p. 71–6.

26. Antonovsky A. The salutogenic model as a theory to guide health promotion. Health Promot Int. 1996;11(1):11–8. https://doi.org/10.1093/heapro/11.1.11.

27. Tan KK, Vehvilainen-Julkunen K, Chan SW. Integrative review: salutogenesis and health in older people over 65 years old. J Adv Nurs. 2014;70(3):497–510. https://doi.org/10.1111/jan.12221.

28. Mellqvist M, Wiktorsson S, Joas E, Ostling S, Skoog I, Waern M. Sense of coherence in elderly suicide attempters: the impact of social and health-related factors. Int Psychogeriatr. 2011;23(6):986–93. https://doi.org/10.1017/S1041610211000196.

29. Wiesmann U, Hannich H-J. A salutogenic view on subjective Well-being in active elderly persons. Aging Ment Health. 2008;12(1):56–65. https://doi.org/10.1080/13607860701365998.

30. Read S, Aunola K, Feldt T, Leinonen R, Ruoppila I. The relationship between generalized resistance resources, sense of coherence, and health among Finnish people aged 65-69. Eur Psychol. 2005;10(3):244–53. https://doi.org/10.1027/1016-9040.10.3.244.

31. Wiesmann U, Hannich H-J. A salutogenic analysis of healthy aging in active elderly persons. Res Aging. 2010;32(3):349–71. https://doi.org/10.1177/0164027509356954.

32. Wiesmann U, Hannich H-J. The contribution of resistance resources and sense of coherence to life satisfaction in older age. J Happiness Stud. 2013;14(3):911–28. https://doi.org/10.1007/s10902-012-9361-3.

33. Chiang HH, Lee TS. Family relations, sense of coherence, happiness and perceived health in retired Taiwanese: analysis of a conceptual model. Geriatr Gerontol Int. 2018;18(1):154–60. https://doi.org/10.1111/ggi.13141.

34. Lee C, Payne LL, Berdychevsky L. The roles of leisure attitudes and self-efficacy on attitudes toward retirement among retirees: a sense of coherence theory approach. Leis Sci. 2020;42(2):152–69. https://doi.org/10.1080/01490400.2018.1448025.

35. Monma T, Takeda F, Okura T. Physical activities impact sense of coherence among community-dwelling older adults. Geriatr Gerontol Int. 2017;17(11):2208–15. https://doi.org/10.1111/ggi.13063.

36. Söderhamn U, Dale B, Söderhamn O. Narrated lived experiences of self-care and health among rural-living older persons with a strong sense of coherence. Psychol Res Behav Manag. 2011;4:151–8. https://doi.org/10.2147/PRBM.S27228.

37. Borglin G, Jakobsson U, Edberg AK, Hallberg IR. Older people in Sweden with various degrees of present quality of life: their health, social support, everyday activities and sense of coherence. Health Soc Care Community. 2006;14(2):136–46. https://doi.org/10.1111/j.1365-2524.2006.00603.x.

38. Hornby-Turner YC, Peel NM, Hubbard RE. Health assets in older age: a systematic review. BMJ Open. 2017;7(5):e013226. https://doi.org/10.1136/bmjopen-2016-013226.

39. Yamazaki Y, Togari T, Sakano J. Toward development of intervention methods for strengthening the sense of coherence: suggestions from Japan. In: Muto T, Nakahara T, Nam EW, editors. Asian perspectives and evidence on health promotion and education. Tokyo: Springer Japan; 2011. p. 118–32.

40. Seah B, Espnes GA, Ang ENK, Lim JY, Kowitlawakul Y, Wang W. Achieving healthy ageing through the perspective of sense of coherence among senior-only households: a qualitative study. Aging Ment Health. 2020:1–10. https://doi.org/10.1080/13607863.2020.1725805.

41. Seah B, Espnes GA, Ang ENK, Lim JY, Kowitlawakul Y, Wang W. Mobilisation of health assets among older community dwellers residing in senior-only households in Singapore: a qualitative study. BMC Geriatr. 2020;20:411.

42. Super S, Wagemakers MAE, Picavet HSJ, Verkooijen KT, Koelen MA. Strengthening sense of coherence: opportunities for theory building in health promotion. Health Promot Int. 2016;31(4):869–78. https://doi.org/10.1093/heapro/dav071.

43. Arola LA, Barenfeld E, Dahlin-Ivanoff S, Haggblom-Kronlof G. Distribution and evaluation of sense of coherence among older immigrants before and after a health promotion intervention - results from the RCT study promoting aging migrants' capability. Clin Interv Aging. 2018;13:2317–28. https://doi.org/10.2147/CIA.S177791.

44. Hourzad A, Pouladi S, Ostovar A, Ravanipour M. The effects of an empowering self-management model on self-efficacy and sense of coherence among retired elderly with chronic diseases: a randomized controlled trial. Clin Interv Aging. 2018;13:2215–24. https://doi.org/10.2147/CIA.S183276.

45. Musavinasab M, Ravanipour M, Pouladi S, Motamed N, Barekat M. The effect of self-management empowerment model on the sense of coherence among elderly patients with cardiovascular disease. Educ Gerontol. 2015;42(2):100–8. https://doi.org/10.1080/03601277.2015.1078691.

46. Sundsli K, Soderhamn U, Espnes GA, Soderhamn O. Self-care telephone talks as a health-promotion intervention in urban home-living persons 75+ years of age: a randomized controlled study. Clin Interv Aging. 2014;9:95–103. https://doi.org/10.2147/cia.s55925.

47. Tan KK, Chan SW, Wang W, Vehvilainen-Julkunen K. A salutogenic program to enhance sense of coherence and quality of life for older people in the community: a feasibility randomized controlled trial and process evaluation. Patient Educ Counsel. 2016;99(1):108–16. https://doi.org/10.1016/j.pec.2015.08.003.

48. Ericson H, Skoog T, Johansson M, Wahlin-Larsson B. Resistance training is linked to heightened posi-

tive motivational state and lower negative affect among healthy women aged 65-70. J Women Aging. 2018;30(5):366–81. https://doi.org/10.1080/0895284 1.2017.1301720.

49. Kekalainen T, Kokko K, Sipila S, Walker S. Effects of a 9-month resistance training intervention on quality of life, sense of coherence, and depressive symptoms in older adults: randomized controlled trial. Qual Life Res. 2018;27(2):455–65. https://doi.org/10.1007/s11136-017-1733-z.

50. Pakkala I, Read S, Sipila S, Portegijs E, Kallinen M, Heinonen A, et al. Effects of intensive strength-power training on sense of coherence among 60-85-year-old people with hip fracture: a randomized controlled trial. Aging Clin Exp Res. 2012;24(3):295–9. https://doi.org/10.1007/BF03325261.

51. Murayama Y, Ohba H, Yasunaga M, Nonaka K, Takeuchi R, Nishi M, et al. The effect of intergenerational programs on the mental health of elderly adults. Aging Ment Health. 2015;19(4):306–14. https://doi.org/10.1080/13607863.2014.933309.

52. Tan KK, Chan SWC, Vehviläinen-Julkunen K. Self-care program for older community-dwellers: protocol for a randomized controlled trial. Cent Eur J Nurs Midwifery. 2014;5(4):145–55. https://doi.org/10.15452/cejnm.2014.05.0010.

53. Langeland E, Riise T, Hanestad BR, Nortvedt MW, Kristoffersen K, Wahl AK. The effect of salutogenic treatment principles on coping with mental health problems a randomised controlled trial. Patient Educ Couns. 2006;62(2):212–9. https://doi.org/10.1016/j.pec.2005.07.004.

54. Langeland E, Wahl AK, Kristoffersen K, Hanestad BR. Promoting coping: salutogenesis among people with mental health problems. Issues Ment Health Nurs. 2007;28(3):275–95. https://doi.org/10.1080/01612840601172627.

55. United Nations. World population aging 2017-highlights. New York: United Nations, Department of Economic and Social Affairs; 2017. Contract No.: ST/ESA/SER.A/397.

56. Chan A, Yap MT. Baby-boomers survey Singapore: National University of Singapore. 2009. www.nas.gov.sg/archivesonline/data/pdfdoc/.../baby_boomer_survey_7jan09.pdf. Accessed 16 Feb 2019.

57. Soon GY, Tan KK, Wang W, Lopez V. Back to the beginning: perceptions of older Singaporean couples living alone. Nurs Health Sci. 2015;17(3):402–7. https://doi.org/10.1111/nhs.12203.

58. Thang LL. Living independently, living well: seniors living in housing and development Board Studio Apartments in Singapore. Senri Ethnol Stud. 2014;87:59–78.

59. Wong YS, Verbrugge LM. Living alone: elderly Chinese Singaporeans. J Cross Cult Gerontol. 2009;24(3):209–24. https://doi.org/10.1007/s10823-008-9081-7.

60. Ministry of Social and Family Development. Families and households in Singapore, 2000-2017. Singapore: Ministry of Social and Family Development, Strategic Planning, Research and Development Division; 2019.

61. Ministry of Health. In: Health Mo, editor. I feel young in my Singapore: action plan for successful ageing. Singapore: Ministry of Health; 2016.

62. Singapore Department of Statistics. Population trends, 2018. Singapore: Ministry of Trade & Industry; 2018.

63. Schneider JK, Cook JH Jr. Planning psychoeducational groups for older adults. J Gerontol Nurs. 2005;31(8):33–8. https://doi.org/10.3928/0098-9134-20050801-12.

64. Moore SL, Metcalf B, Schow E. The quest for meaning in aging. Geriatr Nurs. 2006;27(5):293–9. https://doi.org/10.1016/j.gerinurse.2006.08.012.

65. Haber D. Life review: implementation, theory, research, and therapy. Int J Aging Hum Dev. 2006;63(2):153–71. https://doi.org/10.2190/da9g-rhk5-n9jp-t6cc.

66. Reker G, Wong P. Personal meaning in life and psychosocial adaptation in the later years. In: Wong P, editor. The human quest for meaning: theories, research and applications. 2nd ed. New York: Routledge; 2012. p. 433–56.

67. McAdams D. Meaning and personality. In: Wong P, editor. The human quest for meaning: theories, research and applications. 2nd ed. New York: Routledge; 2012. p. 107–23.

68. Hupkens S, Machielse A, Goumans M, Derkx P. Meaning in life of older persons: an integrative literature review. Nurs Ethics. 2016;25(8):973–91. https://doi.org/10.1177/0969733016680122.

69. Idan O, Eriksson M, Al-Yagon M. The salutogenic model: the role of generalized resistance resources. In: tThe handbook of Salutogenesis [Internet]. Cham: Springer; 2016. https://www.ncbi.nlm.nih.gov/books/NBK435841/. Accessed 2 Feb 2020.

70. Hirst SP, Lane A, Stares R. Health promotion with older adults experiencing mental health challenges: a literature review of strength-based approaches. Clin Gerontol. 2013;36(4):329–55. https://doi.org/10.1080/07317115.2013.788118.

71. Saleebey D. Introduction: power in the people. In: Saleebey D, editor. The strengths perspective in social work practice. 5th ed. New York: Pearson; 2009. p. 1–23.

72. Cooperrider DL, Whitney D, Stravros JM. Appreciative inquiry handbook: for leaders of change. 2nd ed. Brunswick: Crown Custom Publishing; 2008.

73. Gottlieb LN, Gottlieb B. Strengths-based nursing: a process for implementing a philosophy into practice. J Fam Nurs. 2017;23(3):319–40. https://doi.org/10.1177/1074840717717731.

74. Ratner H, George E, Iveson C. Solution focused brief therapy. London: Routledge; 2012.

75. Iveson C, George E, Ratner H. Scales. In: Brief coaching: a solution focused approach. London: Routledge; 2012. p. 79–98.

76. Leplege A, Gzil F, Cammelli M, Lefeve C, Pachoud B, Ville I. Person-centredness: concep-

tual and historical perspectives. Disabil Rehabil. 2007;29(20–21):1555–65. https://doi.org/10.1080/09638280701618661.

77. McCormack B, Dulmen AM, Eide H, Skovdahl K, Eide T. Person-centredness in healthcare policy, practice and research. In: Person-centred healthcare research. Hoboken: Wiley; 2017. p. 3–17.

78. Rogers CR. On becoming a person: a therapist's view of psychotherapy. Boston: Houghton Mifflin; 1961.

79. Hakansson Eklund J, Holmstrom IK, Kumlin T, Kaminsky E, Skoglund K, Hoglander J, et al. "Same same or different?" A review of reviews of person-centered and patient-centered care. Patient Educ Couns. 2019;102(1):3–11. https://doi.org/10.1016/j.pec.2018.08.029.

80. McCormack B. A conceptual framework for person-centred practice with older people. Int J Nurs Pract. 2003;9(3):202–9. https://doi.org/10.1046/j.1440-172X.2003.00423.x.

81. Thorarinsdottir K, Kristjansson K. Patients' perspectives on person-centred participation in healthcare: a framework analysis. Nurs Ethics. 2014;21(2):129–47. https://doi.org/10.1177/0969733013490593.

82. Wilberforce M, Challis D, Davies L, Kelly MP, Roberts C, Clarkson P. Person-centredness in the community care of older people: a literature-based concept synthesis. Int J Soc Welf. 2017;26(1):86–98. https://doi.org/10.1111/ijsw.12221.

83. Payne M. Chapter two: ideas informing narrative therapy. In: Narrative therapy: an introduction for coun-sellors [Internet]. London: SAGE; 2006. p. 18–36. http://sk.sagepub.com/books/narrative-therapy-2e.

84. Eriksson M, Lindström B. Bringing it all together: the salutogenic response to some of the most pertinent public health dilemmas. In: Morgan A, Davies M, Ziglio E, editors. Health assets in a global context: theory, methods, action. New York: Springer; 2010. p. 339–51.

85. Morgan A, Ziglio E. Revitalising the evidence base for public health: an assets model. Promot Educ. 2007;14(2_Suppl):17–22. https://doi.org/10.1177/10253823070140020701x.

86. Whiting L, Kendall S, Wills W. An asset-based approach: an alternative health promotion strategy? Community Pract. 2012;85(1):25–8.

87. Miller VJ, Fields NL, Adorno G, Smith-Osborne A. Using the eco-map and ecosystems perspective to guide skilled nursing facility discharge planning. J Gerontol Soc Work. 2017;60(6–7):504–18. https://doi.org/10.1080/01634372.2017.1324548.

88. Li Z, Liu T, Han J, Li T, Zhu Q, Wang A. Confrontation as a mediator between sense of coherence and self-management behaviors among elderly patients with coronary heart disease in North China. Asian Nurs Res. 2017;11(3):201–6. https://doi.org/10.1016/j.anr.2017.08.003.

89. Stevens-Ratchford RG. Occupational engagement: motivation for older adult participation. Top Geriatr Rehabil. 2005;21(3):171–81.

Health Promotion in the Community Via an Intergenerational Platform: Intergenerational e-Health Literacy Program (I-HeLP)

24

Vivien Xi WU

Abstract

The increase in life expectancy and emphasis on self-reliance for older adults are global phenomena. As such, living healthily in the community is considered a viable means of promoting successful and active aging. Existing knowledge indicates the prevalence of health illiteracy among the older population and the impact of poor health literacy on health outcomes and health care costs. Nevertheless, e-health literacy is a critical issue for a rapidly aging population in a technology-driven society. Intergenerational studies reported that older adults enjoy engaging with younger people and benefit from the social stimulation by improved social behaviours, intergenerational social network, and participation.

An *Intergenerational e-health Literacy Program* (I-HeLP) is developed to draw upon the IT-savvy strength of the youth, and teach older adults to seek, understand and appraise health information from electronic sources and apply knowledge gained to address the health problem. I-HeLP is an evidence-based program, which provides comprehensive coverage on relevant health-related e-resources.

I-HeLP aims to engage youth volunteers to teach older adults regarding e-health literacy, and enhance older adults' sense of coherence, e-health literacy, physical and mental health, cognitive function, quality of life, and intergenerational communication. I-HeLP promotes social participation, health, and wellbeing of older adults, and empowers the younger generation to play an active role in society. Furthermore, I-HeLP aligns with the 'Smart Nation' initiative by the Singapore government to empower citizens to lead meaningful and fulfilled lives with the use of technology.

Keywords

Attitude towards the older generation
Community-dwelling older adults · e-Health literacy · Empathy · Empower younger generation · Health promotion in the community · Intergenerational communication
Reliable health-related e-resources
Salutogenesis · Youth volunteer

24.1 Introduction

Improved living conditions, medical technology, and health services increase the life expectancy of people. The United Nations [1] reported that

V. X. WU (✉)
Alice Lee Centre for Nursing Studies, Yong Loo Lin School of Medicine, National University of Singapore, Singapore, Singapore
e-mail: nurwux@nus.edu.sg

© The Author(s) 2021
G. Haugan, M. Eriksson (eds.), *Health Promotion in Health Care – Vital Theories and Research*,
https://doi.org/10.1007/978-3-030-63135-2_24

only 8% of the world's population were aged 60 and above in 1950; it increased to 12% by 2013, and is expected to rise to 21% by 2050. The global increase in life expectancy has made aging a political and economic issue as increased longevity raises social concerns about rising health care costs. Community-dwelling older adults are defined by those aged 60 years and above and living independently in a community [2]. Some older adults may live healthily in a community, but others may suffer from a large variety of health care problems, ranging from just getting older to specific medical conditions such as stroke, diabetes, osteoarthritis, or dementia.

World Health Organisation's active aging framework encourages the public and practitioners to 'support and value the process of optimising opportunities to maintain and enhance physical, mental, and social health as well as independence and quality of life over the life course' [3]. In this emerging paradigm, there is increasing pressure on older adults to keep themselves active and independent—physically, mentally and socially—in their communities, and cope with chronic health conditions and other challenges in late life [4]. The increase in life expectancy and emphasis on self-reliance for older adults are global phenomena. As such, living healthily in the community is considered a viable means of promoting successful and active aging.

24.2 Background and Literature Review

24.2.1 Benefits of Intergenerational Interaction

Intergenerational studies reported that older adults enjoy engaging with younger people, and that they benefit from the social stimulation [5]. Research indicates that older adults often participate in lifelong learning programs based on their interest and interaction with others [6]. These are often similar motivations for older adults who choose to engage in intergenerational learning projects [7]. Emerging evidence shows that intergenerational programs are significantly associated with subjective wellbeing in terms of

boosting the quality of life, health status and life satisfaction [8]. Jenkins' study [8] shows that participation in these programs brings intrinsic enjoyment and provides opportunities to get out and socialise. The results of the intergenerational study indicate improved social behaviours, intergenerational social network scores and intragenerational social support, and increased social participation [9].

24.2.2 E-Health Literacy

Health literacy is the degree to which individuals have the capacity to obtain, process, and understand basic health information and services needed to make appropriate health decisions [10]. Building on this definition, the concept of e-health is being promoted intensively with the wide use of information technology. E-health literacy is the ability to seek, find, understand and appraise health information from electronic sources and apply the knowledge to address a health problem [11]. Existing knowledge indicates the prevalence of health illiteracy among the older population and the impact of poor health literacy on health outcomes and health care costs. Nevertheless, e-health literacy is a critical issue for a rapidly aging population in a technology-driven society. Literatures illustrate that intergenerational programs could contribute to the wellbeing of older adults holistically [9]. Herein, we describe an intergenerational e-health literacy program developed to draw upon the IT-savvy strength of youth teaching older adults to enhance their abilities to seek and appraise electronic health information.

24.2.3 Empathy and Attitudes Towards Older Adults

Empathy is the ability to identify and share emotions of others, and feel concerns when others are in distress [12]. Regardless of age, empathy is one of the key factors that affects one's social interaction and communication with other people [13, 14]. Rapid growth of aging population changes socio-structural dynamics [15]. Enlarged aging population might increase intergenerational prejudice and tension between younger and older generation [15]. Negative stereotypes towards older adults do exist, including the portraying of older adults as being lack of independence, less contributing, more fragile and forgetful [16]. Gradually, the older adults tend to accept the stereotypes and may develop low self-esteem [16]. During the process of self-stereotyping, older adults may experience failing memory, decreasing cognition, frailty, and even cardiovascular symptoms as a result of feeling stressed [17].

As a reflection, the younger generation may develop negative attitudes towards older adults due to the stereotypes, even despite having initially had positive attitudes towards the older generation [18]. Studies reported both younger and older generation could experience negative feelings during intergenerational communications and interactions [19, 20]. However, with more contact with older adults, youth has been shown to develop more empathy and positive attitudes towards older adults [21]. Hence, intergenerational programs could also reshape the attitude and perception of the younger people towards older generation.

24.3 Conceptual Framework

The salutogenesis health model focuses on promoting individuals' health rather than the traditional risk and prevention focus which are central in the pathogenesis paradigm [22]. The salutogenic approach leads to a profound understanding through reflection on life situations and review of available resources and active adaptation to a stress-rich environment [23]. The key concepts in salutogenesis consists of Generalized Resistant Resources (GRRs) and Sense of Coherence (SOC). GRRs are protective factors, such as knowledge and social support. The individual could better cope with life stressors with enhanced GRRs [24]. By interacting with youth volunteers during e-health literacy program, community-dwelling older adults can improve their mental and cognitive wellbeing, as well as their intergenerational communication. The e-health literacy program creates opportunities for older adults to have more social contact

and make commitments [25, 26]. It promotes the sense of belonging and social inclusion for older adults, which could lead to a greater sense of life's meaningfulness [27].

SOC is a dispositional orientation of life described as perceived as comprehensive, manageable and meaningful, influencing how people think and behave by utilising the resources they have [24]. SOC comprises three core components: comprehensibility, manageability and meaningfulness. An individual with well-developed SOC is able to enhance his/her health by reducing the exposure to emotional and physiological stressors. SOC could be developed over time through empowering people with knowledge, experience, and perceived meaning-in-life, and utilising appropriate resources to minimise negative impacts on health [23]. The e-health literacy program provides a platform for older adults to access to GRRs, which is positively related to SOC, health condition and quality of life [26]. SOC plays an important role in the mental health and quality of life of older adults.

An *Intergenerational e-health Literacy Program* (I-HeLP) will be developed and evaluated. I-HeLP aims to promote intergenerational interaction between older adults and youth volunteers who teach them e-health. I-HeLP is an innovative program as it is guided by the salutogenic framework and integrates the concept of e-health literacy and intergenerational interaction which promotes social participation, health and wellbeing of older adults, and empowers the younger generation to play an active role in the society. Furthermore, I-HeLP aligns with the 'Smart Nation' initiative by the Singapore government to empower citizens to lead meaningful and fulfilled lives with the use of technology [44]. The notion of 'Smart Nation' opens up new possibilities to enhance the way we live, work and interact, and supports better living and stronger communities. Health and enabled aging are identified as one of the key domains, and government has put in place the infrastructure, policies, and enablers to encourage innovation [44].

In summary, salutogenesis promotes health in the community. Besides benefiting for the older adults, I-HeLP provides a platform for the youth to work with older adults and empowers

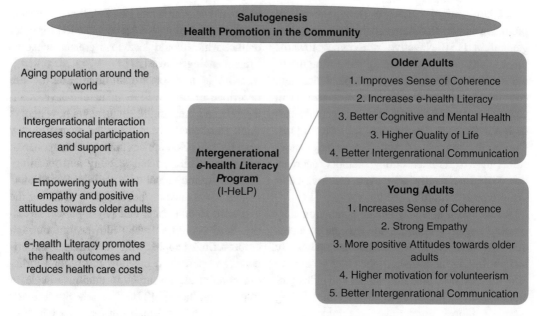

Fig. 24.1 Conceptual framework—salutogenesis

the youth with empathy and positive attitudes towards older adults. In a long run, the e-health literacy program promotes health outcomes and reduces health care costs. The impact of I-HeLP is twofold: (1) for older adults— improves sense of coherence, cognitive and mental health, increase e-health literacy, quality of life, and intergenerational communication; (2) for young adults—improves sense of coherence, more positive attitudes towards older adults, increase empathy, motivation for volunteerism, and intergenerational communication (Fig. 24.1).

24.4 Formative Design of the Intervention: I-HeLP

This intervention is designed through a three-phase iterative, client-centred participatory action research process [28]. First, a front-end analysis is conducted via focus groups and literature search to identify the unique health care needs of older adults and to formulate initial design ideas. Second, a preliminary design of the intervention is developed from literatures and focus group results. Finally, revisions and refinements are iteratively

incorporated based on client-centred feedback which has been collected during usability sessions.

24.4.1 Phase 1: Front-End Analysis

A comprehensive search and evaluation of the existing e-health literacy interventions are carried out. The evaluation from the evidence-based literatures provides the fundamental understanding of current interventions. The research team conducts focus groups with older adults to explore their needs with regards to e-health. As an initial step, the research team in the university and the management team of Senior Activity Centres (SAC) had regular meetings and discussed the preliminary contents of I-HeLP and the methods of delivery.

24.4.2 Phase 2: Design and Development

The evaluation of literatures and focus groups findings in Phase 1 are centred on developing the contents of I-HeLP. Information gleaned from focus groups with older adults, and team design meetings are applied for the development of I-HeLP. Based on client-centred design suggestions, the following principles guide the development of I-HeLP: (1) the intervention must be designed for older adults; (2) content must be related to the specific e-health deficits that were identified during focus group and literature evaluations; (3) the content needs to be delivered in a brief and bite-size format to fit the attention span and cognitive capabilities of the older adults. A Content Expert Committee is formed which consists of two SAC managers who specialise in elder care, two researchers and one Advance Practice Nurse who specialises in Geriatrics. The Content Expert Committee reviewed the contents of I-HeLP and provided comments and feedback. The research team revised the contents based on the feedback.

24.4.2.1 Pedagogical Considerations

Pedagogical decisions are driven by unique needs revealed in Phase 1 focus groups. The intervention is designed to provide a platform for older adults to seek, find, understand and appraise health information from electronic sources and apply the knowledge to address their health problem. It is imperative to include instruction that promotes self-efficacy and motivation for the older adults. Interactive game sessions are used as a platform for hands-on practice to help the older adults to revise the contents. These features of I-HeLP meet the need of older adults and engage content that are not overly didactic in nature. In addition, the concepts of universal design for learning are applied to cater to the needs of the older adults. Not only is information presented in multiple formats and mediums (e.g. video, interactive content, imagery, and games), participants are also able to use various outlets of expression and/or action throughout the intervention.

24.4.3 Phase 3: Formative, User-Centred Evaluation

Formative evaluation takes the form of multi-modal usability testing [29, 30] which seeks to elicit feedback on applicability, content, ease-of-use, acceptance, and time to completion of modules. We collect feedback on the usage of information

from the participants during the development of the intervention and during usability testing, which subsequently are used to further extend and refine the intervention [31]. The formative evaluation generates inputs regarding revisions and modifications that inform the design and development of I-HeLP.

24.5 Outline of Intergenerational e-Health Literacy Program

I-HeLP is developed to promote older adults' intellectual activities and engagement with youth regularly and cyclically through weekly learning and interacting session. The contents of the program are developed based on literature reviews [32, 33]. The outline of I-HeLP is illustrated in Table 24.1.

Table 24.1 Outline of the intergenerational e-health literacy program (I-HeLP)

Session	Types of activity/ duration	Expected learning outcomes
1	• Computer and Internet basics • Access health information websites • Practice	• Master the basic knowledge of operating a computer and accessing the Internet • Use the internet to search for health-related information on the recommended websites, e.g. Ministry of Health, Health Promotion Board, and the various hospitals • Navigate those recommended health-relevant websites • Search for a health-related topic • Find answers to health-related questions
2	• Browse through health information websites FAQs, Videos Quizzes • How to use Health-related Apps on mobile devices • Practice	Learn how to: • Use the Frequently Asked Questions, • Search for the videos and view the appropriate video • Download and use of Health-related Apps • Use the quizzes and practice the questions

(continued)

Table 24.1 (continued)

Session	Types of activity/ duration	Expected learning outcomes
3	• Browse through Ministry of Health, and Health Promotion Board, Health Hub, Singapore websites • Practice	Learn how to: • Find information about doctors, hospitals and clinics • Search for health care cost • Search for health care schemes and subsidies • Search for healthy choices food • Search for physical activities program • Use the various health screening program
4	• Evaluating the reliability of the health information websites • Practice	Learn to recognise • Reliable health information websites • Purpose of a health information website • Reviewers of a health information website • Most recent update of health information • Clues about the accuracy of health information website • Contacts for a health information website

24.5.1 Implementation Plan

I-HeLP is delivered over a period of 4 weeks. The program consists of preparation of the youth volunteers and implementation of the *I*ntergenerational *e-h*ealth *L*iteracy *P*rogram.

24.5.1.1 Part 1: Preparation of the Youth Volunteers

The workshop aims to equip the youth volunteers with knowledge and skills to function as trainers to conduct teaching for older adults. Subsequently, the youth volunteers can carry out hands-on practical sessions to guide the older adults to access and browse through the relevant health-related websites. The intensive workshop for the youth volunteers focuses on relevant health-related websites, communication skills to promote effective intergenerational

interactions with older adults, basic knowledge of older adults' usual life, and rules and regulations as a volunteer. Two Junior College students have joined the research team as interns and they have brought in a significant perspective in the development of the contents for the youth volunteer training workshop, since they are of the same age group as the youth volunteers.

24.5.1.2 Part 2: Intergenerational e-health Literacy Program

I-HeLP is carried out for the subsequent 4 weeks, one session (2 h) per week, whereby the youth volunteers will visit SAC in groups of 5–6. During the sessions, they will teach and guide the older adults to access, understand and appraise health information from reliable health-related websites.

Mode of Delivery

Face-to-face workshops are conducted for the older adults during the training program at the SAC. The youth volunteers would conduct a short teaching on the specific topic for each session, which is followed by individual guidance and practice with the older adults. Interactive games are utilised throughout the session to keep the older adults engaged. The workshop applies small group teaching technique to meet the learning needs of the older adults. Each session engages 8–10 older adults and 5–6 youth volunteers (with the ratio of 1 volunteer to 2 older adults, providing close guidance). During the face-to-face sessions, the older adults could interact with their peers, the youth, and provide inputs about the program with the researchers.

24.5.2 Plan for Program Evaluation

Self-reported survey questionnaires will be used for the program evaluation. Outcome measures are used before and after the program to evaluate the effects of the I-HeLP. The outcome measures for older adults will include sense of coherence [34], e-health literacy [35], physical health, mental health (depression, anxiety) [36, 37], cognitive function [36], quality of life [38], and intergenerational communication [39]. Outcome measures for youth volunteers will include sense of coherence [34], empathy [40], attitudes towards older people [41], volunteerism [42], and intergenerational communication [43]. I-HeLP is planned to be conducted in the last quarter of 2020. Currently, the team is working on the development and refinement of the program. Data will be collected before and after the I-HeLP, and results of the research will be reported and published later.

24.6 Conclusion

I-HeLP aims to contribute to building capabilities in population health research and foster collaboration with the goal of translating evidence into action, offer important insights into the need for more intergenerational volunteer programs not only to promote social participation, health and wellbeing of older adults, but also to empower younger generation to play an active role in the society. The evaluation of I-HeLP will assist in understanding the effectiveness of such program in enhancing older adults' sense of coherence, e-health literacy, physical, mental health, cognitive function, quality of life, and intergenerational communication. I-HeLP may potentially be extended to a larger-scale in the community-living environment.

Take Home Messages
- I-HeLP aligns with the 'Smart Nation' initiative by the Singapore government [44] to empower people to lead meaningful and fulfilled lives with the use of technology.
- I-HeLP aims to use technology to support the 'Smart Nation' initiative [44] to promote healthy and active aging and enhance the wellbeing of the older adults.

- I-HeLP develops partnerships among researchers, schools, communities, and health care organisations, which is critical to the successful adoption and implementation of health promotion programs.
- The partnership with SACs and schools represents an unprecedented opportunity to inform practice and policy at school, community and at national levels to promote healthy and active lifestyles among older adults, and thereby contribute to health and wellbeing of the elderly population in Singapore.

References

1. United Nations. Global issues: aging United Nations. 2017. http://www.un.org/en/sections/issues-depth/ageing/.
2. Steultjens EMJ, Dekker J, Bouter LM, Jellema S, Bakker EB, Ende CHMVD. Occupational therapy for community dwelling elderly people: a systematic review. Age Ageing. 2004;33:453–60.
3. Butler-Jones D. The chief public health officer's report on the state of public health in Canada, 2010: growing older-adding life to years; 2010.
4. Narushima M, Liu J, Diestelkamp N. The association between lifelong learning and psychological wellbeing among older adults: implications for interdisciplinary health promotion in an aging society. Act Adapt Aging. 2013;37(3):239–50.
5. Dauenhauer J, Steitz DW, Cochran LJ. Fostering a new model of multigenerational learning: older adult perspectives, community partners, and higher education. Educ Gerontol. 2016;42(7):483–96.
6. Brady EM, Cardale A, Neidy JC. The quest for community in Osher Lifelong Learning Institutes. Educ Gerontol. 2013;39(9):627–39.
7. Underwood HL, Dorfman LT. View from the other side. J Intergener Relationsh. 2006;4(2):43–60.
8. Jenkins A. Participation in learning and wellbeing among older adults. Int J Lifelong Educ. 2011;30(3):403–20.
9. Fujiwara Y, Sakuma N, Ohba H, Nishi M, Lee S, Watanabe N, et al. Reprints: effects of an intergenerational health promotion program for older adults in Japan. J Intergener Relationsh. 2009;7(1):17–39.
10. Services USDoHaH, editor. Healthy people 2010: understanding and improving health. Washington, DC: U.S. Department of Health and Human Services; 2000.

11. Norman CD, Skinner HA. Eheals: the ehealth literacy scale. J Med Internet Res. 2006;8(4):e27.

12. Gould ON, Gautreau SM. Empathy and conversational enjoyment in younger and older adults. Exp Aging Res. 2014;40:60–80.

13. Bailey PE, Henry JD, Von Hippel W. Empathy and social functioning in late adulthood. Aging Ment Health. 2008;12:499–503.

14. Beedle J, Brown V, Keady B, Tranel D, Paradiso S. Trait empathy as a predictor of individual differences in perceived loneliness. Psychol Rep. 2012;110:3–15.

15. North MS, Fiske ST. An inconvenienced youth? Ageism and its potential intergenerational roots. Psychol Bull. 2012;138(5):982–97.

16. Nelson TD. Ageism: prejudice against our feared future self. J Soc Issues. 2005;61(2):207–21.

17. Levy BR, Leifheit-Limson E. The stereotype-matching effect: greater influence on functioning when age stereotypes correspond to outcomes. Psychol Aging. 2009;24(1):230–3.

18. Cesario J, Plaks JE, Higgins ET. Automatic social behavior as motivated preparation to interact. J Pers Soc Psychol. 2006;90:893–910.

19. Williams A, Giles H. Intergenearaional conversations: young adults' retrospective accounts. Hum Commun Res. 1996;23:220–50.

20. Williams A, Garrett P. Communication evaluations across the life span: from adolescent storm and stress to elder aches and pains. J Lang Soc Psychol. 2002;21:101–26.

21. Schwalbach E, Kiernan S. Effects of an intergenerational friendly visit program on the attitudes of fourth graders towards elders. Educ Gerontol. 2002;28(3):175–87.

22. Antonovsky A. Health, stress and coping: new perspectives on mental and physical Well-being. San Francisco: Jossey-Bass; 1979.

23. Tan KK, Vehvilainen-Julkunen K, Chan WCS. Integrative review: salutogenesis and health in older people over 65 years old. J Adv Nurs. 2014;70:497–510.

24. Lindstrom B, Eriksson M. Contextualizing salutogenesis and Antonovsky in public health development. Health Promot Int. 2006;21(3):238–44.

25. Idan O, Eriksson M, Al-Yogon M. The salutogenic model: the role of generalized resistance resources. In: Mittelmark MB, Sagy S, Eriksson M, Bauer GF, Pelikan JM, Lindström B, et al., editors. The handbook of salutogenesis. Cham: Springer; 2017.

26. Koelen M, Erikkson M, Cattan M. Older people, sense of coherence and community. In: Mittelmark MB, Sagy S, Eriksson M, Bauer GF, Pelikan JM, Lindström B, et al., editors. The handbook of salutogenesis. Cham: Springer; 2016.

27. Murayama Y, Ohba H, Yasunaga M, Nonaka K, Takeuchi R, Nishi M, et al. The effect of intergenerational programs on the mental health of elderly adults. Aging Ment Health. 2015;19(4):306–14.

28. Branch RM, Kopcha TJ. Instructional design models. In: Spector JM, Merrill MD, Elen J, Bishop MJ, editors. Handbook of research on educational communications and technology. New York: Springer; 2014. p. 77–87.

29. Krug S. Rocket surgery made easy: the do-it yourself guide to finding and fixing usability problems. New Riders: Canada; 2010.

30. Nielsen J. Usability engineering. Boston: Academic Press; 1994.

31. Dick W, Carey L. The systematic design of instruction. 3rd ed. Harper-Collins: New York; 1990.

32. Tse MM, Choi KC, Leung RS. E-health for older people: the use of technology in health promotion. Cyberpsychol Behav. 2008;11(4):63–71.

33. Xie B. Improving older adults' e-health literacy through computer training using NIH online resources. Libr Inf Sci Res. 2012;34(1):63–71.

34. Eriksson M, Lindstrom B. Validity of Antonovsky's sense of coherence scale: a systematic review. J Epidemiol Community Health. 2005;59(6): 460–6.

35. Chung SY, Nahm ES. Testing reliability and validity of the eHealth Literacy Scale (eHEALS) for older adults recruited online. Comput Inf Nurs. 2015; 33(4):150.

36. Brown LM, Schinka JA. Development and initial validation of a 15-item informant version of the geriatric depression scale. Int J Geriatr Psychiatry. 2005;20(10):911–8.

37. Pachana NA, Byrne GJ, Siddle H, Koloski N, Harley E, Arnold E. Development and validation of the geriatric anxiety inventory. Int Psychogeriatr. 2007;16:103–14.

38. Power M, Quinn K, Schmidt S. World Health Organization quality of life -OLD group. Development of the WHOQOL-old module. Qual Life Res. 2005;14:2197–214.

39. Keaton SA, McCann RM, Giles H. The role of communication perceptions in the mental health of older adults: views from Thailand and the United States. Health Commun. 2017;32(1):92–102.

40. Spreng RN, Mckinnon MC, Mar RA, Levine B. The Toronto Empathy Questionnaire: scale development and initial validation of a factor-analytic solu-

tion to multiple empathy measures. J Pers Assess. 2009;91(1):62–71.

41. Kogan N. Attitudes toward older people: the development of a scale and an examination of correlates. J Abnorm Soc Psychol. 1961;2(1):44–54.

42. Clary EG, Snyder M, Ridge RD, Copeland J, Stukas AA, Haugen J, et al. Understanding and assessing the motivations of volunteers: a functional approach. J Pers Soc Psychol. 1998;74:1516–30.

43. McCann RM. Intra- and intergenerational communication in the workplace: perspectives from Thailand and the United States of America; 2003.

44. Singapore SN. 2017. https://www.smartnation.sg/about-smart-nation.

Coping and Health Promotion in Persons with Dementia

25

Anne-S. Helvik

Abstract

For those who receive the diagnosis of dementia, their daily life is turned upside down. Dementia represents daily challenges in many aspects, cognitively, socially, emotionally and functionally. Most commonly, the dementia disorder is progressive, and currently there is no cure or treatment to stop it. Emphasizing coping and health-promotion among individuals having dementia is fundamental to obtain wellbeing as well as finding meaning-in-life. This chapter focuses on coping strategies among persons with dementia, how these are related to health-promotion, wellbeing and meaning-in-life and how nurses and health professionals can promote health and wellbeing in persons with dementia.

Keywords

Activity · Balancing life · Close family · Cognitive resources · Cognitive impairment · Dementia disorder · Dementia friendly environment · Next of kin · Participation · Sense of humour

A.-S. Helvik (✉)
Department of Public Health and Nursing, NTNU Norwegian University of Science and Technology, Trondheim, Norway

Norwegian National Advisory Unit on Ageing and Health, Vestfold Hospital Trust, Tønsberg, Norway
e-mail: anne-sofie.helvik@ntnu.no

25.1 Introduction

Dementia is caused by various brain disorders, among which Alzheimer's disease is the most frequent [1, 2]. Dementia is common in aged populations (≥65 years) [3–5], but does also occur before the age of 65 years (early onset dementia) [2]. The prevalence of dementia globally, is reported to 46.8 million [1, 6]. Furthermore, due to the aging population worldwide, the number of people living with dementia is estimated to nearly double every 20 years [7, 8]. In most cases, dementia is progressive and characterized by cognitive impairment, changes in behaviour and/or social function and impaired activities of daily living (ADL) [9].

During progression of the functional declines, need for help from others are necessary [10]. In order to promote meaning-in-life, wellbeing and health, professional health care is essential. In the early phase, there may be a need of information and support to maintain activities of daily living, social relationships, as well as to support the individual's coping with their situation. With further functional decline, informal carers and/or formal care providers naturally must extend the scope of care and support. The health-promoting actions will aim towards compensating for loss of functioning and facilitating for change to maintain meaningful aspects in life. In the late, severe stage of dementia, the person will be fully dependent on others and will eventually die [11,

G. Haugan, M. Eriksson (eds.), *Health Promotion in Health Care – Vital Theories and Research*,
https://doi.org/10.1007/978-3-030-63135-2_25

12]. Independent of phase of dementia development, treatment and care must be provided in accordance to people with dementia's own needs and fundamental human rights and resources. In all phases of the disorder, knowledge about how people with dementia experience and cope with their current and future life situation is important for health professionals to contribute to wellbeing and meaning-in-life. There must be a shift from solely focusing on the symptoms, disabilities and restrictions related to dementia, towards capabilities and potential of persons having dementia. Despite having dementia, the individuals have resources which are fundamental to their wellbeing and health. A health-promoting perspective and approach to care is crucial and essential to fulfil these requirements.

Health-promotion utilizes a biographical approach; viewing the individual as a whole person, embedded in his or her gender, culture, identity and society [13]. Moreover, health-promotion theory focuses on resources and capabilities in and around the person. How you cope with life stressors and challenges is affected by the available internal and external resources. Personal coping resources may facilitate and contribute to resist stress and promote health [14]. In the salutogenic health model, these personal coping characteristics are termed general resistant resources (GRR) and sense of coherence (SOC) [14]. SOC is a general expression of an individual's ability to comprehend the whole situation and the capacity to use the resources available to move in a health-promoting direction [15]. SOC reflects the extent to which a person finds life to be meaningful (a motivational and emotional disposition), manageable (readiness to control and influence) and comprehensible (a cognitive disposition) [14, 15]. The way people are able to perceive structures, create coherence and manage change in a meaningful manner has a central impact on health [16].

25.2 Methods

This chapter builds on a previously published systematic meta-synthesis of studies on coping among persons with dementia [17]. This meta-synthesis was based on international published qualitative studies referring to the person with dementia's own experiences regarding coping. In total, 74 articles were found by use of a systematic and computerized search of qualitative internationally published articles between 2004 and 2019 in AgeLine, CHINDAL Complete, Embase, Medline and PsycINFO motors. The 74 articles were included based on a quality assessment by means of the CASP criteria; studies evaluated to moderate and high quality were included. The search terms are reported in the meta-synthesis [17].

25.3 Coping with Life When Having Dementia

Coping is how people face and handle challenging experiences and situations. In health-promoting theory, coping is interconnected with salutogenic processes and wellbeing [18]. Successful coping is health-promoting and may contribute to an experience of hope, meaning-in-life and a sense of coherence [14, 18]. Knowledge about how persons with dementia cope with their challenges due to their diagnosis and life changes will assist nurses, other health professionals and informal care takers to support and empower the person with dementia as well as to create health-promoting surroundings.

Only two qualitative studies have explicitly aimed to explore coping strategies in persons with dementia [19, 20]. However, several qualitative studies aiming to explore other phenomena than coping describe coping actions persons living with dementia use as well as how coping actions and strategies affect their life. This chapter focuses on vital coping strategies in the face of challenges and stress related to living with dementia [17]. Dementia may affect individuals differently; the progress of the disease as well as coping resources available will vary among the individuals. Thus, the coping strategies and actions used will also vary considerably in persons having dementia. Coping strategies are defined as cognitive and behavioural efforts to master, reduce or tolerate internal or external demands created by challenges and stress [21]. The choice of coping strategies is affected by the person's experience of internal and external resources [22]. In general, people use problem-focused strategies (strategies aiming to alter stressful situations) and emotional-focused strategies (strategies aiming to regulate emotional stress associated with the situation) and alternate between these, but in severe situations all available strategies are trigged in a global response [22].

The qualitative meta-synthesis on coping among persons with dementia [17] found several coping strategies which were grouped into four overall categories: (1) The first category of coping strategies was related to keep going and holding on to life as usual, (2) the second category was related to adapting and adjusting to the demands resulted from the disease, while (3) the third category were related to accepting the situation, followed by the (4) fourth category which was to avoid difficult situations.

25.3.1 Coping Strategies: Keep Going and Holding on to Life as Usual

This category of coping strategies among persons with dementia aims to keep going and holding on to activities, roles and relationships as usual [17]. This strategy seems most often to be used in early phases of dementia before the progression of the disease reduces the individual's abilities severly. This category of coping strategies included actions which contribute to (a) preserving the person s' identity, (b) normalization of the situation and (c) participating in the society.

25.3.1.1 Preserving Identity
The first set of coping actions supporting the individuals with dementia to keep going aims to *preserve their identity*. It refers to holding on to the identity that defines them as a person [17]. For example, they remind themselves and others by telling stories from their past life [23, 24]; this includes recalling known characteristics and strengths of one's personality [23, 25], past achievements [26], experiences from pre-

vious occupations [27] and happy memories in general [28], as well as referring to difficult times they have mastered before [29]. Drawing on past roles and status contributes to preserve identity and self-esteem. By holding on to past aspects of themselves, individuals having dementia maintain their sense of self [17]. Past roles and achievements remind them of who they are, despite their new strange situation.

In a health-promoting perspective, preserving identity and self-esteem helps to find meaning-in-life and keep going. Perceived meaning-in-life and self-esteem are important to handle challenges and thereby reduce stress; finding meaning-in-life in the midst of dementia may contribute to a renewed understanding of themselves. Thus, preserving identity is health-promoting. Knowledge about such identity-preserving actions and their health-promoting potential is fundamental for the nursing professionals using the nurse–patient interaction as a resource for preserving and strengthening these individuals' identity and self-esteem. As severity of dementia increases, talking about or recalling one's personal characteristics, past roles, previous hobbies, activities and past achievements may prove difficult. Consequently, the health professionals when caring for persons with dementia should initiate and utilize communication contributing to preserving identity and wellbeing. Pictures from previous times and written histories can be used to facilitate for such communication, which is termed "health-promoting nurse–patient interaction" (see [30], Chap. 10 in this book). It is therefore important that health personnell ask for such material and for the life story in an early phase of dementia. In cases where dementia has progressed, next of kin and close family members may contribute with such information. Such identity supporting communication could for example take place during regular care interaction.

25.3.1.2 Maintaining Normality
The second set of coping actions to keep going is *maintaining normality*. The person with dementia seeks to reduce his/her worries due to the diagnosis [17]. The above-mentioned meta-

synthesis [17] revealed that they maintained normality by keeping up with activities, roles and relationships they had before. They normalize the new situation by trying to go on as usual [31]. Individuals having dementia made extra efforts to appear in accordance with the social norms and thus avoid negative reactions and problems [32]. These coping actions preserving their previous way of living released will-power and hope for a good life in the future [33]. Moreover, memory loss was explained by high age rather than dementia, which facilitated normalization and thereby an experience of maintaining normality, decreased worries and increased wellbeing [34, 35]. Additionally, normality was maintained by using high age and loss of interest rather than dementia to explain giving up one's occupation or common activities [27] and keep going focusing on aspects of one's life which are still manageable. By keep telling oneself that the dementia and experiences related to it were of minor importance for their overall situation [23], they could keep going 'as usual'. Also, comparing themselves with others having poorer health conditions made them feel that what they lived through was not that special [35].

Normalization may be a way the person with dementia use to experience control. Normalization strategies facilitate manageability as well as comprehensibility (both SOC) and thereby wellbeing and health. It is normal to stop with activities when these are no longer of any interest. So, when you as a nurse or health professional experience that persons with dementia explain lack of interest or use age as reasons for stopping with previous interesting activities, it may be an attempt to normalize the situation. However, it may also be a natural change. Even so, it may be that the specific activity is stressful by representing challenges which they are not able to handle anymore because of their dementia. Thus, health professionals should be supportive and understand such attempts to normalize their situation, actions and priorities. Health professionals may ask if tailored ways to participate in activities etc. are of interest; that is to check if any support such as going together with them,

support driving, or provide what is needed could make the activity manageable. In other words, if someone in the society such as a volunteer or significant other could arrange or contribute, a person with dementia could find the activities still manageable and pleasant. This means that individuals with dementia may still be able to perform the activities which they like, but these activities do now include specific challenges calling for assistance. Therefore, health professionals' role could be to inform next of kin and relevant others about recent change in interest and its reasons, and eventually their possibility to facilitate for participating in activities, etc.

Coping actions directing normalization intend to maintain activities which the individuals are used to, since such continuation gives meaning and wellbeing as well as hope for the future. Meaningfulness, identifying solutions and having resources to solve challenges are essential to sense of coherence (SOC) [14, 15], which is central for health-promoting processes contributing to wellbeing. Moreover, prevailing normality may represent a general resistance resource (GRR); when the person with dementia experience to cope with challenges, this contributes to satisfaction, self-confidence and joy [36], all of which are important health-promotion processes [16]. The role of the health professionals' is to explain the positive gains by normalization to family members and others, and eventually to facilitate for participating in activities for an extended period of time.

25.3.1.3   Contribute to the Society

The third set of coping actions that persons with dementia use to keep going and holding on to life as before is aiming to *contribute to the society* in the way they can. It refers to the value of still being able to do meaningful activities and being useful [17]. However, their way of contributing to others may differ from before. Individuals having dementia search for new ways to be useful [24] and ways to use their remaining abilities to contribute in a larger context. They search for ways to contribute in the family and household [37], to be useful for others [38], doing something practical to help another person [27] and engage in voluntary work to the best for the society [27, 38, 39]. The influence of utilizing such coping strategies include a feeling of being someone to others and to oneself [27] and having purpose in life [39]. Thus, despite having dementia, being someone who contributes to the society provides a sense of meaning-in-life as well as coherence between the person with dementia, his/her surroundings and the society.

Accordingly, nurses and health professionals' health-promotion initiatives among people with dementia, especially in the early phase, should ensure that these individuals can support, contribute and feel valuable to their family, friends as well as to the society. However, such health-promotion initiatives must be based on knowledge about the individual as a person and what he/she wants. Suggestions and activities should be built upon his/her previous experiences and knowledge as well as interests and available resources. Such support can be implemented in an out-patient clinic consultation and in a home visit when planning future actions for retaining health and promoting wellbeing. Counselling of the person with dementia, the next of kin and other informal care givers should preferably incorporate information about that contributing to others and the society may represent a vital salutary resource for wellbeing. Dementia friendly families, neighbourhoods and societies represent environments where persons with dementia can contribute in the society and maintain normality. As a result, they are enabled and empowered to keep on going, holding on to activities, roles and relationships 'as usual' for an extended period, which provides wellbeing and quality of life. Furthermore, health-promoting initiatives and dementia friendly environments may facilitate for adaption and adjustment to the situation and demands.

25.3.2 Coping Strategies: Adapting and Adjusting to the Demands

Adapting and adjusting to the demands is the second category of coping strategies that was found in the meta-synthesis [17]. These strate-

gies describe how people adapt and adjust their own expectations toward themselves and activities which they can perform. The different coping actions involve being active, planning and making changes to handle the situation. This category of coping strategies includes actions aiming at (a) *Taking control and compensate* and (b) *Reframing the identity*.

25.3.2.1 Taking Control and Compensate

This first set of coping actions, *taking control and compensate*, includes what persons with dementia do to continue being active, both physically and cognitively [17]. Furthermore, coping actions directing the need of information, compensation for loss of functionality, and planning to reduce stress, are central.

Being physically and cognitively active includes doing life-long hobbies and continue with previous habits to provide enjoyment [40]. Maintaining meaningful activities were seen as helpful to cope with symptoms of dementia and contributed to an experience of control [34]. Continuing one's daily routines helped to stay in control of the situation and to preserve identity [41]. Participating in leisure activities was a part of counteracting development of disease, it helps keeping the mind active and supports a sense of meaningfulness [34]. Correspondingly, physical activity was experienced to delay deterioration [42], but also to develop social attributes and avoiding being defined only by their dementia [29]. In times of stress, relying on religion and life-values was important for a sense of control and comfort [20]. Moreover, involvement in music could give persons with dementia a sense of empowerment and control [43].

The overall coping category termed 'keep going and holding on to life' which was described firstly in this chapter, may also involve decisions to not participate in specific activities. The persons with dementia reasoned their change of participation to increased age and loss of interest rather than difficulties due to dementia [27]. This means that emotional coping strategies were used to regulate emotional stress associated with the situation rather than solving the problems or challenges caused by the situation. Persons continuing taking part in activities, also when experiencing challenges, strived to take control [17]. In this matter, problem-solving rather than emotional coping strategies seem sufficient; by taking control and compensate for loss of functionality the challenges could be handled. Participation in these specific activities was seen as meaningful [34]. Taking control over challenges imply both identifying solutions and having resources (either internal and/or external) to solve the challenges which represent two of three essential elements in SOC [14, 15]. The third aspect of SOC is finding such activities meaningful [14, 15]. A strong SOC is important for the health-promoting processes contributing to wellbeing. Thus, nurses and other health professionals should inform next of kin about the importance of persons with dementia taking control by being physically and cognitively active and facilitating for participation in such activities when indicated.

The persons with dementia adjusted to the new demands by putting extra effort into preparations and accomplishment to partake in activities [17]. They developed strategies to *compensate for the impairment* [44] in order to avoid mistakes due to memory loss. Utilizing such strategies and investing time and effort into planning and organizing to better meet difficulties and memory loss were part of taking control and adapting to the situation [40, 45]. Strategies such as writing notes [44], use of external memory aids [35], use of technology to keep control [46] and asking for assistance from others [42] e.g. external services, friends and family [47] were used to compensate for memory loss, to remember routines and to provide a sense of control and meaningfulness. Also, cognitive exercise was used to improve memory [47] and some actions contributed to maintain autonomy. Holding on to autonomy could be managed by for example going to familiar places so they could handle the activity by themselves [48] or avoiding concerns of their partner and others [44].

The coping actions described here show how persons with dementia compensate for reduced cognitive functioning and handle challenges to be active. They put time and effort into planning activities, use technical tools to assist them as well as asking for help from others to compensate for loss of capacity. Trying to adapt to their new life situation caused by dementia, they described coping strategies which supported a sense of control and autonomy. The various coping actions are based in available resources, strength to stand strains (resilience) [49], a wish to overcome obstructions and finding meaning by doing so, all of which are salutogenic factors promoting wellbeing and health [14, 15].

As shown, individuals having dementia use available personal resources as well as resources in their social network, environment and provided by professionals when necessary. If properly met, asking for help is health-promoting. By means of counselling, empowerment as well as health-promoting interaction, nurses and other health professionals can support coping strategies which improve control, adaption and adjustment to their situation. A sense of control, adaption and adjusting represent vital resources for wellbeing and health [50].

Planning for the future, i.e. being proactive in managing dementia is a part of the adapting and adjusting coping strategies [17]. Such planning might include contacting internet support groups to get knowledge of dementia, finding ideas about how to make appropriate changes [47], to contact health care services when you know help will be needed in the future [51] or accessing groups with other people having dementia [52].

As shown above, the described coping actions aim at taking control and adapt to the situation by looking ahead to future needs. To master their situation here-and-now as well as preparing for the coming challenges, they searched for relevant knowledge and external resources. To master their situation, individuals having dementia took initiative regarding planning their finances, place of living, and their last will. Such planning contributes to wellbeing and hope for a good life also during the times of more severe dementia which they know will come.

The evidence presented so far in this chapter highlights the importance of planning the future while necessary resources still are available. Hence, health professionals should initiate a dialogue with the person having dementia, provide information as well as practical and emotional support to promote such planning, which may include to educate the informal caregivers. Information, counselling or dialogue in support groups as well as the utilization of future planning may prepare for changes, contribute to adaption, adjustment, wellbeing and health. The timing of such information, counselling or dialogue is essential. The person having dementia needs to be mentally ready or prepared to focus on the future, representing a vulnerable state. Thus, health-promoting nurse–patient interaction including acknowledgement, respect, emotional support and sensitivity for the individual's situation, experiences and feelings is an important resource supporting coping and wellbeing [30]. Health-promoting nurse–patient interaction is also an important tool for identifying when the person having dementia and his/her family are ready to focus on planning for the future.

25.3.2.2 Reframing Identity

The second set of coping actions refers to *reframing the identity* [17]. It includes how a person encourages identity by thinking differently about oneself [37]. By comparing themselves with those who were worse off, persons with dementia affirm their own identity and self-worth [24, 29, 37]. Reframing one's identity contributes to hope and satisfaction in life [53]. Reframing the identity can also include decision-making, for instance decisions of whether to ask for help or not [25, 37]. A decision of informing others about one's disease is seen as a key element in the process of coming to terms with the diagnosis of dementia and constructing a new sense of self [54].

Preserving, affirming and reframing identity are different coping actions to cope with changed health resources. Reframing actions help to adapt to the diminished resources caused by the dementia. Both preserving and reframing actions are emotional-focused coping strategies contributing to wellbeing. Adaption to change and reframing strategies are linked to resilience and self-transcendence [50, 55]. Self-transcendence (see Chap. 9 in this book) holds adaption to changes in life as one of the key resources for wellbeing in vulnerable populations [50]. Adaption to changes is an integral process involved in the intra-personal aspect of self-transcendence [56]. Participation in groups of peers arranged by day-care centres or other resource groups may support identity reframing. Nurses or other health professionals should provide information about such groups available.

How people with dementia adapt and adjust their expectations toward themselves and their capacities, represent one of four overall strategies of coping among persons with dementia. The next coping category is termed accepting the situation, which is also a key aspect of intra-personal self-transcendence (see Chap. 9).

25.3.3 Coping Strategies: Accepting the Situation

Accepting one's situation includes acknowledgement and acceptance of the changed situation characterized by the dementia diagnosis and loss of memory. The accepting coping strategies are based in understanding of their capabilities; that is, what they can perform independently and when they need assistance from others [17].

25.3.3.1 Position in Life

This set of coping strategies includes actions to have *a position in life* [17]. When the individuals having dementia accept their changed situation, they simultaneously deny dementia to rule one's life [57]. The focus is shifting from seeing dementia as a disease towards living well with the resources they still possess [58]. Thus, they highlight the possibilities which they still have in life [28, 59–61], maintaining a positive view of oneself [59] and appreciating the present moment [34]. These positive approaches add both hope for a good life in the future and meaning-in-life regardless of the future prospect [34, 60, 62].

When the persons with dementia are accepting the changes and refind a position in life, they do not combat the consequences of their disease, but search for ways of living well with the dementia and the resources they still possess combined with asking for support from others when needed. These coping strategies support hope and meaningfulness, and thereby promote health and wellbeing among the person with dementia. Furthermore, coping actions reflecting acceptation of change are linked to self-transcendence. Self-transcendence is strengthened both by adaption to change in life (as said above) and acceptation of this change [50].

Health care professionals' knowledge about various kinds of coping actions and their possible gains is important to initiate a dialogue supporting the individuals to adapt and accept the changed life situation caused by dementia. By means of counselling, nurses and other health professionals can promote quality of life and wellbeing, independently of context and whether the counselling dialogue is with the person with dementia or those staying close to the person.

25.3.4 Avoiding Coping Strategies

This last coping category includes how individuals having dementia directly and indirectly avoid situations which cause stress and challenges due to the disease [17]. Hence, these strategies include *direct resistance and indirect resistance (distraction) of the disease.*

25.3.4.1 Direct Resistance of the Disease

The set of coping actions termed *direct resistance of the disease* involves actions to resist change, adaption or help from others to hinder accepting the diagnosis and its progression over time [17, 47]. The aim of these actions is to prevent themselves from thinking about the disease, its consequences and the future life with dementia [62–64].

The resistance actions intend to avoid focusing on the realities of the dementia [65], and are used to fight stigma related to the disease and treats of identity [47]. Direct resistance actions include withdrawing from participation in different settings and concealing difficulties from others, which lead to isolation [65]. Consequently, the use of these coping strategies may actively avoid situations requiring support by others, and assistance or information from others might be escaped [66]. Furthermore, to avoid focusing on the realities of dementia they elude situations where they may meet others with dementia or those with a further progression of dementia than themselves [38]. Moreover, linguistic strategies aiming for emotionally distancing themselves from the disease are also seen as part of such avoiding coping strategies [65].

25.3.4.2 Distracting from the Disease

The *distracting from the disease-actions* aims to distract themselves from dementia and its consequences [17]. Thus, they distract themselves from being confronted with symptoms and changes due to reduced cognitive abilities.

Distracting coping actions are understood as indirect avoiding strategies. Such actions may be to keep busy, active and fully occupied to escape the realities of dementia [67, 68]. For example, being actively partaking in social settings may be a way to get distance between themselves and dementia [20].

However, these coping actions aiming for resistance and distracting may give a short relief from the stress, challenges and difficulties caused by the disease. Thus, these strategies are mainly utilized to reduce overwhelming stress and challenges. The dementia itself and thoughts of the potential consequences of dementia put tremendous demands on a person. People with dementia may experience that available resources in themselves or in their context are limited. Accordingly, both resistance and distraction strategies may be a natural as well as a rational reaction in the context of a crisis. However, their challenges will not be solved or disappear by these strategies; therefore, over time such strategies will not be health-promoting.

Health-promoting approaches applied by nurses and other health professional should include emotional support and guidance. Despite the person with dementia may resist the changes, emotional support can help to release some pressure, strain and stress and thereby release health resources. Furthermore, over time emotional support may support adaption and acceptance of their situation, which is key to wellbeing and health. By means of counselling, health professionals should provide the family with knowledge about normal reactions to crises and possible important factors for health and wellbeing. Such knowledge is important to empower the person with dementia as well as his/her family. Such counselling must be based on the readiness of the person having dementia. Thus, the content and method will depend on the situation and the actual persons involved. Empowerment is an important resource to strengthen coping and wellbeing [69].

25.4 A Life with Dementia - An Art of Balance

Persons with dementia are seen to utilize four overall categories of coping strategies [17]. The use of these coping strategies is not based in a chronological order or a linear process starting with avoidance and ending in acceptance of the situation. These strategies should rather be seen as potential ways to meet stress and challenges following dementia [17]; that is, balancing the life with dementia. As previously mentioned, the strategies chosen will depend on the appraisals of the challenges as well as the available resources. Therefore, one person may respond differently to a challenge than another in the same situation, as well as showing a different reaction the next time he or she encounter approximately the same challenge. One alternates between the available strategies depending of what is deemed the best solution in the specific context. Furthermore, in severe situations, a global coping response is triggered including use of all available strategies simultaneously to handle the challenge [22].

Persons with dementia use coping strategies to balance life with dementia independently of limitations in health resources. Coping strategies handling stress and challenges enhance hope and meaning-in-life [17].

How you respond to challenges is, as previously appointed, not only dependent on the challenges but also on the available resources. These are resources within the person self, within close family and next of kin as well as in the environment outside the family.

Firstly, a person's inner strength to handle strain and challenges, i.e. the persons resilience [49], may differ, but is essential for coping and health [70]. Resilience includes abilities to regain inner strength and coping resources while facing different kinds of hardship [70]. A sense of humour is another positive personal quality for coping pointed out by persons with dementia [17]. A sense of humour represents the ability to see the humorous aspects of a situation which reduces stress and elicits positive emotions [17].

Secondly, close family and close social relations are vital resources in peoples' lives, especially in phases of vulnerability. Therefore, such relationships are crucial resources for individuals having dementia in the face of stress. Having vital social relations affects how he or she appraises the stressors and the challenges. Next of kin and close family may give emotional support, backing and practical help [17]. The family's resources may differ with personal health, socioeconomic status, but also regard to knowledge about dementia. Empowerment by means of counselling the close family, i.e. by providing knowledge about dementia and health-promotion, is essential. Empowering courses are sometimes offered online, by peers providing volunteer groups for close family or coping courses arranged by the local health care service or by health agencies. Support from family has also been linked not only to coping, but also directly to meaning-in-life [71] among persons with dementia.

Lastly, coping strategies to reduce and alter stress and challenges are affected by environmental factors. For example, staying in a dementia friendly neighbourhood and society may support coping strategies promoting balance in life, wellbeing and health. The World Health Organization's 'age-friendly' policy movement [1] and dementia awareness campaign [72], underline the importance of supporting environments which facilitate empowerment of persons with dementia and thereby making it possible for them to take part in the society. There must be a shift in the perspective of dementia from only focusing on symptoms, disabilities and restrictions towards capabilities, resources and potential of persons with dementia, not only in health care services but also in public planning. Dementia friendly environment principles involve high safety, good structure and familiarity which are meant to reduce stress and challenges and thereby promote coping and participation in the society [73–76].

25.5   Conclusion

This chapter focuses on coping strategies defined as cognitive and behavioural efforts to master, reduce or tolerate internal or external demands created by challenges and stress and how persons with dementia cope with challenges due to the disorder. How persons with dementia themselves express use of coping strategies has been reported in qualitative studies, and a meta-synthesis of these studies found that persons with dementia used four overall categories of coping strategies: (1) The first category was related to keep going and holding on to life as usual, (2) the second category included adapting and adjusting to the demands resulting from the disease, while (3) the third category embraced accepting the situation, followed by the (4) fourth category centering on avoiding difficult situations. The present chapter describes these coping strategies, how they are linked to health-promotion, wellbeing and meaning-in-life and how persons with dementia use these coping strategies to balance their life with dementia. In treatment and care of persons with dementia, there must be a shift from primarily focusing on symptoms, disabilities and restrictions towards coping and health-promotion, including emphasize on capabilities, resources and potential of persons having dementia.

Nurses and health professionals can promote health and wellbeing in persons with dementia: in the early phase of dementia, information and support to maintain activities of daily living, coping and social relationships are needed. With further functional decline, informal carers and/or formal care providers naturally must extend the scope of care and support. The health-promoting actions aim to compensate for loss of functioning and to facilitate meaningfulness in life.

Take Home Messages
- There must be a shift in dementia care from only focusing on symptoms, disabilities and restrictions towards capabilities, resources and potential of persons with dementia.
- Knowledge about dementia based in an integrated understanding of pathogenesis and salutogenesis, represents a basis for high-quality dementia care.
- Coping strategies such as 'keep going and holding on to life', 'adapting and adjusting to the situation and demands', and 'accepting the situation' contribute to meaningfulness and wellbeing.
- Persons with dementia chose coping strategies and actions dependent on the stressors and challenges they experience and available personal and external resources.
- Coping aims to balance one's life with dementia.

References

1. World Health Organization. World report on ageing and health. Geneva: World Health Organization; 2015.
2. Engedal K, Haugen P. Demens - sykdommer, diagnostikk og behandling. Tønsberg: Forlaget aldring og helse - akademisk; 2018; [Norwegian].
3. Ferri CP, et al. Global prevalence of dementia: a Delphi consensus study. Lancet. 2005;366(9503):2112–7.
4. Berr C, Wancata J, Ritchie K. Prevalence of dementia in the elderly in Europe. Eur Neuropsychopharmacol. 2005;15(4):463–71.
5. Shi Z, et al. Prevalence and clinical predictors of cognitive impairment in individuals aged 80 years and older in rural China. Dement Geriatr Cogn Disord. 2013;36(3–4):171–8.
6. Prince M, et al. World Alzheimer Report 2015. An analysis of prevalence, incidence, cost and trends. London: Alzheimer's Disease International; 2015.

7. Prince M, et al. The global prevalence of dementia: a systematic review and metaanalysis. Alzheimers Dement. 2013;9(1):63–75 e2.
8. Sosa-Ortiz AL, Acosta-Castillo I, Prince MJ. Epidemiology of dementias and Alzheimer's disease. Arch Med Res. 2012;43(8):600–8.
9. Potkin SG. The ABC of Alzheimer's disease: ADL and improving day-to-day functioning of patients. Int Psychogeriatr. 2002;14(Suppl 1):7–26.
10. van der Steen J, et al. White paper defining optimal palliative care in older people with dementia: a Delphi study and recommendations from the European Association for Palliative Care (EAPC). Palliat Med. 2014;28(3):197–209.
11. Engedal K, et al. Demens. Fakta og utfordringer : Lærebok. Tønsberg: Forlaget Aldring og helse; 2009. 424 s.
12. World Health Organization. Dementia: a public health priority. Geneva: World Helth Organization; 2012.
13. Naidoo J, Wills J. Health studies: an introduction. Hampshire: Palgrave; 2001.
14. Antonovsky A. Unraveling the mystery of health. San Francisco: Jossey-Bass; 1987.
15. Lindstrom B, Eriksson M. Salutogenesis. J Epidemiol Community Health. 2005;59(6):440–2.
16. Eriksson M, Lindström B. A salutogenic interpretation of the Ottawa Charter. Health Promot Int. 2008;23(2):190–9.
17. Bjørkløf GH, et al. Balancing the struggle to live with dementia: a systematic meta-synthesis of coping. BMC Geriatr. 2019;19(1):295.
18. Eriksson M. The sense of coherence in the salutogenic model of health. In: Mittelmark MB, Sagy S, Eriksson M, Bauer GF, Pelikan JM, Lindström B, Espnes GA, editors. The handbook of salutogenesis. New York: Springer; 2017.
19. Sharp BK. Stress as experienced by people with dementia: an interpretative phenomenological analysis. Dementia (London). 2019;18(4):1427–45.
20. Frazer S, Oyebode J, Cleary A. How older women who live alone with dementia make sense of their experiences: an interpretative phenomenological analysis. Dementia. 2011;11(5):677–93.
21. Folkman S. Personal control and stress and coping processes: a theoretical analysis. J Pers Soc Psychol. 1984;46(4):839–52.
22. Lazarus RS, Folkman S. Stress, appraisal and coping. New York: Springer; 1984.
23. Dalby P, Sperlinger D, Boddington S. The lived experience of spirituality and dementia in older people living with mild to moderate dementia. Dementia (London). 2012;11(1):75–94.
24. Clare L, et al. The experience of living with dementia in residential care: an interpretative phenomenological analysis. Gerontologist. 2008;48(6):711–20.
25. Nowell Z, Thornton A, Simpson J. The subjective experience of personhood in dementia care settings. Dementia. 2013;12(4):394–409.
26. Hedman R, et al. How people with Alzheimer's disease express their sense of self: analysis using rom Harré's theory of selfhood. Dementia. 2013;12(6): 713–33.
27. Öhman A, Nygård L. Meanings and motives for engagement in self-chosen daily life occupations among individuals with Alzheimer's disease. OTJR. 2005;25(3):89–97.
28. Mjørud M, et al. Living with dementia in a nursing home, as described by persons with dementia: a phenomenological hermeneutic study. BMC Health Serv Res. 2017;17(1):93.
29. Tolhurst E, Weicht B. Preserving personhood. The strategies of men negotiating the experience of dementia. J Aging Stud. 2017;40:29–35.
30. Haugan G. Nurse-patient interation - a vital salutary resource in nursing home care. In Haugan G, Eriksson M. Health promotion in health care - vital theories and research. Chapter 10, Springer Scientific Publisher; 2021.
31. Bronner K, et al. Which medical and social decision topics are important after early diagnosis of Alzheimer's disease from the perspectives of people with Alzheimer's disease, spouses and professionals? BMC Res Notes. 2016;9:149.
32. Mazaheri M, et al. Experiences of living with dementia: qualitative content analysis of semi-structured interviews. J Clin Nurs. 2013;22(21–22):3032–41.
33. Rostad D, Hellzen O, Enmarker I. The meaning of being young with dementia and living at home. Nurs Rep. 2013;3(1):12–7.
34. Genoe MR, Dupuis SL. The role of leisure within the dementia context. Dementia (London). 2014;13(1):33–58.
35. Lee SM, Roen K, Thornton A. The psychological impact of a diagnosis of Alzheimer's disease. Dementia (London). 2014;13(3):289–305.
36. Johannessen A, et al. "To be, or not to be": experiencing deterioration among people with young-onset dementia living alone. Int J Qual Stud Health Wellbeing. 2018;13(1):1490620.
37. Genoe M, et al. Honouring identity through mealtimes in families living with dementia. J Aging Stud. 2010;24(3):181–93.
38. MacRae H. Self and other: the importance of social interaction and social relationships in shaping the experience of early-stage Alzheimer's disease. J Aging Stud. 2011;25(4):445–56.
39. Tak SH, et al. Activity engagement: perspectives from nursing home residents with dementia. Educ Gerontol. 2015;41(3):182–92.
40. Gilmour JA, Huntington AD. Finding the balance: living with memory loss. Int J Nurs Pract. 2005;11(3):118–24.
41. van Zadelhoff E, et al. Good care in group home living for people with dementia. Experiences of residents, family and nursing staff. J Clin Nurs. 2011;20(17–18):2490–500.

42. Hedman R, et al. How people with Alzheimer's disease express their sense of self: analysis using Rom Harre's theory of selfhood. Dementia (London). 2013;12(6):713–33.

43. Sixsmith A, Gibson G. Music and the wellbeing of people with dementia. Ageing Soc. 2007;1:127–45.

44. Derksen E, et al. Impact of diagnostic disclosure in dementia on patients and carers: qualitative case series analysis. Aging Ment Health. 2006;10(5):525–31.

45. Chaplin R, Davidson I. What are the experiences of people with dementia in employment? Dementia (London). 2016;15(2):147–61.

46. Nygard L. Meaning of everyday technology as experienced by people with dementia who live alone. Dementia. 2008;7(4):481–502.

47. Genoe MR, et al. Adjusting to mealtime change within the context of dementia. Can J Aging. 2012;31(2):173–94.

48. Brorsson A, et al. Accessibility in public space as perceived by people with Alzheimer's disease. Dementia. 2011;10(4):587–602.

49. Nygren B, et al. Recillience, sence, of coherence, purpose in life and self-tracendence in relation to perceived physical and mental health among the oldest old. Aging Ment Health. 2005;9(4):354–62.

50. Nordberg A, et al. Self-transcendence (ST) among very old people—its associationas to social and medical factors and development over five years. Arch Gerontol Geriatr. 2015;61(2):247–81.

51. Stephan A, et al. Barriers and facilitators to the access to and use of formal dementia care: findings of a focus group study with people with dementia, informal carers and health and social care professionals in eight European countries. BMC Geriatr. 2018;18(1):131.

52. Read S, Toye C, Wynaden D. Experiences and expectations of living with dementia: a qualitative study. Collegian. 2017;24(5):427–32.

53. Wolverson Radbourne EL, Clarke C, Moniz-Cook E. Remaining hopeful in early-stage dementia: a qualitative study. Aging Ment Health. 2010;14(4):450–60.

54. Weaks D, Wilkinson H, McLeod J. Daring to tell: the importance of telling others about a diagnosis of dementia. Ageing Soc. 2015;35(4):765–84.

55. Rutter M. Resilience in the face of adversity: protective factors and resistance to psychiatric disorder. Br J Psychiatry. 1985;147(6):598–611.

56. Haugan G. Life satisfaction in cognitively intact long-term nursing home patients: symptoms, distress, wellbeing and nurse-patient interaction. In: Sarracino IM, editor. Beyond money—the social roots for health and wellbeing. New York: NOVA Scientific Publisher; 2014. p. 165–211.

57. Langdon SA, Eagle A, Warner J. Making sense of dementia in the social world: a qualitative study. Soc Sci Med. 2007;64(4):989–1000.

58. Hillman A, et al. Dualities of dementia illness narratives and their role in a narrative economy. Sociol Health Illn. 2018;40(5):874–91.

59. Borley G, Hardy S. A qualitative study on becoming cared for in Alzheimer's disease: the effects to women's sense of identity. Aging Ment Health. 2017;21(10):1017–22.

60. Pesonen HM, Remes AM, Isola A. Diagnosis of dementia as a turning point among Finnish families: a qualitative study. Nurs Health Sci. 2013;15(4):489–96.

61. Hulko W. From 'not a big deal' to 'hellish': experiences of older people with dementia. J Aging Stud. 2009;23(3):131–44.

62. Clemerson G, Walsh S, Isaac C. Towards living well with young onset dementia: an exploration of coping from the perspective of those diagnosed. Dementia (London). 2014;13(4):451–66.

63. de Witt L, Ploeg J, Black M. Living on the threshold: the spatial experience of living alone with dementia. Dementia. 2009;8(2):263–91.

64. de Witt L, Ploeg J, Black M. Living alone with dementia: an interpretive phenomenological study with older women. J Adv Nurs. 2010;66(8):1698–707.

65. Aldridge H, Fisher P, Laidlaw K. Experiences of shame for people with dementia: an interpretative phenomenological analysis. Dementia (London). 2019;18(5):1896–911.

66. Svanström R, Sundler AJ. Gradually losing one's foothold—a fragmented existence when living alone with dementia. Dementia (London). 2015;14(2):145–63.

67. MacKinlay E. Using spiritual reminiscence with a small group of Latvian residents with dementia in a nursing home: a multifaith and multicultural perspective. J Relig Spiritual Aging. 2009;21(4):318–29.

68. Vernooij-Dassen M, et al. Receiving a diagnosis of dementia: the experience over time. Dementia. 2006;5(3):397–410.

69. Tveiten S, Knutsen I. Empowering dialogues—the patients' perspective. Scand J Caring Sci. 2011;25:333–40.

70. Wolin S, Wolin S. The resilient self. New York: Villard Books; 1993.

71. Eriksen S, et al. The experience of relations in persons with dementia: a systematic meta-synthesis. Dement Geriatr Cogn Disord. 2016;42:342–68.

72. World Health Organization. Dementia: a public health priority. Geneva: World Health Organization; 2012.

73. Day K, Carreon D, Stump C. The therapeutic design of environments for people with dementia a review of the empirical research. Gerontologist. 2000;40(4):397–416.

74. Marquardt GP, Bueter KMA, Motzek TM. Impact of the design of the built environment on people with dementia: an evidence-based review. HERD. 2014;8(1):127–57.

75. Calkins MP. Evidence-based long term care design. NeuroRehabilitation. 2009;25(3):145–54.

76. van Hoof J, et al. Environmental interventions and the design of homes for older adults with dementia: an overview. Am J Alzheimers Dis Other Dement. 2010;25(3):202–32.

Part IV

Closing Remarks

Future Perspectives of Health Care: Closing Remarks

26

Gørill Haugan and Monica Eriksson

Abstract

The Covid-19 pandemic has demonstrated the vulnerability of our health care systems as well as our societies. During the year of 2020, we have witnessed how whole societies globally have been in a turbulent state of transformation finding strategies to manage the difficulties caused by the pandemic. At first glance, the health promotion perspective might seem far away from handling the serious impacts caused by the Covid-19 pandemic. However, as health promotion is about enabling people to increase control over their health and its determinants, paradoxically health promotion seems to be ever more important in times of crisis and pandemics. Probably, in the future, pandemics will be a part of the global picture along with the non-communicable diseases. These facts strongly demand the health care services to reorient in a health promoting direction.

The IUHPE Global Working Group on Salutogenesis suggests that health promotion competencies along with a reorientation of professional leadership towards salutogenesis, empowerment and participation are required. More specifically, the IUHPE Group recommends that the overall salutogenic model of health and the concept of SOC should be further advanced and applied beyond the health sector, followed by the design of salutogenic interventions and change processes in complex systems.

Keywords

Health promotion · Pandemics · Non-communicable diseases · Reorienting the health-care services · Salutogenesis · Salutary factors

G. Haugan (✉)
Department of Public Health and Nursing, NTNU Norwegian University of Science and Technology, Trondheim, Norway

Faculty of Nursing and Health Science, Nord University, Levanger, Norway
e-mail: gorill.haugan@ntnu.no, gorill.haugan@nord.no

M. Eriksson
Department of Health Sciences, University West, Trollhattan, Sweden
e-mail: monica.eriksson@hv.se

26.1 Future Perspective

The present condition gives us directions in which to look forward; the year of 2020 is the year of the Covid-19 pandemic. Lately, entire cities, regions and countries have been sealed off, travelling has been banned, universities have been closed, along with shops, restaurants etc. all over the world. We have witnessed that economic, cultural and social

G. Haugan, M. Eriksson (eds.), *Health Promotion in Health Care – Vital Theories and Research*,
https://doi.org/10.1007/978-3-030-63135-2_26

activities have come to a stop, resulting in big challenges to a great number of people around the globe. Thus, health concerns have become the prevailing concern that takes precedence over all other issues. In the years to come, the health services globally will need to collaborate on handling pandemics such as the Covid-19 pandemic ruling the world during the writing process of this book. Facing the serious impacts caused by the Covid-19 pandemic, at first sight, this pandemic and the world's response to it might seem far away from the health promotion perspectives. However, in a recently published Editorial in Health Promotion International, Van den Broucke [1] (p. 181) highlights the important role of health promotion in the time of crisis and pandemics by saying "...*Enabling people to increase control over their health and its determinants is at the core of health promotion. As such, health promotion may paradoxically be more important in this time of crisis than ever before*". Probably, in the future pandemics will be a part of the global picture along with the so-called non-communicable diseases (NCD) which covers chronic illnesses such as cancer, dementia, heart failure, diabetes as well as mental health issues. In this book, we have highlighted the need of health promotion as an integrated aspect of the treatment and care of patients with various NCDs. NCD Countdown 2030 [2] is an independent collaboration to inform policies that aim to reduce the worldwide burden of NCDs, and to ensure accountability towards this aim. In 2016, an estimated 40.5 million (71%) of the 56.9 million worldwide deaths were from NCDs. Of these, an estimated 1.7 million (4% of NCD deaths) occurred in people younger than 30 years of age, 15.2 million (38%) in people aged between 30 years and 70 years, and 23.6 million (58%) in people aged 70 years and older. An estimated 32.2 million NCD deaths (80%) were due to cancers, cardiovascular diseases, chronic respiratory diseases, and diabetes, and another 8.3 million (20%) were from other NCDs [2]. These facts strongly demand the health care services to reorient in a health promoting direction. As Van den Broucke [1] argued in his editorial, the pandemic has shown how vulnerable health care services may be, and not only the health care sector;

whole societies are in a turbulent state of transformation in need of ways and strategies to manage.

To return to the health care sector, the IUHPE Global Working Group on Salutogenesis states in a position article that one way is to position health promotion competencies as an essential framework to reorient health care services [3] (p. 9). In addition, the professional leadership must be reoriented towards salutogenesis, empowerment and participation. To move forward with the concept of salutogenesis as a sound scientific base for health promotion, some suggestions have been given:

1. To advance the overall salutogenic model of health
2. To advance the concept of SOC
3. To define and design salutogenic interventions and change processes in complex systems
4. To apply salutogenesis beyond the health sector [3]

26.1.1 Advancing the Overall Salutogenic Model of Health

The IUHPE Group states that the salutogenic model of health needs an additional positive health continuum and a path of positive health development linking resources to this new continuum [3]. During the last decades, a broader literature on the ease-end of the health continuum has emerged emphasizing among others the importance of developing individuals' personal potential and functioning, supporting people's perception of self-fulfillment, purpose and meaning-in-life, thriving, social attractiveness and making a valuable contribution to society [4–6]. Considering these developments, the IUHPE group recommends the addition of a positive health continuum to Antonovsky's original salutogenic model [3]. Furthermore, the IUHPE Group underscores the importance of linking resources to this new continuum of positive health development; "...*Resources not only immediately help people to cope better with stress (and surviving). Also, over time personal and environmental resources can help with recovery and healing... Beyond healing and recovery, resources can directly promote health, wellbeing and thriving—even in the absence of current or previous adversarial life situations*" [3] (p. 3). Consequently, in line with the Health Development Model [7] which proposes that pathogenesis and salutogenesis are two complementary perspectives on health development, GRRs and SRRs[1] are seen to facilitate and nurture positive health; thus direct paths of positive health development have been added to the salutogenic health model [3].

26.1.2 Advancing the Concept of SOC

The second point underscores a need for advancing the SOC concept; many translations of the Orientation to Life Questionnaire (OLQ) and the evidence on SOC have provided confidence that the SOC construct is measurable. However, the substance, content, wording and dimensionality of the SOC construct have yet to be explored. Research on SOC utilizing other methodological approaches than Antonovsky used accompanied by a replicability of Antonovsky's qualitative analyses and findings are highly welcome [3] (p. 4). Further, there is a need of developing new questionnaires for measuring salutary factors for health and wellbeing. Some attempts can be found, for example The Salutogenic Health Indicator Scale (SHIS) [8]. In Sweden, an ongoing research study has developed and tested a new scale, adapted for nurses' work situation and to be used in health care, The Salutogenic Survey on Sustainable Working life—Nurses (SalWork-N) (www.hv.se).

26.1.3 Salutogenic Interventions and Change Processes

Thirdly, strengthening the SOC through health promotion intervention is key. Purposefully designed salutogenic interventions and change processes are needed; therefore, explicit salutogenic intervention theories building on and inte-

grating key elements of salutogenesis should be developed [3]. Antonovsky stated that SOC [9] is formed by three kinds of life experiences: (1) consistency (strengthening comprehensibility), (2) underload–overload balance (strengthening manageability), and (3) participation in socially valued decision making (strengthening meaningfulness). Accordingly, further knowledge about these kinds of life experiences and how they can be assessed (quantitatively and qualitatively) in different contexts as well as on different system levels are required [3] (p. 5). To reorient health care, it is important to capture factors and initiatives that nurses along with other health professionals consider health promoting resources in their everyday clinical practice. We must learn from their experiences and integrate this new knowledge in education for health professionals.

26.1.4 Applying Salutogenesis Beyond Health Sector

Finally, applying salutogenesis and SOC to other fields beyond the individual health issues might be valuable as we can learn from other fields for health research. For instance, intergroup relations are vital in peoples' daily life at work, in leisure, in the communities and the municipalities, etc. Therefore, we need to more fully examine the differential benefits and potential harm of SOC on the individual, group and intergroup as well as organizational and system levels [3]. In a public health perspective, such knowledge seems fruitful for the development of health promoting workplaces, health promoting hospitals, health promoting communities, municipalities, schools, kinder gardens, living areas, etc.

26.2 Health Promotion Is About Thriving and Enabling People to Increase Control over Their Health

The health promotion perspective as well as the salutogenic theory of health is based in the idea that every single person has a health, which varies and moves along the health continuum between

---

[1] GRR = Generalized Resistance Resources; SRR = Specific Resistance Resources, central concepts in salutogenesis.

dis-ease and ease. Antonovsky [9] (p. 14) raised the question: *How can we understand movement of people in the direction of the health end of the continuum?'*—note, *all people, wherever they are at any given time, from the terminal patient to the vigorous adolescent—we cannot be content with an answer limited to 'by being low on risk factors'. A salutogenic orientation, then, as the basis for health promotion, directs both research and action efforts to encompass all persons, wherever they are on the continuum, and to focus on salutary factors.* Beyond survival, health promotion is about thriving and enabling people to increase control over their health [10]. The salutogenic model is useful for all fields of health care and therefore helpful in the reorienting of the health care services.

26.3 A reorientation of Health Care by Implementing Salutogenesis

We started this book showing a figure (Fig. 1.4) describing the salutogenic umbrella adjusted for health care settings. We also choose to end the book with the same figure (Fig. 26.1). Some of the umbrella concepts are described in this book, whilst some remain to be explored. However, to our knowledge this book is the first one to highlight and emphasize concepts closely related to the sense of coherence (SOC) in general, and to health care systems in particular. There is a need to continue exploring other salutogenic concepts to strengthen the salutogenic theory, but also to contribute to the development of nursing and the health sciences. Among others, concepts such as empathy, humour, learned optimism and learned hopefulness, would be interesting.

Moreover, the implementation of the concepts and the salutogenic approach to health and well-being in a *systematic way* is highly needed. An integration would benefit both staff and patients. Such an effort could begin with an education, i.e. salus education proposed in Chap. 15, continuing with a focus on learning processes to finally end with the development of a new way of working in health care settings, which means that salutary factors are recognized, identified and used in a health promoting manner. In other words, reorienting the health care services according to the

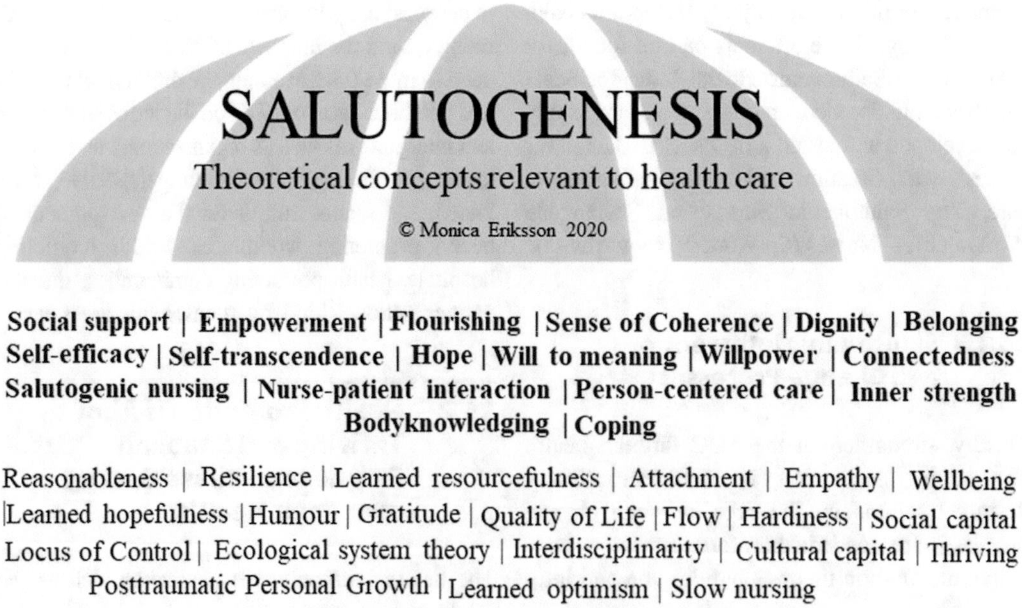

SALUTOGENESIS
Theoretical concepts relevant to health care
© Monica Eriksson 2020

Social support | Empowerment | Flourishing | Sense of Coherence | Dignity | Belonging Self-efficacy | Self-transcendence | Hope | Will to meaning | Willpower | Connectedness Salutogenic nursing | Nurse-patient interaction | Person-centered care | Inner strength Bodyknowledging | Coping

Reasonableness | Resilience | Learned resourcefulness | Attachment | Empathy | Wellbeing |Learned hopefulness | Humour | Gratitude | Quality of Life | Flow | Hardiness | Social capital Locus of Control | Ecological system theory | Interdisciplinarity | Cultural capital | Thriving Posttraumatic Personal Growth | Learned optimism | Slow nursing

Fig. 26.1 The salutogenic umbrella: theoretical concepts relevant to health care. (Reproduced with permission from Folkhälsan Research Center, Lindstrom & Eriksson) [4]

Ottawa Charter for health promotion. Already in the mid-1990s Antonovsky argued the salutogenic orientation as the theoretical basis for health promotion, directing both research and action efforts particularly useful for all fields of health care [9] (p. 18). The progress of new salutogenic models of health has been limited. An attempt to fill this knowledge gap can be seen in an article on "The Synergy Model of Health", which integrates salutogenesis and the assets model in a framework of Bronfenbrenner's ecological theory of human development [11].

When reviewing research on SOC we have become aware of how limited the research on working conditions of health care personnel is. There is a lot of research by nurses and other health professionals on different patient groups including measuring the SOC. However, salutogenic research on how health professionals' health and wellbeing can be maintained and developed is scarce. The same applies to knowledge about health professionals' SOC. For instance, have nurses forgotten themselves in their quest to do good for the patients? We here argue that research must also focus on the work environment and salutary factors for developing a sustainable working life for nurses and other health professionals. However, some attempts to fill this knowledge gap can be seen. A longitudinal study on the influence of a health promoting work environment [12] as well as a study on work-related SOC and its longitudinal relationship with work engagement and job satisfaction [13] were recently conducted in Norwegian nursing homes. Correspondingly, studies focusing on the working culture in nursing homes have shown empowerment, participation and influence over the work situation to be vital aspects for care quality [14, 15]. Moreover, SOC was newly measured among Swedish hospital nursing staff [16]. They found that on a national level, nurses reported weaker SOC than the general population, but stronger in an international comparison of nurses. Nurses found their work difficult to manage, but meaningful. Many nurses want to leave their workplaces and even the profession, as they found the work situation too stressful for their health. This is a worldwide dilemma. Another Swedish study among hospital nurses explored salutary factors for a sustainable working life [17]; having fun at work, being acknowledged, feeling togetherness in the team, having varying tasks with a manageable workload, good interaction between colleagues and patients, doing good work, feeling committed to and pride in the professional role, and having a balance between work and leisure time were found to be factors that made them stronger, which in turn explained why they stayed. Similar findings have been seen in Norway [18, 19]. Further research on salutary factors is needed.

26.4 Closing Remarks

In this book, we have highlighted the need to work to promote health in both hospitals and the municipality health care; treatment and care of patients with chronic diseases and the so-called non-communicable diseases (NCD) will be fundamental in the years to come. Our point of departure has been to focus attention on health promotion and salutogenesis in health care settings. We argue the salutogenic theory of health to be appropriate to guide health promotion in the health services. In a lecture at the Nordic School of Public Health (NHV) Antonovsky lectured about salutogenesis and health [20]. He called on to think salutogenically and act salutogenically. To use his own words, *"the key lies in a society and in people who care about others"* [20]. Nurses and the other health care professions are just such people who cares!

References

1. Van den Broucke S. Why health promotion matters to the COVID-19 pandemic, and vice versa. Health Promot Int. 2020;35:181–6.
2. NCD Countdown 2030 Collaborators. NCD Countdown 2030: worldwide trends in non-communicable disease mortality and progress towards Sustainable Development Goal target. Lancet. 2018;22(392):1072–88.
3. Bauer GF, Roy M, Bakibinga P, Contu P, Downe S, Eriksson M, et al. Future directions for the concept of salutogenesis: a position article. Health Promot Int. 2019;2019:1–9.

4. Lindström B, Eriksson M. The Hitchhiker's guide to salutogenesis. Salutogenic pathways to health promotion. Helsinki: Folkhälsan Research Center; 2010.

5. Commers MJ. Determinants of health: theory, understanding, portrayal, policy. Dordrecht: Springer; 2002.

6. Pelikan JM. Understanding differentiation of health in late modernity—by use of sociological system theory. In: McQueen DV, Kickbusch I, Potvin L, Pelikan JM, Balbo L, Abel T, editors. Health and modernity: the role of theory in health promotion. New York: Springer Scientific Publisher; 2007. p. 74–102.

7. Bauer GF, Davies JK, Pelikan JM. The EUHPID health development model for the classification of public health indicators. Health Promot Int. 2006;21:153–9.

8. Bringsén Å, Andersson HI, Ejlertsson G. Development and quality analysis of the Salutogenic Health Indicator Scale (SHIS). Scand J Publ Health. 2009;37(1):13–9.

9. Antonovsky A. The salutogenic model as a theory to guide health promotion. Health Promot Int. 1996;11(1):11–8.

10. WHO. The Ottawa Charter for health promotion: an international conference on health promotion. The Move towards a New Public Health. Copenhagen; 1986.

11. Pérez Wilson P, Marcos Marcos J, Morgan A, Eriksson M, Lindström B, Alvarez Dardet C. "The synergy model of health"—an integration of salutogenesis theory and health assets model. Health Promot Int. 2020; in press.

12. Grødal K, Innstrand ST, Haugan G, Andre B. Affective organizational commitment among nursing home employees: a longitudinal study on the influence of a health-promoting work environment. Nurs Open. 2019;6(4):1414–23.

13. Grødal K, Innstrand ST, Haugan G, Andre B. Work-related sense of coherence and longitudinal relationships with work engagement and job satisfaction. Scand J Work Organ Psychol. 2019;4(1): 1–11.

14. Andre B, Sjøvold E. What characterizes the work culture at a hospital unit that successfully implements change—a correlation study. BMC Health Serv Res. 2017;17:486.

15. Andre B, Sjøvold E, Rannestad T, Ringdal GI. The impact of work culture on quality of care in nursing homes—a review study. Scand J Caring Sci. 2014;28(3):449–57.

16. Eriksson M, Kerekes N, Brink P, Pennbrant S, Nunstedt H. The level of sense of coherence among Swedish nursing staff. J Adv Nurs. 2019;75: 2766–72.

17. Nunstedt H, Eriksson M, Ayman O, Hillström L, Truong A, Pennbrant S. Salutary factors explaining why hospital nurses remain in work and the profession. BMC Nurs. 2020; in review.

18. Hauvik S, Haugan G. The influence of rotation work on nursing home nurses' health and quality of life. Geriatr Nurs. 2016;20(2):26–35.

19. Hauvik S, Haugan G. The importance of the turn for nurses' work situation and quality of life in nursing homes. Geriatr Nurs. 2017;2017(3):5–13.

20. Antonovsky A. Some salutogenic words of wisdom to the conferees. Lecture held at the Nordic School of Public Health (NHV), 1993. Gothenburg.

Printed in the United States
by Baker & Taylor Publisher Services